Color Atlas of Microsurgical Anatomy

Surgical Flaps of the Limbs

COLOR ATLAS OF MICROSURGICAL ANATOMY

SURGICAL FLAPS OF THE LIMBS

Color Atlas of Microsurgical Anatomy

Surgical Flaps of the Limbs

Editors

Zheng Heping
Associate Professor
Institute for Orthopaedics
Fuzhou General Hospital of Nanjing Military Area Command
Fuzhou, China

Zhang Fahui
Professor
Institute for Orthopaedics
Fuzhou General Hospital of Nanjing Military Area Command
Fuzhou, China

Lin Jianhua
President
Professor of Orthopaedics
First Affiliated Hospital of Fujian Medical University
Fuzhou, China

CBS Publishers & Distributors Pvt Ltd
New Delhi • Bengaluru • Chennai • Kochi • Kolkata • Mumbai
Bhubaneswar • Hyderabad • Jharkhand • Nagpur • Patna • Pune • Uttarakhand

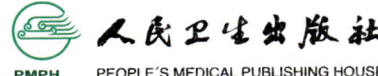

PMPH PEOPLE'S MEDICAL PUBLISHING HOUSE

Book Title: Color Atlas of Microsurgical Anatomy: Surgical Flaps of the Limbs
显微外科解剖学实物图谱：四肢组织瓣

ISBN: 978-93-86827-76-0

CBS Edition: 2019

This edition has been published by CBS Publishers & Distributors under arrangement with People's Medical Publishing House

Copyright © 2007 by People's Medical Publishing House. All rights reserved. No part of this publication may be reproduced, stored in a database or retrieval system, or transmitted in any form or by any electronic, mechanical, photocopy, or other recording means, without the prior written permission of the publisher.

First published: 2007

PMPH   ISBN: 978-7-117-09200-5/R . 9201

Not for sale outside India, Pakistan, Nepal, Bhutan and Sri Lanka.

Cataloguing in Publication Data:
A catalog record for this book is available from the CIP-Database China

Published by Satish Kumar Jain and produced by Varun Jain for

CBS Publishers & Distributors Pvt Ltd
4819/XI Prahlad Street, 24 Ansari Road, Daryaganj, New Delhi 110 002, India.
Ph: 23289259, 23266861, 23266867   Website: www.cbspd.com
Fax: 011-23243014   e-mail: delhi@cbspd.com; cbspubs@airtelmail.in.

Corporate Office: 204 FIE, Industrial Area, Patparganj, Delhi 110 092
Ph: 4934 4934   Fax: 4934 4935   e-mail: publishing@cbspd.com; publicity@cbspd.com

Branches

• **Bengaluru:** Seema House 2975, 17th Cross, K.R. Road, Banasankari 2nd Stage, Bengaluru 560 070, Karnataka, India
  Ph: +91-80-26771678/79   Fax: +91-80-26771680   e-mail: bangalore@cbspd.com

• **Chennai:** 7, Subbaraya Street, Shenoy Nagar, Chennai 600 030, Tamil Nadu, India.
  Ph: +91-44-26680620, 26681266   Fax: +91-44-42032115   e-mail: chennai@cbspd.com

• **Kochi:** 42/1325, 1326, Power House Road, Opposite KSEB Power House, Ernakulam 682 018, Kochi, Kerala, India.
  Ph: +91-484-4059061-65   Fax: +91-484-4059065   e-mail: kochi@cbspd.com

• **Kolkata:** 6/B, Ground Floor, Rameswar Shaw Road, Kolkata-700 014, West Bengal, India
  Ph: +91-33-22891126, 22891127, 22891128   e-mail: kolkata@cbspd.com

• **Mumbai:** 83-C, Dr E Moses Road, Worli, Mumbai-400018, Maharashtra, India
  Ph: +91-22-24902340/41   Fax: +91-22-24902342   e-mail: mumbai@cbspd.com

Representatives

| • Bhubaneswar | 0-9911037372 | • Hyderabad | 0-9885175004 | • Jharkhand | 0-9811541605 | • Nagpur | 0-9021734563 |
| • Patna | 0-9334159340 | • Pune | 0-9623451994 | • Uttarakhand | 0-9716462459 | | |

Printed at Nutech Print Services, Faridabad, India

CONTRIBUTORS

Tao Shengxiang, Ph.D.
Vice-Director Surgeon
Department of Orthopaedics
Zhongnan Hospital of Wuhan University
Wuhan, China

Wang Wanming, Ph.D.
Professor and Director
Department of Orthopaedics
Fuzhou General Hospital of Nanjing Military Area Command
Fuzhou, China

Wang Wei, Ph.D.
Professor and Director
Department of Anatomy
Fujian Medical University
Fuzhou, China

Xian Ronghua
Associate Professor
Fuzhou General Hospital of Nanjing Military Area Command
Fuzhou, China

Xie Yun, Ph.D.
Attending Physician
Department of Orthopaedics
First Affiliated Hospital of Fujian Medical University,
Fuzhou, China

Xu Yongqing, Ph.D.
Professor and Director
Institute of Orthopedic Surgery
Kunming General Hospital of Chengdu Military Region
Kunming, China

Xu Weihong, M.D.
Professor, Director Surgeon
Department of Orthopaedics
First Affiliated Hospital of Fujian Medical University,
Fuzhou, China

Zhan Wang, Ph.D.
Professor and Director
Institute of Orthopedic Surgery
Hainan People's Hospital
Haikou, China

Zhang Chaochun
Associate Professor
Department of Orthopaedics
Fuzhou General Hospital of Nanjing Military Area Command
Fuzhou, China

Zhang Guodong, Ph.D.
Attending Physician
Affiliated Hospital of Putian College
Putian, China

Zheng Xiaohui, Ph.D.
Vice-Director Surgeon
Institute of Orthopaedics
Affiliated Hospital of Putian College
Putian, China

TRANSLATOR

Huang Youqi
Professor
Foreign Languages Department of the Pre-clinical Medicine College of Fujian Medical University
Fuzhou, China

FOREWORD

In the introduction of this atlas, the editors have reviewed all the authorities in the very field before they came up with some new ideas to compile the Anatomic Atlas of Compound Bone Flaps in their own way. This is a rare atlas in that the dissection of flaps mimics the anatomy of layer structures in clinical surgery, in that all the specimen are made out of fresh body specimens and in that all figures are illustrated in a concise and precise language. It seems to me that among all the dermovascular specimens that I have seen, the ones collected in this atlas are the best in designs, process and interpretations. They might make a deep impression on the intended readers, both scientifically and artistically. I am sure that the atlas would be very helpful for those who are engaged in the clinical anatomy.

As is known, the participants in the job are experts in the modern clinical anatomy and microsurgery. Among them is Zheng Heping, an associate professor, who is an industrious and intelligent scholar and researcher. In the past decade, he has overcome all the difficulties, solved all the encountered problems and compiled this atlas. Although I was once a teacher of those editors, I do not think that I should take the credit of honorary editor. Nor do I believe that disciples should be less wise than their master. It is only a matter of time and effort.

Prof. Zhong Shizhen
Membership of China's Academy of Engineering
Chief Editor of Journal Clinical Anatomy
Director of the Clinical Anatomy Institute of
Southern Medical University
Guangzhou, Spring 2007

V

PREFACE

Microsurgery is one of the newly emerging branches of surgery. It is brimming over with such vigor and vitality that the microsurgical technique has found a wide application in diseases treatment, tissues or organ transplantation, especially function restoration and orthopedics. It helps make the wounded able humans and the invalid valid ones, which was once beyond the reach of the conventional surgery under the naked eye. The 21st century will witness the rapid development and popularization of this new technique. This atlas will prove its theoretical and clinical significance in promoting microsurgery.

In the late 1970s, modern clinical anatomy came on the scene and made surgery a chief subject for research. In the due course of its development and perfection, theoretical researches on the application of microsurgery have played a grounding role, with the publications of clinical authorities: *Microscopical Anatomy, Bases of Microscopical Anatomy, Clinical Anatomy of Microsurgery, Applied Anatomy of Bone Defect Restoration and the Illustration of Transferring Compound Flaps with Vascular Pedicles,* for example. But there are few atlases that are made out of fresh body specimens.

All the figures in the atlas are made out of fresh body specimens perfused with red gelatin and taken with digital cameras so that they could demonstrate the anatomic layer structures explicitly with concise and precise literal interpretations of flap vasculature and the main aspects of clinical anatomy. They are really more authentic and definitive, more vivid and colorful than the conventional diagrams. The atlas is unique in that the dissection of flaps mimics the dissection of the really layer structures in clinical operation. It is more understandable and instructive in that it is divided into two parts: the compound limb flaps and the skull (including neurosurgery and dentofacial surgery which will come out soon). Each section is subdivided into applied anatomy and mimic dissection. The former is based on the figures of fresh body specimens to demonstrate the courses, branches and distributions of the vessels whereas the latter is based on the body positions identical to the clinical operations to make it as authentic as possible. This atlas is initiated to bridge the gap between the basic knowledge and the clinical practice for those surgeons majored in microsurgery or orthopedics. It turns out to be a useful referent book for those surgeons, but the size of each flap was designed smaller than that needed for the clinical application in case unnecessary damage should be done to the adjacent donor sites of the specimens. Besides, due to the limitations of the editors' knowledge, there might be deficiencies here and there that require criticism.

We have not been alone in this venture of atlas compilation. There has been our teacher Zhong Shizhen, famous professor of clinical anatomy, who encouraged and supported us to do more and who has written the preface of this atlas for us. Another person who played vital role was professor Xu Dachuan, without whose careful review and revision this atlas would not have been accomplished. There has been the Funding Committee of Fujian Natural Science (No. C0120001) that has sponsored the *Color Atlas of Microsurgical Anatomy: Surgical Flaps of the Limbs.* Finally we must give our thanks to the People's Medical Publishing House for its firm support.

Zheng Heping
August 2007

Contents

Chapter I
Skin Flaps

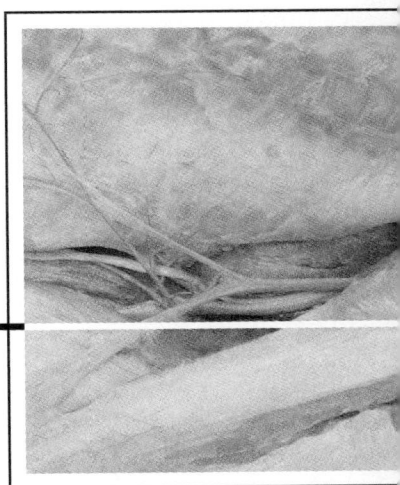

Classification of Skin Flaps

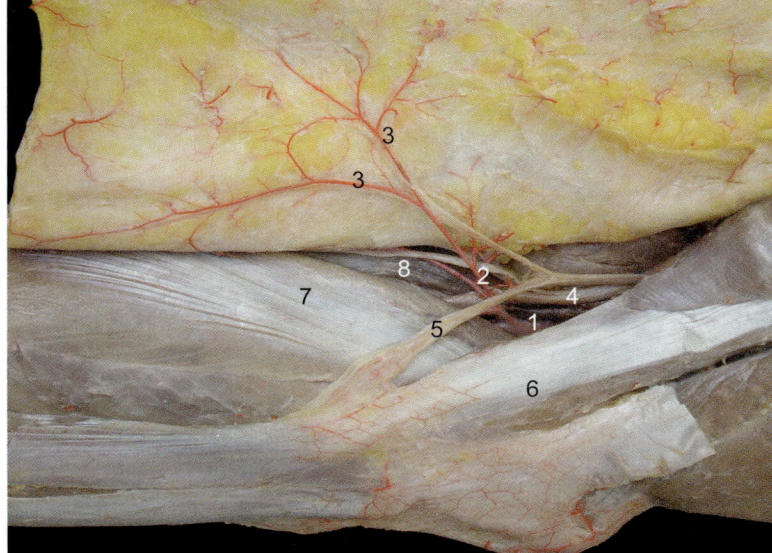

1. Popliteal artery
2. Lateral sural cutaneous artery
3. Cutaneous branch
4. Tibial nerve
5. Common peroneal nerve
6. Biceps femoris muscle
7. Lateral head of gastrocnemius muscle
8. Medial head of gastrocnemius muscle

Figure 1-1   Direct cutaneous artery flap

The vascular main trunk from which the cutaneous artery emerges is situated superficial to the skin or located in the spatium intermusculare. The cutaneous artery has no connections to the surrounding muscles and does not give any muscular branches. It then passes from the fissure of the deep fascia, running parallel to the skin surface with a sufficient length in the subcutaneous tissue, and finally sends small branches to form vascular net to nourish the subcutaneous tissue and the overlying skin.

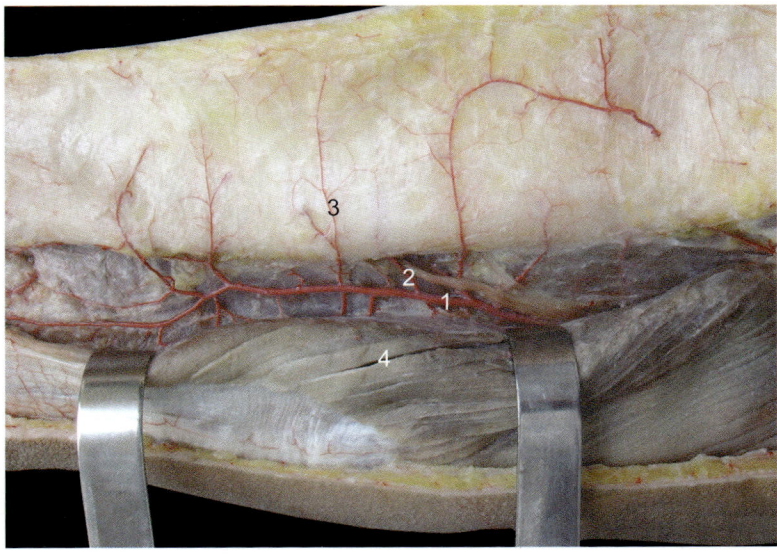

1. Radial collateral artery
2. Muscular branch
3. Cutaneous branch
4. Triceps brachii muscle

Figure 1-2   Intermuscular cutaneous artery flap

The main vascular trunk is located deep, and its cutaneous branch has to run a distance in the septum between different muscle bellies before it perforates through the deep fascia layer. The septal vessels nay also send small branches to nourish the surrounding muscles. After perforating through the deep fascia, the cutaneous artery fans out over the surface of the deep fascia, forms a dense superior fascial vascular net, and then gives branches to the overlying subcutaneous fat and the skin.

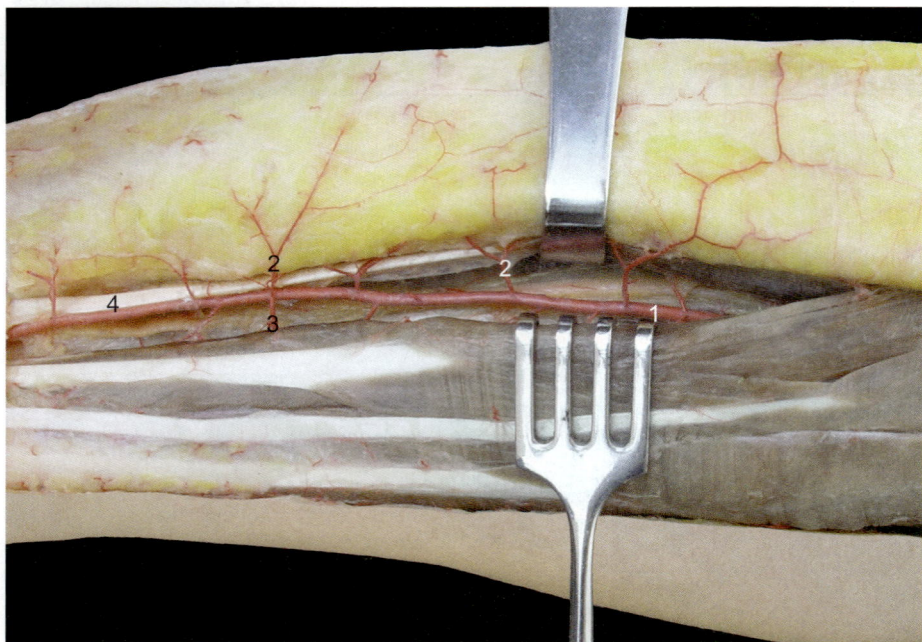

1. Ulnar artery
2. Cutaneous branch
3. Muscular branch
4. Flexor carpi ulnaris muscle

Figure 1-3   **Flap based on the arterial trunk and its branches**

One main artery extends through the donor region of the flap, and along its course, it sends many small branches to nourish the flap. When this type of flap is being transferred, either free or pedicled, a segment of the main vascular trunk should be harvested carrying with it some small branches.

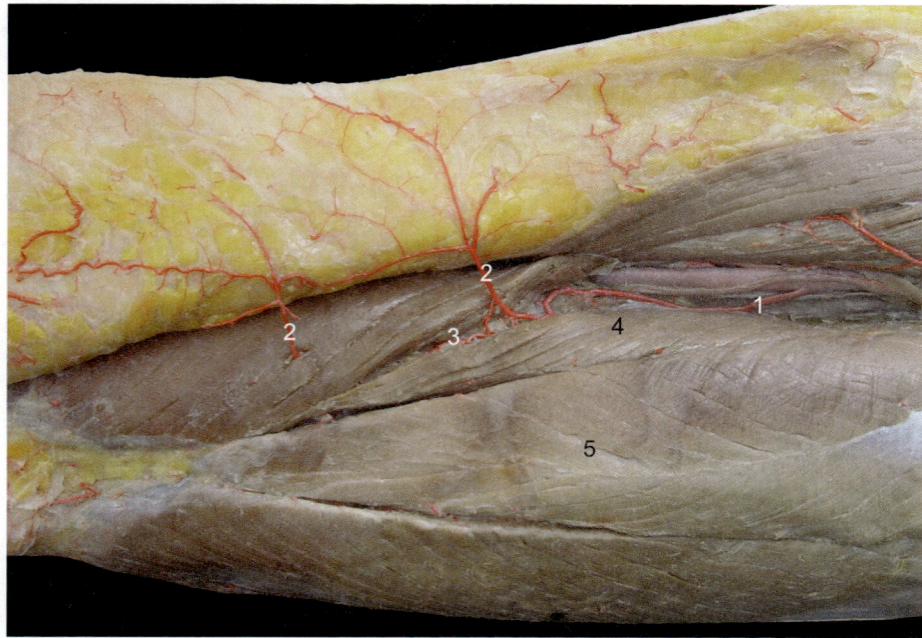

1. Artery of vastus medialis muscle
2. Perforating branch
3. Muscular branch
4. Medial vastus muscle
5. Rectus femoris muscle

Figure 1-4   **Musculocutaneous artery flap**

Musculocutaneous flap, or myocutaneous flap, is a compound flap containing the deep muscle and its overlying fascia and skin. It is based on the musculocutaneous vessel, which originates from the deep main artery trunk and enters the muscle at its deep surface. A musculocutaneous vessel usually gives three kinds of branches, the muscular branch to nourish the muscle, the cutaneous perforating branch, and the direct cutaneous limb (marginal branch).

Scapular Flap

The axial artery in the scapular flap is the vascular axis of the infrascapular artery (circumflex scapular artery) the trilateral cutaneous branches. It is characterized as donor site cosmetics by direct closure, and flap hairlessness. Its vascular pedicles are large in diameter and constant in the anatomical position. The scapular flap has a variety of clinical applications. This type of flap with a pedicle of the scapular artery can be transferred to relieve the scar contracture of the axillary fossa or to restore a soft tissue defect of the superior-middle arm. The compound flap pedicled with a piece of the scapular bone can be transferred to restore an osseous defect at the proximal humerus.

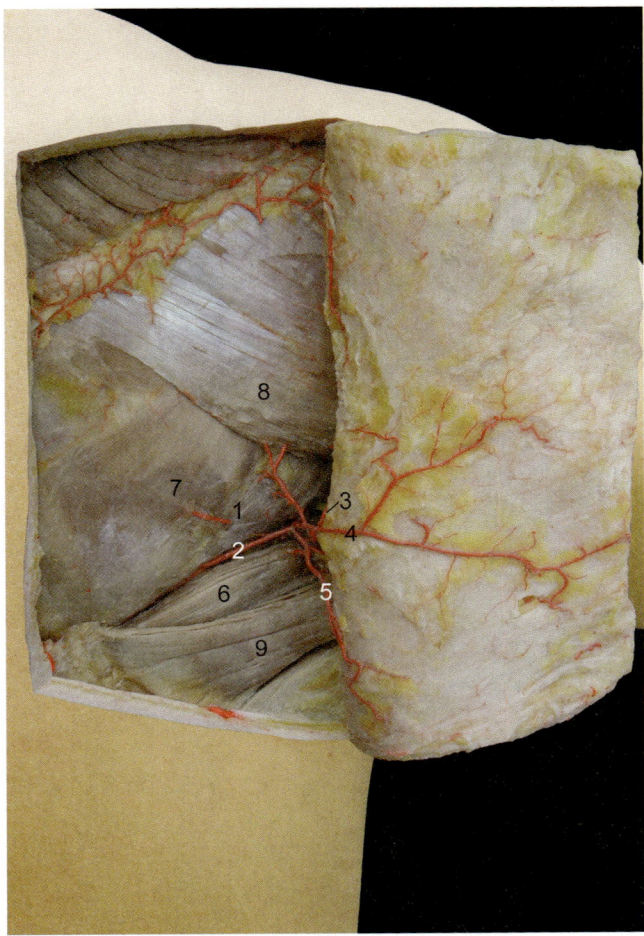

1. Teres minor muscle
2. Inferior cornus branch
3. Ascending branch
4. Transverse branch
5. Descending branch
6. Teres major muscle
7. Infraspinatus muscle
8. Deltoid muscle
9. Latissimus dorsi muscle

Figure 1-5	**Applied anatomy**

The circumflex scapular artery, in most cases (80%), emerges from the infrascapular artery. In a few cases (20%), it arises from another adjacent artery. The artery extends inferiorly along the teres minor muscle in the trilateral space. The circumflex scapular artery divides into the infraspinous fossa muscle branch, the inferior cornus muscle branch and trilateral cutaneous branch at the scapular axillary edge. The trilateral cutaneous branch perforates through the deep fascia to divide further into the ascending, the transverse and the descending branches. The small ascending branch extends superiorly to fan out over the adjacent region of the scapular spine; the small transverse branch extends medially to fan out over the adjacent region of the medial scapular edge; the large descending branch is actually the main part of the trunk of the trilateral cutaneous artery. It continues inferiorly to fan out over a vast cutaneous region extending for 3-4 cm to the distal scapula. The subscapular artery is 4.5 mm in diameter and the subscapular vein 5.5 mm; the circumflex scapular artery is 3.0 mm in diameter and the circumflex scapular vein 4.0 mm; the trilateral cutaneous artery is 1.0 mm in diameter and the trilateral cutaneous vein 1.7 mm.

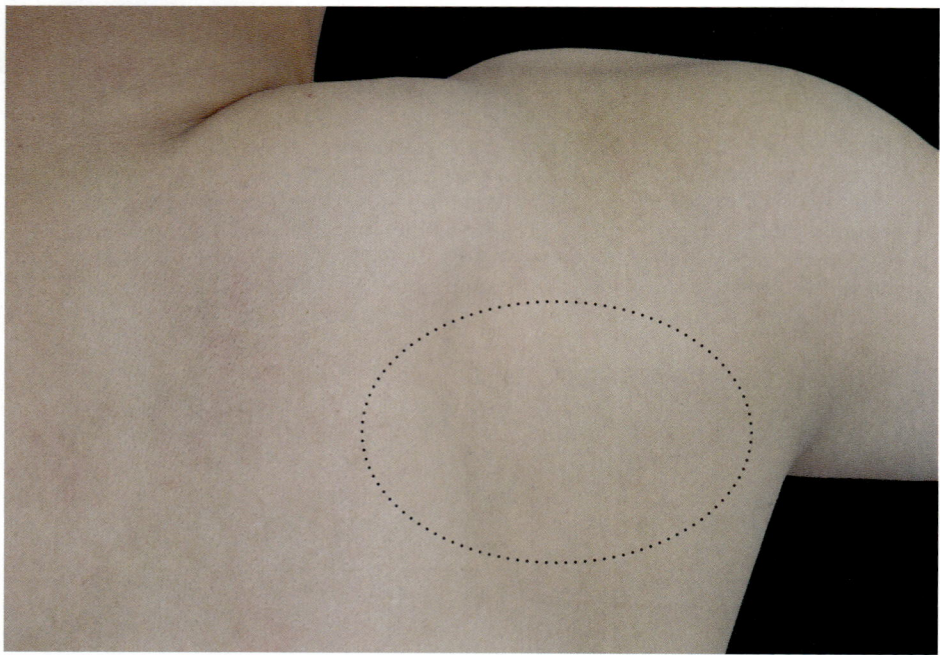

Figure 1-6   Design of the flap

A transverse scapular flap should be designed medially with a pedicle of the transverse artery. A longitudinal scapular flap should be designed inferiorly with a pedicle of the desending artery. The pivot point of the two flaps should be located at the junction of two lines. Besides, that of the transverse one should also be located at 2 cm above the margin of the posterior axillary wall and that of the longitudinal one along the margin of the lateral scapula.

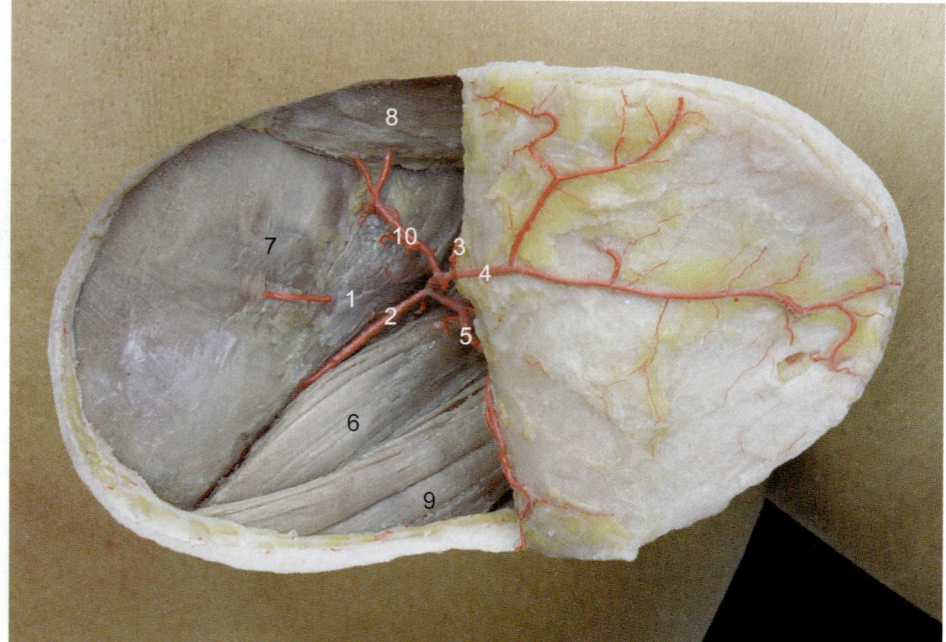

1. Teres minor muscle
2. Inferior cornus branch
3. Ascending branch
4. Transverse branch
5. Descending branch
6. Teres major muscle
7. Infraspinatus muscle
8. Deltoid muscle
9. Latissimus dorsi muscle
10. Muscular branch

Figure 1-7   Dissection of the flap

The flap should first be dissected from distal to proximal and then turned from the muscular sheath towards the vascular pedicle.

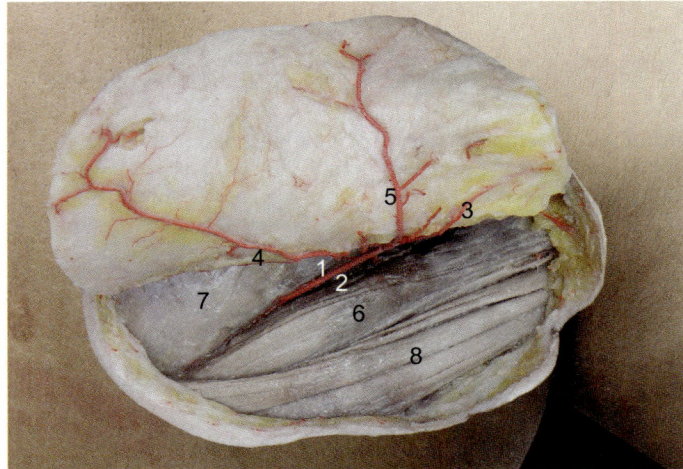

1. Teres minor muscle
2. Inferior cornus branch
3. Ascending branch
4. Transverse branch
5. Descending branch
6. Teres major muscle
7. Infraspinatus muscle
8. Latissimus dorsi muscle

| **Figure 1-8** | **Elevation of the flap** |

The flap should be dissected along the scapular axillary border, attaching closely to the muscle. The muscular branches should be cut and ligated. The dissection continues laterally along the cutaneous artery.

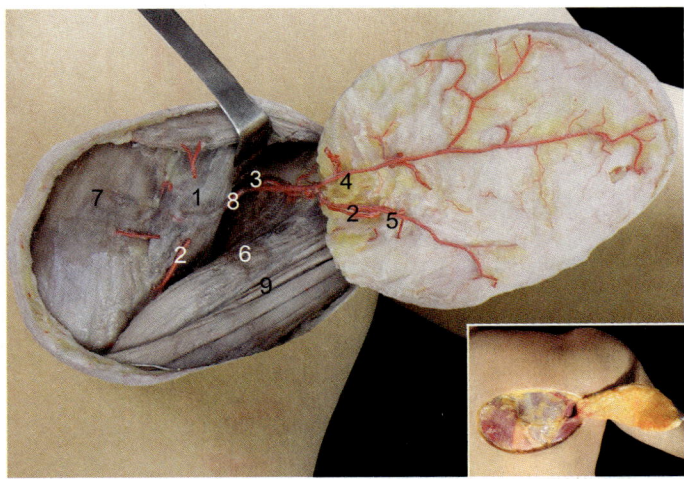

1. Teres minor muscle
2. Inferior cornus branch
3. Circumflex scapular artery
4. Transverse branch
5. Descending branch
6. Teres major muscle
7. Infraspinatus muscle
8. Infraspinatus fossa branch
9. Latissimus dorsi muscle

| **Figure 1-9** | **Transposition of the flap** |

The vascular pedicle should be confirmed with blunt dissection in the trilateral intermuscular space. The flap should then be completely raised in an island with the circumflex scapular cutaneous artery. It could be transferred by rotation to its adjacent defects.

Key points in applied anatomy

Firstly, the anatomical trilateral space is clear and easy to be separated, whose skin surface projection might fall at 7.0 cm below the midpoint of the scapular spina. Secondly, since the trilateral cutaneous branches are too small (about 1.0 mm in diameter) and the vascular pedicles too short for microsurgical anastomosis, the incision of the flap might extend to the upper part of the trilateral cutaneous branch. After the inferior cornual branch and the infraspinous fossa branch are cut and ligated, the flap might be harvested with a pedicle of the circumflex scapular artery. The pedicle is generally 6.0 cm in length and 3.0 mm in diameter. If a longer and larger pedicle is needed, the thoracodorsal artery should be cut and ligated and the subscapular artery adopted. Thirdly, if the posterior branches of the 2nd-4th thoracic nerves are identified and anastomosed, a flap with the sensory nerve may be possible. The operation should be done with great care, since the vascular and the nervous pedicles are located neither in the same position nor in the same direction. Moreover, the nerve branches are small in transverse diameter (1.0 mm in general).

Lateral Superior Brachial Flap

The superior lateral brachial flap is located on the lateral superior part of the upper arm. Its axial vessels comprise the posterior circumflex brachial artery and the superior lateral brachial cutaneous artery. The flap might have a skin of good quality and carry a cutaneous nerve. The donor site might be more cosmetic than the forearm flap. It might be transferred to restore a skin defect on the proximal arm, the shoulder or the axilla. It might also be used as a free flap.

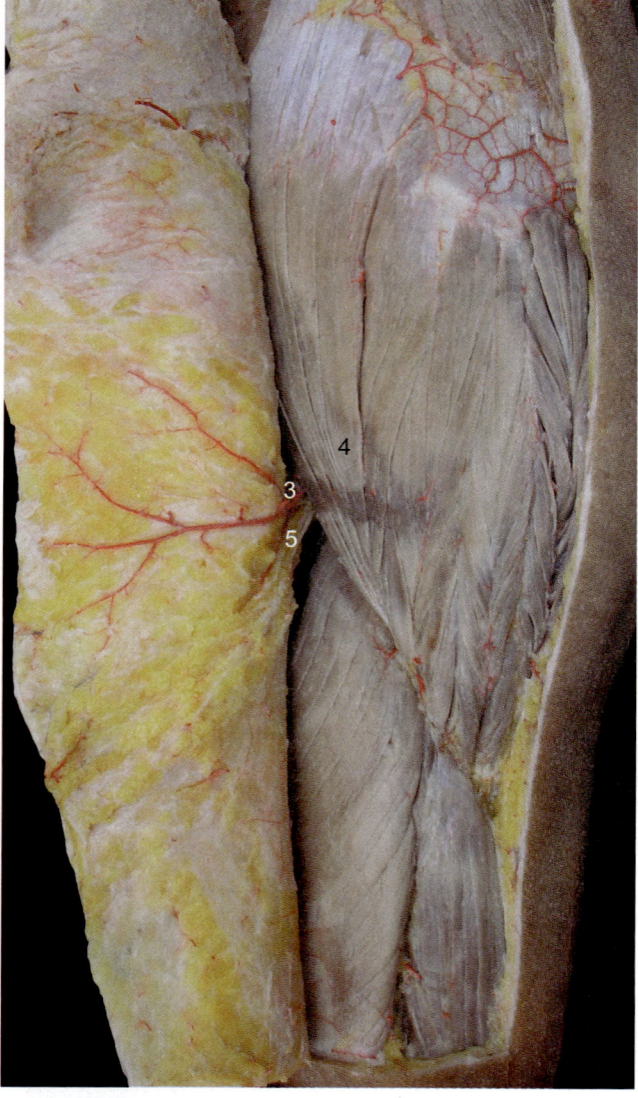
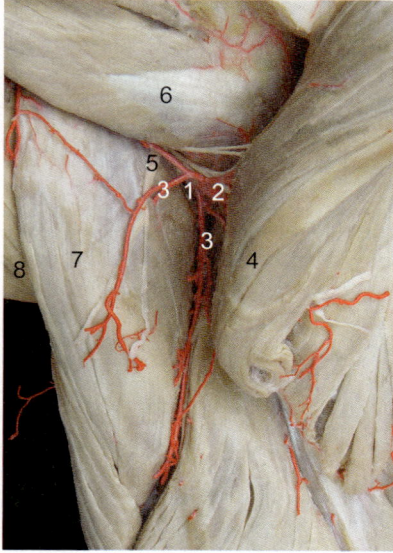

1. Posterior circumflex brachial artery
2. Muscular branch
3. Cutaneous branch (superior lateral brachial cutaneous artery)
4. Deltoid muscle
5. Superior lateral brachial cutaneous nerve
6. Teres minor muscle
7. Long head of triceps brachii muscle
8. Teres major muscle

Figure 1-10   **Applied anatomy**

The posterior circumflex brachial artery arises from the axillary artery, passes through the quadrilateral space and reaches the deep surface of the deltoid muscle. The artery trunk is 3.8 mm in diameter. The posterior circumflex brachial artery gives several relatively large muscular branches and 1-2 relatively small cutaneous branches at the posterior quadrilateral space. The muscular branches enter the deltoid muscle together with their accompanying veins. The superior lateral brachial cutaneous artery passes through the posterior deltoid muscle, accompanied by the superior lateral brachial cutaneous nerves, which originate from the axillary nerve. These vascular branches pass through the postero-inferior deltoid muscle (0.8-1.0 mm in diameter), and fan out over the deep fascia of the superior lateral brachial region. The vascular pedicles are about 5cm in length.

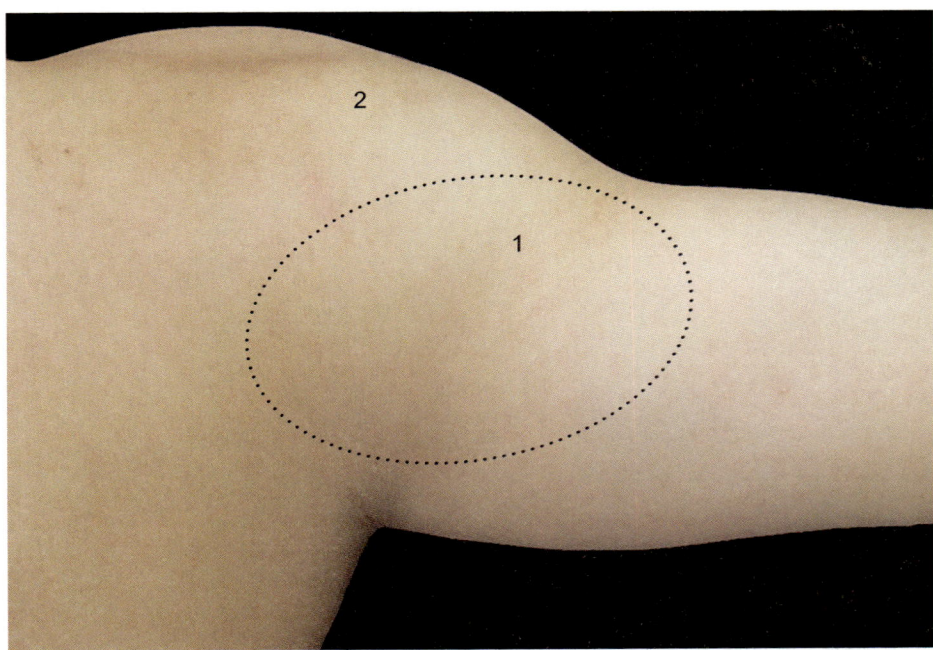

1. Deltoid muscle
2. Acromion

Figure 1-11   Design of the flap

The Core point of the flap might fall on the superficial point of the superior lateral brachial cutaneous artery, which should be confirmed with the Doppler pre-operatively. Its pivot point should be located at the quadrilateral space, which is usually located at 7 cm below the acromion. The flap might be extended to 5 cm above the olecranon.

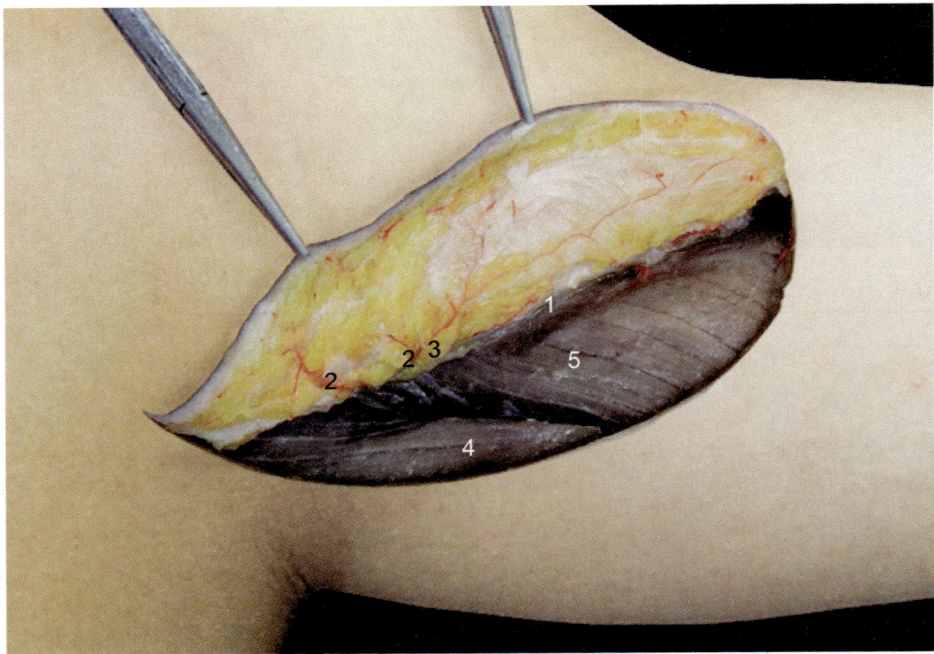

1. Deltoid muscle
2. Superior lateral brachial cutaneous artery
3. Superior lateral brachial cutaneous nerve
4. Long head of triceps brachii muscle
5. Lateral head of triceps brachii muscle

Figure 1-12   Dissection of the flap

The flap should be dissected from its posterior border to its anterior and elevated under the deep fascia until it overlies the posterior deltoid muscle. The superior lateral brachial cutaneous artery and the homonymous nerve that may be identified at the posterior deltoid muscle should be kept intact.

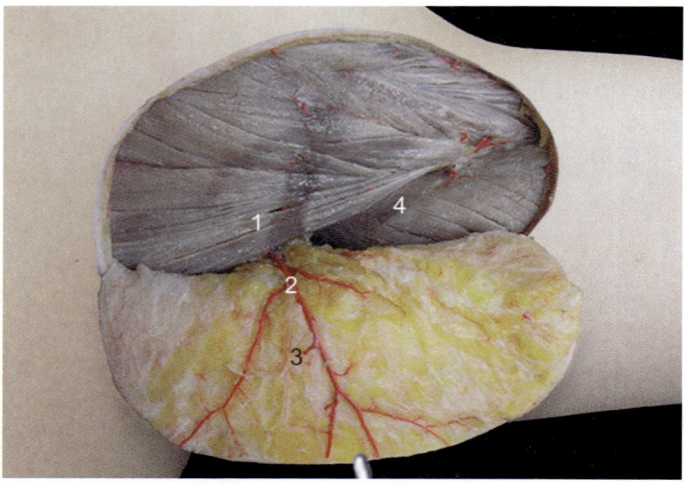

1. Deltoid muscle
2. Superior lateral brachial cutaneous artery
3. Superior lateral brachial cutaneous nerve
4. Lateral head of triceps brachii muscle

Figure 1-13   **Exposure of the vessel**

The flap should be incised from its anterior border and dissected retrogradely to the quadrilateral space along the superior lateral brachial cutaneous artery to expose the trunk of the posterior circumflex brachii artery.

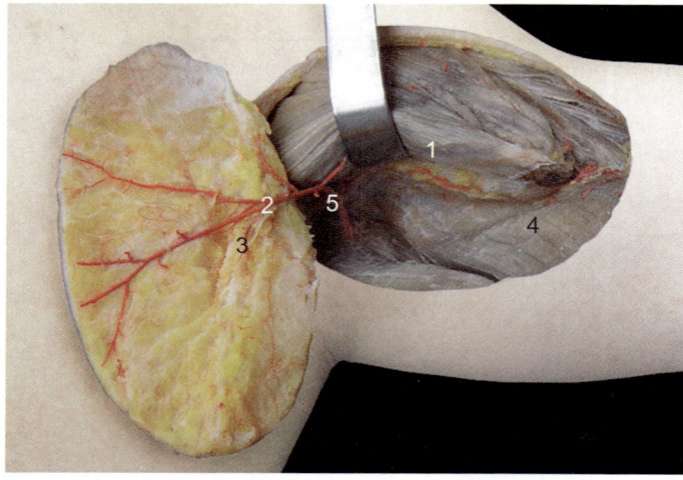

1. Deltoid muscle
2. Superior lateral brachial cutaneous artery
3. Superior lateral brachial cutaneous nerve
4. Lateral head of triceps brachii muscle
5. Posterior circumflex brachii artery

Figure 1-14   **Transposition of the flap**

The posterior border of the deltoid muscle should be elevated to observe the course of the vessels in the deep muscular surface. The flap should be dissected as has been designed with a pedicle of the posterior circumflex brachii artery. Then it might be transferred to restore a nearby wound.

Key points in applied anatomy

Firstly, the anatomic point at which the superior lateral brachial cutaneous artery and nerve perforate through the deep fascia might fall on the intersection of the two lines, one is between the acromion and the olecranon, and the other is the posterior border of the deltoid muscle. This point should be confirmed with the Doppler. Secondly, when the operation is being performed, the posterior deltoid muscle should be elevated to expose the vascular and nervous pedicles. Therefore, the skin incision should begin medial to the posterior deltoid muscle and extend to the posterior axillary fold. The flap should be elevated from posterior to anterior under the deep fascia. Thirdly, when the flap is being transferred, the cutaneous artery and nerve should be traced back to and cut at the posterior circumflex brachii artery (in some cases to the common trunk of the deltoid muscular branch) or the axillary nerve. Both the artery and the nerve are about 1.5-2.0 mm in diameter. They are large enough to be microsurgically anastomosed.

Lateral Middle Brachial Flap

The flap is located at the lateral middle part of the upper arm. Its axial vessel is the lateral brachial cutaneous artery. The flap has a skin of good quality and its donor site is more cosmetic than the forearm flap. But there are no proper cutaneous nerves in the flap to be anastomosed. The flap might be used with a pedicle for the restoration of a skin defect on the proximal arm or for a free transposition.

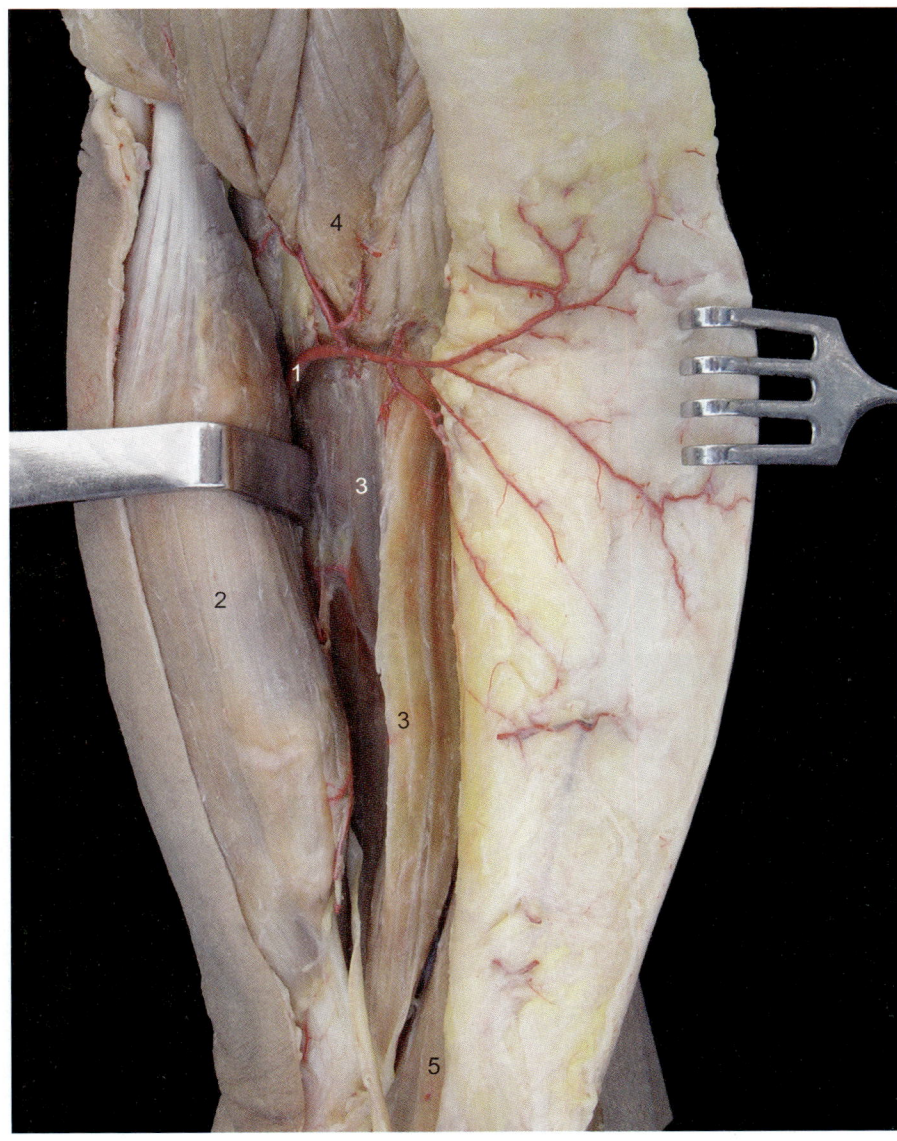

1. Lateral brachial cutaneous artery
2. Brachialis muscle
3. Biceps brachii muscle
4. Deltoid muscle
5. Triceps brachii muscle

Figure 1-15	Applied anatomy

The lateral brachial cutaneous artery originates from the trunk of brachial artery or from the muscular branch of biceps brachii muscle of the brachial artery. In most cases (90%), it emerges from 2 cm under the anterior axillary fold. It extends in the septum between the biceps brachii muscle and the brachialis muscle, and continues under the terminal edge of the deltoid muscle to fan out over the lateral middle skin region of the upper arm. The artery is 1.5 mm in diameter at the origin of the brachial artery. It is 0.8-1.0 mm in diameter and 3-4 cm in length at the deep fascia where it runs superficially. The flap is about 12× 8cm in size. There are veins running through the flap: the accompanying vein that is as large in diameter as the artery, and the cephalic vein that is large in diameter.

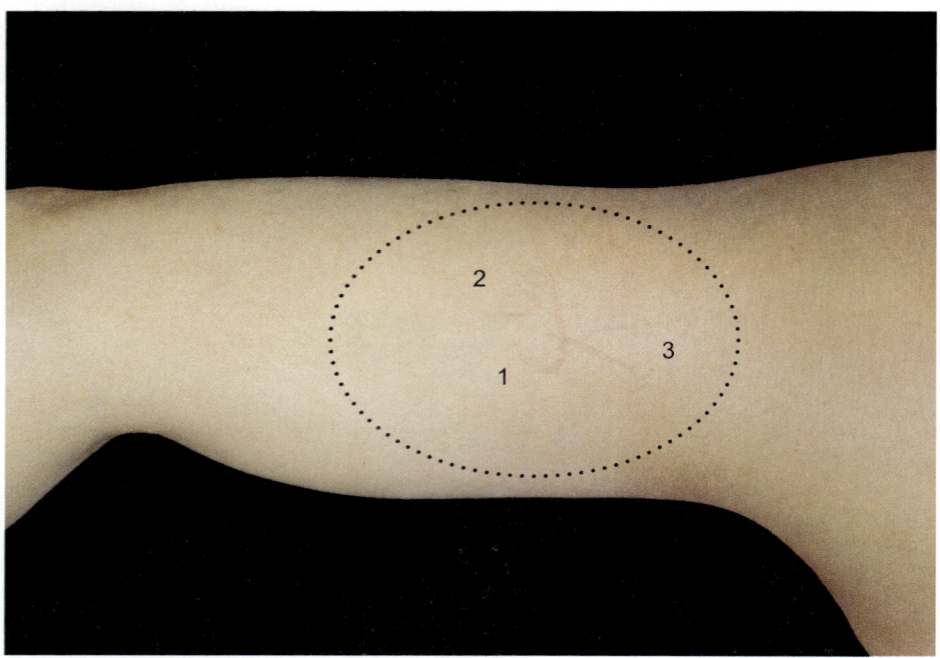

Figure 1-16   Design of the flap

The flap should be designed with its pivot point falling on the intersection between the septum of the brachialis muscle and the biceps brachial muscle, and the terminal edge of the deltoid muscle. This point can be confirmed with the Doppler.

1. Brachialis muscle
2. Biceps brachii muscle
3. Deltoid muscle

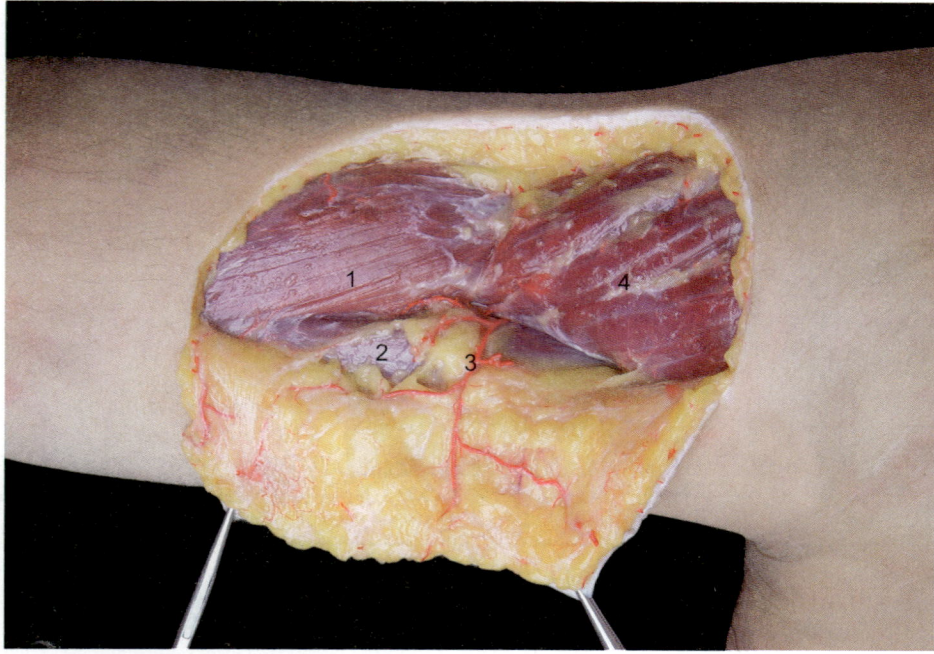

1. Brachialis muscle
2. Biceps brachii muscle
3. Lateral brachial cutaneous artery
4. Deltoid muscle

Figure 1-17   Dissection of the flap

The flap should be dissected firstly from its posterior border and then elevated anteriorly from under the deep fascia to the septum between the brachialis muscle and the biceps brachii muscle.

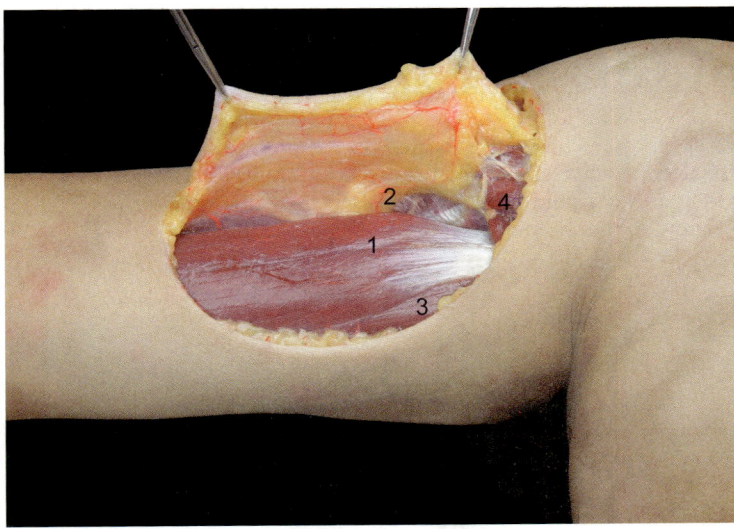

1. Long head of biceps brachii muscle
2. Lateral brachial cutaneous artery
3. Short head of biceps brachii muscle
4. Deltoid muscle

Figure 1-18   **Elevation of the flap**

After the posterior dissection, the anterior border of the flap should be incised. The dissection should be performed posteriorly under the deep fascia and traced to the septum between the biceps brachii muscle and the brachialis muscle, where the axial vessels are visualized.

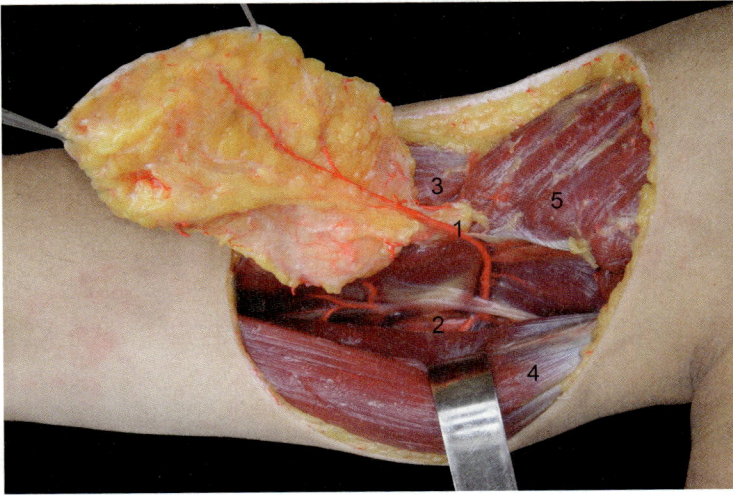

1. Lateral brachial cutaneous artery
2. Brachial artery
3. Brachialis muscle
4. Long head of biceps brachii muscle
5. Deltoid muscle

Figure 1-19   **Transposition of the flap**

The flap then should be dissected in a peripheral to central manner along the lateral brachial cutaneous artery to its origin. It might be transferred to restore an adjacent skin defect or used as a free graft.

Key points in applied anatomy

Firstly, the flap should be based on the middle part of the upper arm with its axial line falling along the spatium intermusculare of the lateral arm. It should not be larger than 10×5cm in size. Secondly, the operation might become easier if the dissection is done in the septum between the biceps brachii muscle and the brachialis muscle. The vascular pedicle under the marginal deltoid muscle should be given great attention to avoid getting it damaged, since the vessel might be closely attached to the periosteal surface in some cases, or it might perforate through the humeral muscular fibers in other cases.

5 Lateral Inferior Brachial Flap

The flap is commonly termed as the lateral arm flap in clinics. It is located on the lateral lower part of the upper arm. Its axial artery comprises the deep brachial artery and the posterior branch of the radial collateral artery. The vascular pedicle is long and constant. The pedicled flap might be transferred either anterogradely to restore a shoulder region, or retrogradely to cover an elbow wound.

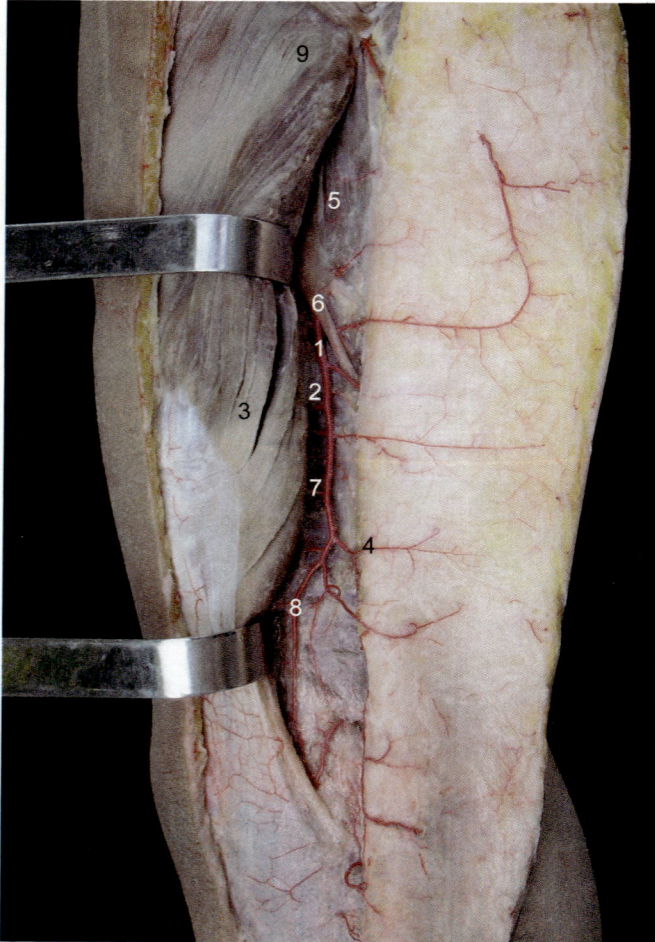
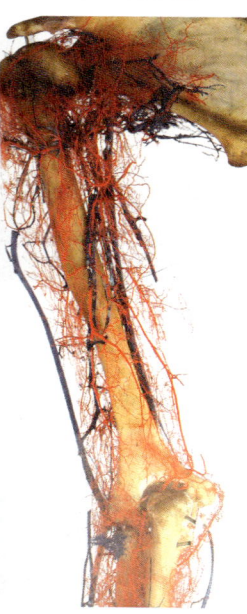

1. Radial collateral artery
2. Brachioradial muscle
3. Triceps brachii muscle
4. Cutaneous branch
5. Biceps brachii muscle
6. Radial nerve
7. Muscular branch
8. Periosteal branch
9. Deltoid muscle

Figure 1-20   Applied anatomy

The radial collateral artery emerges from the deep brachial artery at the insertion plane of the deltoid muscle. It then bifurcates into the anterior and the posterior branches at 4 cm under the terminal plane. The anterior branch extends with the radial nerve in the lateral spatium intermusculare of the upper arm and continues in the deep septum between the brachialis muscle and the triceps brachii muscle. The anterior branch has little to do with the blood supply of the flap. The posterior branch attaches closely to the lateral posterior septum of the upper arm and extends distally along the septum brachioradialis muscle and the triceps brachii muscle. It continues superficially to the posterior lateral groove of the elbow and anastomoses with the radial recurrent artery to form the arterial net of the cubital articulation. Along the course, it gives 1-6 cutaneous branches to fan out over the lateral skin of the arm. The artery has its own accompanying vein and cutaneous nerve. The cutaneous nerve sends small superior branches (inferior lateral brachial cutaneous nerves, 2.0 mm in transverse diameter) and large inferior branches (posterior antebrachial cutaneous nerves, 2.5 mm in transverse diameter). The radial collateral artery is 1.3 mm in diameter. There are two venous systems in the flap: the radial collateral veins of the deep group that accompanying the arteries, and the cephalic vein of the superficial group.

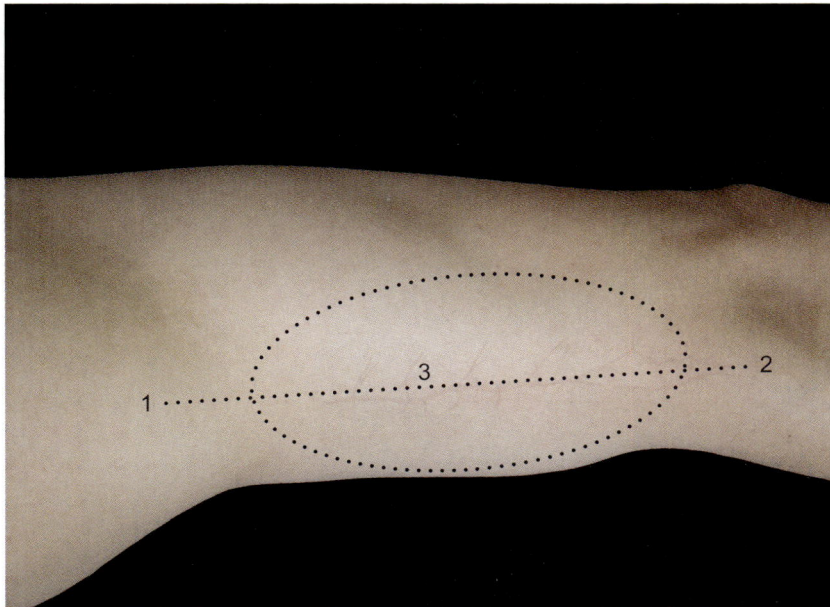

1. Terminal point of the deltoid muscle
2. Lateral epicondyle of humerus
3. Posterior branch of radial collateral artery

Figure 1-21   Design of the flap

The flap should be designed with its axial line falling along the surface project line of the lateral spatium intermusculare, which represents the posterior branch of the radial collateral artery. The body surface project line should be determined by the connection between the insertion point of the deltoid muscle and the lateral epicondyle of the humerus. The flap size should be adjusted to that of the defect. Its superior border might extend to 5.0 cm above the insertion of the deltoid muscle, its lateral to the posterior midline, its medial to the anterior arm and its inferior to the cubital transverse line.

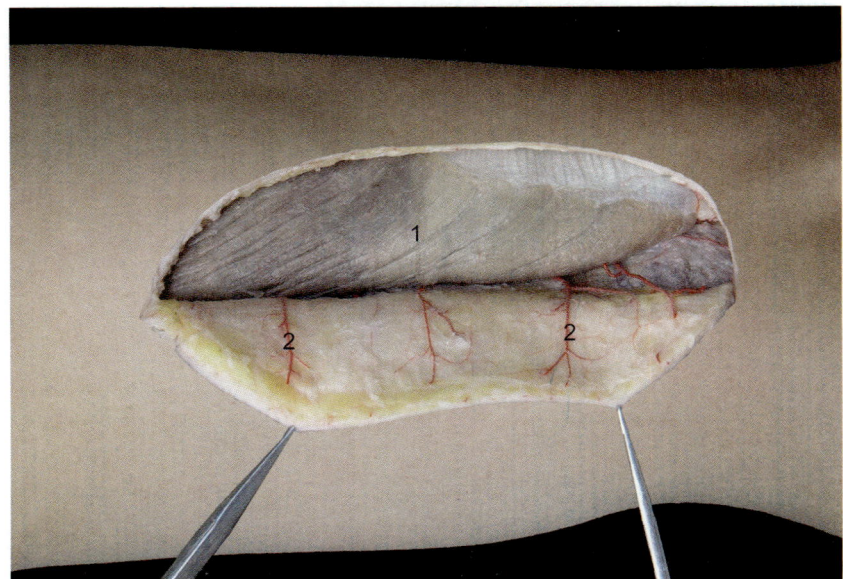

1. Triceps brachii muscle
2. Cutaneous branch

Figure 1-22   Dissection of the flap

As has been designed, the dissection of the flap should begin with its posterior border. Then the flap should be elevated anteriorly from under the deep fascia to the septum between the triceps brachii muscle and the biceps brachii muscle to expose the small vascular branches that perforates through the spatium intermusculare to enter the flap.

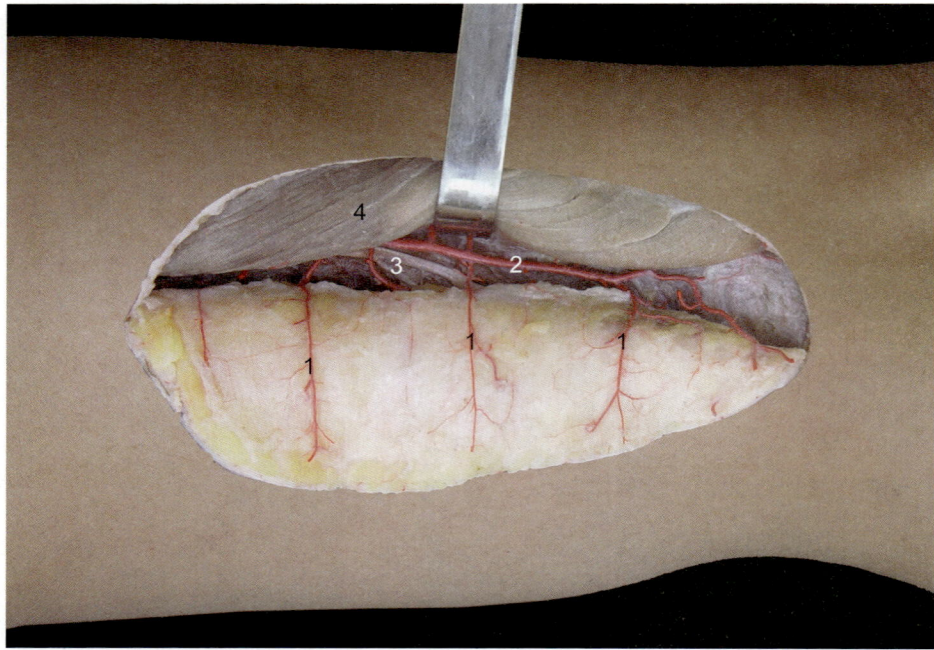

1. Cutaneous branch
2. Radial collateral artery
3. Inferior lateral brachial cutaneous nerve
4. Triceps brachii muscle

| **Figure 1-23** | **Exposure of the vessels** |

The spatium intermusculare should be incised open and the dissection continues in the septum along the cutaneous branch to expose the posterior branch of the radial collateral artery, which is situated deep in the spatium intermusculare.

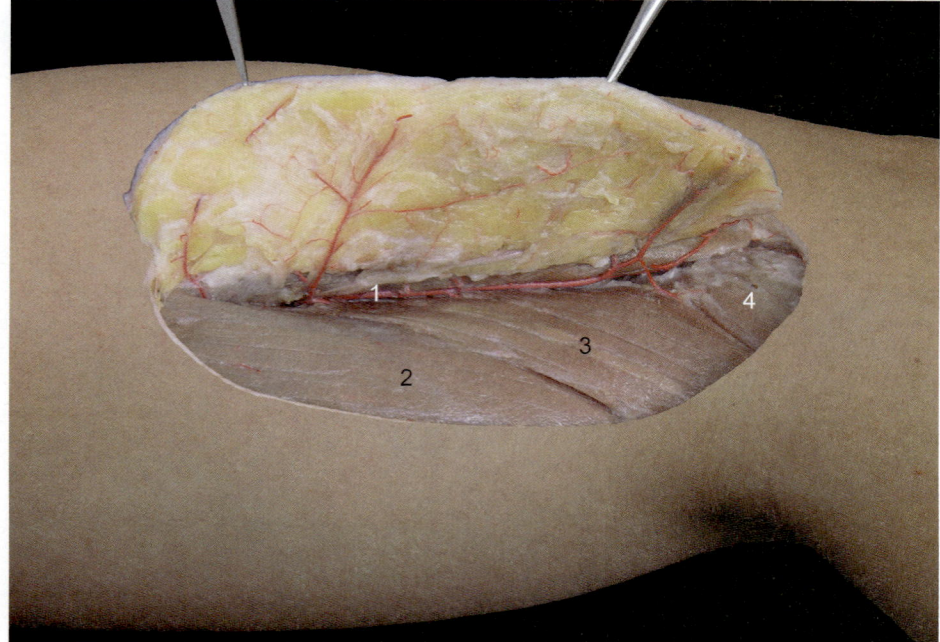

1. Radial collateral artery
2. Biceps brachii muscle
3. Brachioradial muscle
4. Extensor carpi radialis longus muscle

| **Figure 1-24** | **Elevation of the flap** |

Then the flap should be pulled back to where it was located and temporarily sutured. Then its anterior border should be opened and the dissection performed posteriorly under the deep fascia and traced to the lateral spatium Limtermusculare.

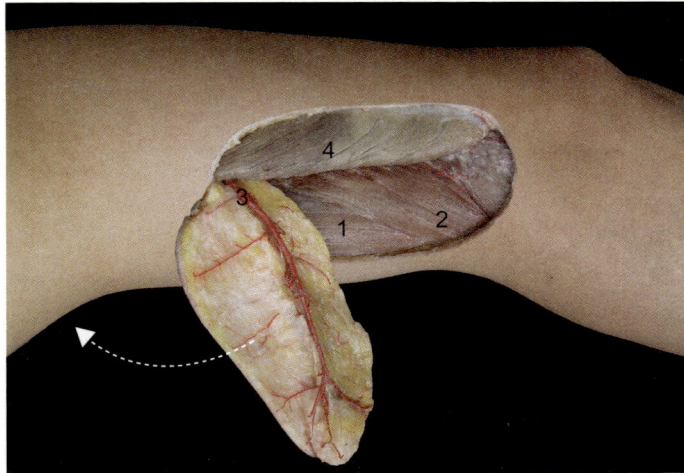

1. Biceps brachii muscle
2. Brachioradial muscle
3. Radial collateral artery
4. Triceps brachii muscle

Figure 1-25   Anterograde transposition of the flap

The posterior branch of the radial collateral artery should be cut at the distal end of the flap. The incision should continue proximally until the vascular pedicle is long enough to guarantee a tension-free transposition. An antegrade-flow lateral arm flap pedicled with the radial collateral artery might be transferred to cover an adjacent would on the shoulder region.

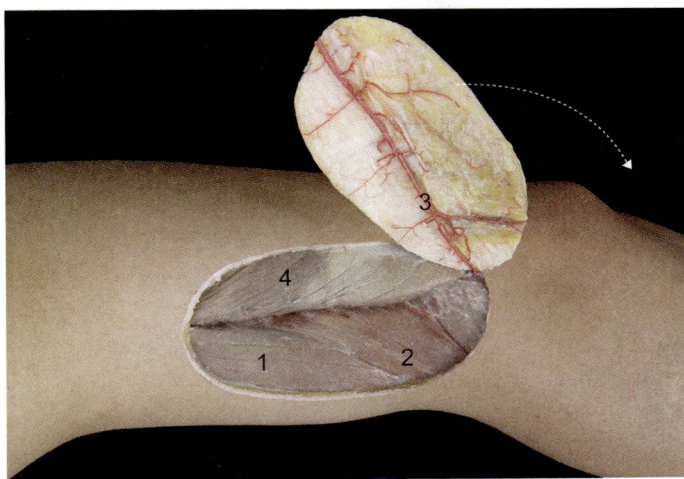

1. Biceps brachii muscle
2. Brachioradial muscle
3. Radial collateral artery
4. Triceps brachii muscle

Figure 1-26   Retrograde transposition of the flap

The posterior branch of the radial collateral artery should be cut at the proximal end of the flap. The incision should continue distally until the vascular pedicle is longer enough to guarantee a proper transposition. A retrograde-flow lateral arm flap pedicled with the radial collateral artery might be transferred to cover a wound on the elbow region.

Key points in applied anatomy

Firstly, the radial collateral neurovascular pedicles should be located in the lateral spatium intermusculare of the arm. Surgical dissection might be easy when the septum is confirmed and the vessel bundle identified long and constant. Secondly, the radial collateral artery is the final branch of the deep brachial artery. It might be separated proximally along the lateral spatium intermusculare of the upper arm to harvest the deep brachial artery if a long vascular pedicle is needed. Thirdly, the inferior lateral brachial cutaneous nerve in the superior donor region, which gives small branches, is preferable to the posterior antebrachial cutaneous nerve when a sensory flap is needed. The latter runs through the donor region but do not innervate the flap. Fourthly, the lateral arm flap might be designed and raised with the forearm skin as a composite flap, as there are constant vascular connections between the lateral arm and the proximal radial forearm.

Medial Brachial Flap

The medial arm flap is located on the middle-distal part of the medial arm. At the donor site, the skin is elastic, fine and thin with little fat. The flap is located on the concealed site. It has two pivot points with two axial arteries: the superior ulnar collateral artery and the ulnar recurrent artery. It might be transferred locally to cover a wound in the axillary fossa or on the elbow. It might also be used as a free flap to restore a skin defect on the frontal head or the cheek.

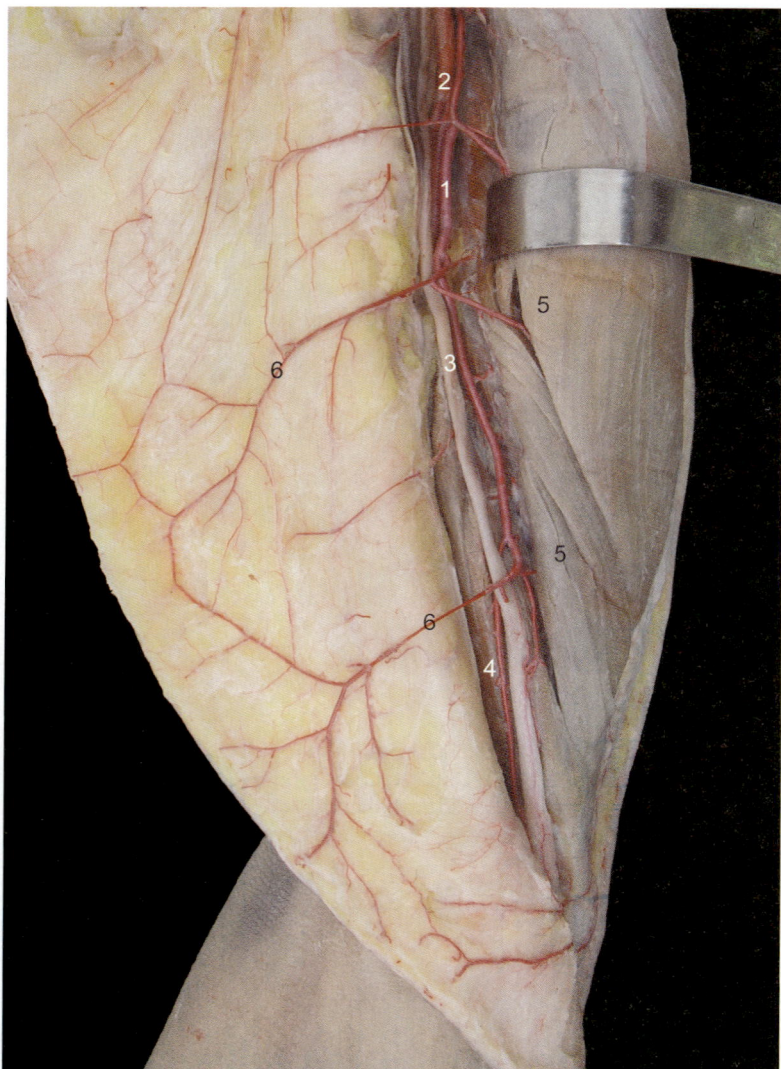

1. Superior ulnar collateral artery
2. Brachial artery
3. Ulnar nerve
4. Brachialis muscle
5. Triceps brachii muscle
6. Cutaneous branch

Figure 1-27   **Applied anatomy**

The superior ulnar collateral artery arises from the brachial artery at the inferior border of the major pectoral muscle. It descends with the ulnar nerve along the medial spatium intermusculare of the arm. The artery is 1.7 mm in diameter and 9 cm in length. In the proximal forearm, the ulnar recurrent artery emerges from the ulnar artery and sends two branches upward: the anterior branch and the posterior branch. The posterior branch extends posteriorly to the medial epicondyle and ascends between the two heads of the flexor carpi ulnar muscle. It then accompanies the ulnar nerve to anastomose with the superior ulnar collateral artery. Along its course, it gives 5-6 cutaneous branches in the spatium intermusculare between the brachialis muscle and the triceps brachii muscle to nourish the medial arm skin. Based on these arteries, a flap might be harvested with a pedicle of either the superior ulnar collateral artery or the ulnar recurrent artery.

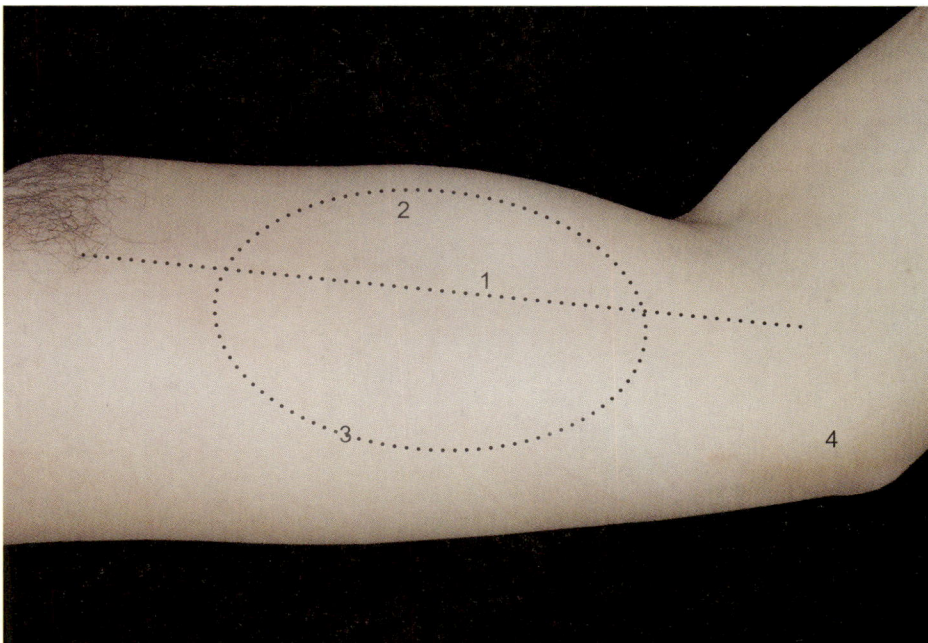

1. Medialis sulcus
2. Biceps brachii muscle
3. Triceps brachii muscle
4. Medial epicondyle

Figure 1-28   Design of the flap

The flap should be designed with its axial line falling on the medialis sulcus of the biceps brachii muscle, where the cutaneous arteries pass through. The central point could be confirmed with the Doppler. The anterior and the posterior margins of the flap might extend to the anterior and the posterior midlines. Its proximal margin extends to the axillary fossa and its distal margin above the medial epicondyle of the humerus.

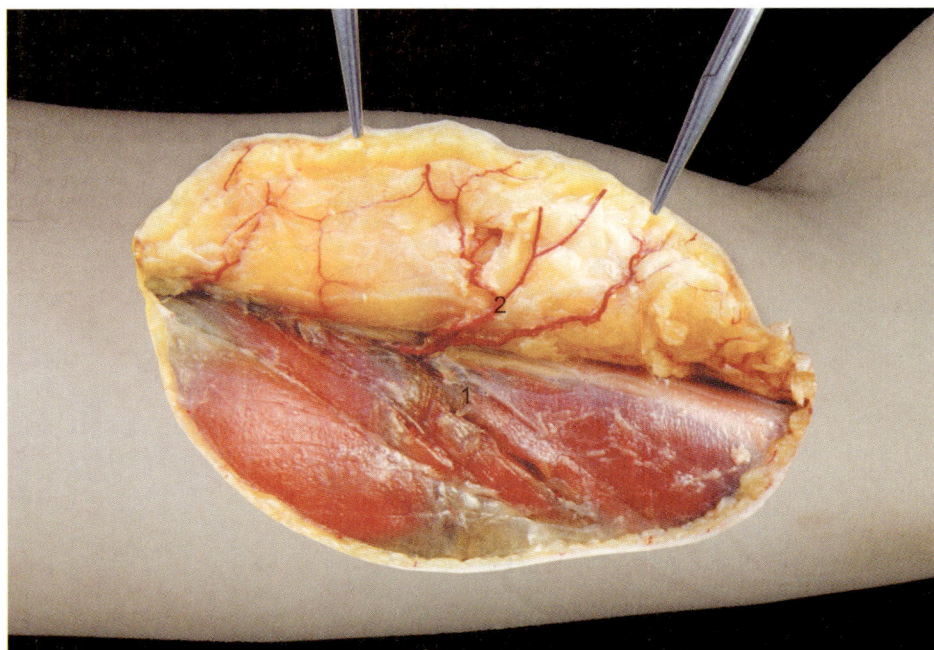

1. Brachialis muscle
2. Cutaneous branch

Figure 1-29   Dissection of the flap

The flap should be first incised at its posterior border and elevated anteriorly from under the deep fascia to expose the cutaneous branches that pass through the spetum between the biceps brachii muscle and the brachialis muscle.

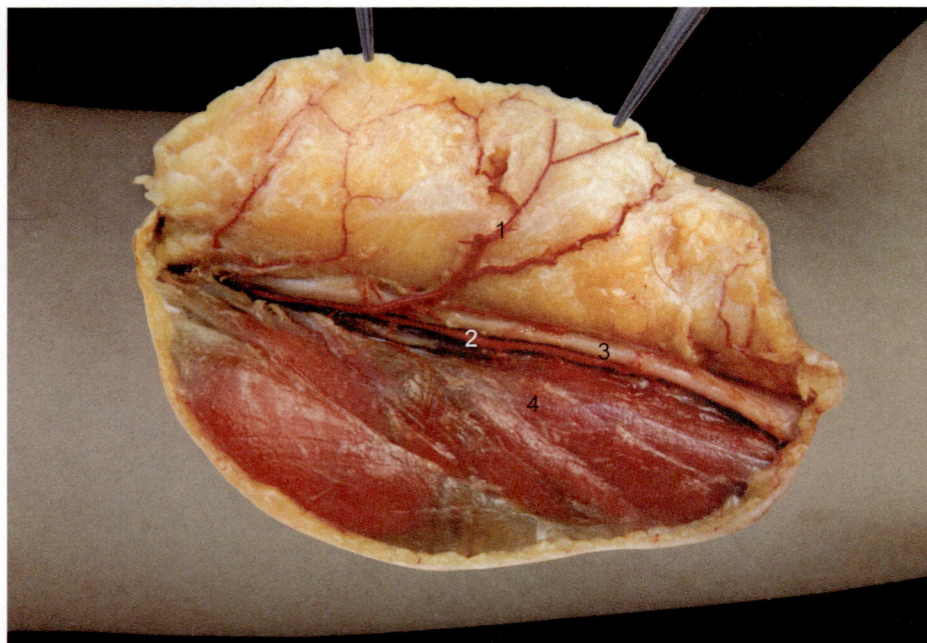

1. Cutaneous branch
2. Superior ulnar collateral artery
3. Ulnar nerve
4. Brachialis muscle

Figure 1-30   Exposure of the artery

The spatium intermusculare should be incised and the dissection continue along the cutaneous branch to the deep anatomical plane of the spatium intermusculare to expose the superior ulnar collateral artery (or the ulnar recurrent artery) and the ulnar nerve.

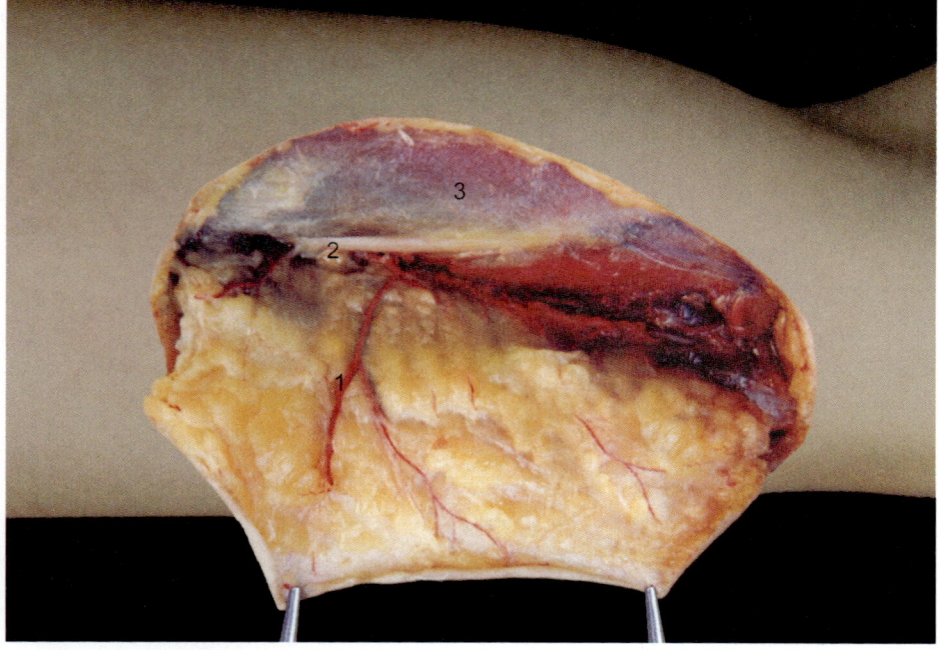

1. Cutaneous branch
2. Median nerve
3. Biceps brachii muscle

Figure 1-31   Elevation of the flap

The anterior border of the flap should be incised and the dissection continue posteriorly from under the deep fascia to the medial spatium intermusculare.

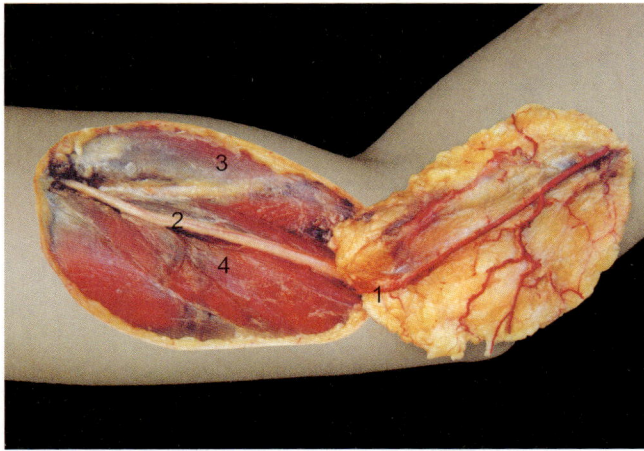

1. Superior ulnar collateral artery
2. Ulnar nerve
3. Biceps brachii muscle
4. Brachialis muscle

Figure 1-32   Retrograde transposition of the flap

The superior ulnar collateral artery should be cut at the proximal end of the flap and the vascular pedicle separated towards the distal end until it is as long as has been expected. A medial arm flap with an ulnar recurrent artery pedicle might be transferred distally to cover a wound on the elbow.

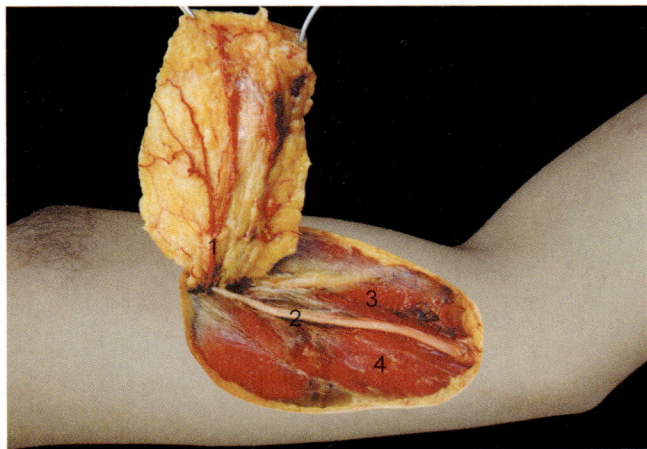

1. Superior ulnar collateral artery
2. Ulnar nerve
3. Biceps brachii muscle
4. Brachialis muscle

Figure 1-33   Anterograde transposition of the flap

The ulnar recurrent artery should be cut at the distal end of the flap and the vascular pedicle separated towards the proximal end until it is as long as has been expected. A medial arm flap with superior ulnar collateral artery pedicle might be transferred proximally to cover a wound on the axillary fossa.

Key points in applied anatomy

Firstly, the donor region of the flap is large. Its superior margin extends to the hairy region of the axillary fossa, its inferior to the plane of the cubitus fossa, its anterior and posterior to the midlines of the arm. The flap has a size of 20×8cm at most. Secondly, the flap should be elevated anteriorly with ease to the medial spatium intermusculare of the arm. With the recognizable ulnar nerve as the mark, it is easy to separate the superior ulnar collateral artery that accompanies the ulnar nerve and nearby superficial cutaneous nerve of the medial brachialis. However, the flap might not be easily elevated anteriorly backwards and this manner is not recommended. Thirdly, the superior ulnar collateral artery is large in diameter, and its branches are distributed over the nerves and muscles. But in some cases (10%), it gives few or no cutaneous branches. Therefore, whether there do exist cutaneous branches of the superior ulnar collateral artery should be confirmed intra-operatively to avoid affecting the blood circulation in the flap. Fourthly, if a reverse-flow island flap is designed, the basilic vein in the donor region should be excluded from the flap to prevent venous ingress.

Posterior Arm Flap

The posterior brachial cutaneous artery serves as the axial vessel of the posterior arm flap. The flap is located at the concealed donor site where the skin is elastic, fine and thin with little hair and little subcutaneous fat. The color of the skin looks like that of the frontal head and the cheeks and so the posterior arm flap is considered as a good donor for the facial surgery and the hand surgery. The flap might also be transferred locally to restore a tissue defect on the axillary fossa or the acromion part.

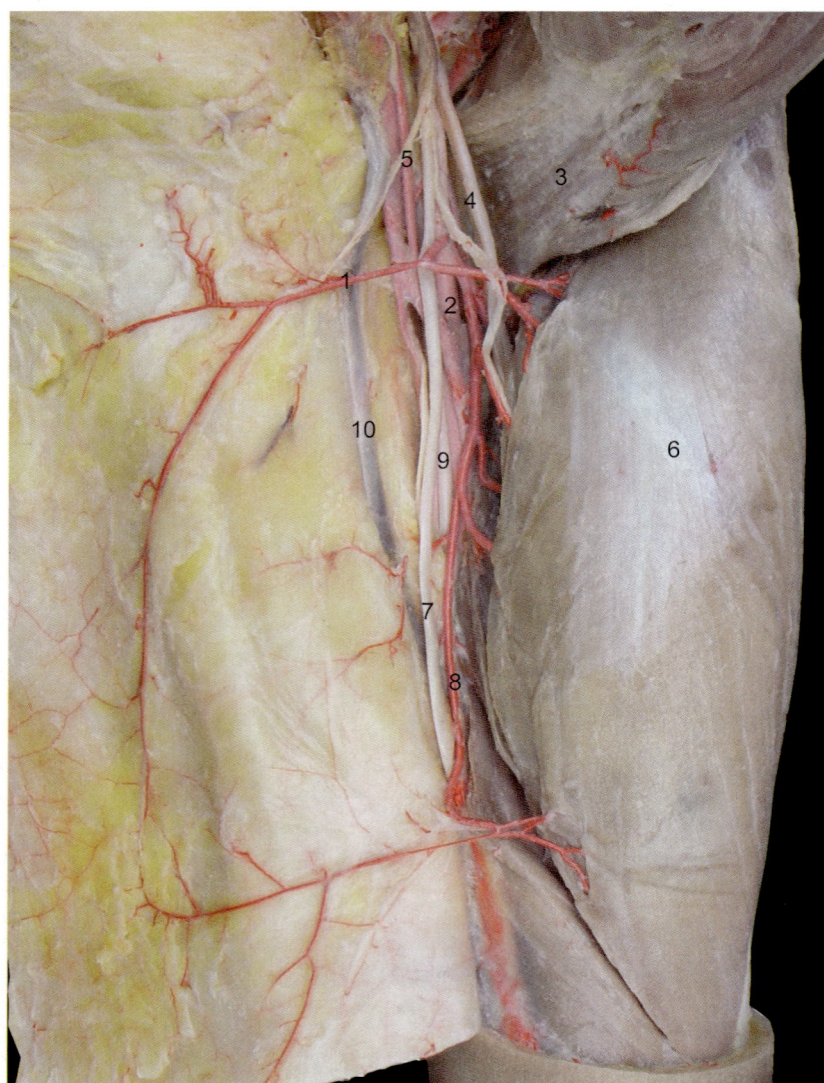

1. Posterior brachial cutaneous artery
2. Brachial artery
3. Latissimus dorsi muscle
4. Radial nerve
5. Posterior brachial cutaneous nerve
6. Long head of triceps brachii muscle
7. Ulnar nerve
8. Superior ulnar collateral artery
9. Median nerve
10. Basilic vein

Figure 1-34	**Applied anatomy**

The posterior brachial cutaneous artery emerges from the brachial artery (77%) and passes constantly through the posterior axillary fold between the latissimus dorsi muscle and the teres major muscle. It then runs with the posterior brachial cutaneous nerve of the radial nerve under the long head of triceps brachii muscle to fan out over the posterior brachial cutaneous region. It nourishes an area of 15×8 cm. The posterior brachial cutaneous artery is 1.5 mm in diameter at its origin. Its pedicle is 3-5 cm long. It has two accompanying veins about 1.8-2.2 mm in diameter and an accompanying nerve about 1.5 mm in transverse diameter.

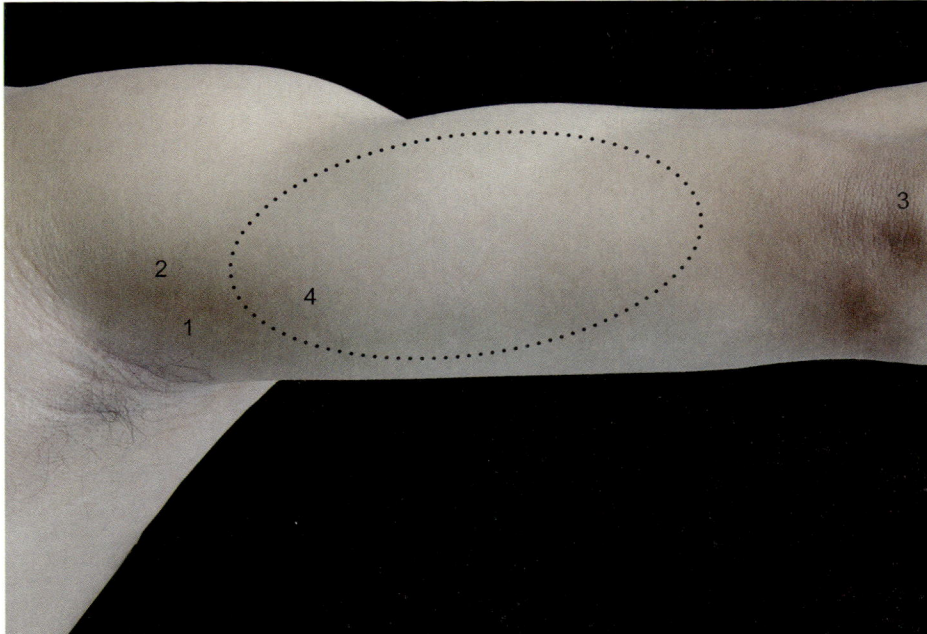

1. Latissimus dorsi muscle
2. Triceps brachii muscle
3. Olecranon
4. Posterior brachial
   cutaneous artery

Figure 1-35   **Design of the flap**

A fusiform flap should be designed with its axial line falling along the body surface projection line of the posterior brachial cutaneous artery. The projection line is based on the superior half of a connecting line from the angular point of the latissimus dorsi muscle and the triceps brachii muscle to the olecranon. The posterior brachial cutaneous artery extends superficially at 2 cm lateral to the angular point of the latissimus dorsi muscle and the triceps brachii muscle.

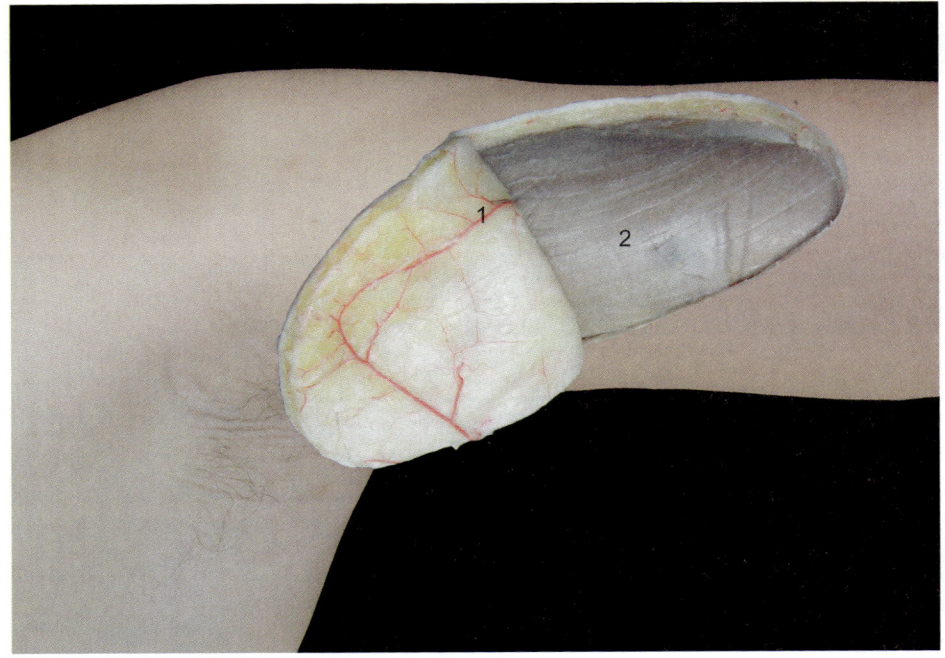

1. Posterior brachial
   cutaneous artery
2. Triceps brachii muscle

Figure 1-36   **Dissection of the flap**

The flap should be first incised from the distal end and elevated at the surface of the muscular sheath from the distal to the proximal to expose the cutaneous artery at about one-third or one-half way.

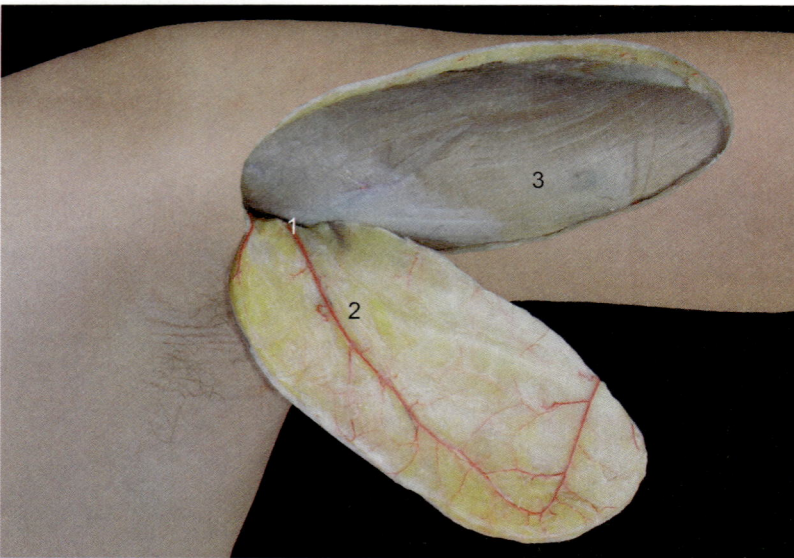

1. Posterior brachial cutaneous artery
2. Posterior brachial cutaneous nerve
3. Triceps brachii muscle

Figure 1-37   Elevation of the flap

The proximal end of the flap should be then incised and the dissection continues to the origin of the posterior brachial cutaneous artery, vein and nerve.

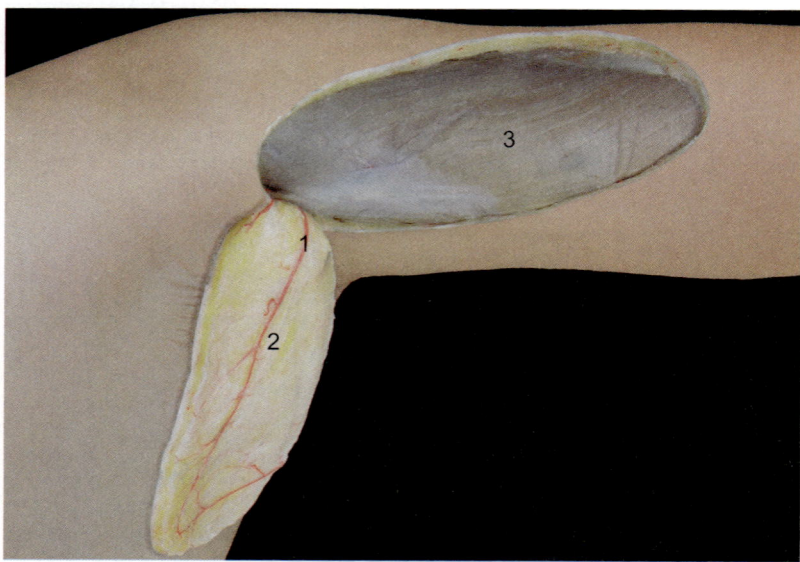

1. Posterior brachial cutaneous artery
2. Posterior brachial cutaneous nerve
3. Triceps brachii muscle

Figure 1-38   Transposition of the flap

The tissue of scar contracture in the recipient region should be removed and the flap transferred to the recipient region either via the subcutaneous tunnel or via the open incision.

Key points in applied anatomy

Firstly, the vascular and nervous pedicles of the flap that pass through the posterior axillary fold are constantly positioned. The tissue near the posterior-inferior axillary fossa is so loose that the pedicles could be easily separated. The muscular branches of the radial nerve that enter the long head of triceps brachii muscle might serve as the anatomic mark, by which the vascular and the nervous bundle that have the common trunk with the muscular branches could be easily found. Secondly, the posterior arm flap might have a size about 15×8 cm.

Radial Forearm Flap

The radial artery might serve as the axial vessel in the radial forearm flap. It is characterized as large in caliber, superficial in location, constant for anatomy, and easy for dissection. The radial forearm flap might be transferred anterogradely or retrogradely to cover wound on the upper limb. Conventionally, a main artery of the hand has to be sacrificed after the flap is dissected. But this shortcoming could be overcome if a cutaneous branch of the radial artery with its deep fascia is included in the flap.

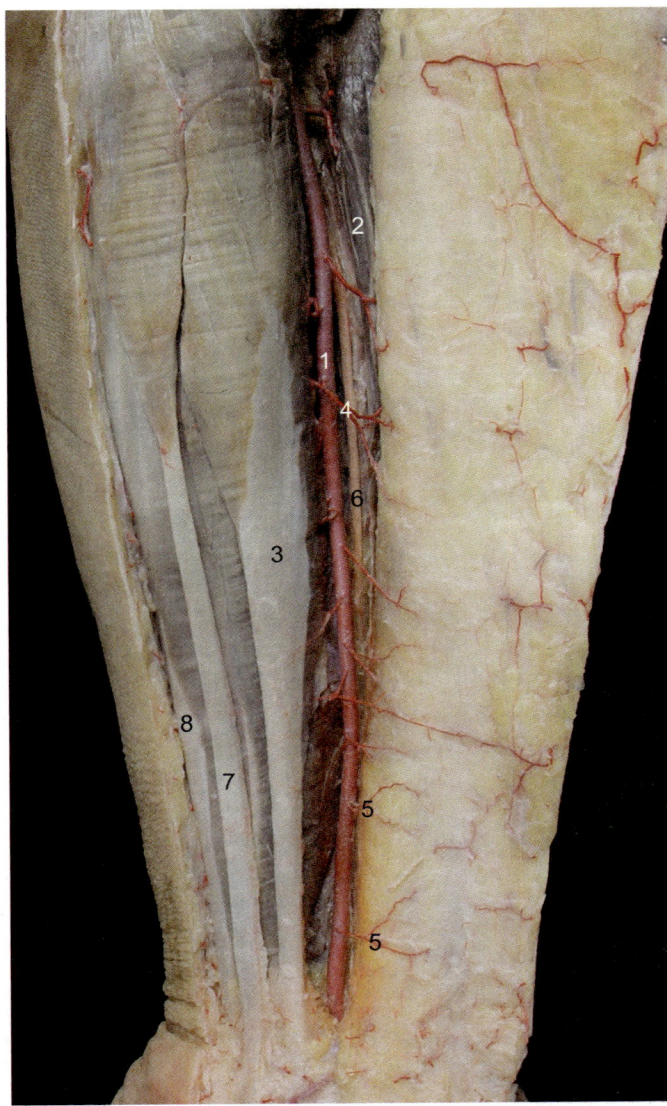

1. Radial artery
2. Brachioradial muscle
3. Flexor carpi radialis
4. Musculocutaneous branch
5. Cutaneous branch
6. Radial nerve
7. Palmaris longus muscle
8. Flexor digitorum superficialis muscle

Figure 1-39	Applied anatomy

The radial artery emerges from the cubitus fossa, descends distally along the radial border and hides itself under the brachioradial muscle at the proximal 2/3 of the forearm. The distal 1/3 of the radial artery runs superficial in the septum between the brachioradialis muscle and the flexor carpi radialis muscle, covered merely by the overlying skin and fascia. The radial artery gives 1-3 musculocutaneus branches at its proximal segment (1/3), 2-3 cutaneous branches at its middle segment (1/3) and 3-7 cutaneous branches at its distal segment (1/3). If a flap with a pedicle of the distal radial artery is transferred retrogradely to restore a wound on the hand, the ulnar artery supplies it via the volar arterial arches.

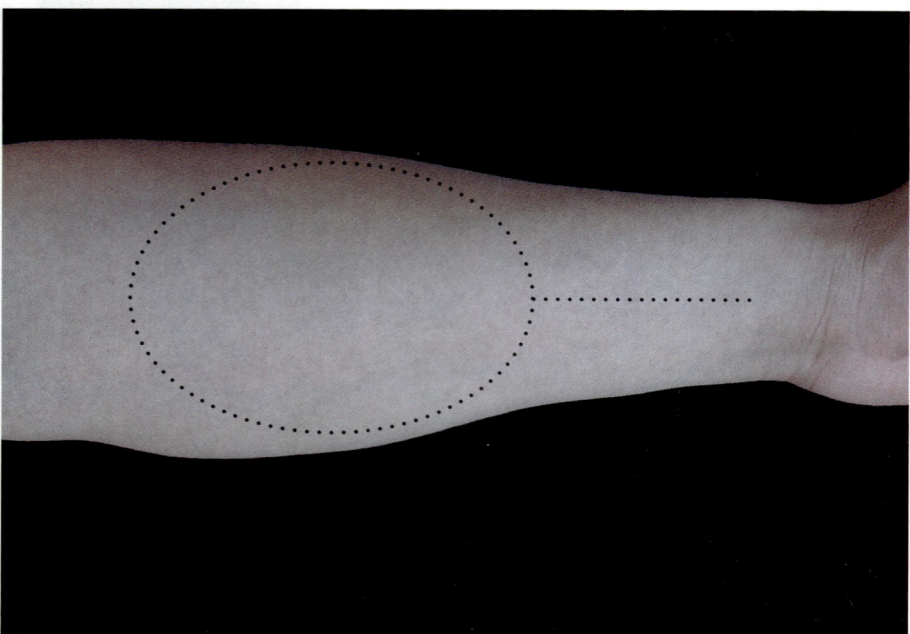

Figure 1-40   **Design of the flap**

The flap might be designed with its axial line falling on the connecting line between the central point of the cubitus fossa and the pulsating point of the carpal radial artery. Its pivot point can be located at the origin of the cubital radial artery if the flap was to be transferred proximally to repair a wound on the upper arm or on the elbow. Its pivot point should be located at the pulsating point of the carpal radial artery if the flap was to be transferred distally to repair a wound on the hand. A bat-like flap might be designed on the radial forearm.

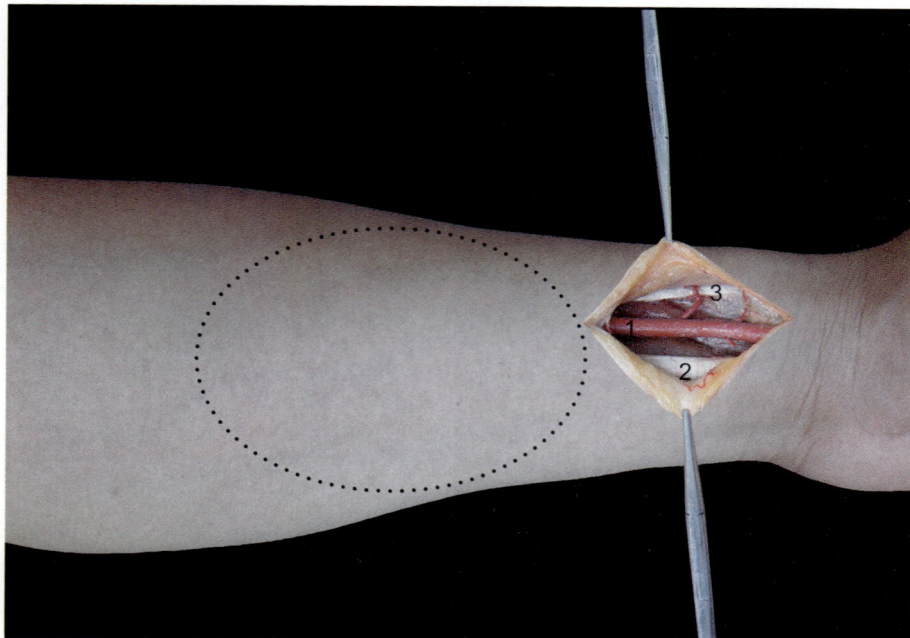

1. Radial artery
2. Brachioradial muscle
3. Flexor carpi radialis muscle

Figure 1-41   **Exposure of the vessels**

The base of the pedicle should be incised to expose the radial artery and the concomitant radial veins between the flexor carpi radialis muscle in the ulnar side and the brachioradial muscle in the radial side. The vascular bundle should be given great attention to keep them intact.

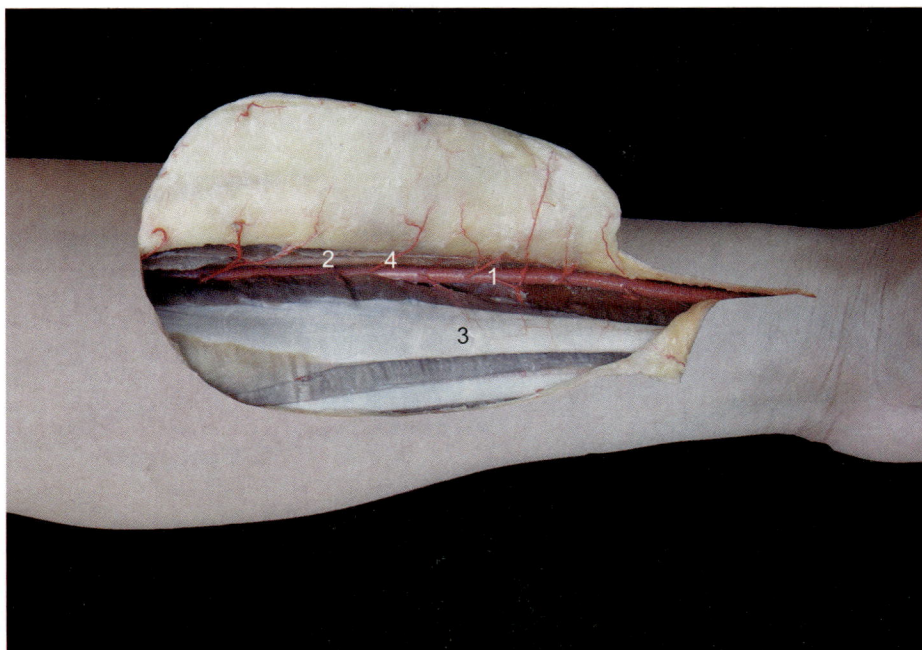

1. Radial artery
2. Brachioradial muscle
3. Flexor carpi radialis muscle
4. Cutaneous branch

Figure 1-42   **Dissection of the flap**

As has been designed, the dissection of the flap should begin with its medial border and continue downwards to the deep fascia, and the flap elevated as a fasciocutaneous one. The central part of the flap should be dissected sharply, and the part near the septum between the brachioradial muscle and the flexor carpi radialis muscle dissected under the tunica muscularis to avoid damaging the small cutaneous branches from the radial artery. The branches in the deep tissue that the radial artery gives should be ligated.

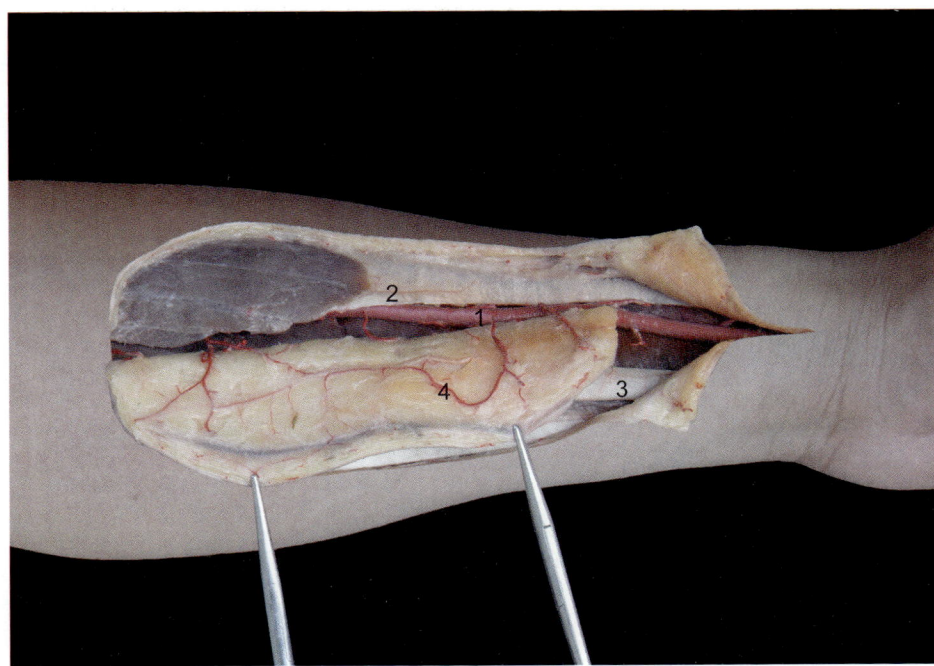

1. Radial artery
2. Brachioradial muscle
3. Flexor carpi radialis muscle
4. Cutaneous branch

Figure 1-43   **Elevation of the flap**

As has been designed, the flap should be incised from its lateral border and separated from lateral to medioinferior under the deep fascia. Then it should be completely elevated.

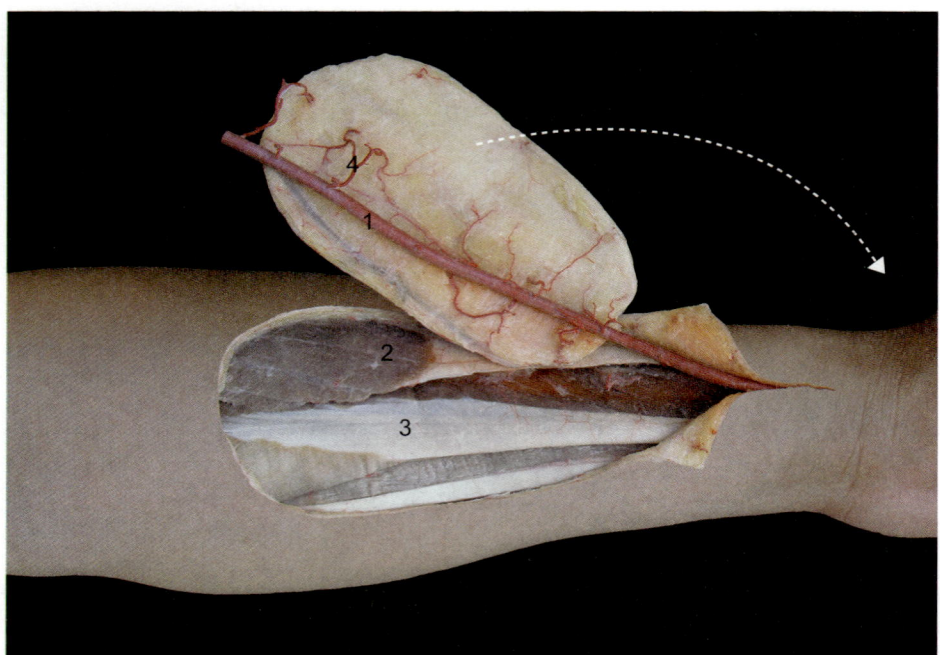

| **Figure 1-44** | **Transposition of the flap** |

When the flap has been elevated completely, the radial artery and the radial vein in the proximal flap should be interrupted with vascular clamps before the pneumatic tourniquet is released. The blood circulation in the hand and in the flap should be monitored and so should the pulsation of the distal radial artery. If nothing is abnormal, the vascular bundles should be ligated and cut at the proximal end to make an island flap with pedicles of the distal radial artery and veins. A flap of this type might be transferred to repair a wound on the hand.

1. Radial artery
2. Brachioradial muscle
3. Flexor carpi radialis muscle
4. Cutaneous branch

Key points in applied anatomy

Firstly, the trunk of the radial artery might serve as the vascular pedicle of the radial forearm flap. It gives bilaterally cutaneous branches and runs superficially through the spatium intermusculare to enter the subcutaneous tissue. Since its trunk is rather long, the size of the flap might be determined as is expected. If a small one is needed, only the exposed part of the artery should be cut; if a large one is needed, both the exposed and the hidden parts should. Thirdly, the flap should be incised and dissected from either the anterior or the posterior edge to the spatium intermusculare. The superficial part of the cutaneous branch should be separated cautiously together with the deep fascia, incorporating the radial vessel en bloc. The muscular branches should be ligated one after another. Fourthly, since the cutaneus branches of the arteries anastomose extensively with one another, it is not necessary that the arterial pedicle be as long as the flap itself..

Ulnar Forearm Flap

9

The ulnar forearm flap is based on the ulnar artery, the ulnar vein and the basilic vein as its axial vessels. A flap of this type might be classified into the category—flaps with pedicles of a main trunk and some branches. Compared to the radial forearm flap, the ulnar flap has a relatively cosmetic donor site. But it has its own disadvantages: the donor size is small and the ulnar artery has to be sacrificed.

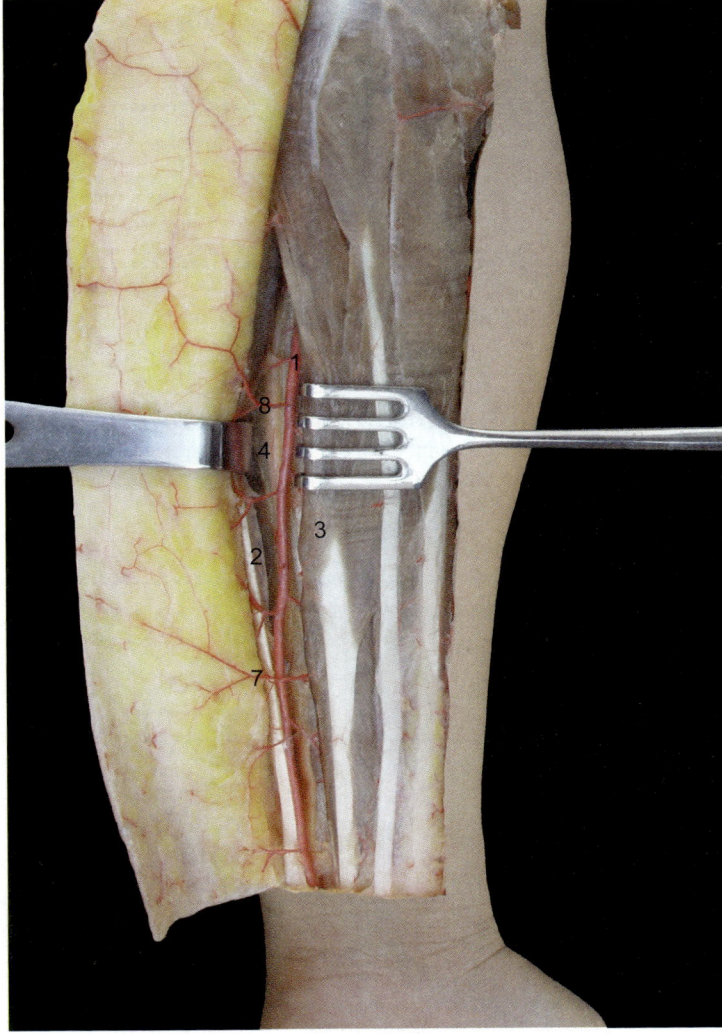
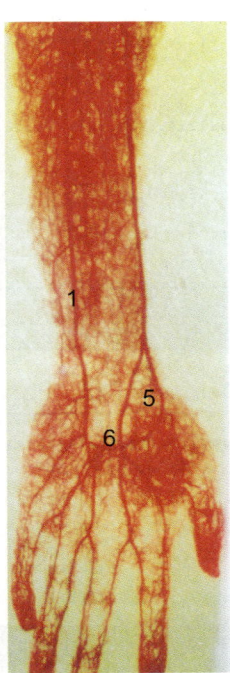

1. Ulnar artery
2. Flexor carpi ulnaris muscle
3. Flexor digitorum superficialis muscle
4. Ulnar nerve
5. Superficial branch of radial artery
6. Superficial volar arch
7. Cutaneous branch of ulnar artery
8. Musculocutaneous branch of ulnar artery

Figure 1-45	Applied anatomy

The ulnar artery arises from the brachial artery at the elbow and extends distally in the spatium intermusculare between the superficial and deep flexors of the forearm and reaches the flexor carpi ulnaris muscle (at about the mid-point of the forearm). It continues distally in the septum of the flexor carpi ulnaris muscle and the flexor digitorum superficialis muscle. It has two accompanying ulnar veins and one ulnar nerve. Its final branch anastomoses with the branch of the radial artery to form a superficial volar arch. The course of the ulnar artery in the forearm might be divided into two parts: the exposed segment and the hidden segment. The hidden segment is located deep between the flexor superficialis muscle and the flexor profundus muscle, and the exposed segment between the flexor carpi ulnaris muscle and the flexor digitorum profundus muscle. The ulnar artery is 21.6 cm long on average and the hidden segment is as long as the exposed one, in which most cutaneous branches of the ulnar artery gather.

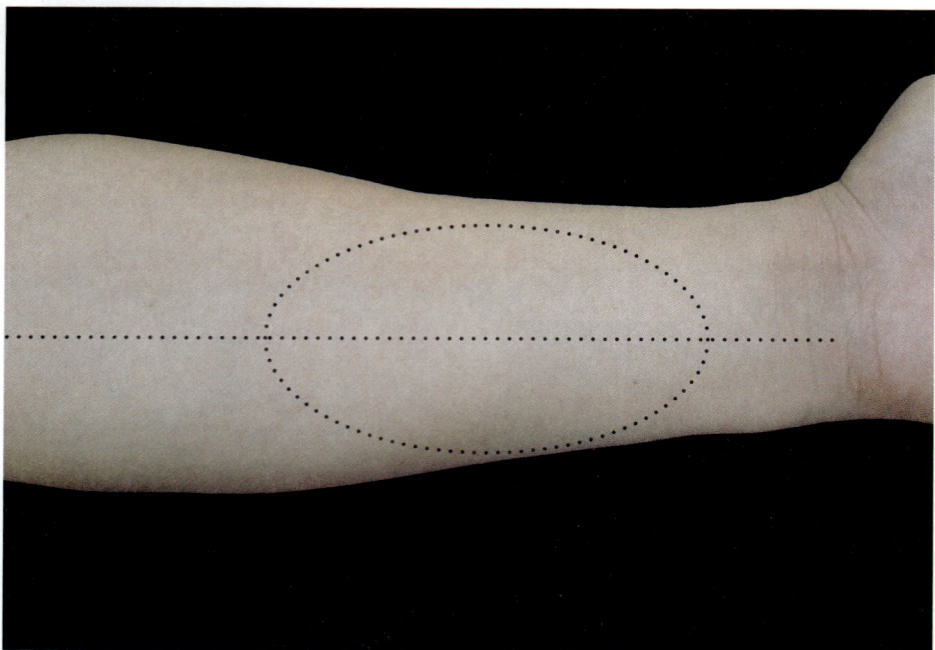

| **Figure 1-46** | **Design of the flap** |

The flap should be designed with its axial line along the ulnar artery. Its proximal edge might extend to the middle-superior segment (1/3) of the forearm, its distal to the transverse carpal line, its lateral to the radial artery and its medial to the posterior ulna.

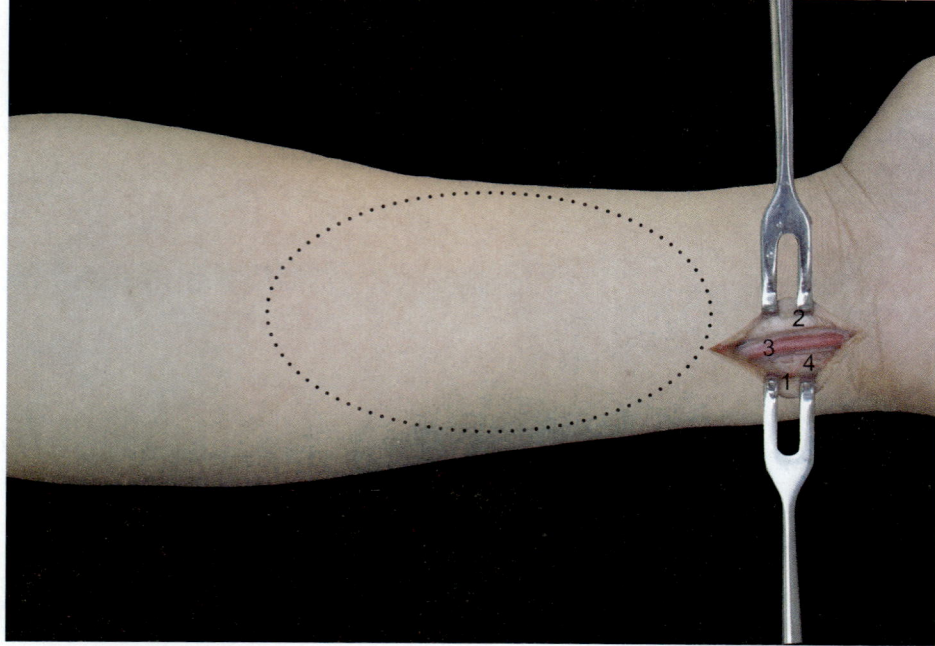

1. Flexor carpi ulnaris muscle
2. Flexor digitorum superficialis muscle
3. Ulnar artery
4. Ulnar nerve

| **Figure 1-47** | **Exposure of the vessels** |

The wrist should be first incised down to the deep fascia, the flexor carpi ulnaris muscle or tendon then drawn ulnarly, and the flexor digitorum superficialis muscle drawn radially to expose the ulnar neurovascular bundle including the artery, the vein and the nerve.

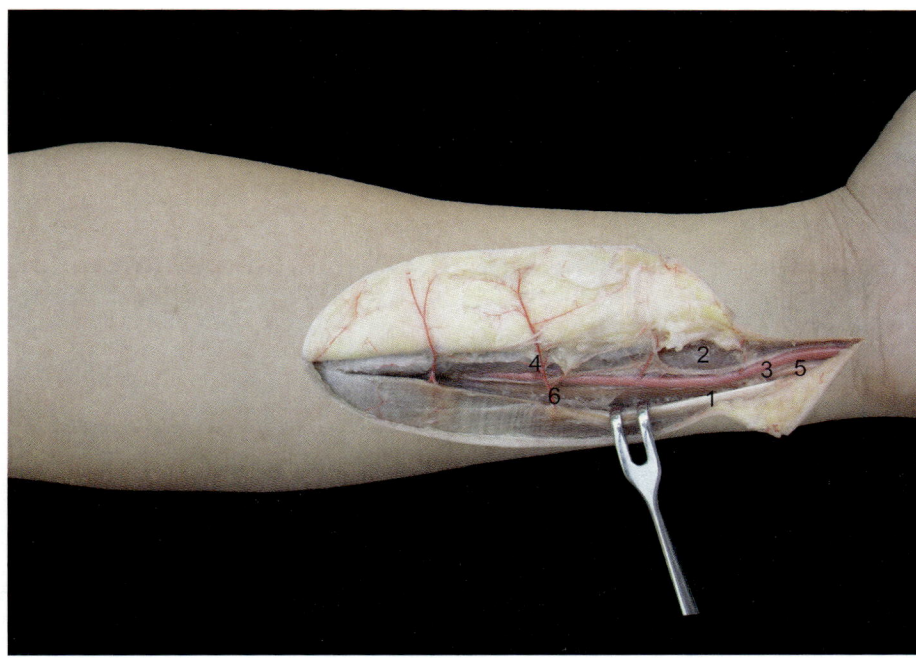

1. Flexor carpi ulnaris muscle
2. Flexor digitorum superficialis muscle
3. Ulnar artery
4. Cutaneous branch of ulnar artery
5. Ulnar nerve
6. Muscular branch of ulnar artery

Figure 1-48   Dissection of the flap

As has been designed, the flap should be incised from its medial border. The incision extends under the deep fascia. The central part of the flap should be dissected sharply near the septum between the flexor carpi ulnaris muscle and the flexor digitorum superficialis muscle to include the vascular bundle (the artery, the vein and the nerve).

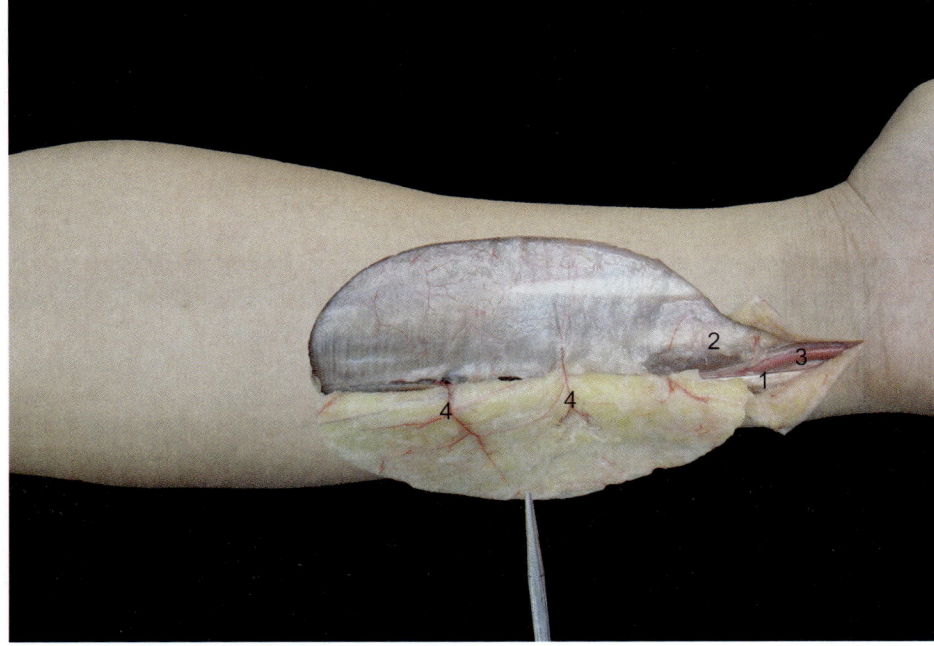

1. Flexor carpi ulnaris muscle
2. Flexor digitorum superficialis muscle
3. Ulnar artery
4. Muscular branch of ulnar artery

Figure 1-49   Elevation of the flap

As has been designed, the flap should be incised from the lateral border, dissected from lateral to medioinferior under the deep fascia and then elevated completely.

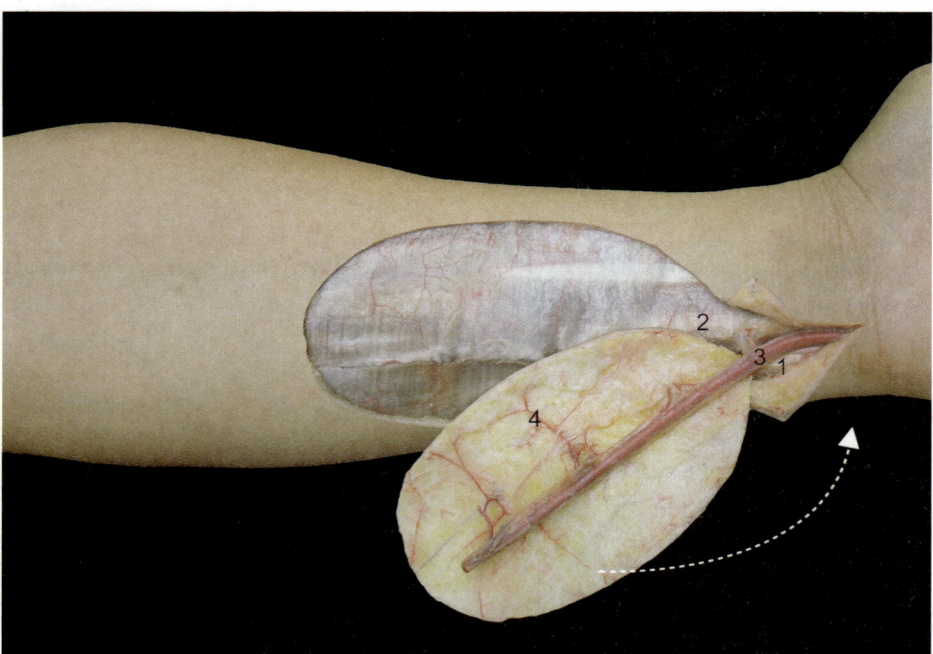

| **Figure 1-50** | **Transposition of the flap** |

After the flap has been elevated completely, the proximal end of the ulnar artery should be interrupted with vascular clamps before the pneumatic tourniquet is released. The blood circulation in the hand and in the flap should be monitored and so should the pulsation of the distal ulnar artery. Nothing abnormal, the vascular bundles should be ligated and cut at the proximal end to make an island flap with pedicles of the distal ulnar artery and veins. A flap of this type might be transferred to cover a wound on the hand.

1. Flexor carpi ulnaris muscle
2. Flexor digitorum superficialis muscle
3. Ulnar artery
4. Muscular branch of ulnar artery

Key points in applied anatomy

Firstly, the skin of the ulnar flap is of good quality, but the location of it is not concealed. Since the flap is made at the cost of the ulnar artery, a main trunk vessel to the hand, the indications of the flap should be strict in some specific cases. A flap of this type might be transferred to reconstruct such important organs as the tongue and the penis. Secondly, since the axial arteries of the flap comprise the trunk of the ulnar artery and its small branches, the trunk is preferable as the vascular pedicle. Since the trunk is large in diameter and adequate in blood pressure, a large region of the flap might have its compensatory circulation via the collateral branches. Therefore the trunk artery with a limited length might be strong enough to stimulate the blood circulation in the concealed segment of the artery. Thirdly, there are abundant communicating branches in the space between the two accompanying veins in the deep layer of the donor region but no venous valves inside the communicating branches. It has been proven in experimental researches and clinical applications that the forearm island flap could be transferred retrogradely to restore defects on the hand with no occurrence of venous return problems. The reason is that the valves in the concomitant veins are not strong and the communicating branches of the veins of the two groups have no valves. A valve incompetent mode or crossover and bypass mode fulfils the venous return.

10

Dorsal Forearm Flap

The dorsal forearm flap is based on the pedicle of the arteriae interossea dorsalis. It might be transferred retrogradely to repair a wound on the hand without damaging the main artery on the forearm or affecting blood supply for the hand.

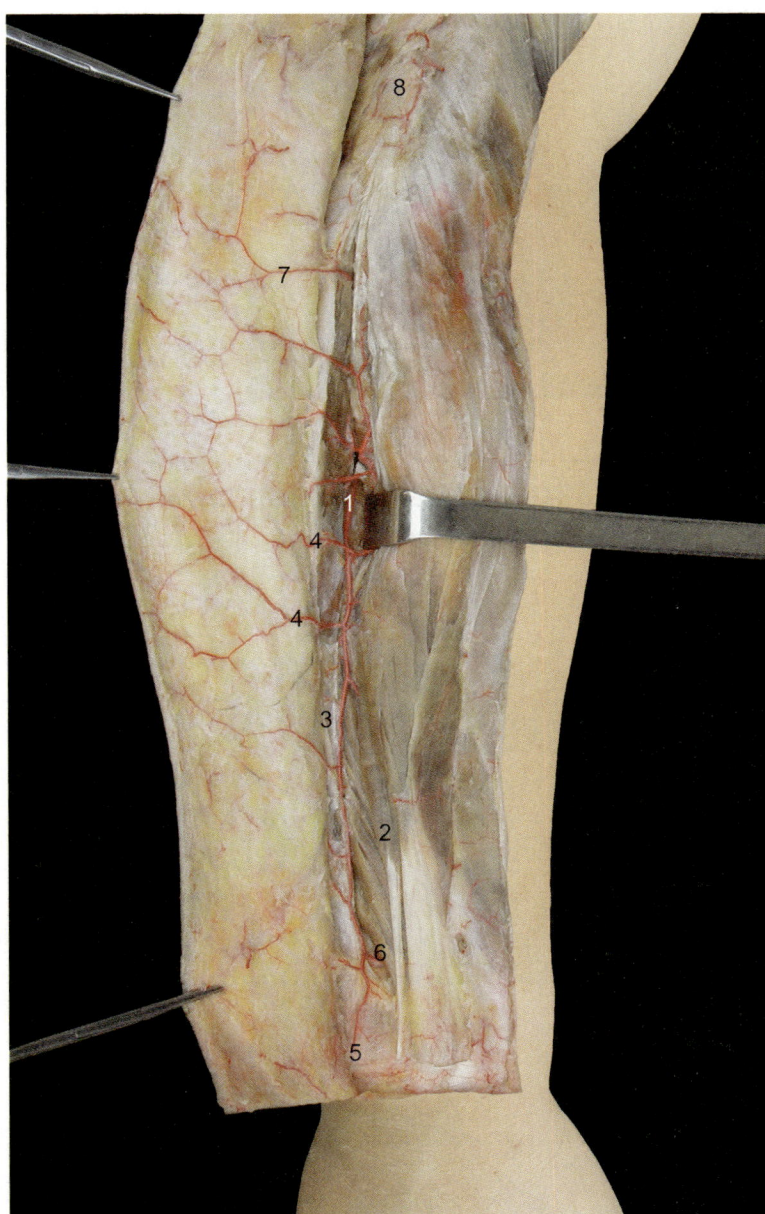

1. Arteriae interossea dorsalis
2. Extensor digiti minimi muscle
3. Extensor carpi ulnaris muscle
4. Cutaneous branch
5. Styloid process of ulna
6. Anastomotic branch
7. Cutaneous branch of interosseous recurrent artery
8. Lateral epicondyle of humerus

Figure 1-51   **Applied anatomy**

The arteriae interossea dorsalis perforates through the interosseous membrane in the proximal part to reach the dorsal forearm. It extends in the septum between the anconeus muscle and the abductor pollicis longus muscle and then between the deep and the superficial extensors to accompany the posterior interosseous nerve. Then it descends along the septum between the extensor digiti minimi muscle and the extensor carpi ulnaris muscle. Along the course, it gives 5-13 cutaneous branches to nourish the adjacent skin. The terminal branch of the arteriae interossea dorsalis anastomoses with the dorsal perforator of the anterior interosseous artery at about 2.5 cm proximal to the carpal crease.

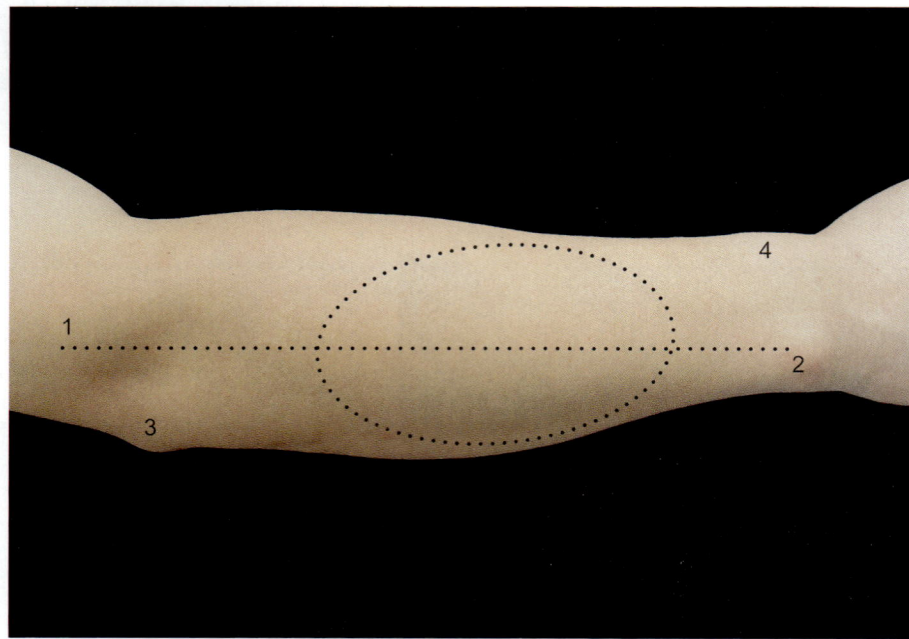

1. External epicondyle of humerus
2. Short head of ulna
3. Ulnar olecranon
4. Styloid process of radius

Figure 1-52   Design of the flap

The flap should be designed according to the size of the recipient and its pedicle length adjusted to the distance between the pivot point and the recipient. Its axial line should fall on the connecting line between the lateral epicondyle of the humerus and the radial side of the ulna head. If the flap is transferred retrogradely, its pivot point should be located at 2.5 cm above the styloid process of the ulna. If it is transferred antegradely, its pivot point should be located at 7 cm to the olecranon tip.

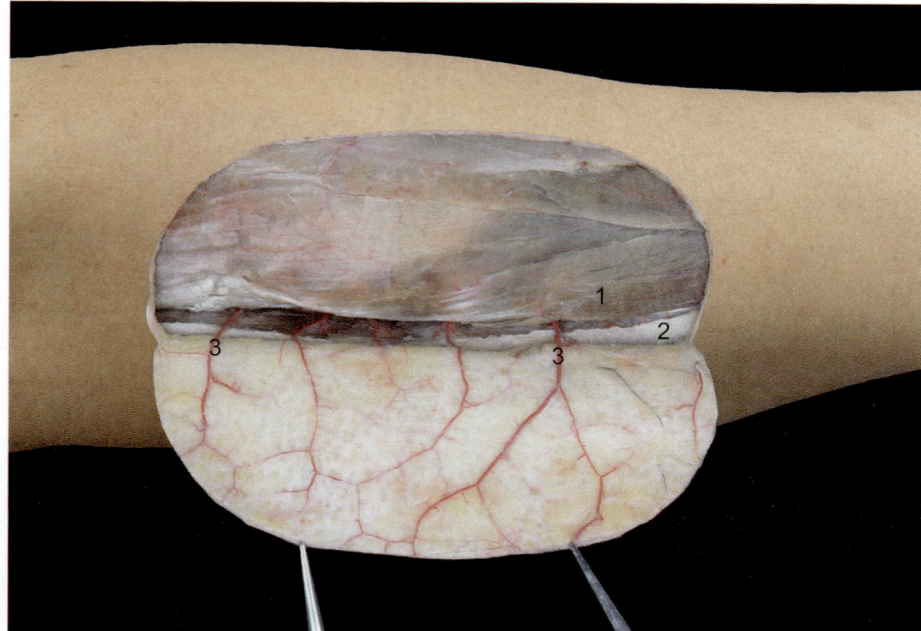

1. Extensor digiti minimi muscle
2. Extensor carpi ulnaris muscle
3. Cutaneous branch

Figure 1-53   Dissection of the flap

The flap should be first incised at the radial side and elevated from under the deep fascia to the ulnar side to expose the cutaneous branches near the septum between the extensor digiti minimi muscle and the extensor carpi ulnaris muscle. These cutaneous branches perforate through the spatium intermusculare to enter the flap.

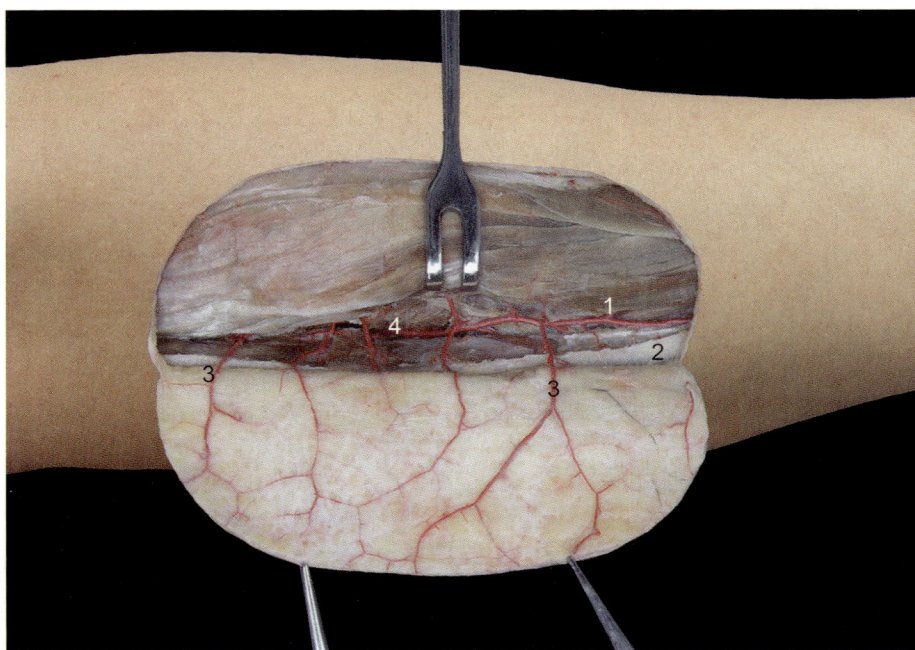

1. Extensor digiti minimi
   muscle
2. Extensor carpi ulnaris
   muscle
3. Cutaneous branch
4. Arteriae interossea
   dorsalis

Figure 1-54   **Exposure of the vessels**

The spatium intermusculare should be incised and the dissection continue along the cutaneous branch down to the septum between the extensor digiti minimi muscle and the extensor carpi ulnaris muscle to expose the arteriae interossea dorsalis. The dissection should be done under the tunica muscularis to keep the cutaneous branches intact.

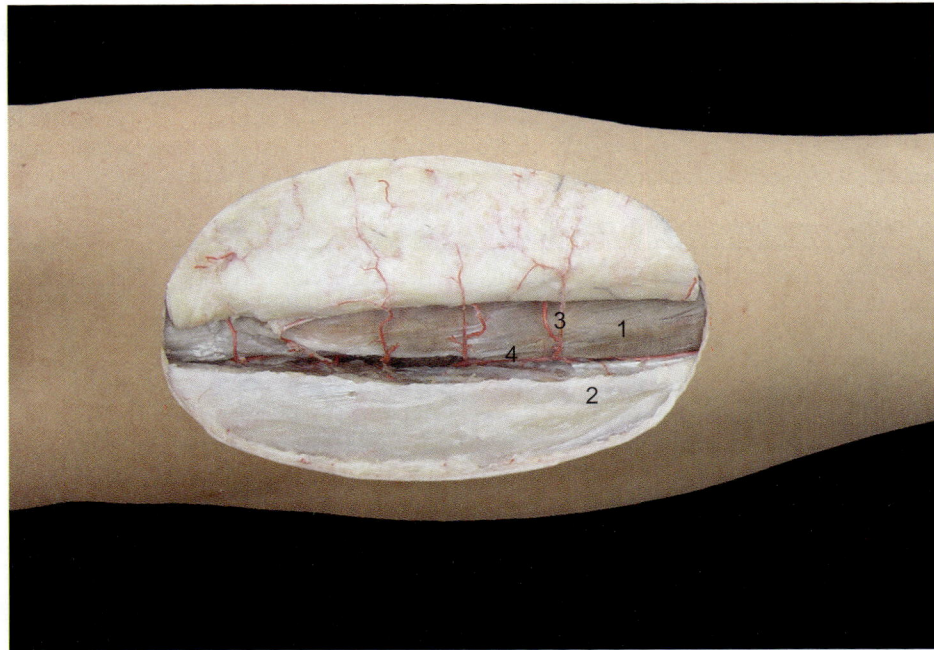

1. Extensor digiti minimi
   muscle
2. Extensor carpi ulnaris
   muscle
3. Cutaneous branch
4. Arteriae interossea
   dorsalis

Figure 1-55   **Elevation of the flap**

After the dissection in the radial side, the flap should be pulled back and sutured temporarily. The flap should be then incised at the ulnar border, dissected under the deep fascia and traced radially to the vascular axis of the spatium intermusculare.

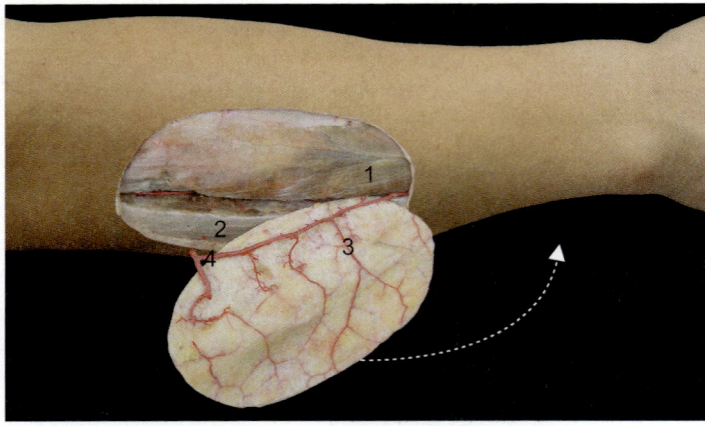

1. Extensor digiti minimi muscle
2. Extensor carpi ulnaris muscle
3. Cutaneous branch
4. Arteriae interossea dorsalis

Figure 1-56   **Retrograde transposition of the flap**

The superior segment of the dorsal interosseous vascular bundle, together with the perivascular spatium intermusculare, should be separated from the extensor muscles of the deep and the superficial groups. The proximal end of the vascular pedicle is then cut. The dissection should continue along the vessel until the required length of the pedicle is satisfied. A flap of this type might be transferred retrogradely to cover a distal wound on the dorsal hand.

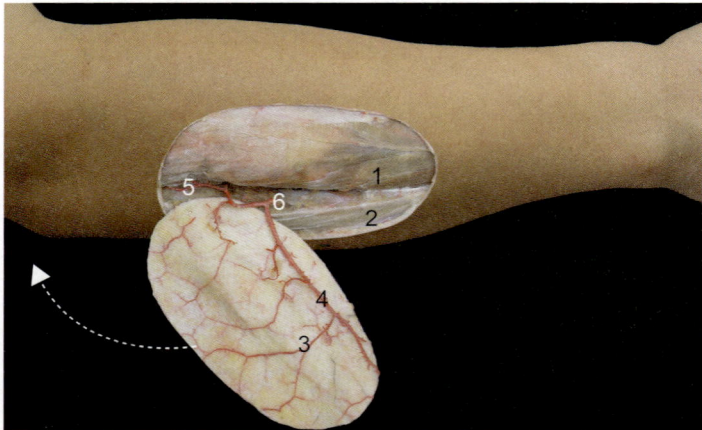

1. Extensor digiti minimi muscle
2. Extensor carpi ulnaris muscle
3. Cutaneous branch
4. Arteriae interossea dorsalis
5. Recurrent branch of arteriae interossea dorsalis
6. Trunk of arteriae interossea dorsalis

Figure 1-57   **Anterograde transposition of the flap**

The distal dorsal interosseous vascular bundle should be cut at the distal end of the flap and the dissection of the pedicles continue towards the proximal end of the pedicle until the required length is satisfied. A flap with a proximal pedicle of arteriae interossea dorsalis might be transferred anterogradely to cover a proximal wound on the elbow. If the posterior interosseous vascular pedicle is too tense and too short, a variant mode might be created by ligating its main trunk before it sends the recurrent branch so that a flap pedicled with the recurrent branch could be made.

Key points in applied anatomy

Firstly, the point from which the interosseous recurrent artery emerges and through which the cutaneous branch perforates should be confirmed with the Doppler. Secondly, the cutaneous branch is situated in the septum between the cubitus muscle and the extensor carpi ulnaris muscle and perforates through the spetum to enter the subcutaneous tissue. The vascular pedicle should be separated proximally to the spatium intermusculare and then raised with the septum and the bilateral muscular cuffs (0.5 cm) to keep the pedicle and the cutaneous branch intact. Thirdly, if the flap is pedicled with the anastomotic branch of the interosseous recurrent artery and the radial recurrent artery, its pivot point should be located at the superficial surface of Frohse's arch. The dorsal interosseous nerve should be given great attention to avoid getting it damaged.

Retrograde Dorsal Forearm Flap

The flap based on the posterior interosseous artery of the dorsal forearm might be transferred retrogradely to cover a wound on the hand. Its main advantage is that no main vessels of the forearm should be sacrificed, nor should the blood supply of the hand be affected.

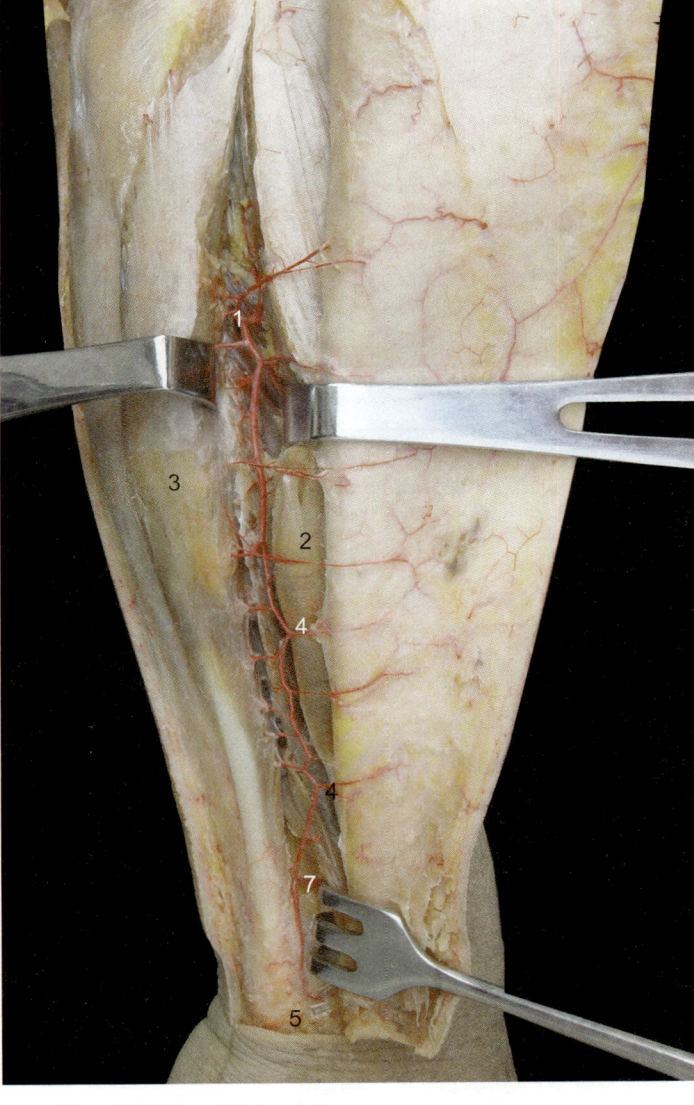

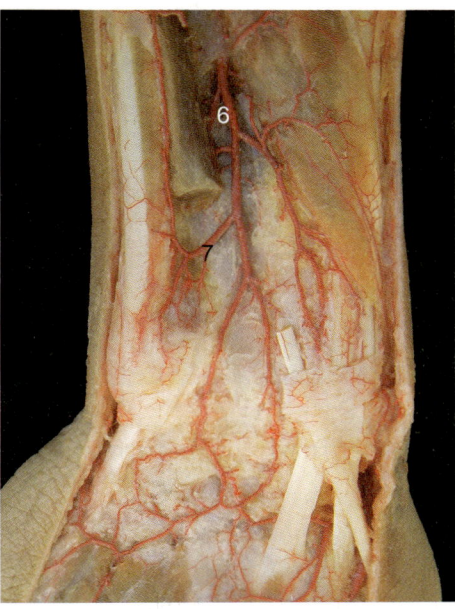

1. Arteriae interossea dorsalis
2. Extensor digiti minimi muscle
3. Extensor carpi ulnaris muscle
4. Cutaneous branch
5. Styloid process of ulna
6. Dorsal perforator of anterior interosseous artery
7. Anastomotic branches

| Figure 1-58 | Applied anatomy |

The posterior interosseous artery perforates through the proximal interosseous membrane to reach the dorsal region. It extends in the septum between the anconeus muscle and the abductor pollicis longus muscle and accompanies the posterior interosseous nerve through the septum between the deep and the superficial extensors. The neurovascular bundle descends along the septum between the extensor digiti minimi muscle and the extensor carpi ulnaris muscle. Along the course, the artery gives 5-13 cutaneous branches to nourish the adjacent skin. There is a constant anastomotic branch at 2.5cm above the styloid process of the ulna that connects the terminal branch of the posterior interosseous artery with the dorsal carpi perforator of the anterior interosseous artery. The anastomosis between the posterior and anterior interosseous artery makes the vascular basis of the retrograde-flow arteriae interossea dorsalis flap for hand coverage.

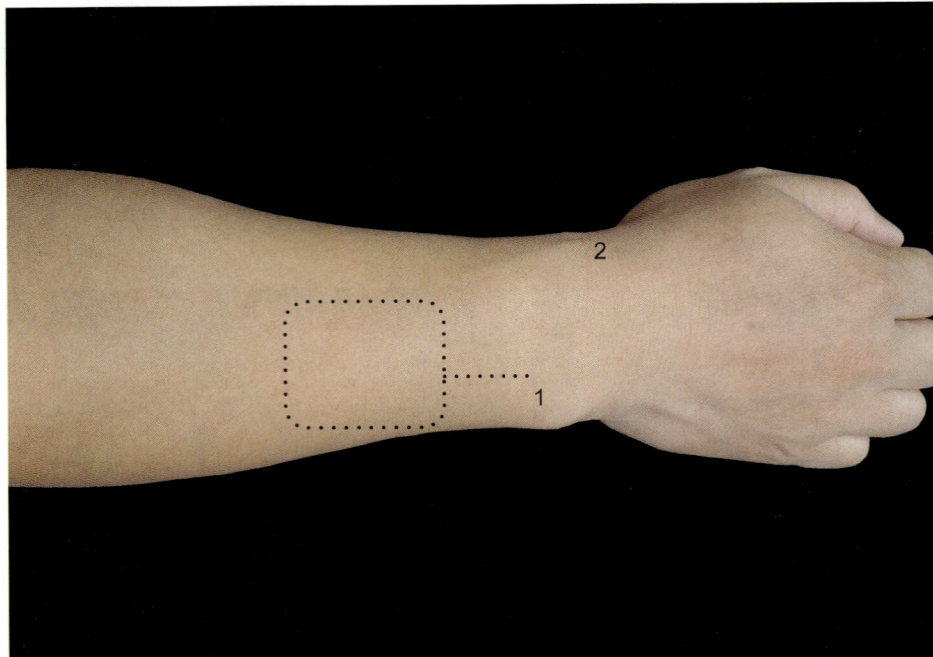

1. Ulna head
2. Styloid process of radius

| **Figure 1-59** | **Design of the flap** |

The flap should be designed with its axial line falling on the connection between the lateral epicondyle of humerus and the radial side of the ulnar head. Its pivot point should be located at 2.5 cm above the styloid process of ulna. The size of the flap should be adjusted to that of the recipient region and the length of its pedicle to the distance between the pivot point and the recipient region.

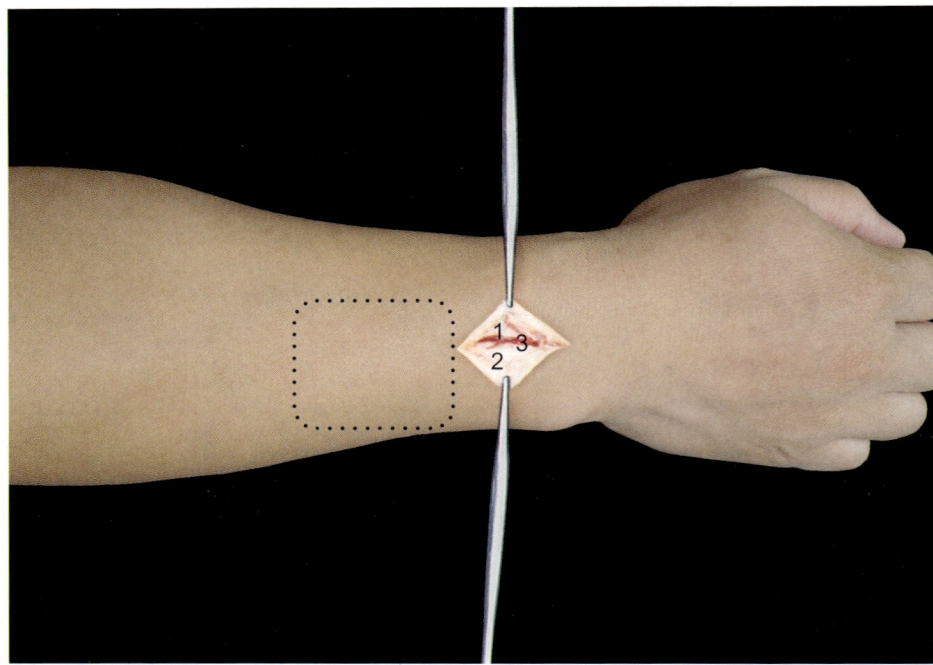

1. Extensor digiti minimi muscle
2. Extensor carpi ulnaris muscle
3. Dorsal interosseous vessels

| **Figure 1-60** | **Exposure of the vascular pedicle** |

After an incision is made down to the deep fascia at the distal pedicle, the skin, the subcutaneous tissue and the antebrachial fascia should be opened to expose the dorsal interosseous vessels in the septum between the extensor digiti minimi muscle and the extensor carpi ulnar muscle.

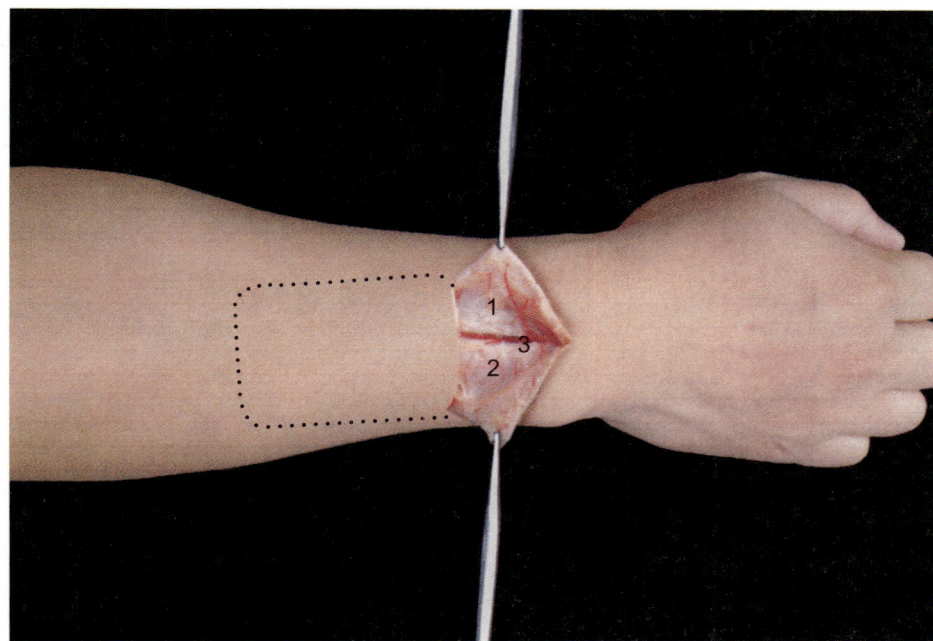

1. Extensor digiti minimi muscle
2. Extensor carpi ulnaris muscle
3. Dorsal interosseous vessels

Figure 1-61   Elevation of the vascular pedicle

The dorsal interosseous vascular bundle, together with the septum, should be dissected and elevated with some deep fascia pedicle (1.5 cm wide).

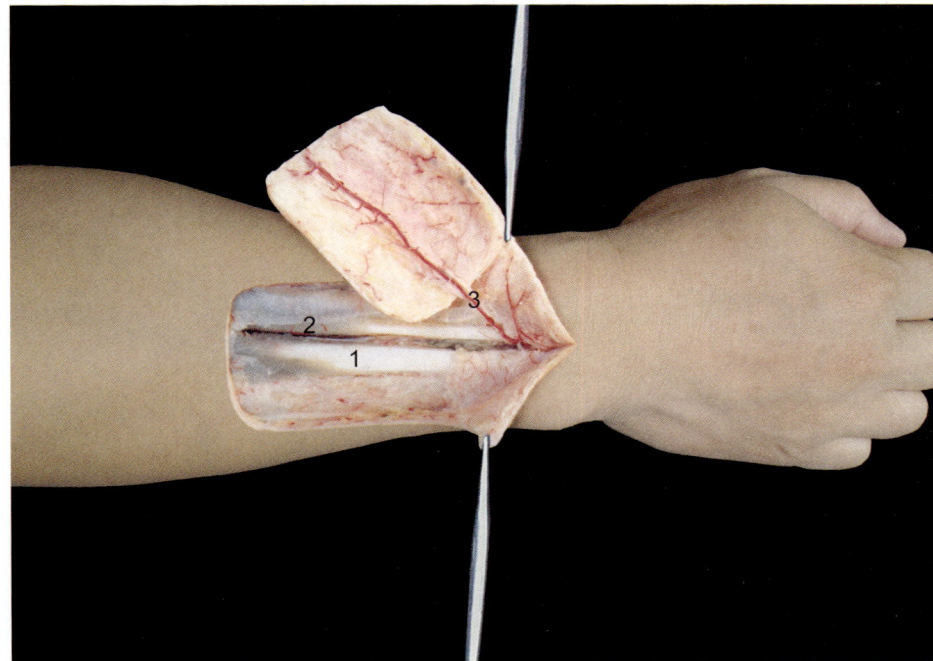

1. Extensor digiti minimi muscle
2. Extensor carpi ulnaris muscle
3. Dorsal interosseous vessels

Figure 1-62   Dissection of the flap

As has been designed, the flap should be incised bilaterally and separated sharply in the space between the deep fascia and the tunica muscularis. While the separation continues, some stitches should be put into hold the deep fascia and the skin together. The flap should be elevated bilaterally and the separation continue proximally along the vascular pedicle to expose the proximal segment of the dorsal interosseous vascular bundle and its attaching spatium intermusculare. The cutaneous branch should be given great attention to avoid getting it damaged.

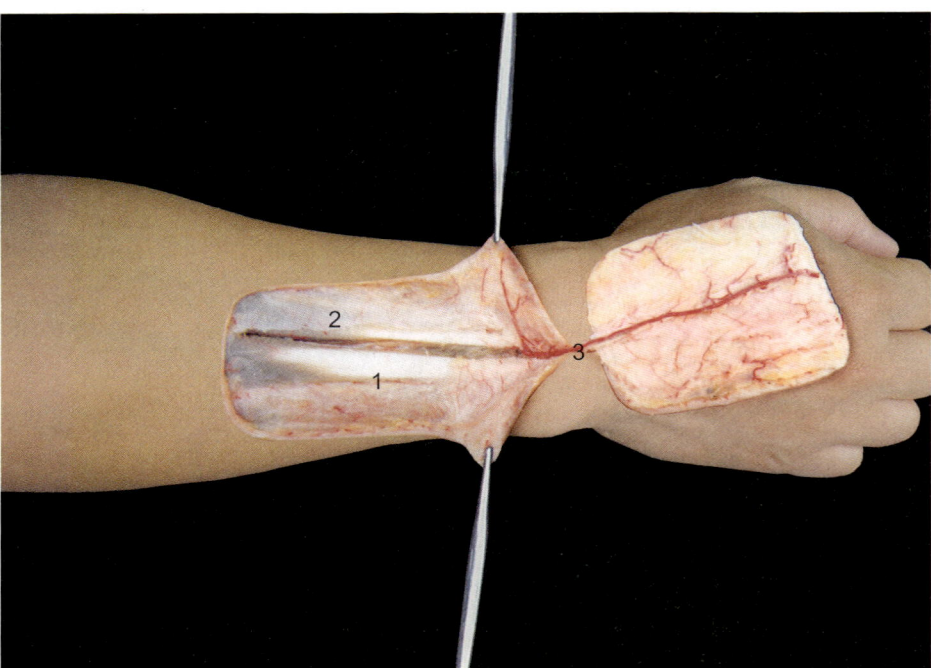

Figure 1-63   **Transposition of the flap**

The flap should be transferred retrogradely via a subcutaneous or an open tunnel to reach the defect in the hand.

1. Extensor digiti minimi muscle
2. Extensor carpi ulnaris muscle
3. Dorsal interosseous vessels

Key points in applied anatomy

The retrograde island flap from the dorsal forearm is actually an island flap with a pedicle of the dorsal perforator of the anterior interosseous artery. It is one of the pedicled flaps frequently used in hand surgery. Its pivot point should be located at 3.5cm above the midpoint of the dorsal carpal transverse line, where the dorsal branch of the anterior interosseous artery perforates through the superior border of the pronator quadratus muscle. Its axial line should fall on the connecting line between this point and the lateral epicondyle of humerus, which represents the anastomotic channel of the perforating branch of the anterior interosseous artery and the cutaneous branch of the posterior interosseous artery. The flap might have a size of 16×10cm.

Dorsoulnar Forearm Flap

12

The radial and the ulnar forearm flaps have a common shortcoming—both have to sacrifice a main artery of the hand. The shortcoming does not exist in a dorsoulnar forearm flap with the cutaneous branch of carpal ulnar artery .

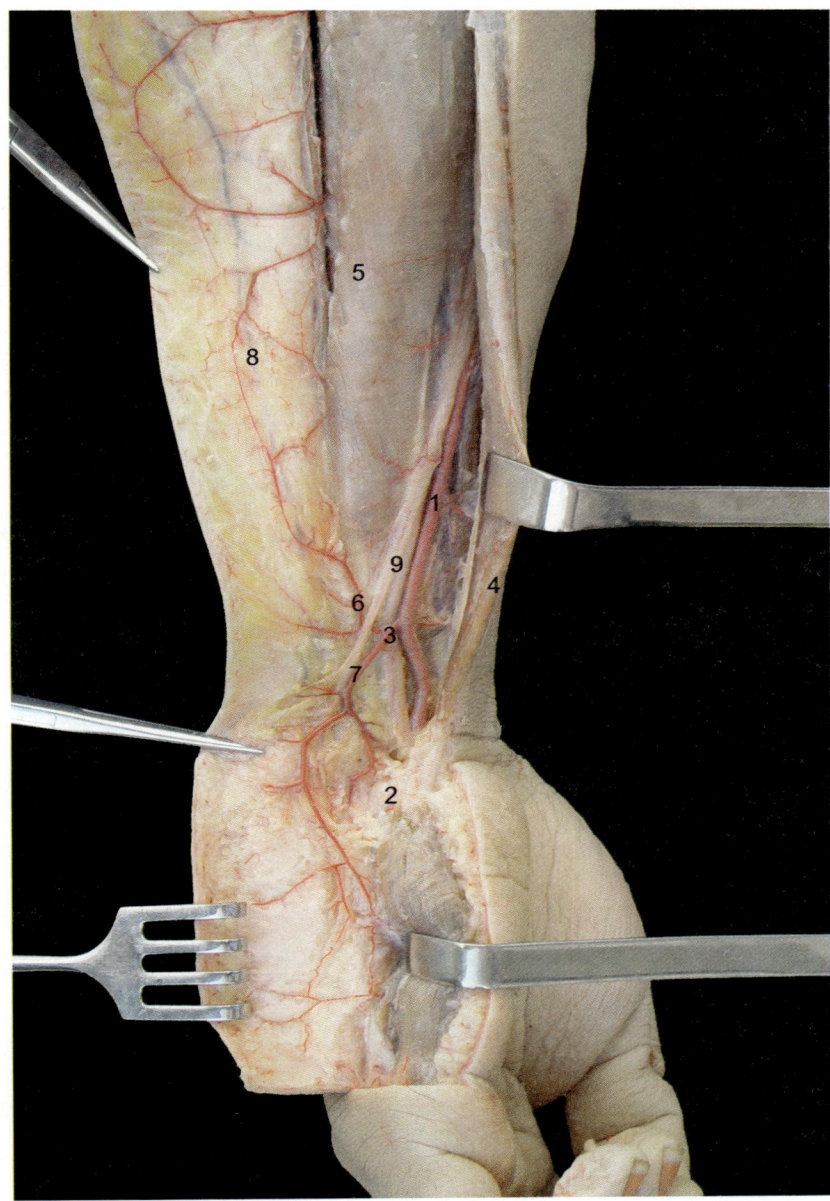

1. Ulnar artery
2. Pisiform bone
3. Superior carpal cutaneous branch of ulnar artery
4. Flexor carpi ulnar muscle
5. Extensor carpi ulnar muscle
6. Ascending branch
7. Descending branch
8. Branch of the basilic vein
9. Dorsal branch of carpal ulnar nerve

Figure 1-64   **Applied anatomy**

The ulnar artery gives a constant cutaneous branch at 3.5-4.0cm proximal to the pisiform bone. The trunk of the cutaneous branch is 1.2 cm in length and 1.3 mm in diameter. The cutaneous branch perforates through the septum between the flexor carpi ulnaris muscle and the extensor carpi ulnaris muscle, and gives the ascending branch and the descending branch on the deep fascia surface. The ascending branch, about 8-10 cm long, sends many small branches to anastomose with the adjacent artery to form a vascular net. The venous system of the flap consists of the deep accompanying veins (1.5 mm in diameter) and the superficial basilic vein or its branches. The sensory nerve in the flap is the posterior branch of the medial antebrachial cutaneous nerve.

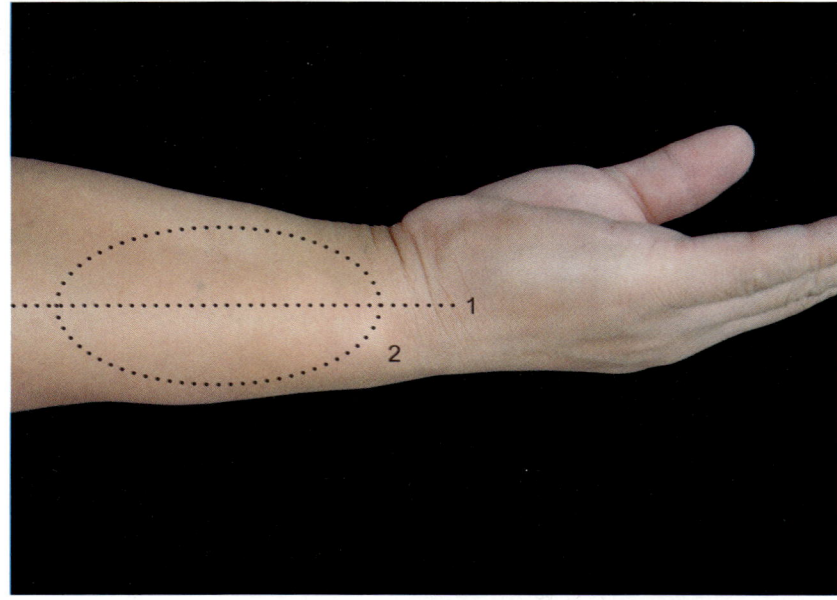

1. Pisiform bone
2. Styloid process of ulna

Figure 1-65   Exposure of the vessels

The flap should be designed according to its vascular anatomy. Its axial line should fall on the connecting line between the medial epicondyle of the humerus and the pisiform. Its pivot point should be located at 4 cm above the pisiform. Its proximal margin might extend to the elbow, its lateral and medial to the midline of the volar and dorsal forearm surface.

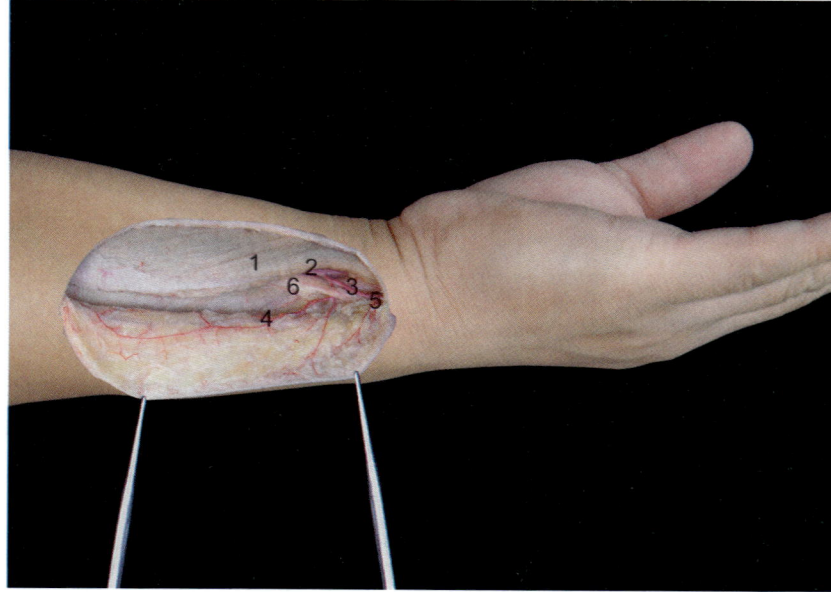

1. Extensor carpi ulnar muscle
2. Ulnar artery
3. Superior carpal cutaneous branch of ulnar artery
4. Ascending branch
5. Descending branch
6. Dorsal carpal branch of ulnar nerve

Figure 1-66   Exposure of the vascular pedicle

A distal incision should be made on the volar forearm down to the deep fascia. The dissection should continue to the radial side of the flexor carpi ulnaris muscle to expose the ulnar artery and its concomitant veins. Care should be taken to avoid damaging the dorsoulnar cutaneous branch that emerges from the ulnar artery within the region of 3-5cm proximal to the pisiform bone. The cutaneous branch extends beneath the tendon of the flexor carpi ulnaris muscle and perforates through the deep fascia to enter the subcutaneous tissue. If necessary, the tendon of the flexor carpi ulnaris muscle should be interrupted (sutured back after operation) to expose the perforator.

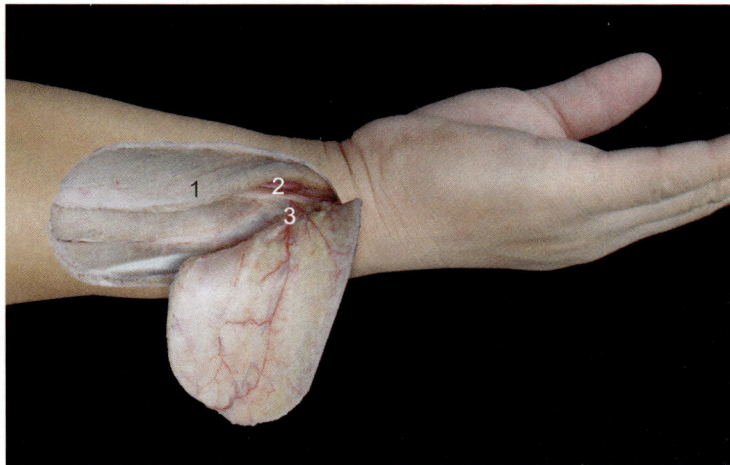

1. Extensor carpi ulnar muscle
2. Ulnar artery
3. Ascending branch

Figure 1-67	Dissection of the flap

The superior carpal cutaneous branch should be confirmed to have been included in the flap before the flap could be dissected from under the tunica muscularis as has been designed. When the distal vascular pedicle is being dissected, the perivascular soft tissue of the cutaneous branch should be retained as much as possible to protect it from damage.

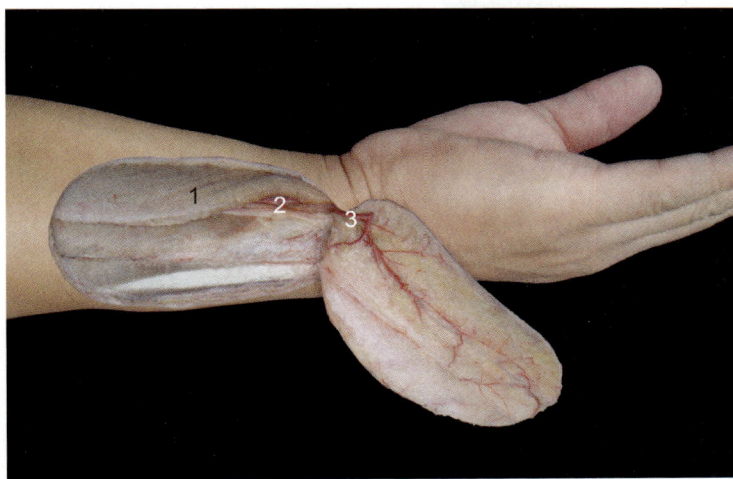

1. Extensor carpi ulnar muscle
2. Ulnar artery
3. Descending branch

Figure 1-68	Transposition of the flap

The island flap with the superior carpal cutaneous branch might be transferred distally to cover a wound on the hand.

Key points in applied anatomy

Firstly, as for the design of the flap, the point at 4cm above the pisiform bone plays a critical role. It is the origin point of the superior carpal cutaneous branch from the ulnar artery and the pivot point of a retrograde island flap. Secondly, the axial line of the flap should fall on the connecting line between the pisiform bone and the medial epicondyle of the humerus. The distal border of the flap might extend to the pisiform bone, its proximal to the medial epicondyle of the humerus and its bilateral to midlines of the anterior and the posterior forearm. Thirdly, the vascular pedicles should be dissected at the surgical plane under the deep surface. Fourthly, although the ascending branch of the superior carpal cutaneous branch of the ulnar artery is only 8-10 cm long, it has been proven clinically if the harvested flap (with the descending branch included) extends for 20-25 cm long. Fifthly, the flap should be transferred as an island flap rather than a free one since the vascular pedicles are very short and very small. Sixthly, if a free flap is needed, it has to include a segment of the ulnar artery (about 1cm) to increase the vascular caliber for anastomosis.

13

Retrograde Flap of the Radial Dorsal Hand

The radial dorsal hand flap with a pedicle of the dorsal metacarpal artery has such advantages as constant vessels, long pedicles and large rotation arch. It might be transferred retrogradely to restore a soft tissue defect on the palm or on the finger. It might also be transferred as a compound one with the extensor tendon and the metacarpal bone.

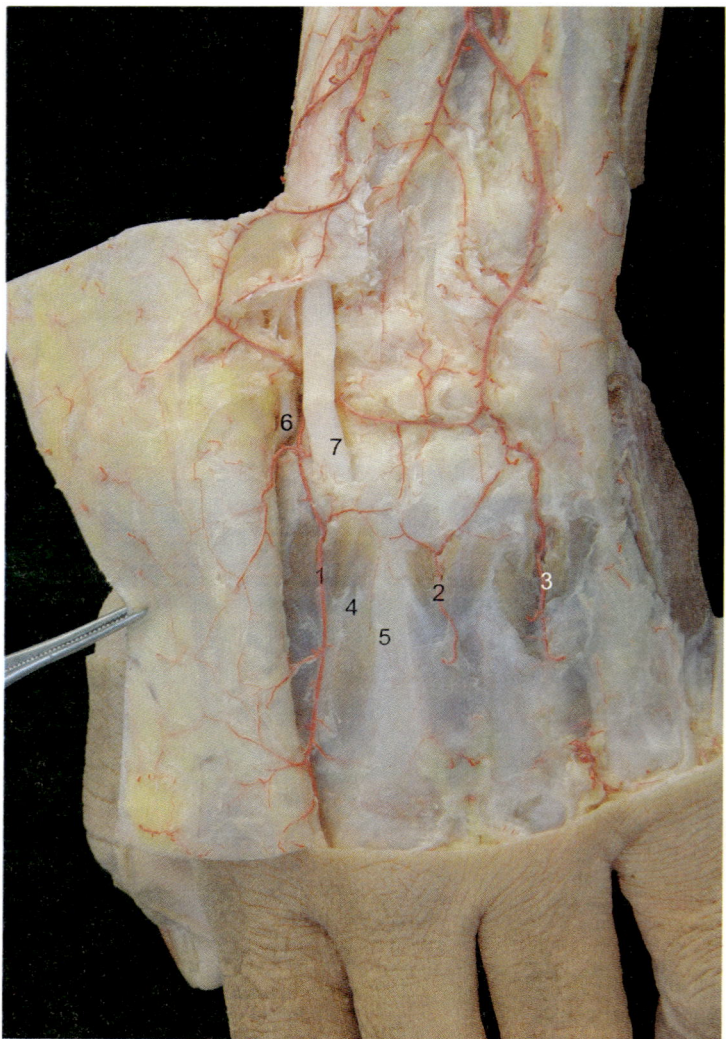

1. 2nd dorsal metacarpal artery
2. 3rd dorsal metacarpal artery
3. 4th dorsal metacarpal artery
4. Dorsal interossei
5. 3rd metacarpal bone
6. Long radial extensor carpal muscle and tendon
7. Short radial extensor carpal muscle and tendon

Figure 1-69   Applied anatomy

There are 4 dorsal metacarpal arteries on the dorsal hand that are located at the deep surface of the extensors and extend along the superficial surface in the dorsal interoseis. These dorsal metacarpal arteries send 2 dorsal digital arteries each at the metacarpal head. The 1st dorsal metacarpal artery arises from the radial artery and extends distally along the radial side of the 2nd metacarpal. The 2nd, 3rd and 4th dorsal metacarpal arteries arise from the deep palmar arch and extend along the corresponding intercarpal spaces. They perforate through the dorsal interosseous muscle and anastomose with the communicating branches of the dorsal carpal arterial net. Along the course, these arteries send branches to nourish the tendons and the metacarpal bones and the overlying skin. There are constant anastomotic branches in the digital palmatures, which connect the dorsal metacarpal arteries with the common palmar digital arteries and their branches. A retrograde island flap should be based on the distal anastomotic branches in the web space. There are dorsal metacarpal nerves extending in the same direction as the vessels.

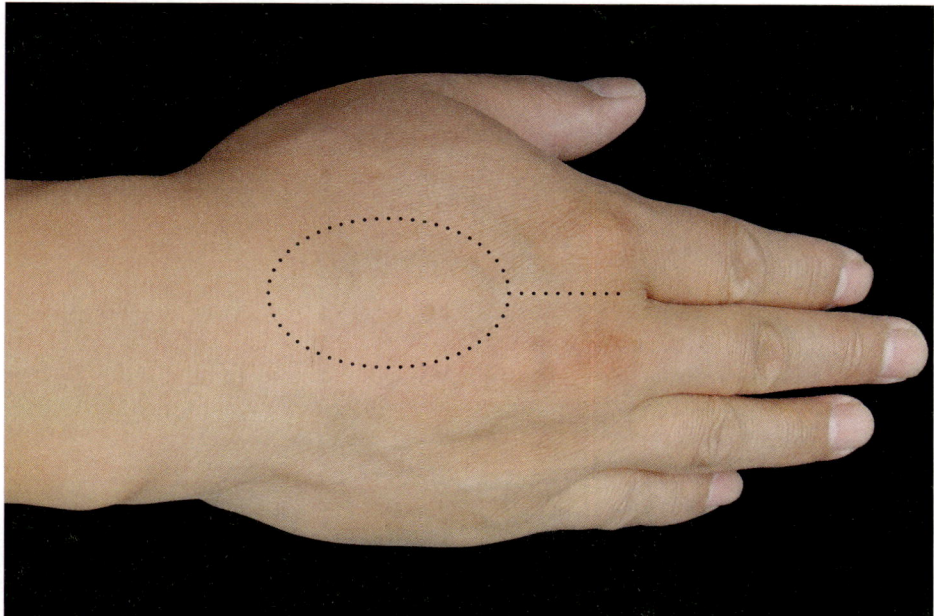

Figure 1-70   **Design of the flap**

The flap should be designed with its axial line falling along the dorsal metacarpal artery. Its pivot point should be located at the web space. Its proximal margin extends to the dorsal carpal transverse crease, its distal to its palmature edge and its bilateral to 2.5 cm from its axis line.

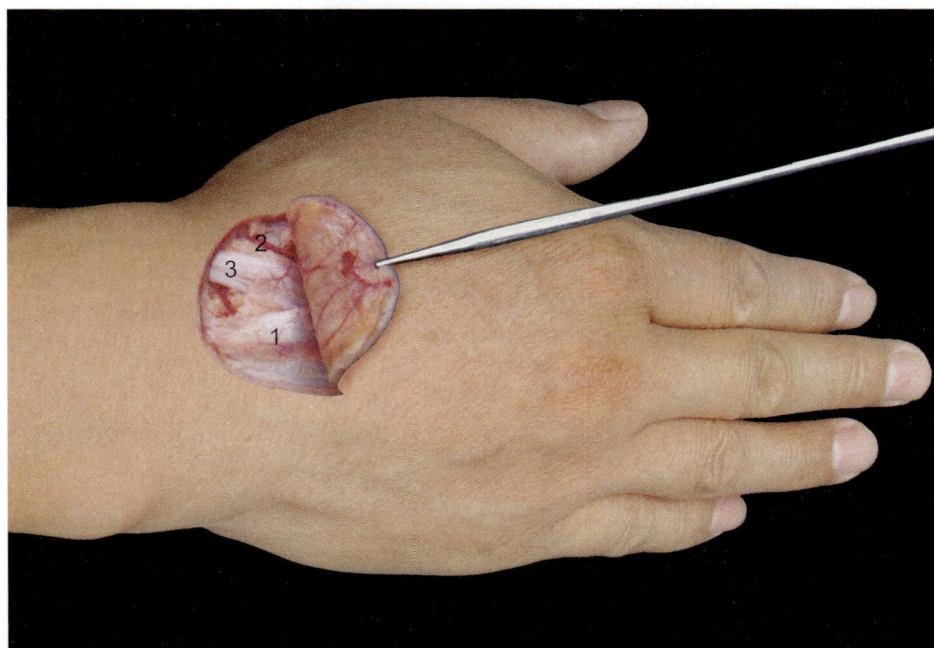

1. Extensor digital tendon
2. Dorsal metacarpal artery
3. Extensor carpi radialis brevis tendon

Figure 1-71   **Exposure of the vessel**

The incision of the flap should begin with its proximal border and extends under the deep fascia to expose the extensor digitorum tendon. The extensor tendons should be drawn bilaterally to expose the dorsal metacarpal artery that is situated in the interosseous space of the 2nd and the 3rd fingers. The proximal perforating artery from the deep palmar arch should be ligated.

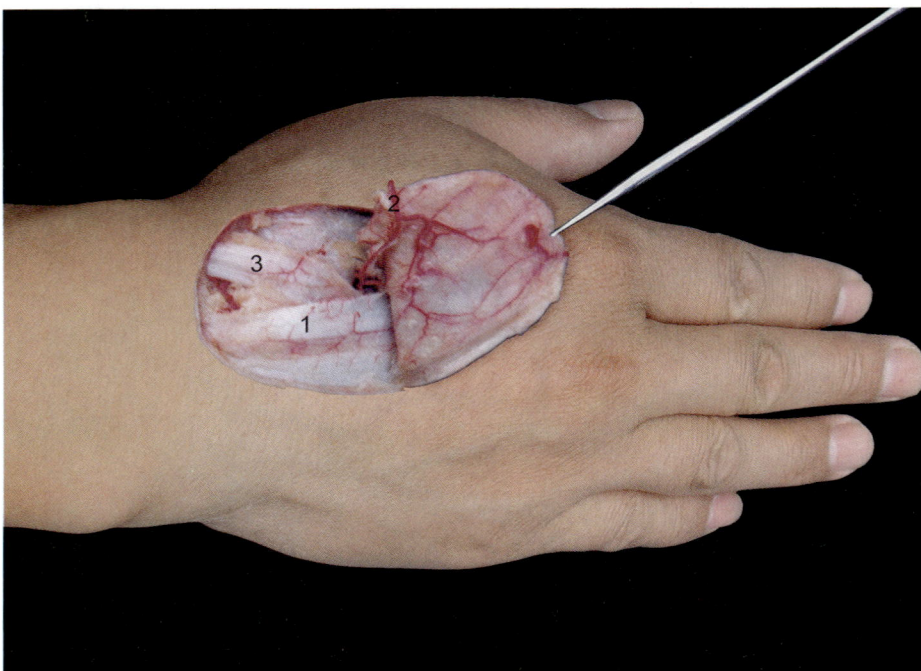

1. Extensor digital tendon
2. Dorsal metacarpal artery
3. Extensor carpi radialis
   brevis tendon

| **Figure 1-72** | **Dissection of the flap** |

The flap should be incised distally from under the deep fascia and traced in the same direction the vesselsrun.

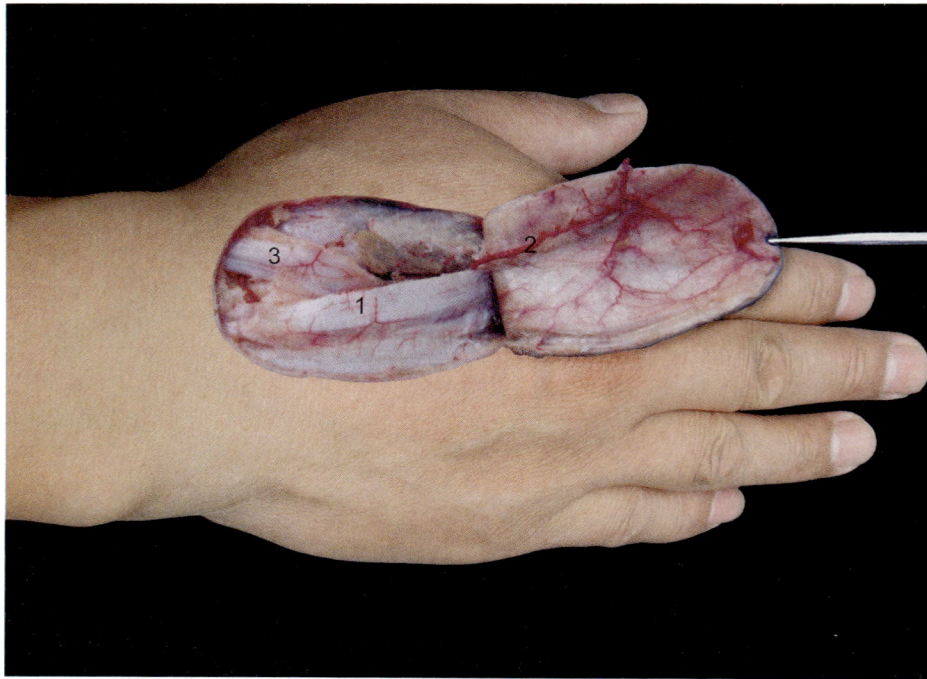

1. Extensor digital tendon
2. Dorsal metacarpal artery
3. Extensor carpi radialis
   brevis tendon

| **Figure 1-73** | **Elevation of the flap** |

The base of the pedicle should be first incised and the dissection continues distally along the dorsal metacarpal artery until it reaches the communicating branch from the common palmar digital artery. In this way, the vascular pedicle might be long enough for the coverage of the wound in the recipient region.

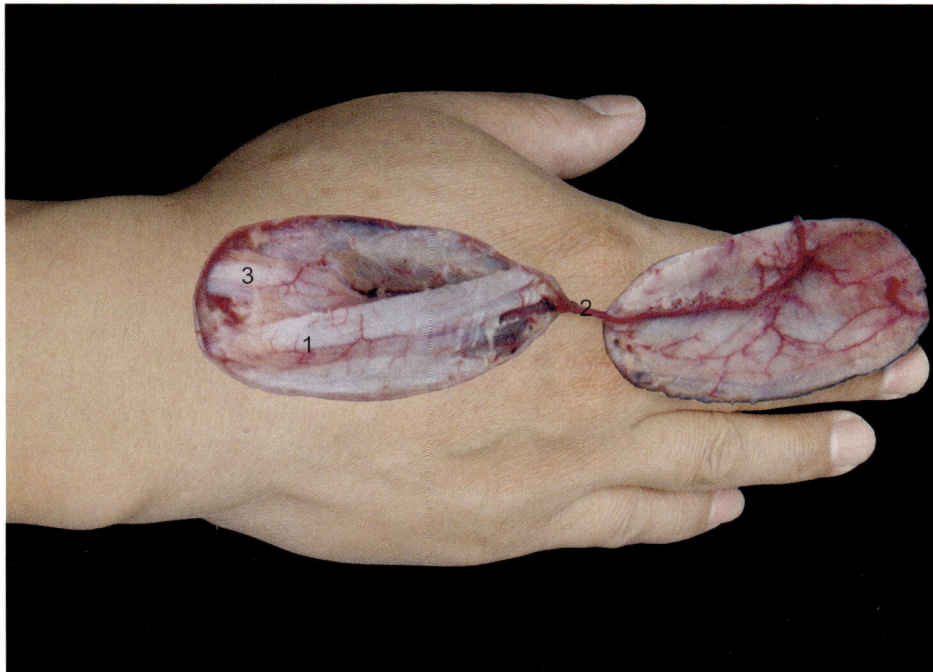

Figure 1-74   **Transposition of the flap**

The flap might be transferred retrogradely to restore a defect on the palm or the finger.

1. Extensor digital tendon
2. Dorsal metacarpal artery
3. Extensor carpi radialis brevis tendon

Key points in applied anatomy

Firstly, when the flap is being dissected, the perivascular tissues should be retained as much as possible to guarantee the venous blood return in the flap. Secondly, since the dorsal metacarpal artery is located in the deep surface of the extensor tendon and the superficial surface of the dorsal interossei, the flap should include a pedicle of the sheath of the dorsal interossei. In some cases, the flap should include the index extensor tendon to guarantee the blood circulation. Thirdly, the cutaneous nerves in the flap should be sutured with the digital nerves in the recipient site to restore the sensory function of the flap.

Dorsal Metacarpal Flap from the Ulnar Hand

The ulnar dorsal metacarpal artery flap is based on the dorsal carpal branch of the ulnar artery and the dorsal carpal branch of the ulnar nerve. It has a good sensory function. It might be transferred anterogradely to cover a wound on the palm or the wrist. It might also be transferred retrogradely to cover a wound on the finger.

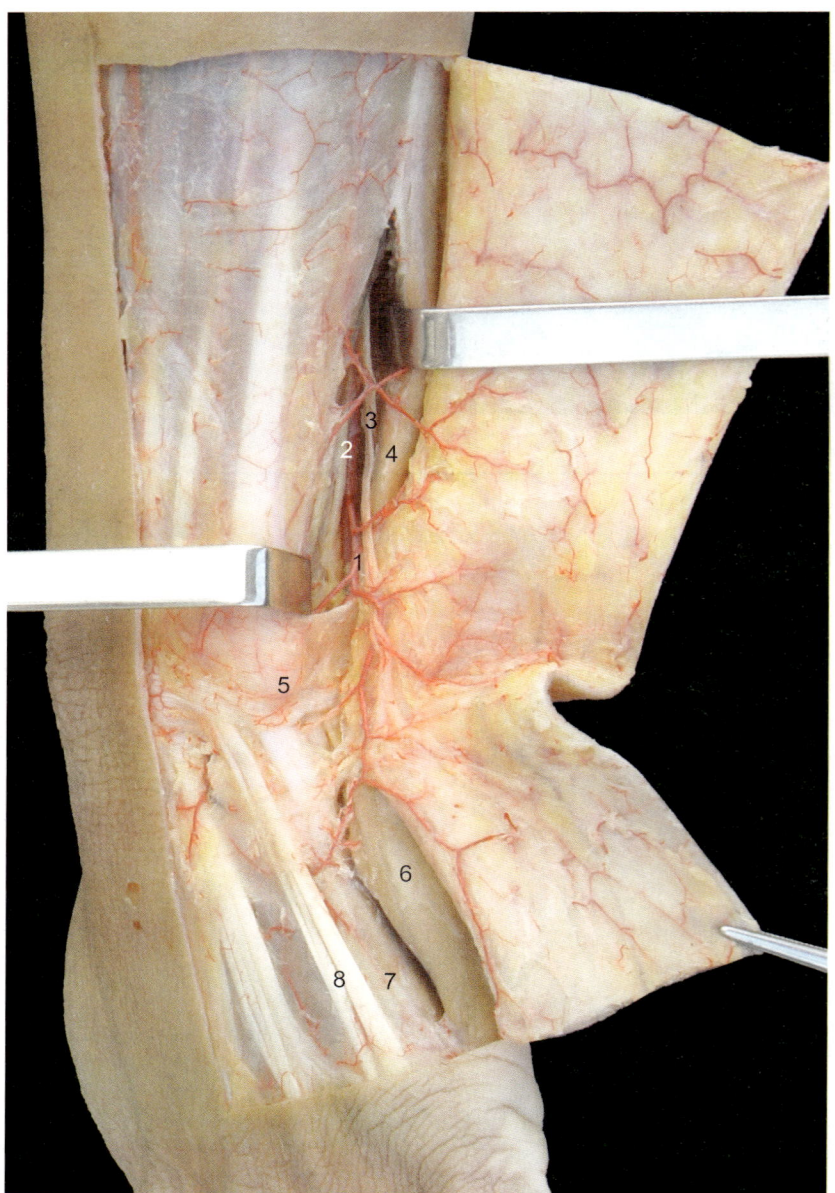

1. Dorsal carpal branch of ulnar artery
2. Ulnar artery
3. Ulnar nerve
4. Flexor carpi ulnaris muscle
5. Styloid process of ulna
6. Hypothenar muscle
7. 5th metacarpal bone
8. Extensor digiti minimi tendon

| Figure 1-75 | Applied anatomy |

The dorsal carpal branch of the ulnar artery arises from the ulnar artery at 4cm proximal to the pisiform. It extends distally via the anterior ulnar nerve (with some exceptions: via the posterior ulnar nerve) and the posterior flexor carpi ulnaris muscle and passes via the anterior styloid process of the ulna to reach the dorsum palm. It descends distally in the space between the hypothenar muscle and the 5th dorsal metacarpal bone to reach the metacarpophalangeal articulation. Along the course, it gives branches to anastomose with the branches of the 4th and the3rd dorsal metacarpal arteries. The artery is accompanied with the dorsoulnar nerves.

A. Anterograde flap

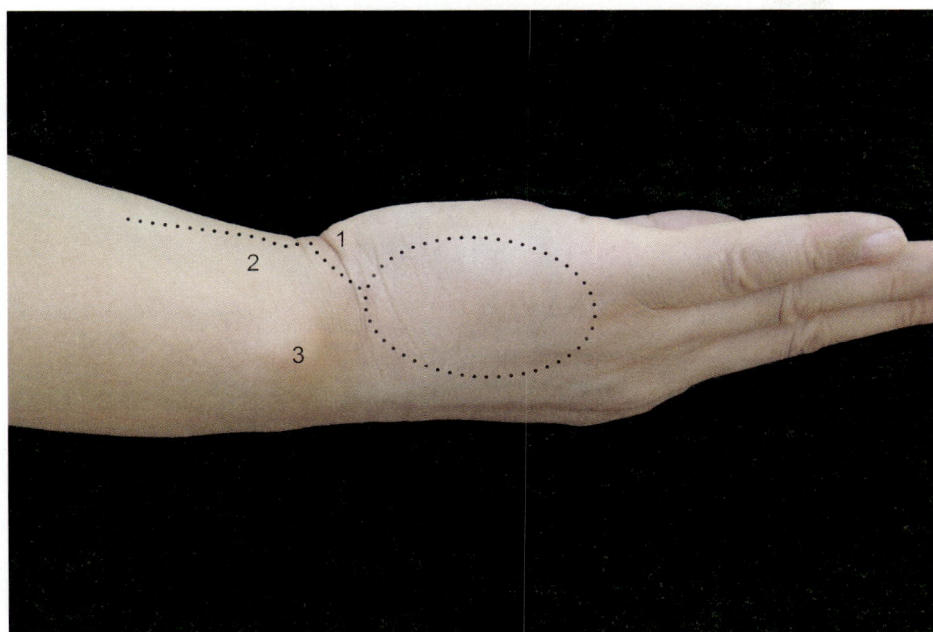

1. Pisiform bone
2. Flexor carpi ulnaris muscle
3. Styloid process of ulna

Figure 1-76   **Design of the flap**

Take the design of a flap for the repair of a wound on the carpal palm. The incision should begin with the proximal border, continue to the proximal pisiform bone, turns to the palm and then extends proximally for 5cm along the radial side of the flexor carpi ulnaris muscle.

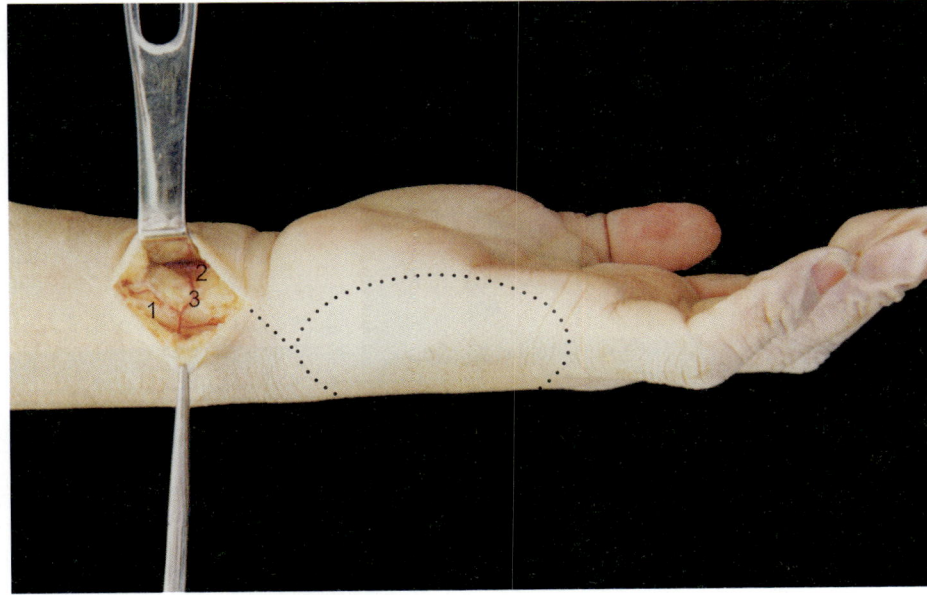

1. Ulnar nerve
2. Ulnar artery
3. Dorsal carpal branch of ulnar artery

Figure 1-77   **Exposure of the vessels**

The incision of the flap should begin with the pedicle portion at the proximal pisiform to expose the ulnar nerve and the ulnar artery. Both of the two might be found in the radial side of the flexor carpi ulnaris muscle. Then the dorsal carpal branch of the ulnar artery and the dorsal palmar branch of the ulnar nerve could be identified.

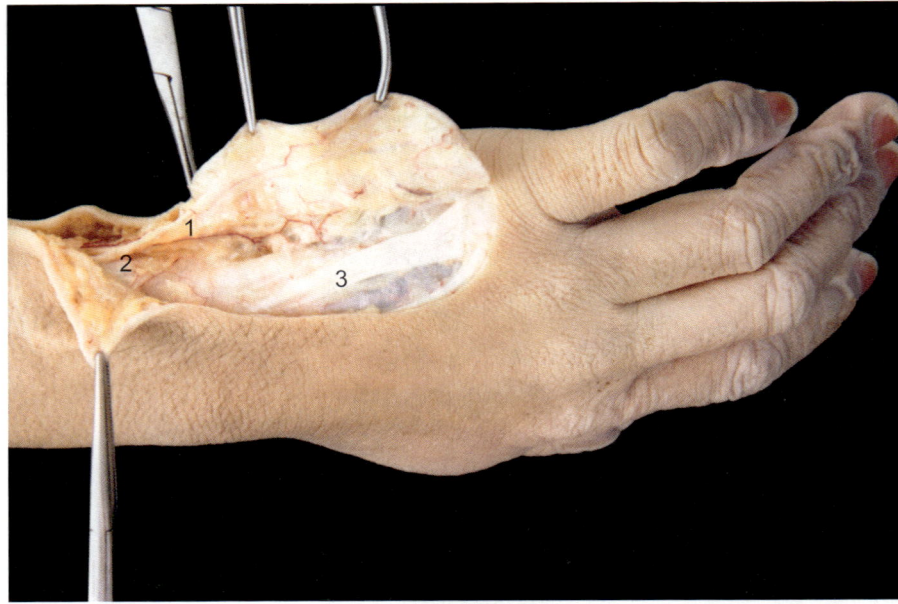

1. Dorsal carpal branch of ulnar artery
2. Dorsal palmar branch of ulnar nerve
3. Extensor digit minimi tendon

Figure 1-78   **Dissection of the flap**

The incision of the dorsal hand should be made along the dorsal carpal branch of the ulnar artery. The pedicles of the ulnar artery and the ulnar nerve should be dissected from proximal to distal. Intraoperatively, the design of the flap should be adjusted to the actual direction of the artery. Then the radial border of the flap should be opened and dissected from under the deep fascia. It is preferable that the 3rd and the 4th dorsal metacarpal arteries and their cutaneous branches be included in the flap to keep the vascular net intact.

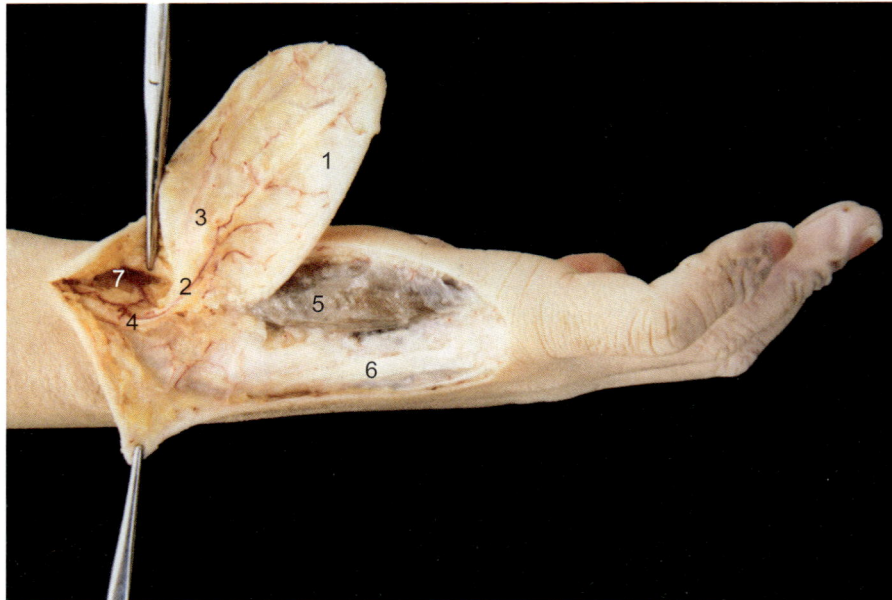

1. Flap
2. Dorsal carpal branch of ulnar artery
3. Basilic vein
4. Dorsal palmar branch of ulnar nerve
5. Hypothenar muscle
6. Extensor digiti minimi tendon
7. Ulnar artery

Figure 1-79   **Elevation of the flap**

The incision of the flap should continue towards the ulnar side until the whole flap is separated, including the dorsal carpal branch of the ulnar artery. The basilic vein should be included at the proximal end of the flap to increase the venous blood returns. After the wound on the recipient region is debrided, the skin between the donor and the recipient site should be opened and the flap transferred to the recipient region by rotation.

B. Retrograde flap

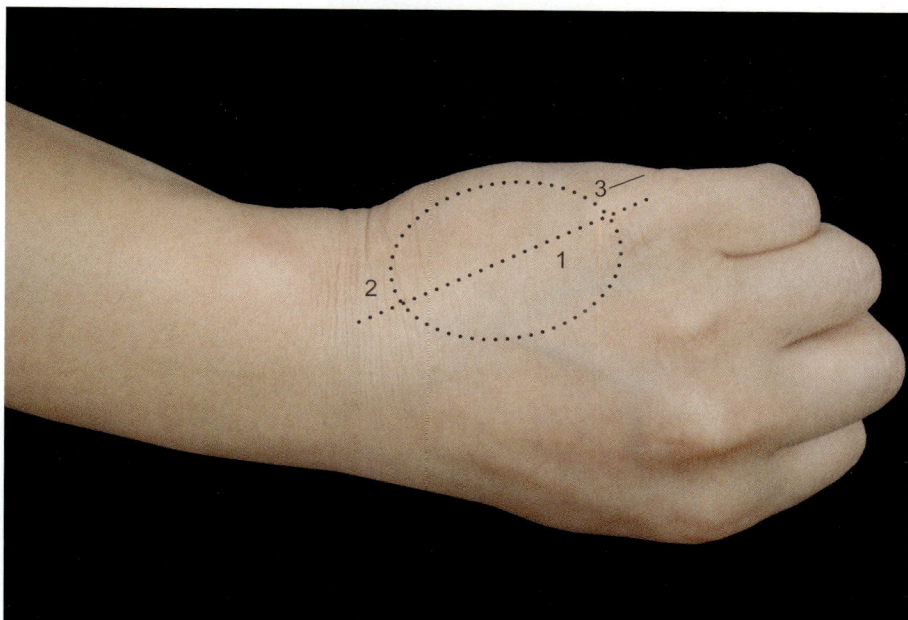

1. 5th metacarpal bone
2. Dorsal carpal transverse line
3. Distal palm print

Figure 1-80   **Design of the flap**

Take the flap for restoration of the finger. The flap should be designed with its axial line falling on the axis of the 5th metacarpal bone and extends bilaterally for 2-2.5 cm wide from the axial line. Its proximal margin extends to the dorsal carpal transverse crease, and its distal margin to the metacarpal head. The flap has a size about 6cm×4cm.

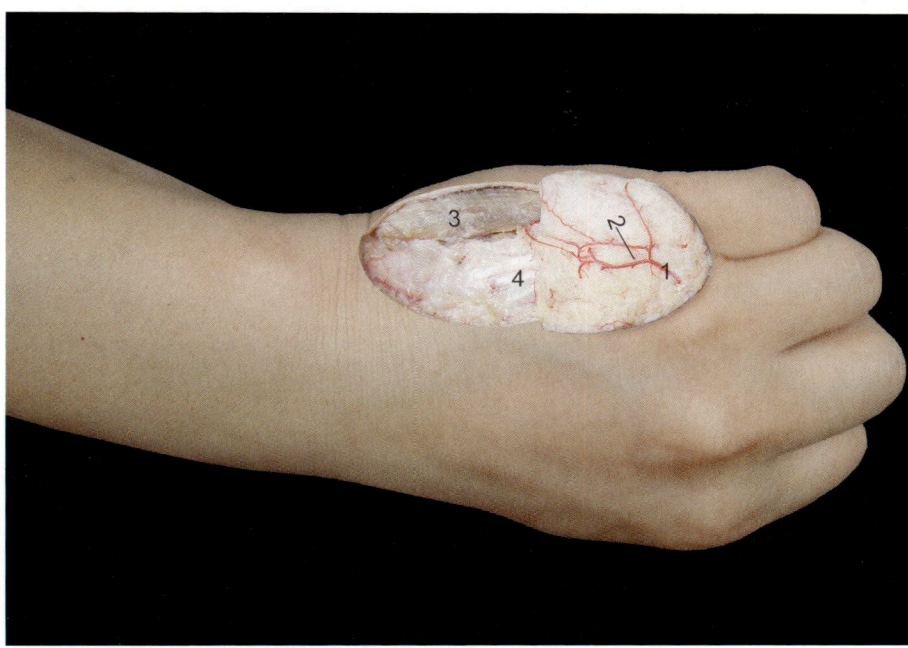

1. Descending branch of the dorsal carpal branch of ulnar artery
2. Dorsal palmar branch of ulnar nerve
3. Hypothenar muscle
4. Extensor digiti minimi tendon

Figure 1-81   **Dissection of the flap**

The proximal margin of the flap should be first incised to expose the descending branch of the dorsal carpal branch of the ulnar artery and the dorsal branch of the ulnar nerve.

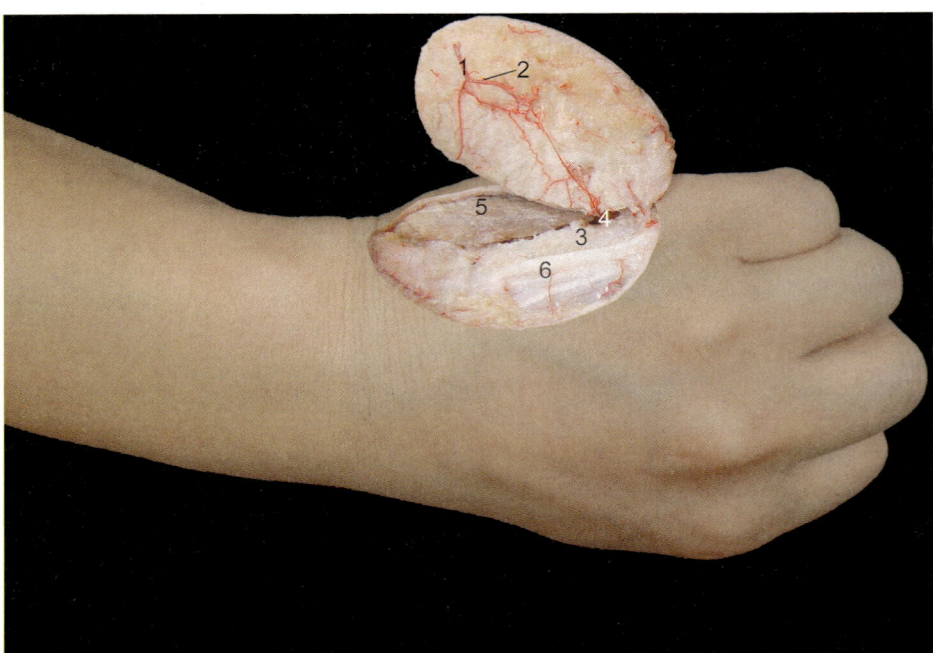

| Figure 1-82 | **Elevation of the flap** |

The flap should be separated from under the deep fascia to include the artery and the nerve. The dissection should extend distally to the pedicle. The flap should be elevated to the region of the head and the neck of the 5th metacarpal bone, generally at 5cm beneath the pisiform, where the anastomotic branch might be identified and dissected with a bilateral fascia cuffs about 1.0-1.5 cm wide.

1. Descending branch of dorsal carpal branch of ulnar artery
2. Dorsal palmar branch of ulnar nerve
3. 5th metacarpal bone
4. Anastomotic branch
5. Hypothenar muscle
6. Extensor digiti minimi tendon

Key points in applied anatomy

Firstly, the flap should be restricted in size with its proximal margin to the dorsal carpal transverse crease, its distal to the metacarpophalangeal articulation, its medial to the dorsal ulnar edge and its lateral to the 3rd metacarpal bone. Secondly, it should be dissected including the perivascular tissues as is necessary to guarantee sufficient blood returns. Thirdly, it should be dissected with the deep fascia to keep intact the descending branch and the perivascular net. Fourthly, the pivot point of the retrograde flap should be located at the head of the 5th metacarpal bone, that is, at 5cm from the pisiform bone. Fifthly, the distal vascular pedicle should be an axial vessel with a wide fascia cuff (1.0-1.5 cm) to guarantee the blood supply. Sixthly, when a retrograde flap is harvested, either the dorsal palmar branch of the ulnar nerve or the extensor digiti minimi tendon should be included. That is, if the flap is based on the ulnar region, it is not necessary to include all the 3 branches of the cutaneous nerve, nor all the extensor tendons. One branch is enough to restore the flap sensation. Seventhly, it is possible that a compound flap with blocks of the 5th and the 4th metacarpal bones be harvested.

The Flap Based on the 1st Dorsal Metacarpal Artery

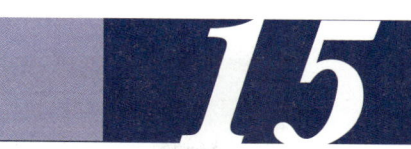

The flap is based on the 1st dorsal metacarpal artery and the connection with the deep branch of the metacarpal radial artery. It might be transferred retrogradely to restore a wound on the thumb or the first web space.

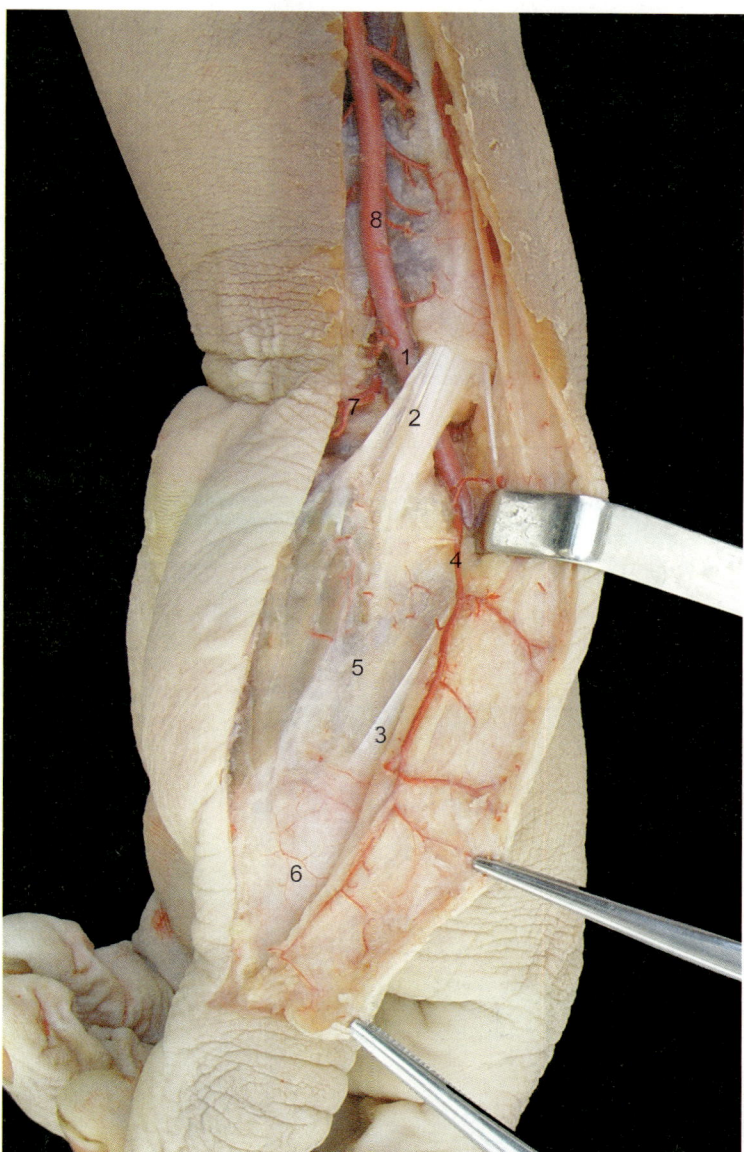

1. Deep branch of radial artery
2. Abductor pollicis longus muscle
3. Abductor pollicis brevis muscle
4. Dorsal pollicis artery
5. 1st metacarpal bone
6. Proximal pollicis joint
7. Superficial branch of radial artery
8. Radial artery

Figure 1-83   **Applied anatomy**

The deep branch of the radial artery runs along the abductor pollicis longus and the extensor pollicis brevis to reach the anatomical snuff-box and gives dorsal pollicis artery. The dorsal pollicis artery sends 1-2 branches near its origin and extends through the extensor pollicis brevis to fan out and nourish the proximal 1/3 of the 1st dorsal metacarpal bone and the overlying skin. Its trunk extends obliquely through the deep surface of the extensor pollicis brevis and sends many small branches to nourish the distal 2/3 of the 1st dorsal metacarpal bone and the overlying dorsal radial skin. The deep branch of the radial artery perforates through the deep surface of the extensor pollicis longus to enter the palm via the two heads of the 1st dorsal interossei and form a profound palmar arch. There are cephalic vein and the dorsal carpal veins that pass through the flap donor area.

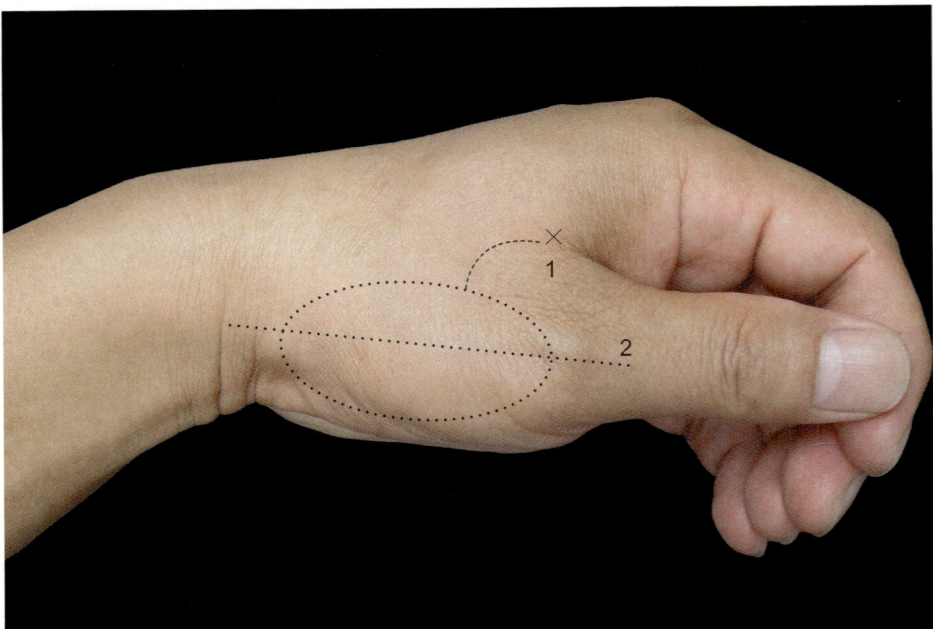

| **Figure 1-84** | **Design of the flap** |

The flap should be designed with its axial line falling on the connection between the snuff-box center and the dorsoradial border of the interphalangeal joint of the thumb. Its pivot point should be located at the point where the deep branch of the radial artery enters the 1st dorsal interossei.

1. Pivot point
2. Axial line

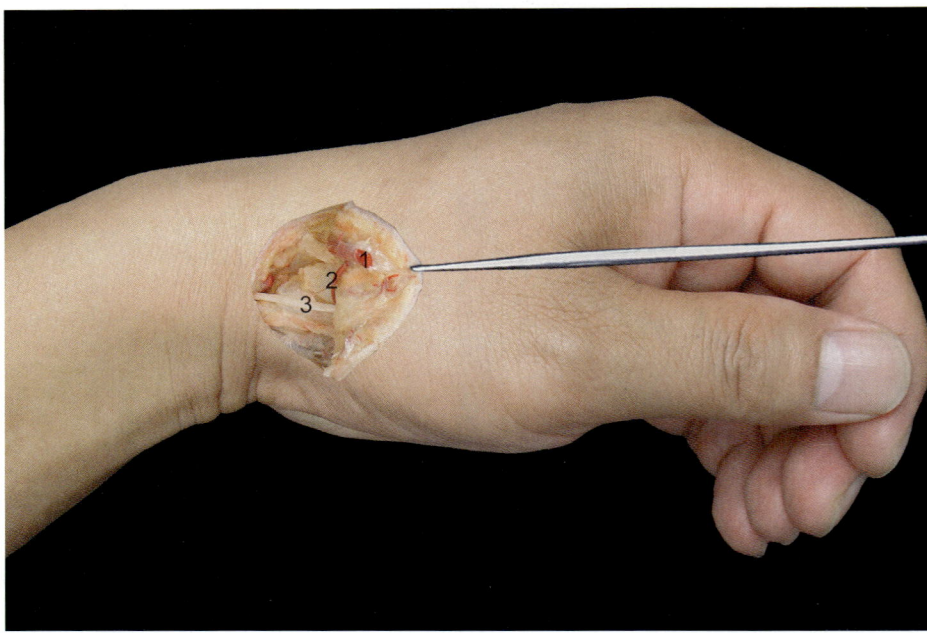

1. Deep branch of radial artery
2. Dorsal pollicis artery
3. Extensor pollicis brevis tendon

| **Figure 1-85** | **Exposure of the vessels** |

The incision of the flap should begin with its proximal border. The cephalic vein that passes through the incision should then be ligated. The dissection continues to the deep anatomical plane of the extensor pollicis brevis until the deep branch of the radial artery is exposed. It is ligated and cut.

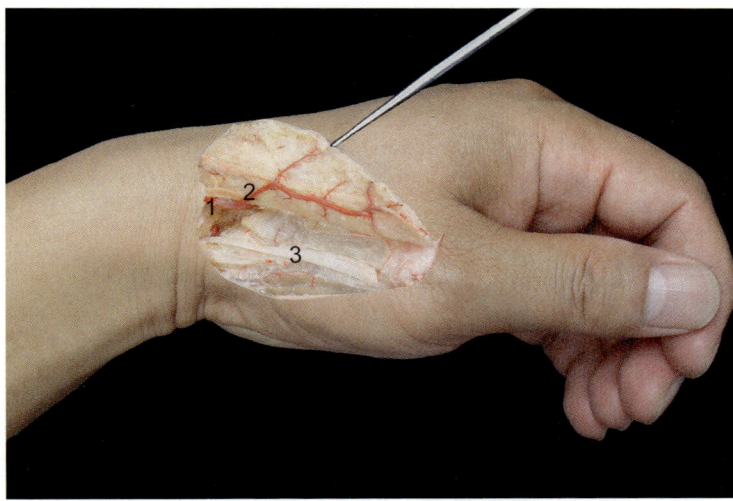

1. Deep branch of radial artery
2. Dorsal pollicis artery
3. Extensor pollicis brevis tendon

Figure 1-86   Dissection of the flap

The flap should be dissected distally along the deep branch of the radial artery. Since the dorsal pollicis artery extends beneath the extensor pollicis brevis tendon, the tendon should be cut at the distal of the flap and pulled out from the proximal part of the flap. The nutrient vessels should be given great attention to keep them intact.

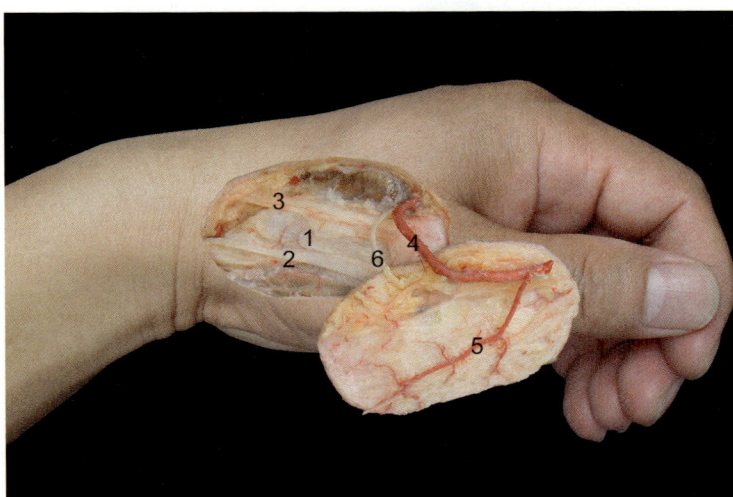

1. 1st metacarpal bone
2. Extensor pollicis brevis tendon
3. Extensor pollicis longus tendon
4. Deep branch of radial artery
5. Dorsal pollicis artery
6. Cephalic vein

Figure 1-87   Elevation of the flap

The Elevation of the flap should be done closely to the surface of the 1st metacarpal bone, tendon and the joint capsule. It should extend distally to the deep branch of radial artery. The flap should be raised as an island with pedicles of the deep branch of the radial artery and the dorsal pollicis artery.

Key points in applied anatomy

Firstly, the point at which the deep branch of the radial artery enters the 1st dorsal interossei should be confirmed preoperatively with the Doppler. Secondly, the cephalic vein and the communicating branch of the dorsal carpal veins should be retained during the operation. Thirdly, the dissected extensor pollicis brevis muscle should be sutured back after the flap is elevated. Fourthly, the flap size is restricted to 10×5cm. Fifthly, the pedicle of the neurovascular bundle should be long enough to avoid tension, kinking, or compression.

16 Dorsal Index Flap

The dorsal index flap is commonly termed as the 2nd dorsal metacarpal flap, or the kite flap. Its blood supply comes from the first dorsal metacarpal artery, the dorsal digital radial artery and the dorsal branch of proper digital artery. It might be transferred to restore a soft tissue defect on the thumb or the first web space, or to reconstruct the thumb.

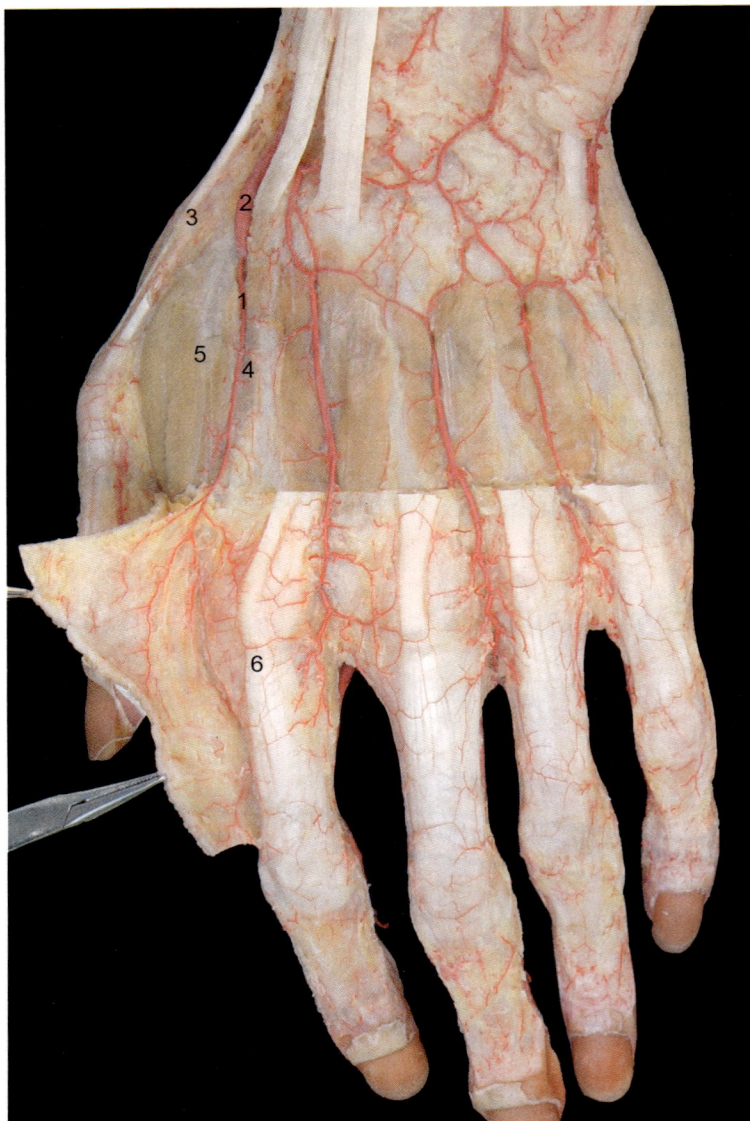

1. 1st dorsal metacarpal artery
2. Radial artery
3. Extensor pollicis longus tendon
4. 2nd metacarpal bone
5. 1st dorsal interossei
6. Index finger

Figure 1-88   **Applied anatomy**

In most cases (70%), the 1st dorsal metacarpal artery emerges from the radial artery in the snuff-box. The skin surface project of the artery origin falls on the cross point of the extensor pollicis longus tendon and the 2nd metacarpal bone. In a few cases (30%), the artery originates from the main pollicis artery. In some other cases, there is not such artery at all. The 1st dorsal metacarpal artery extends distally on the surface of the 1st dorsal interossei, and runs closely to the 2nd metacarpal bone. It gives one branch to the ulnar thumb. Its final branch reaches the proximal dorsal phalanx of the 2nd digit. The venous blood is drained via the dorsal veins of the 2nd digit, which joins the dorsal metacarpal venous network. The dorsal digital nerve of the 2nd digit originates from the superficial branch of the radial nerve

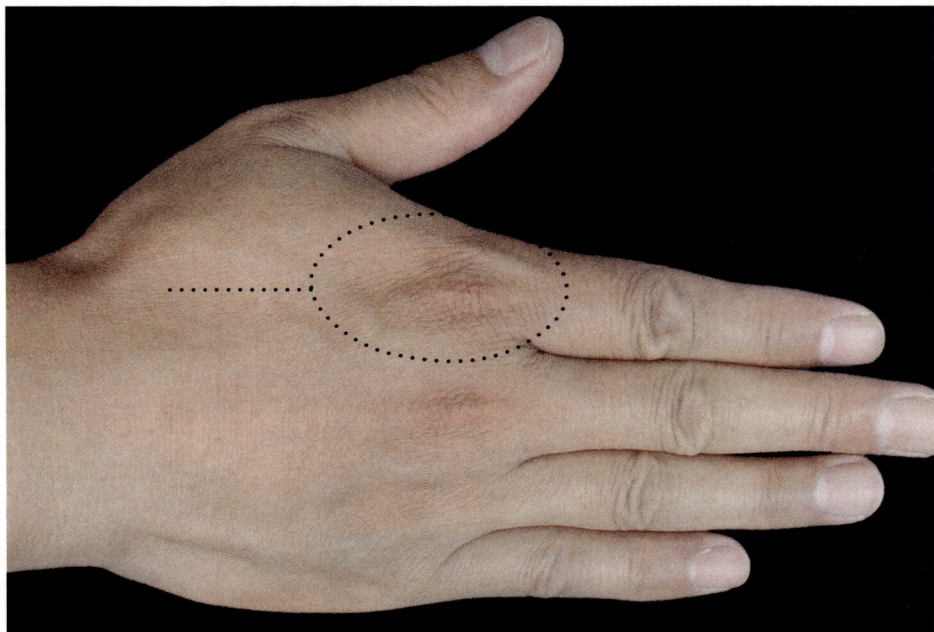

Figure 1-89   Design of the flap

The flap should be designed with its distal margin extending to the proximal interdigital joint, its lateral to the bilateral midline of the digit and its proximal to the dorsal wrist crease if necessary. The flap size should be adjusted to the defect of the thumb.

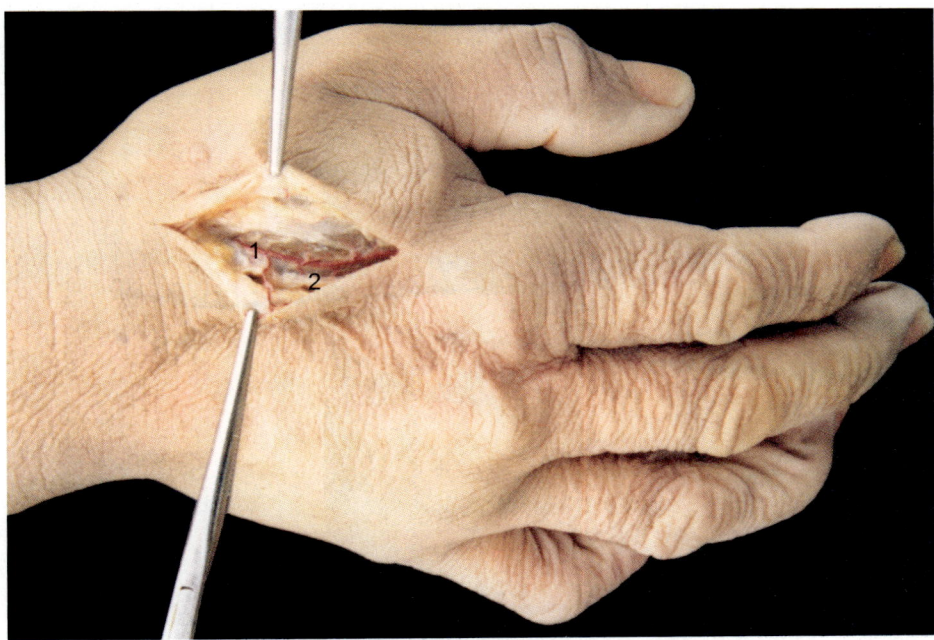

1. 1st dorsal metacarpal artery
2. Extensor digital tendon

Figure 1-90   Elevation of the neurovascular bundle

A vertical incision of the flap should be made between the 1st dorsal interossei and the 2nd metacarpal bone. The flap should be then dissected bilaterally under the dermis to expose the dorsal carpal vein in the subcutaneous tissue. Then the superficial branch of the radial nerve might be identified beneath the subcutaneous vein, and the 1st dorsal metacarpal artery beneath the nerve. The dissection should be done under the muscle sheath from proximal to distal onto the metacarpophalangeal joint. The connective tissues surrounding the artery and the nerve should be kept with the neurovascular bundle.

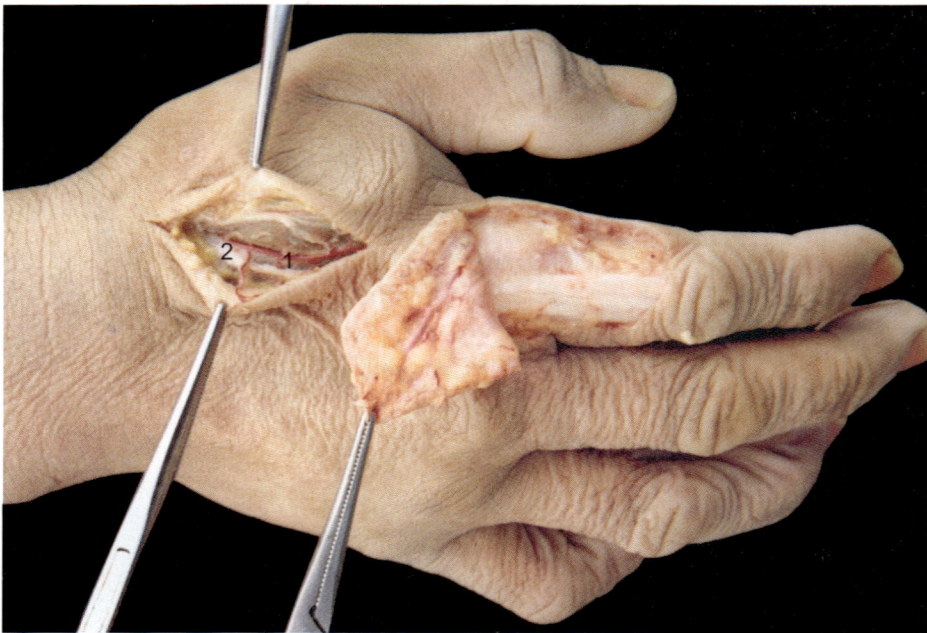

| **Figure 1-91** | **Dissection of the flap** |

The distal margin of the flap should be confirmed and incised. The flap should be elevated from the surface of the extensor tendon of the digit.

1. 1st dorsal metacarpal artery
2. Extensor digital tendon

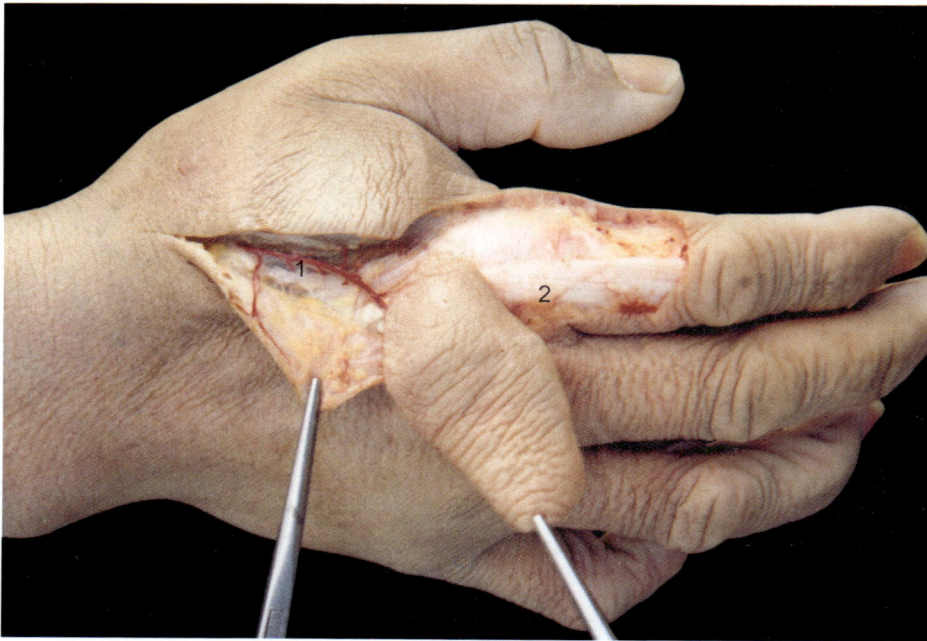

| **Figure 1-92** | **Elevation of the flap** |

The flap should be elevated from distal to proximal.

1. 1st dorsal metacarpal artery
2. Extensor digital tendon

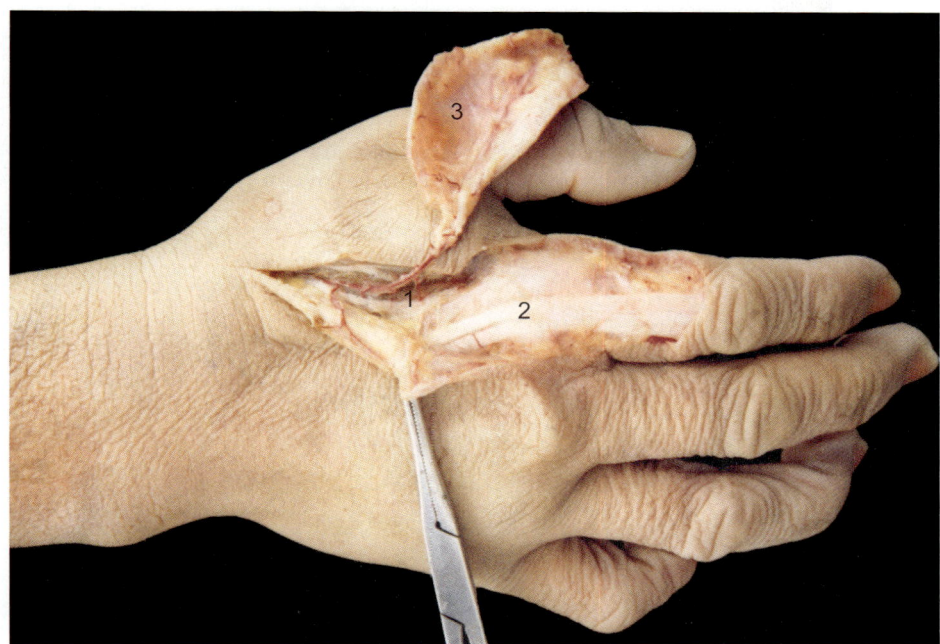

Figure 1-93   **Transposition of the flap**

The flap should be transferred through the subcutaneous tunnel to reach the thumb defect.

1. 1st dorsal metacarpal artery
2. Extensor digital tendon
3. Flap

Key points in applied anatomy

Firstly, since the vessels of the flap are generally small, the vascular spasm tends to occur postoperatively and the flap looks pale. The vascular spasm might be relieved by warm normal saline or by infiltration of lidocaine (2%). Secondly, the subcutaneous tunnel through which the flap is to be transferred should be wide and loose enough to prevent compression. Moreover, the neurovascular pedicles should be long enough to avoid tension and kinking after the transposition.

17

Groin Flap

The groin flap is based on the superficial circumflex iliac artery. The donor site is hidden, and the vessel relatively large in diameter. The flap might be transferred locally to cover a wound on the perineum or the greater trochanter.

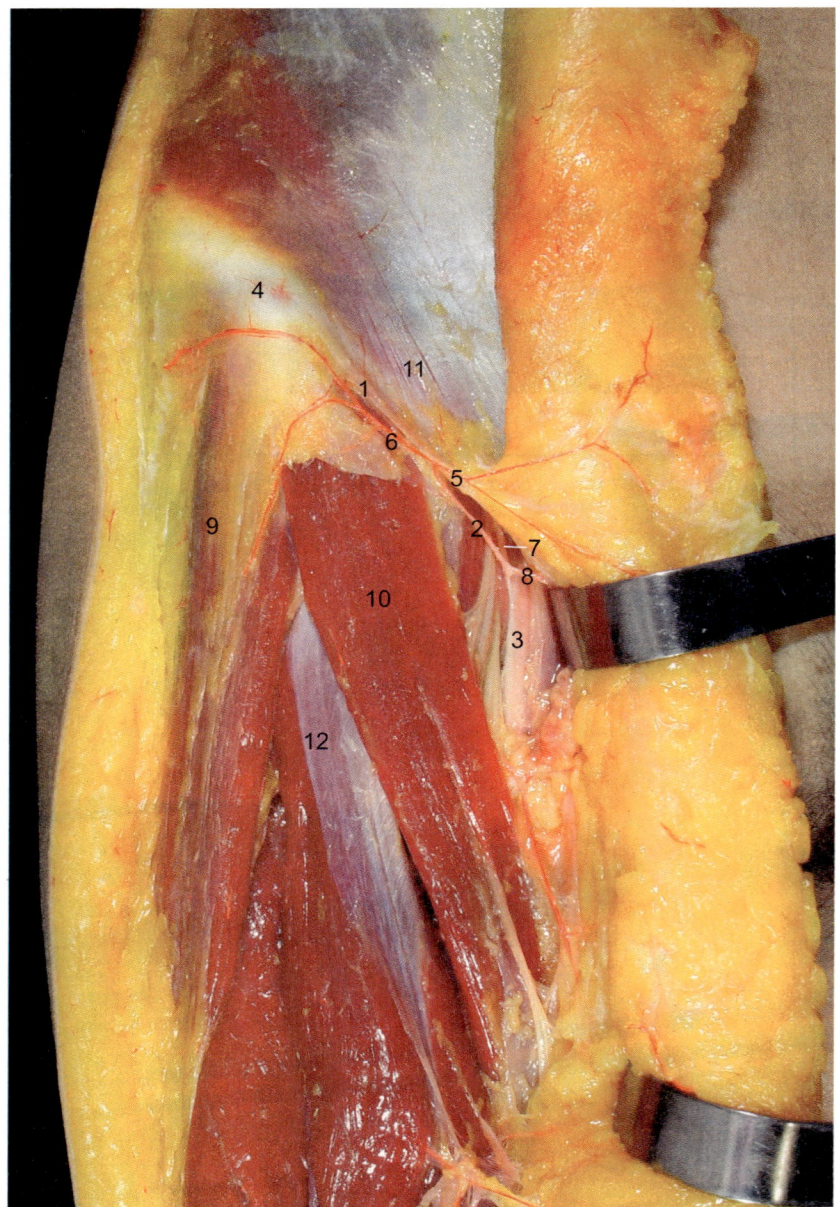

Figure 1-94   **Applied anatomy**

1. Inguinal ligament
2. Superficial circumflex iliac artery
3. Femoral artery
4. Iliac spine
5. Superficial branch
6. Deep branch
7. Superficial epigastric artery
8. Superficial external pudendal artery
9. Tensor fasciae latae muscle
10. Sartorius muscle
11. Aponeurosis of the obliquus externus abdominis
12. Rectus femoris muscle

The superficial circumflex iliac artery is a direct cutaneous artery. It arises from the femoral artery at 1.5cm distal to the midpoint of the inguinal ligament and extends to the anterior superior iliac spine. Its trunk is relatively short, usually less than 1.5mm on average, and soon divides into superficial and deep branches that continue in the same direction. The superficial branch courses for 5mm in the deep layer of the deep fascia and perforates through the fasciae latae to enter the superficial subcutaneous layer. The deep branch courses under the deep fascia and perforates through it at 2cm distal to the anterior superior iliac spine to enter the subcutaneous tissue.

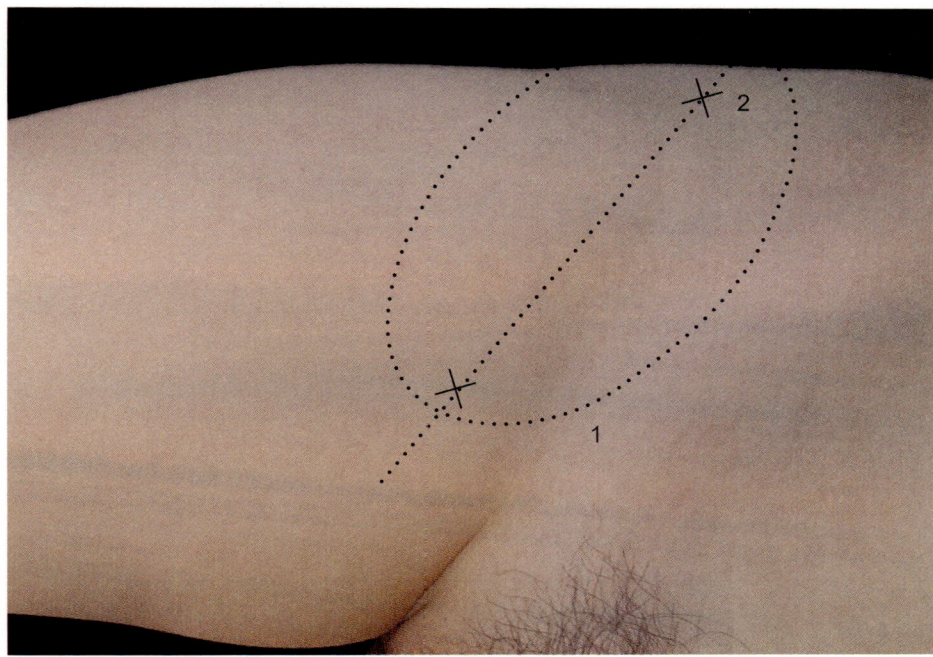

1. Inguinal ligament
2. Superficial circumflex iliac artery

Figure 1-95   Design of the flap

The flap should be designed with its pivot point at 1.5cm distal to the midpoint of the inguinal ligament, and its axial line fall on the connecting line between the anterior superior iliac spine and the pivot point.

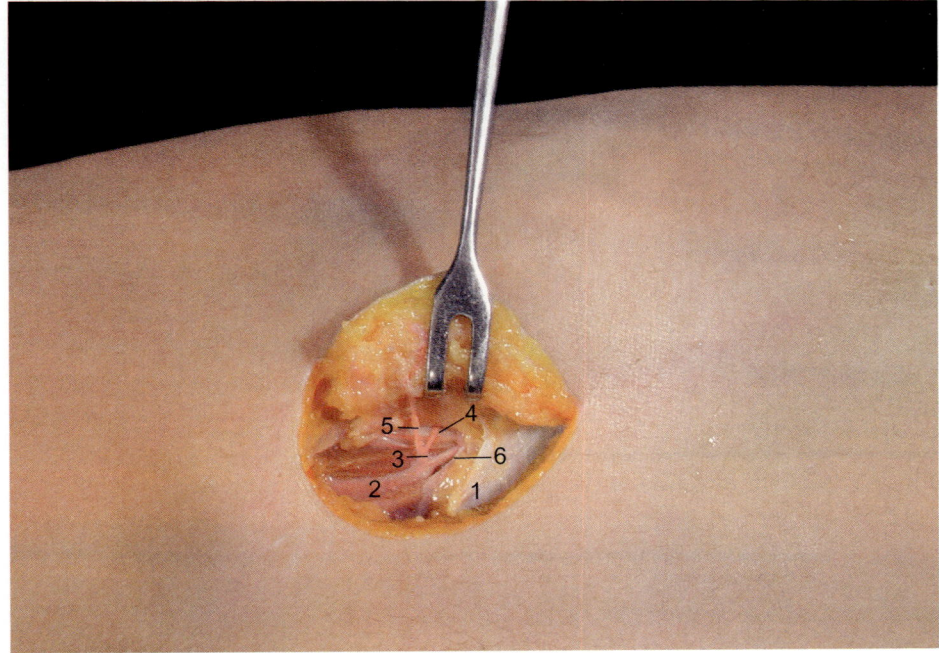

1. Inguinal ligament
2. Femoral artery
3. Superficial circumflex iliac artery
4. Deep branch
5. Superficial branch
6. Superficial epigastric artery

Figure 1-96   Exposure of the vessels

The incision of the flap should begin with its medial border to expose the inguinal ligament and the femoral artery. The dissection should continue along the femoral artery to expose the superficial circumflex iliac artery branch that emerges from the lateral femoral artery wall and extends proximally outwards to the anterior superior iliac spine.

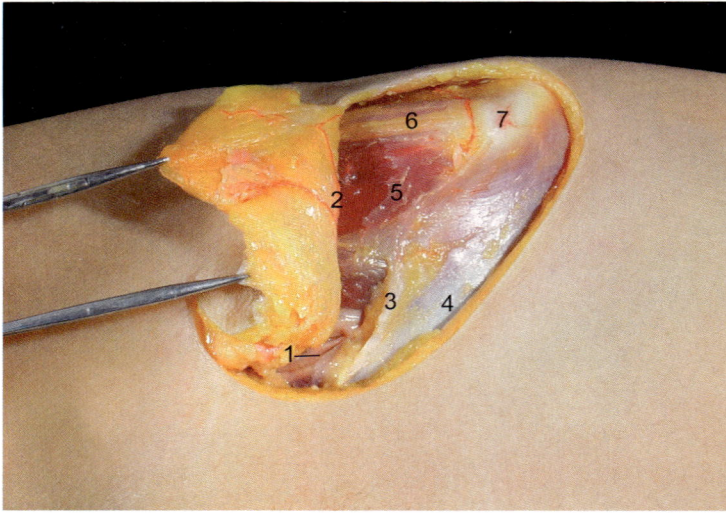

1. Superficial circumflex iliac artery
2. Superficial branch of superficial circumflex iliac artery
3. Inguinal ligament
4. Aponeurosis of obliquus externus abdominis
5. Sartorius muscle
6. Tensor fasciae latae muscle
7. Anterior superior iliac spine

Figure 1-97   **Dissection of the flap**

The flap should be separated laterally along the superficial circumflex iliac artery to the bifurcation of the deep and the superficial branches. The deep branch should be ligated, and the dissection continue from proximal to distal along the superficial branch to harvest the flap. If a larger flap is needed and the deep branch included, the dissection should be done along the deep branch under the deep fascia until it perforates superficially through the subcutaneous tissue.

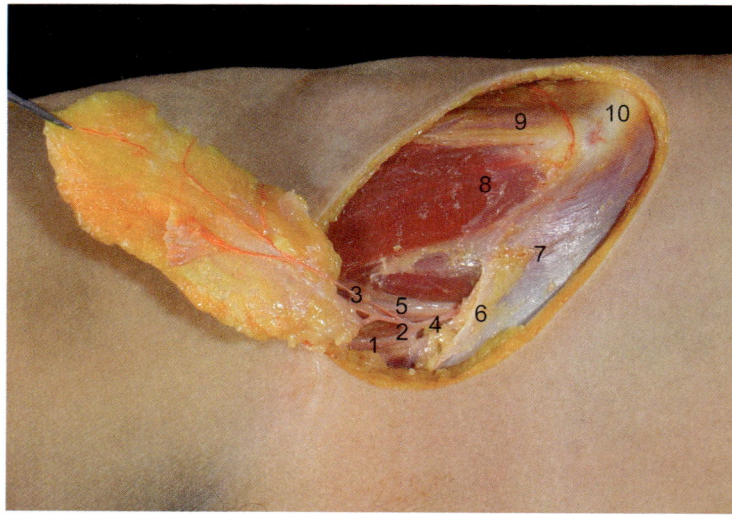

1. Femoral artery
2. Superficial circumflex iliac artery
3. Superficial branch of superficial circumflex iliac artery
4. Superficial epigastric artery
5. Femoral nerve
6. Inguinal ligament
7. Aponeurosis of obliquus externus abdominis
8. Sartorius muscle
9. Tensor fasciae latae muscle
10. Anterior superior iliac spine

Figure 1-98   **Transposition of the flap**

The flap might be transferred locally to repair a wound of the greater trochanter. The donor site could usually be directly sutured at the first stage.

Key points in applied anatomy

Firstly, the groin flap usually includes only the superficial branch of the superficial circumflex iliac artery. But in some cases it might include the deep branch to make it large and augment its vascularization. In that case the flap can become relatively bulky. Secondly, in most cases, the superficial circumflex iliac vein converges into the great saphenous vein or the femoral vein branch, and in about half cases, it courses all the way distal to the inguinal ligament. Therefore it should be given great attention while the flap is being raised.

Anterolateral Thigh Flap

18

The anterolateral thigh flap is located on the anterolateral part of the upper leg. It is based on the descending branch of the lateral circumflex femoral artery and its perforating branch of the musculo-cutaneous artery. The vessels are anatomically constant and large in diameter. The flap might be transferred locally to restore a wound on the greater trochanter, the perineal or the inguinal region. It could be harvesed as a retrograde island flap to cover a genicular defect since the distal artery anastomoses with the lateral superior genicular artery.

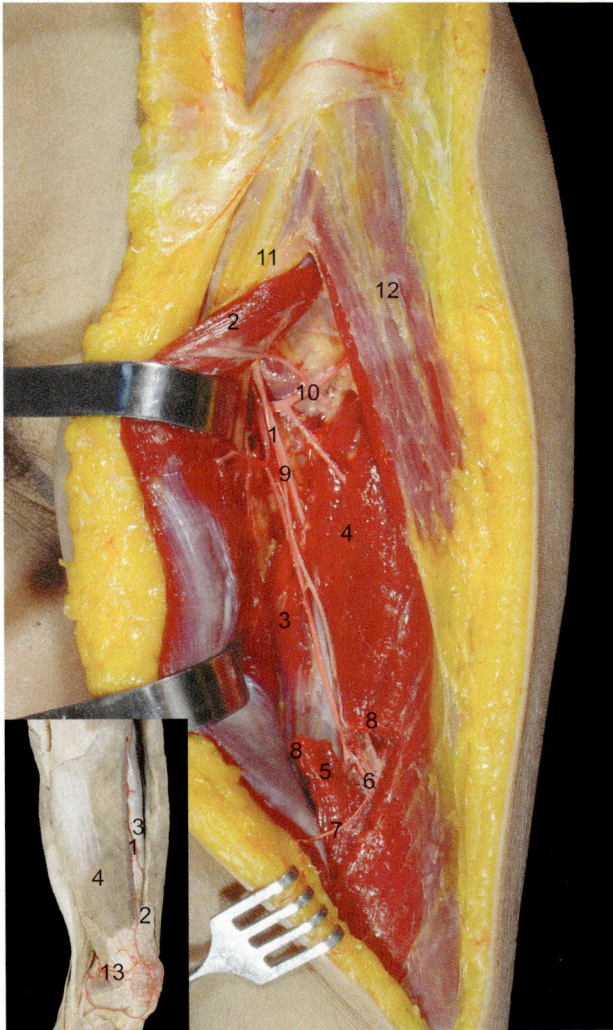

1. Descending branch of lateral circumflex femoral artery
2. Rectus femoris muscle
3. Vastus intermedius muscle
4. Vastus lateralis
5. Medial branch
6. Lateral branch
7. Perforating branch of 1st musculo-cutaneous artery
8. Vastus lateralis (cut to expose the perforating branch)
9. Femoral nerve (muscular branch)
10. Ascending branch of lateral circumflex femoral artery
11. Sartorius muscle
12. Tensor fasciae latae muscle

Figure 1-99	Applied anatomy

The descending branch of the lateral circumflex femoral artery courses laterally in the septum between the rectus femoris muscle and the vastus intermedius muscle. It divides into two branches—the medial branch and the lateral branch in the spatium intermusculare between the vastus lateralis and the rectus femoris muscle. Then the lateral branch extends laterally and sends branches to perforate through the vastus lateralis or the spatium intermusculare to reach the lateral anterior skin. Most of these branches are musculocutaneous perforators, but some are septum cutaneous perforators. The first perforating musculocutaneous artery is the largest and the most important one, which is about 0.5-1.0 mm in diameter. It serves as the main artery in the flap. The medial branch extends distally and gives branches to nourish the adjacent skin. Its final branch anastomoses with the lateral superior genicular artery, and then participates in the formation of the genicular vascular net.

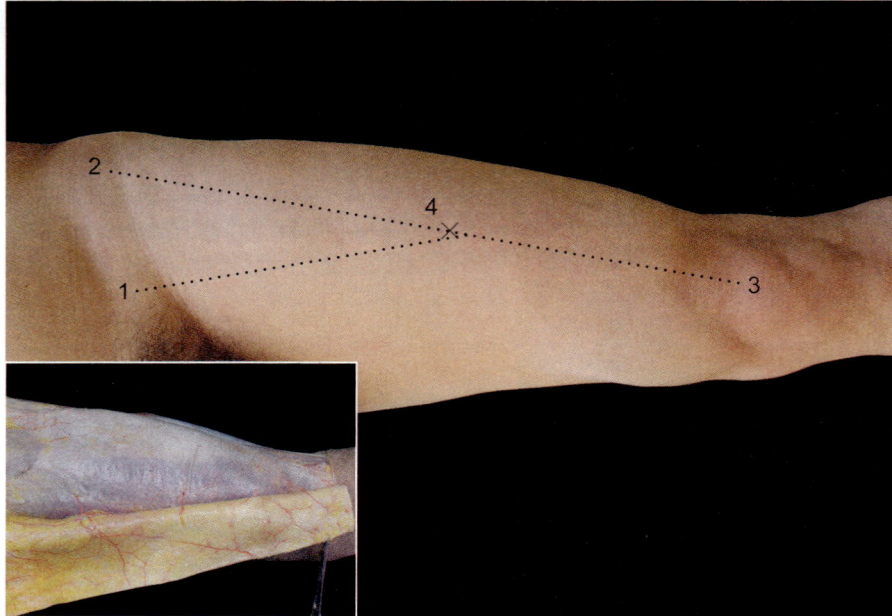

1. Inguinal ligament
2. Anterior superior iliac spine
3. Lateral superior patella
4. Perforating branch of 1st musculo-cutaneous artery

| **Figure 1-100** | **Design of the flap** |

A line should be drawn from the midpoint of the inguinal ligament to the midpoint between the anterior superior iliac spine and the lateral superior patella, and the distal 2/3 represents the body surface projection of the descending branch of lateral circumflex artery. The 1st musculocutaneous perforator might be found near the midpoint of the connecting line between the anterior superior iliac spine and the lateral superior patella. When an anterolateral thigh flap is being designed, the 1st perforating vessel should be located in the center of the flap.

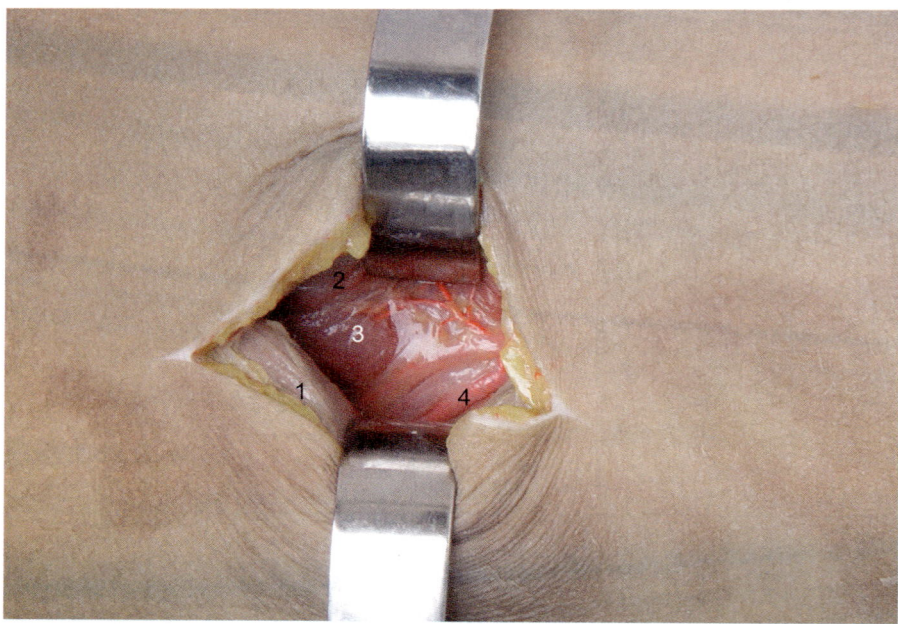

1. Rectus femoris muscle
2. Vastus lateralis
3. Vastus intermedius muscle
4. Descending branch of lateral circumflex femoral artery

| **Figure 1-101** | **Exposure of the vessels** |

The incision of the vascular pedicles should be made along the body surface projection of the descending branch of the lateral circumflex femoral artery. The septum between the rectus femoris muscle and the vastus lateralis should be separated. The muscles should be drawn bilaterally to expose the descending branch along the septum between the rectus femoris muscle and the vastus lateralis and on the superficial surface of the vastus intermedius muscle.

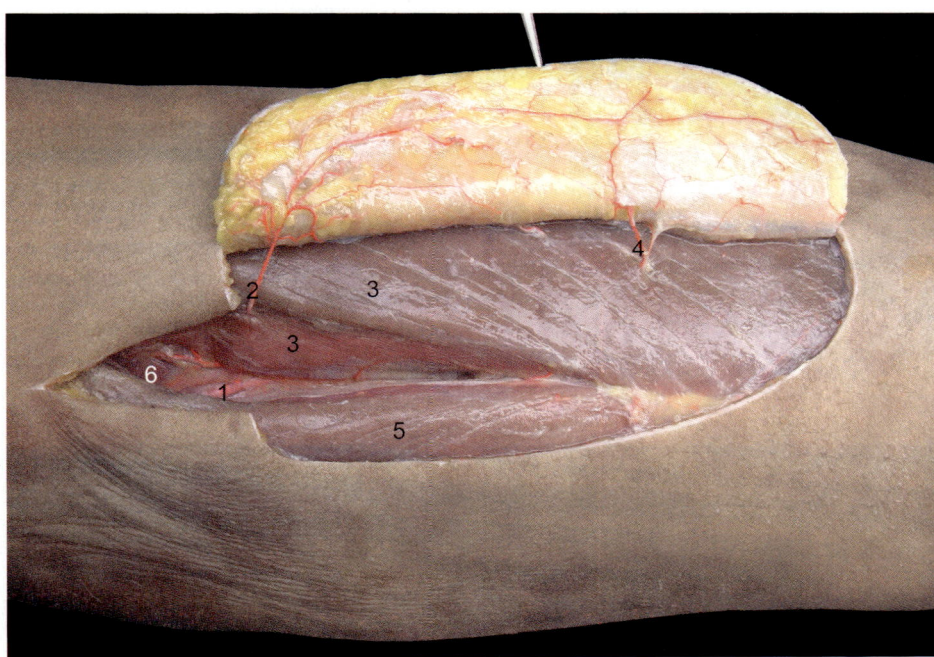

1. Descending branch of lateral circumflex femoral artery
2. Perforating branch of 1st musculo-cutaneous artery
3. Vastus lateralis
4. Perforating branch of 2nd musculo-cutaneous artery
5. Rectus femoris muscle
6. Vastus intermedius muscle

Figure 1-102 **Dissection of the flap**

The descending branch should be separated towards the distal to expose the perforating branch of the 1st musculocutaneous artery. Then most of the descending branch of the lateral circumflex femoral artery enters the vastus lateralis. Some muscular fibers should be separated to expose the perforators until they enter the overlying deep fascia. Some perivascular muscular fibers should be retained to protect the vessels from being damaged. Then the flap should be turned laterally to expose the sequential 2nd and the 3rd musculocutaneous branches to increase the blood supply for the flap.

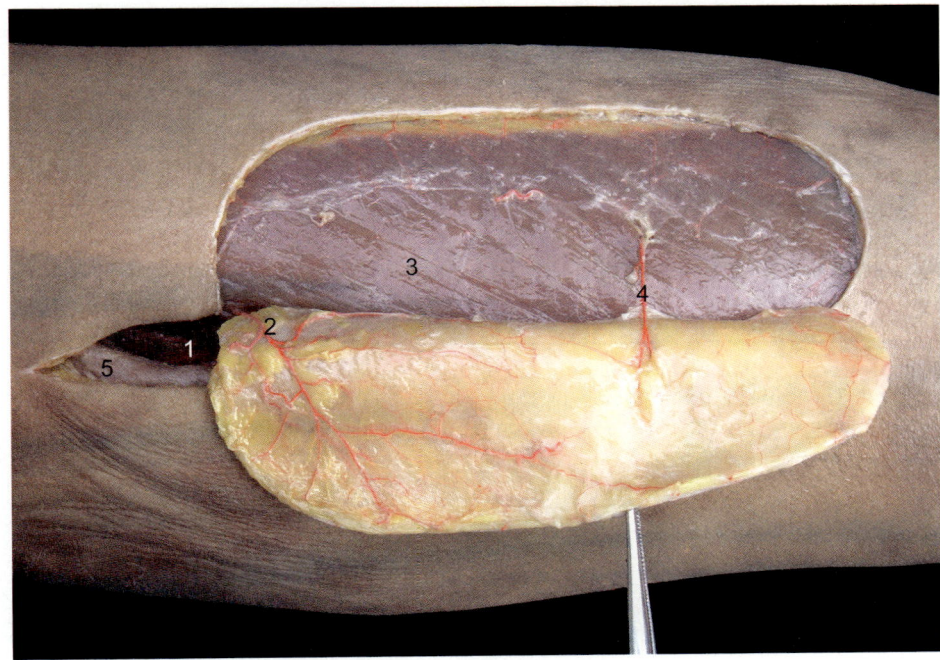

1. Descending branch of the lateral circumflex femoral artery
2. Perforating branch of the 1st musculo-cutaneous artery
3. Vastus lateralis
4. Perforating branch of the 2nd musculo-cutaneous artery
5. Rectus femoris muscle

Figure 1-103 **Elevation of the flap**

After the medial dissection is finished, the lateral border of the flap should be incised and raised together with some of the tensor fasciae latae. The dissection should be carried out medially under the deep fascia.

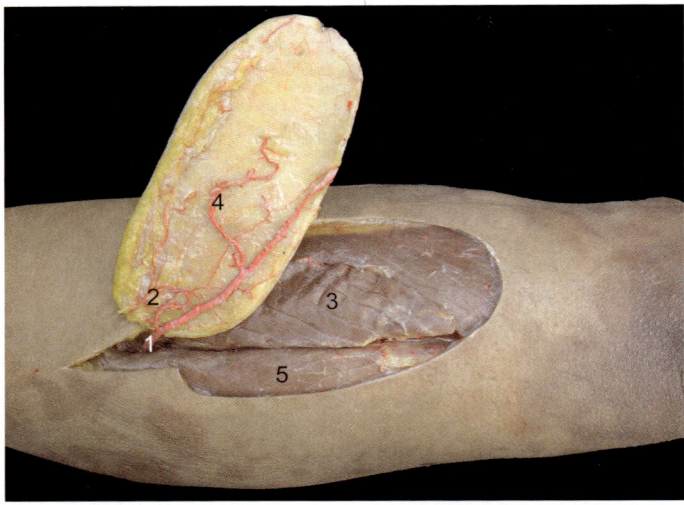

1. Descending branch of lateral circumflex femoral artery
2. Perforating branch of 1ˢᵗ musculo-cutaneous artery
3. Vastus lateralis
4. Perforating branch of 2ⁿᵈ musculo-cutaneous artery
5. Rectus femoris muscle

Figure 1-104   Anterograde transposition of the flap

After the Elevation of the flap, the vessels should be cut off at its distal end and raised along the descending branch of the lateral circumflex femoral artery towards the proximal pedicle. The flap might be transferred to restore a wound on the adjacent region.

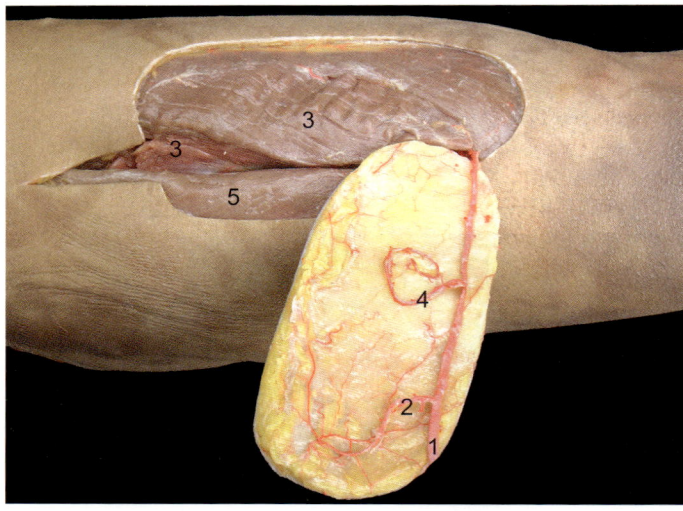

1. Descending branch of lateral circumflex femoral artery
2. Perforating branch of 1ˢᵗ musculo-cutaneous artery
3. Vastus lateralis
4. Perforating branch of 2ⁿᵈ musculo-cutaneous artery
5. Rectus femoris muscle

Figure 1-105   Retrograde transposition of the flap

After the Elevation of the flap, the descending branch of the lateral circumflex femoral artery should be cut and ligated at the proximal end. The flap should be raised distally with the pedicle of the lateral superior genicular artery. Then it might be transferred to cover a wound on the adjacent genicular region.

Key points in applied anatomy

Firstly, the courses of the vessels and the point through which the musculocutaneous artery perforates should be confirmed preoperatively with the Doppler. Secondly, in most cases, the point where the 1ˢᵗ musculocutaneous perforates through the deep fascia could be anticipated within the circle of 3 cm semi-diameter and centered on the midpoint of the connecting line between the anterior superior iliac spine and the lateral superior patella. In general, the perforators are mostly located at the 1/4 lateral inferior sphere. Thirdly, during the operation, the descending branch of the lateral circumflex femoral artery should be sought in the septum between the vastus lateralis and the rectus femoris muscle. The femoral motor nerve branch should be given great attention to avoid getting it damaged. Fourthly, the muscular fibers should be separated to trace the perforating branch until it reaches the subcutaneous tissue.

Anteromedial Thigh Flap

19

The anteromedial thigh flap is based on the medial branch of the lateral circumflex femoral artery. Its vascular pedicle is large and long. It might be transferred to repair a wound on the perineum or in the inguinal groove.

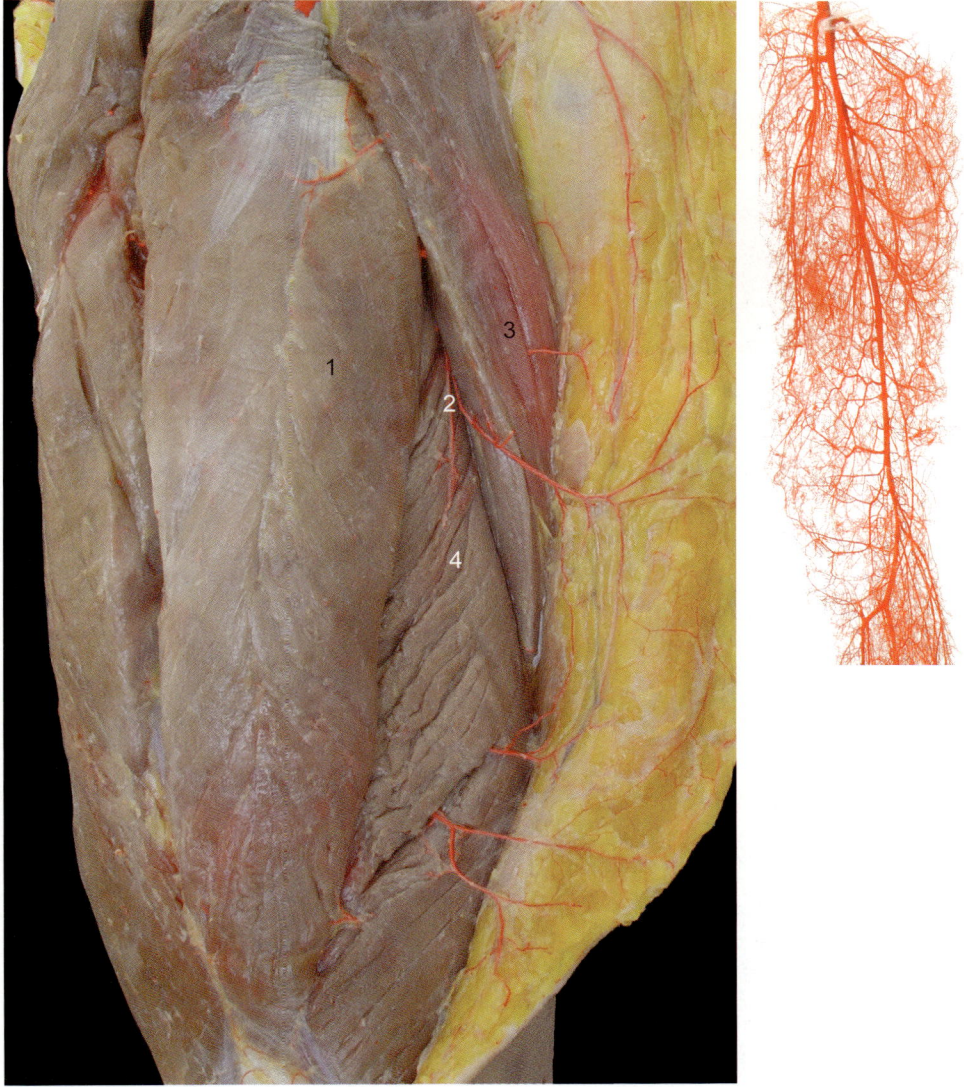

| **Figure 1-106** | **Applied anatomy** |

The descending branch of the lateral circumflex femoral artery gives a medial branch in the deep layer of the rectus femoris muscle. It descends further inwards to the medial rectus femoris muscle and down to the septum between the sartorius muscle and the medial vastus. Its musculocutaneous branch perforates through at the triangular space composed of the sartorius muscle, the rectus femoris muscle and the medial vastus. The vascular pedicle is about 12cm long.

1. Rectus femoris muscle
2. Branch of lateral circumflex femoral artery
3. Sartorius muscle
4. Vastus lateralis

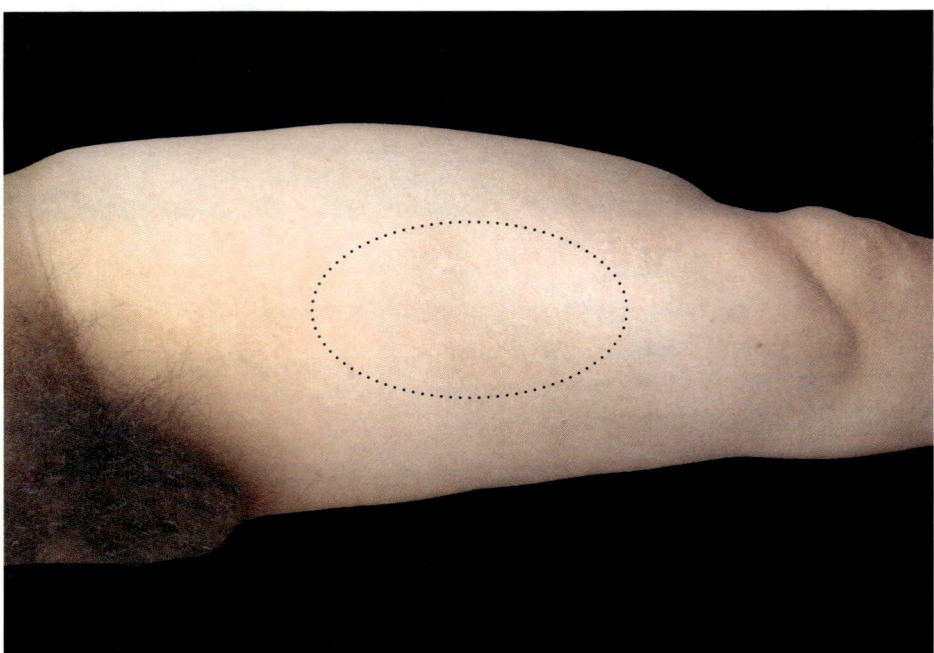

| **Figure 1-107** | **Design of the flap** |

The point through which the cutaneous artery perforates could be probed at the triangular space of the sartorius muscle, the rectus femoris muscle and the medial vastus. The flap should be centered around this point, and its proximal incision drawn to expose the vascular pedicle.

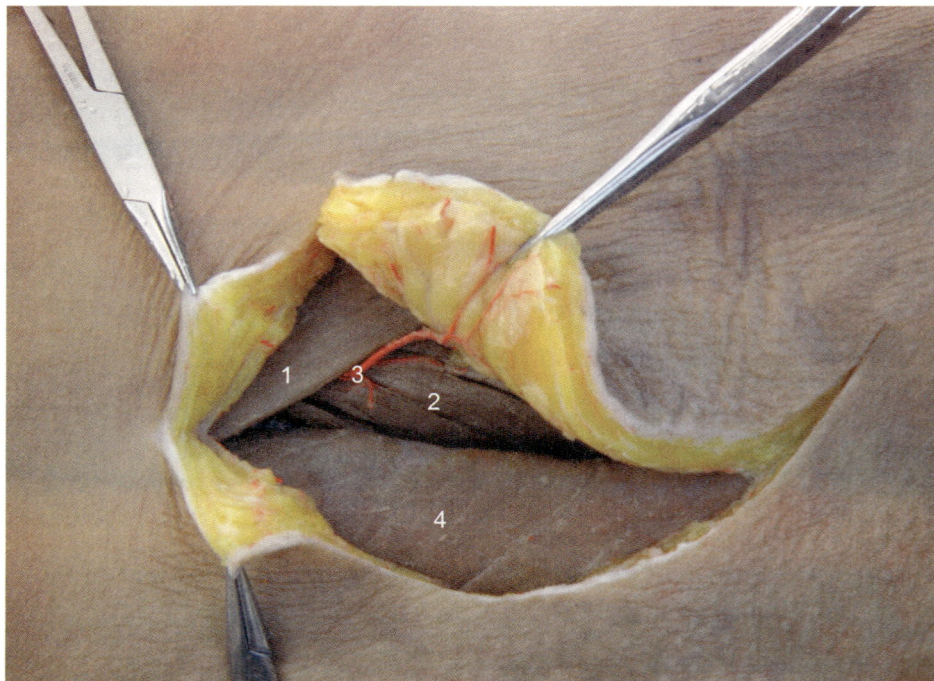

1. Sartorius muscle
2. Rectus femoris muscle
3. Branch of lateral circumflex femoral artery
4. Vastus lateralis

| **Figure 1-108** | **Exposure of the vessels** |

The lateral and the proximal borders of the flap should be incised first to expose the sartorius muscle and the rectus femoris muscle. The sartorius muscle should be tracted medially to expose the medial branch of the lateral circumflex femoral artery. The dissection should continue toward the distal part of the flap to seek the cutaneous artery that enters the flap. The flap should be adjusted to the direction of the cutaneous artery.

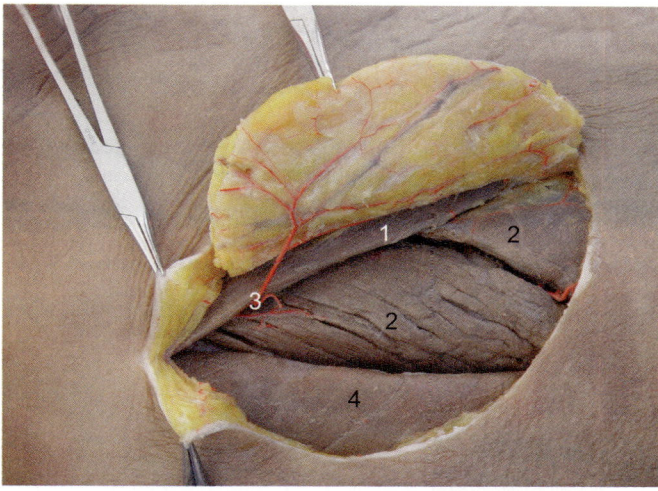

1. Sartorius muscle
2. Rectus femoris muscle
3. Branch of lateral circumflex femoral artery
4. Vastus lateralis

Figure 1-109   Elevation of the flap

Along the cutaneous artery, the flap should be elevated from proximal to distal under the deep fascia.

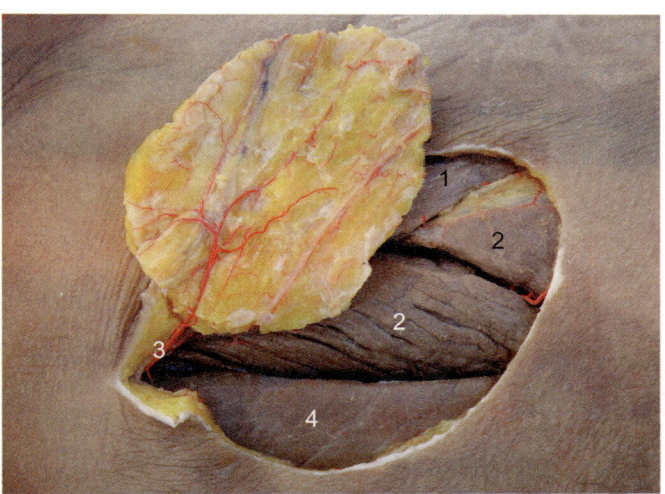

1. Sartorius muscle
2. Rectus femoris muscle
3. Branch of lateral circumflex femoral artery
4. Vastus lateralis

Figure 1-110   Transposition of the flap

The harvested flap might be transferred proximally to repair a wound on the perineum or the inguinal region.

Key points in applied anatomy

Firstly, the flap should be designed with its center falling on the strongest signal point that could be determined with the Doppler. Secondly, since the cutaneous artery bifurcates into a short ascending branch and a long descending branch after it perforates through the deep fascia, the flap should be designed with 1/3 of it above and 2/3 of it below the perforating point. Thirdly, if the designed flap includes the lateral branch as a pedicle, an arch incision should be made first at 3-4cm medial to the signal point and then extend laterally to the sartorius muscle. The vascular pedicle should be located along the lateral border of the sartorius muscle. Fourthly, if the designed flap includes the medial branch as a pedicle, an arc incision should be made first at the lateral side of the sartorius muscle and then extend medially to the medial border of the muscle. Fifthly, the dissection should continue along either the lateral or the medial border of the sartorius muscle to the proximal origin of the cutaneous artery, and a large and long vascular pedicle might be gotten for anastomosis. Sixthly, since there are 3-4 anterior femoral cutaneous nerves running through the superficial layer of the flap, attention should be given to the point where they perforate through the deep fascia. It would be preferable that an adjacent nerve be included to make the flap sensate.

20

Medial Thigh Flap

The medial thigh flap is based on the branches that emerge from the femoral artery and vein. It is located in the middle portion of the medial leg, and has such advantages as fine skin, thin subcutaneous fat and constant vessels. But it has such disadvantages as short pedicles and limited application. The flap could be transferred proximally to restore a wound on the perineum.

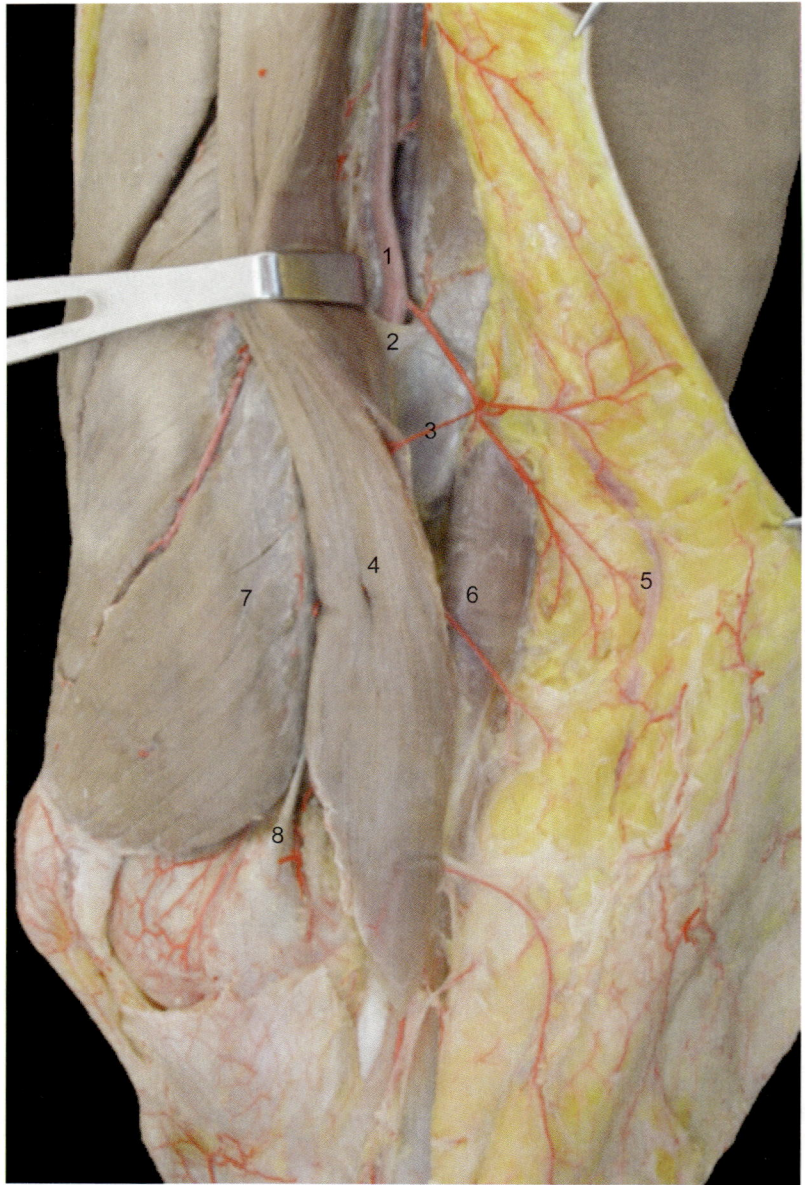

1. Femoral artery
2. Adductor canal
3. Muscular branch (sartorius muscle)
4. Sartorius muscle
5. Greater saphenous vein
6. Gracilis muscle
7. Medial vastus muscle
8. Adductor magnus muscle

Figure 1-111   **Applied anatomy**

The femoral artery gives a constant branch acont the proximal entrance of the adductor canal. The branch extends with the femoral artery for 1-2cm and then gives the muscular branches to nourish the sartorius muscle. The cutaneous trunk runs distally along the medial side of the femoral artery until it perforates through the fasciae latae at the medial border of the sartorius muscle to enter the medial thigh skin. It is 1-2 mm in diameter at its origin. There is the greater saphenous vein running through the flap.

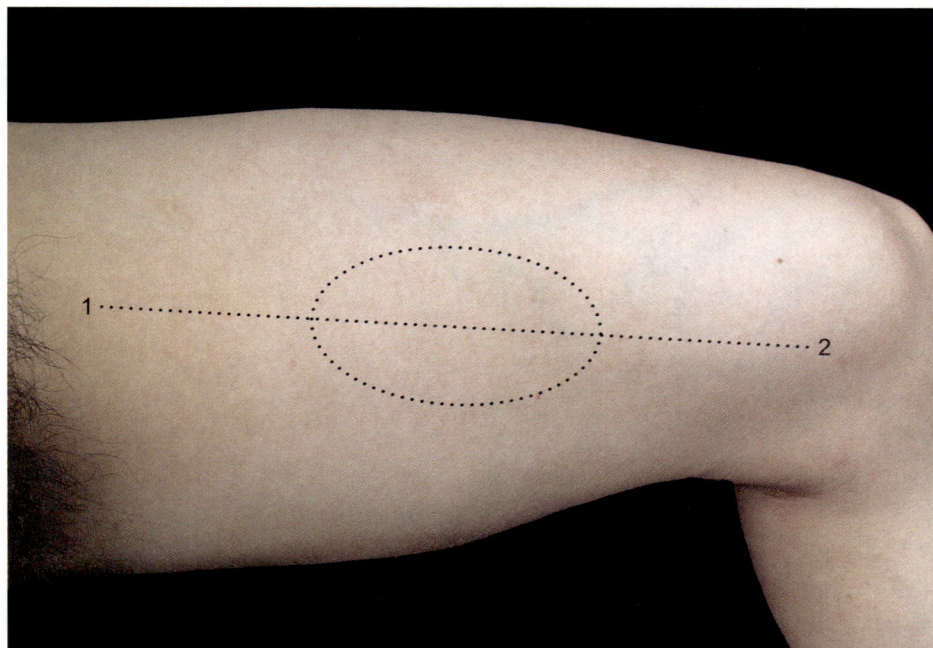

1. Inguinal ligament
2. Condylus medialis femoris

Figure 1-112   **Design of the flap**

The vascular pedicle of the flap is located at 2 cm lateral along a drawing line between the midpoint of the inguinal ligament and the condylus medialis femoris at the middle 1/3. The flap could be designed vertical, oblique or transverse. In practice, it should be adjusted to the cutaneous artery after it is identified intraoperatively.

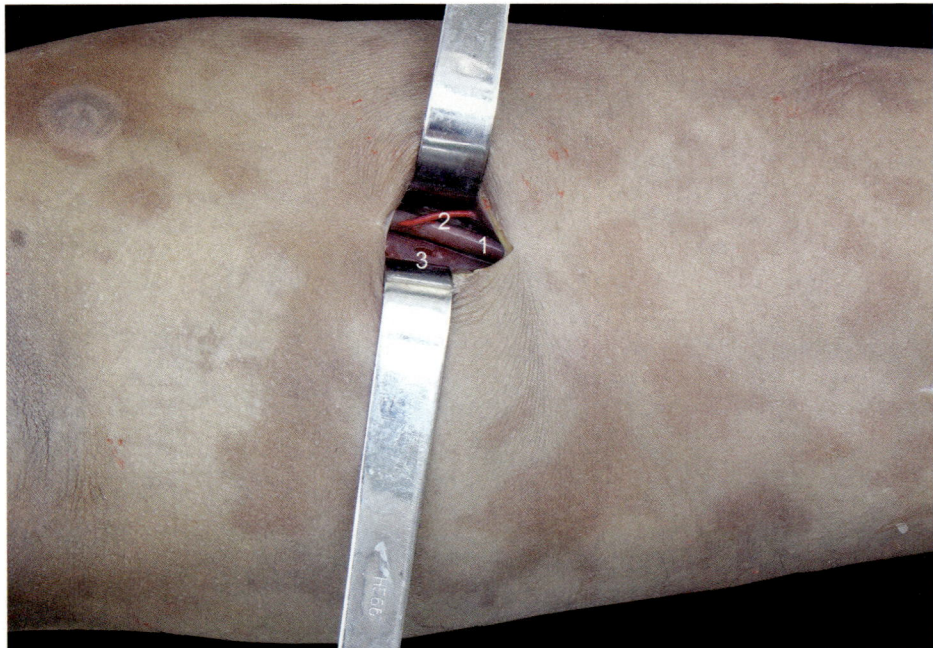

1. Femoral artery
2. Cutaneous artery
3. Medial vastus muscle

Figure 1-113   **Exposure of the vessels**

The pedicle incision should be made first and then the sartorius muscle drawn laterally to expose the femoral artery. The femoral sheath and the adductor canal should be opened to trace the main cutaneous artery of the femoral artery from proximal to the distal. After the cutaneous artery is identified, the design of the flap could be adjusted to its distributing direction.

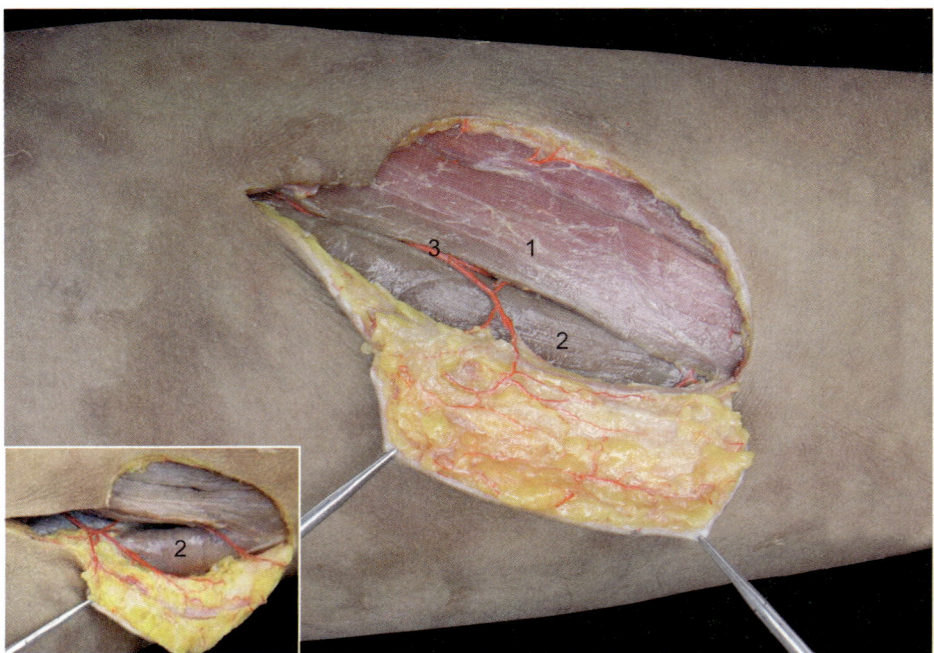

| **Figure 1-114** | **Dissection of the flap** |

The flap should be further incised from lateral to distal and dissected medially on the deep surface of the fasciae latae.

1. Sartorius muscle
2. Gracilis muscle
3. Cutaneous branch

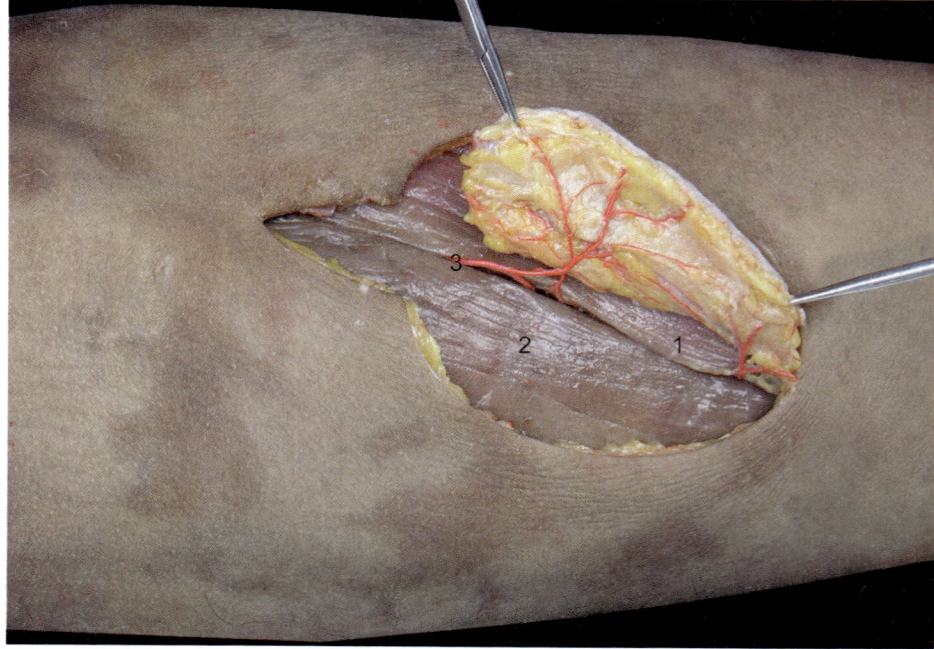

1. Sartorius muscle
2. Gracilis muscle
3. Cutaneous branch

| **Figure 1-115** | **Elevation of the flap** |

The flap should be incised at the medial border and elevated completely from distal to proximal.

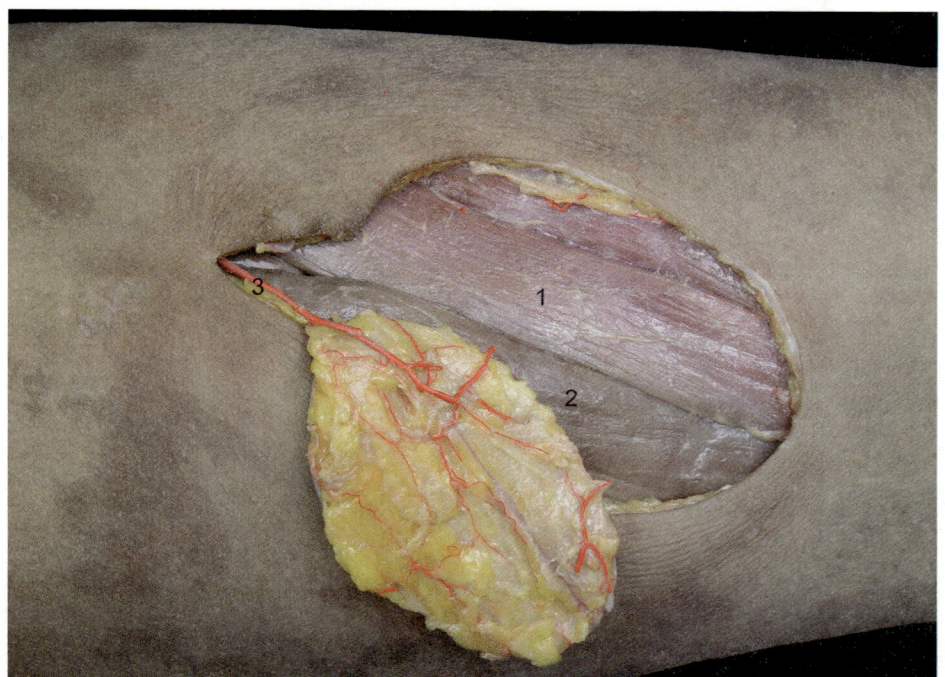

Figure 1-116   **Transposition of the flap**

The flap might be transferred proximally to repair a wound on the perineum.

1. Sartorius muscle
2. Gracilis muscle
3. Cutaneous branch

Key points in applied anatomy

Firstly, the surface position of the sartorius muscle should be confirmed preoperatively since the cutaneous vessels are closely attached to the medial and the lateral borders of the muscle. Secondly, the vascular detection should be confirmed preoperatively with the Doppler along the lateral and the medial border of the sartorius muscle. Thirdly, the flap could be designed with the medial and the lateral vascular pedicles of the sartorius muscle. Its pivot point might fall on the strongest signal point determined by the Doppler. Fourthly, the flap should be designed with 1/3 above the signal point and 2/3 below it. Fifthly, if the designed flap includes the lateral branch as a pedicle, an arch incision should be made first at 3-4cm medial to the signal point and then extend laterally to the sartorius muscle. The vascular pedicle should be located along the lateral border of the sartorius muscle. Sixthly, if the designed flap includes the medial branch as a pedicle, an arc incision should be made first at the lateral side of the sartorius muscle and then extend medially to the medial border of sartorius muscle. The vessels are dissected along the lateral or the medial sartorius muscle to its origin to get a large and long pedicle for easy anastomosis. Seventhly, since there are 3-4 anterior femoral cutaneous nerves running through the superficial layer of the flap, the point where they perforate through the deep fascia should be given great attention. It would be preferable that an adjacent nerve be included to make the flap sensate.

21

Posterior Lateral Thigh Flap

The flap is based on 1st perforating artery of the deep femoral artery. It can be transferred as a pedicle flap to the defects of the greater trochanter region by rotation or advancement.

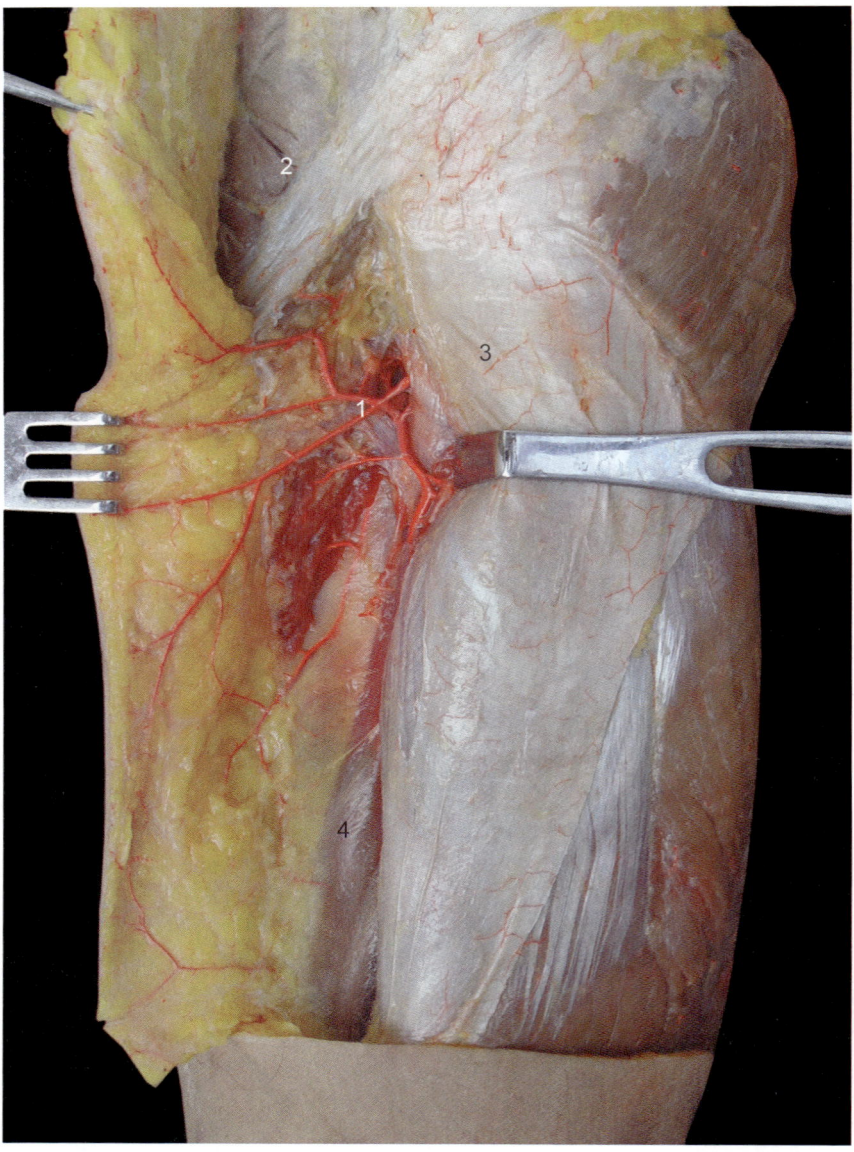

| Figure 1-117 | Applied anatomy |

The 1st perforating artery of the posterior thigh emerges from the deep femoral artery. It extends distally outwards to the lateral spatium intermusculare and enters the subcutaneous tissue under the terminal edge of the gluteus maximus muscle to nourish the skin of the middle 1/3 of the posterolateral thigh (20×10cm in size). The sensory nerve of the flap is the posterior femoral cutaneous nerve, which is situated at 2-2.5cm to the lateral spatium intermusculare.

1. 1st perforating artery
2. Gluteus maximus muscle
3. Vastus lateralis
4. Biceps femoris muscle

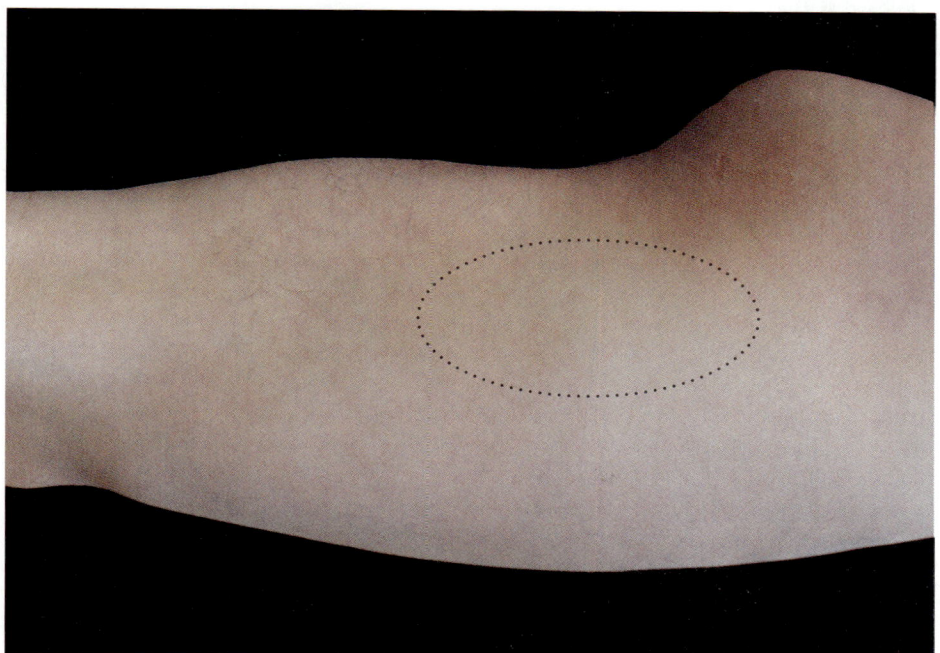

Figure 1-118 **Design of the flap**

The flap should be designed with its center falling on the point in the middle 1/3 portion of the posterolateral thigh where the 1st perforating artery passes through the deep fascia. This point should be confirmed with the Doppler. The size of the flap depends on the defect of the greater trochanter.

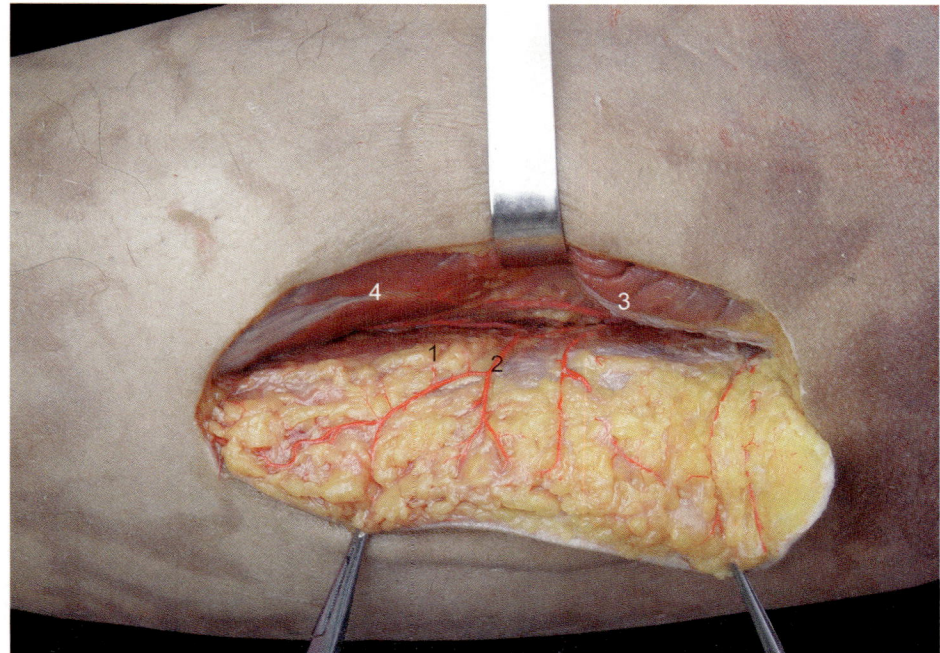

1. Lateral femoral spatium intermusculare
2. Cutaneous branch of 1st perforating artery
3. Gluteus maximus muscle
4. Biceps femoris muscle

Figure 1-119 **Dissection of the flap**

The incision of the flap should begin with its medial border down to the deep fascia. The dissection should extend to the lateral spatium intermusculare. The cutaneous branch that extends superficially to the deep fascia in the lateral spatium intermusculare should be identified and kept intact.

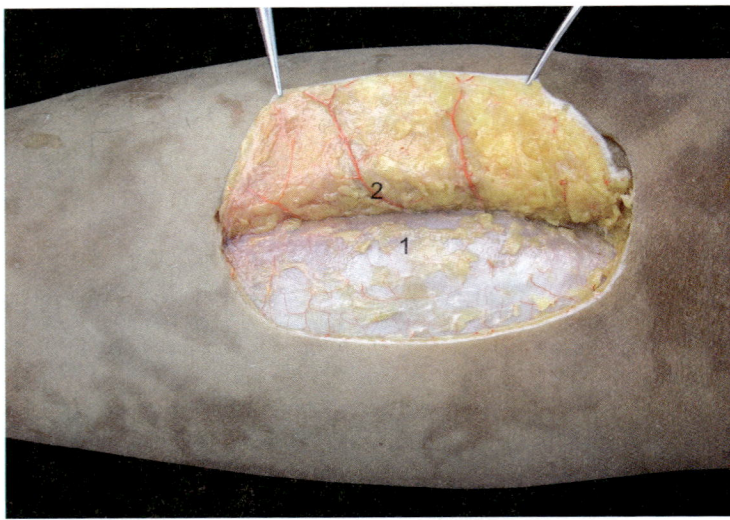

1. Vastus lateralis
2. Cutaneous branch of
   1st perforating artery

| **Figure 1-120** | **Elevation of the flap** |

With the artery identified, the incision of the flap should continue to the lateral spatium intermusculare to get it completely separated so that it could be transferred freely.

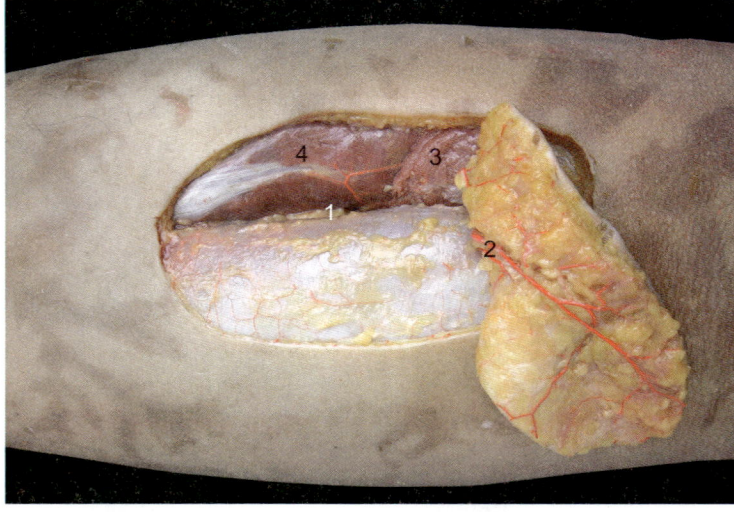

1. Lateral femoral spatium intermusculare
2. 1st perforating artery
3. Gluteus maximus muscle
4. Biceps femoris muscle

| **Figure 1-121** | **Transposition of the flap** |

The flap might be transferred proximally to the greater trochanter, either by rotation or by advancement.

Key points in applied anatomy

Firstly, the septum cutaneous branch of the 1st perforating artery could serve as the main pedicle of the flap. It perforates through the deep fascia at the inferior border of the gluteus maximus muscle to enter the subcutaneous tissue. The incision of the flap should begin vertically at 2 cm medial to the midline of the posterior gluteus maximus muscle. Secondly, the posterior femoral cutaneous nerve passes through the donor site, and so the flap might be a sensate one. Thirdly, the flap should be a fasciocutaneous one and its vascular pedicle could be found at the lateral spatium intermusculare of the thigh under the gluteus maximus. Fourthly, the intermuscular cutaneous artery should be dissected proximally in the septum to trace a longer and larger vascular pedicle for easy transplantation or anastomosis.

Lateral Superior Genicular Artery Compound Flap

22

The flap with a pedicle of lateral superior genicular artery might include parts of the distal femur (or its periosteum), the iliotibial tract and the skin to form a compound one. The lateral superior genicular artery composite flap might be transferred to restore a compound tissue defect on the hand, the distal forearm, the ankle or the dorsal finger. It has such advantages as a long vascular pedicle, a large vessel, constant anatomical cutaneous branches, and rich blood supply to the bone flap. There are loose connections and mobility between the overlying skin flap and the deep bone flap, the skin flap and the iliotibial tract flap. Therefore, a compound flap of the distal lateral thigh might be transferred freely to restore an irregular compound tissue defect due to the different mobility of the flap layers.

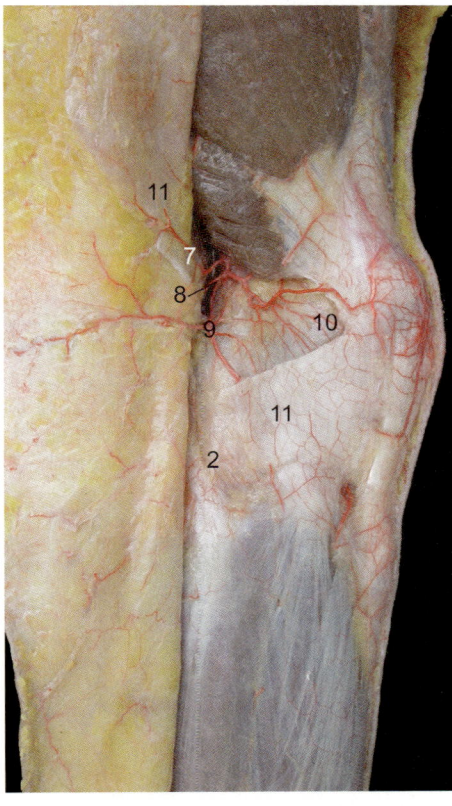
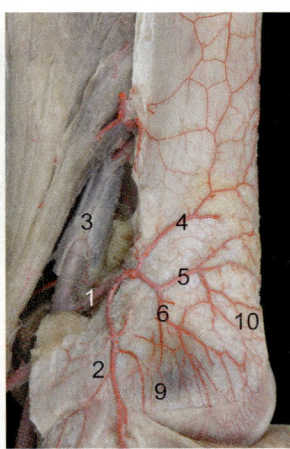

1. Lateral superior genicular artery
2. Lateral epicondyle
3. Popliteal artery
4. Superior periost branch
5. Middle periost branch
6. Inferior periost branch
7. Anterior cutaneous branch
8. Posterior cutaneous branch
9. Distal cutaneous branch
10. Anastomotic branch
11. Iliotibial tract

Figure 1-122	Applied anatomy

The lateral superior genicular artery emerges from the popliteal artery at 2.8cm above the lateral epicondyle of the femur. It extends horizontally outwards along the posterior femur to perforate through the lateral spatium intermusculare. Here it attaches closely to the periosteum and gives three periosteal branches (the superior, the middle and the inferior branches), and three cutaneous branches (the anterior, the posterior and the distal branches). The periosteal branches send many tiny branches to fan out over the lateroanterior segment of the distal femur and anastomose with other periosteal branches that come from the lateral superior genicular artery and the descending genicular artery to form a dense anastomotic net. The net can nourish the bone flap about 8.6×5.4 cm. The anterior cutaneous branch extends anteriorly outwards, and perforates through the iliotibial tract to enter the lateral distal femoral skin. The posterior branch extends laterally from the posterior lateral spatium intermusculare to enter the inferior segment of the lateral posterior femur. The distal branch, upon emerging from the lateral superior genicular artery, extends distally from the posterior lateral spatium intermusculare to enter the lateral inferior femoral skin via the iliotibial tract. Along the course, it gives communicating branches to anastomose with the surrounding articular vascular net. At the same time, the vascular net nourishes the iliotibial tract. The skin flap might account for 17.5×11.0 cm in size. The initiation of the lateral superior genicular artery is 2.1mm in diameter and the trunk is 2.5 cm in length.

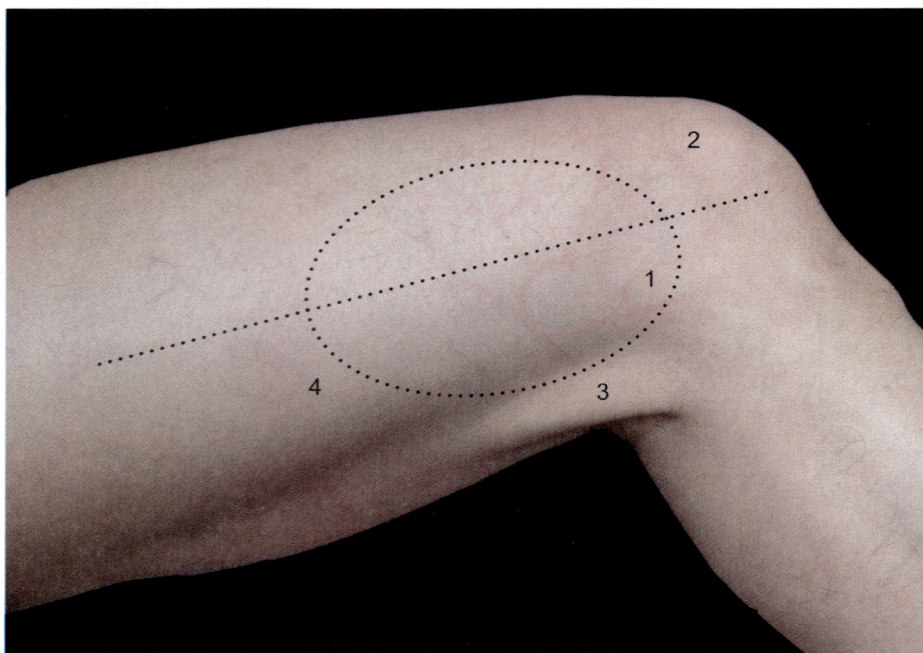

1. Lateral epicondyle of
   femur
2. Patella
3. Biceps femoris muscle
4. Vastus lateralis

Figure 1-123   **Design of the flap**

With the knee in flexion, the flap should be designed with its axial line falling on the lateral midline of the leg. The point at which the cutaneous branch enters the skin should be located at 4cm to the lateral epicondyle of the femur. The anterior border of the flap should fall along the vertical line of the lateral patella, its posterior border along the posterior margin of the biceps femoris muscle, and its inferior margin being the horizontal line from the superior patella. The size of the flap should be adjusted to that of the recipient.

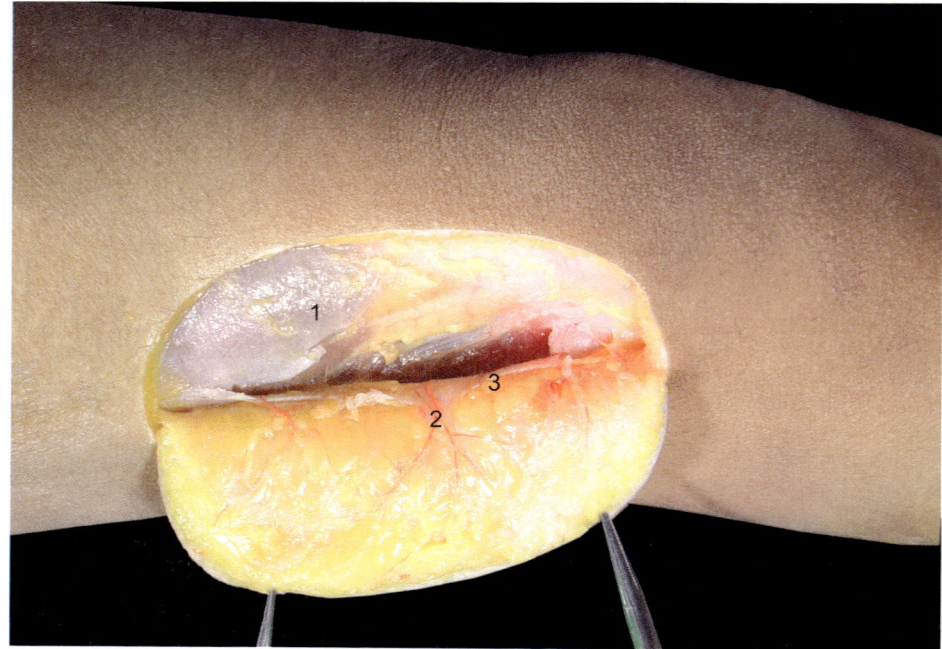

1. Vastus lateralis
2. Anterior cutaneous branch
   of lateral superior
   genicular artery
3. Iliotibial tract

Figure 1-124   **Dissection of the flap**

The flap should first be incised at its anterior border, dissected bluntly from under the deep fascia and raised over the surface of the vastus lateralis to expose the anterior cutaneous branch that enters the skin.

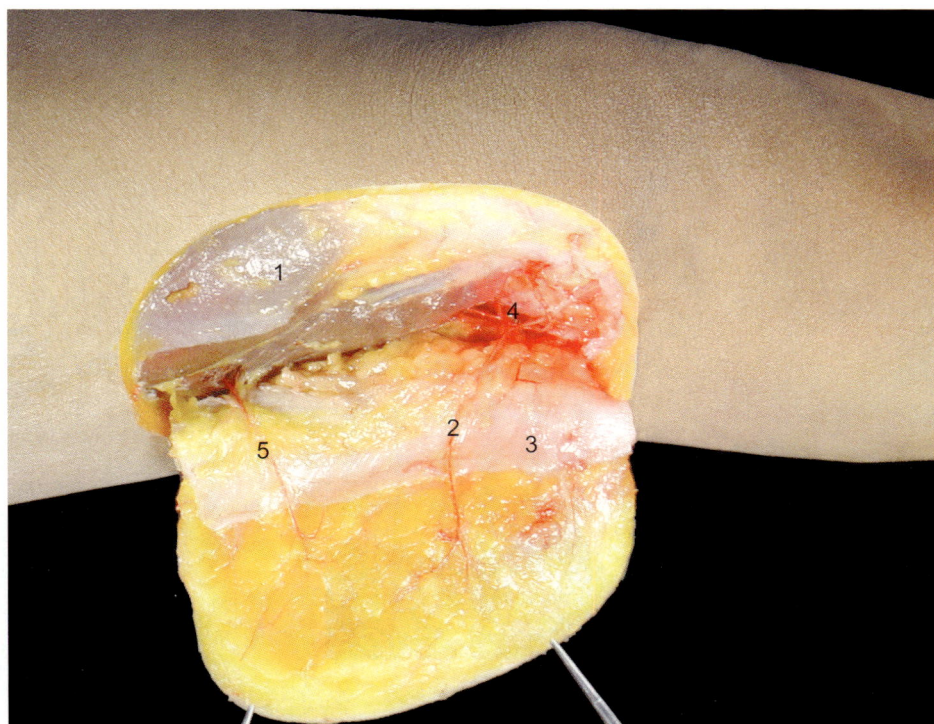

1. Vastus lateralis
2. Anterior cutaneous branch of lateral superior genicular artery
3. Iliotibial tract
4. Lateral superior genicular artery
5. Cutaneous branch of 3ʳᵈ artery

Figure 1-125   **Exposure of the vessel**

The dissection should continue along the anterior branch to the spatium intermusculare, and trace to the trunk of the lateral superior genicular artery. The muscular branches to the vastus lateralis should be ligated.

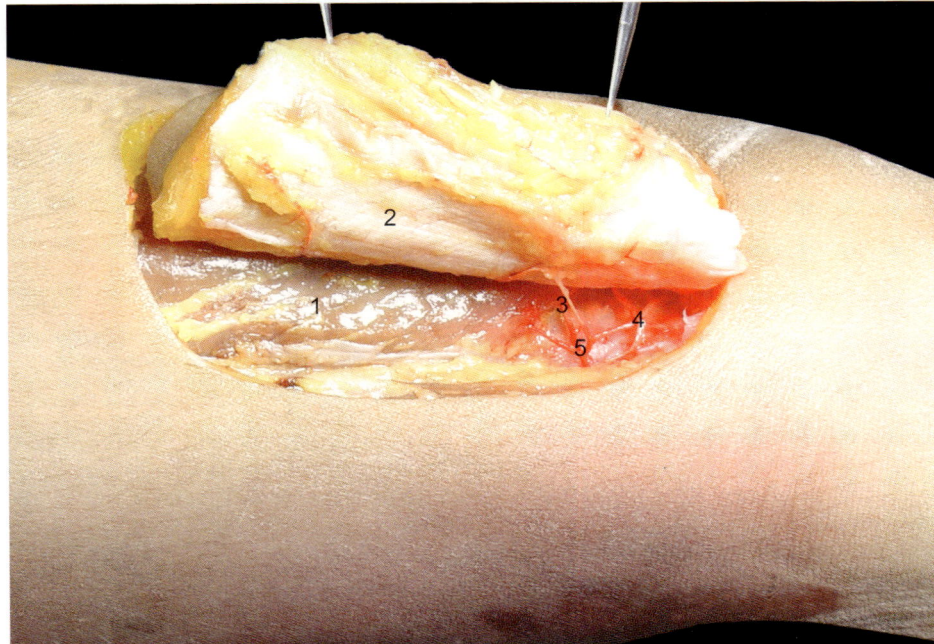

1. Vastus lateralis
2. Iliotibial tract
3. Posterior cutaneous branch of lateral superior genicular artery
4. Distal cutaneous branch of lateral superior genicular artery
5. Periost branch

Figure 1-126   **Elevation of the flap**

The posterior border of the flap should be incised and separated forward from under the deep fascia to the lateral spatium intermusculare to expose the posterior cutaneous branch and then the distal branch. The attachment of the lateral spatium intermusculare to the femur should then be cut and separated to expose the superior, the middle and the inferior periosteal branches.

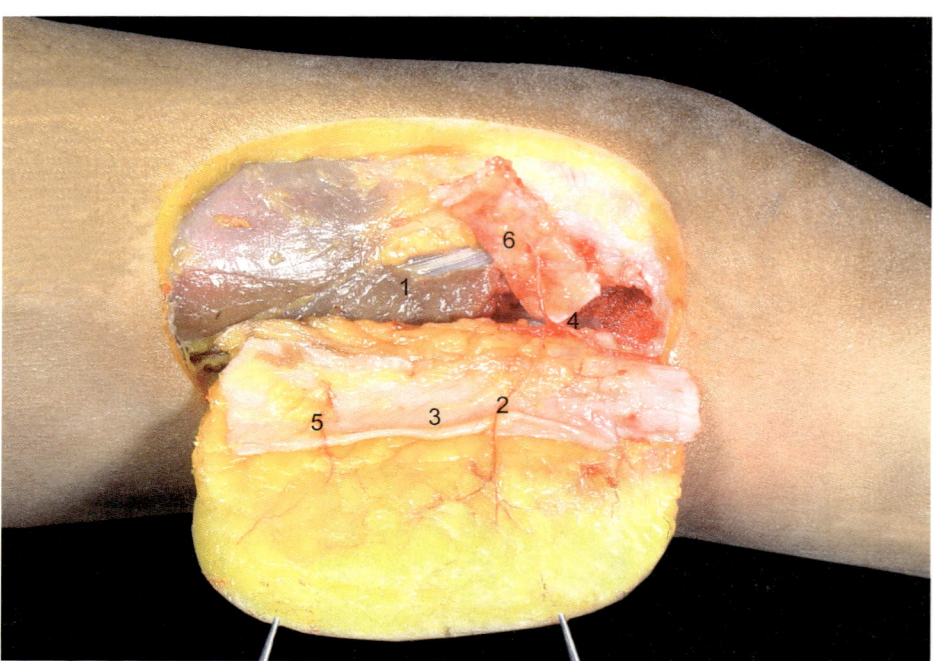

| **Figure 1-127** | **Harvest of the bone flap** |

The bone flap should be harvested along the two lines of the pre-drilled holes with an osteotome or an electric oscillating saw. If a free flap is needed, it is sufficient to include only the anterior cutaneous branch in the flap. If a retrograde flap is needed, it is necessary to include either the distal cutaneous branch or the periosteal branch of the inferior branch in the flap. The flap, with one or two vascular branches, might be transferred to the anterior or the inferior genicular region.

1. Vastus lateralis
2. Anterior cutaneous branch of lateral superior genicular artery
3. Iliotibial tract
4. Lateral superior genicular artery
5. Cutaneous branch of 3rd perforating artery
6. Bone flap

Key points in applied anatomy

Firstly, the anterior border of the flap should be incised down to the deep fascia. The skin and the deep fascia should be sutured together to avoid disconnection of the two. Secondly, the inferior border of the flap should be limited within the horizontal line of the superior patella to avoid motion sequelae of the knee. Thirdly, with the patient in lateral position, the flap should be incised initially from its posterior border, and raised anteriorly to the lateral spatium intermusculare to expose the lateral superior genicular artery. With knee flexion, the biceps femoris muscle should be retracted posteriorly to expose the deep origin of the lateral superior genicular artery. Fourthly, it is preferable to separate the vascular pedicle first, and then harvest the bone flap. Fifthly, in an anterior cruciate ligament reconstruction with a strip of the iliotibial tract band, it would be preferable to include the anterior and the distal cutaneous branches to guarantee a good blood supply for the iliotibial tract. If the anterior branch of the lateral superior genicular artery makes the retrograde rotation of the flap impossible, its vascular pedicle should be traced up to the vastus lateralis to get a longer pedicle. Sixthly, in some cases, vascular variations, such as the supreme genual artery or the 3rd perforating artery, are dominant, and so a composite flap could also be harvested with either of the two vessels as its pedicle.

Inferior Gluteal Posterior Thigh Flap

23

The inferior gluteal posterior thigh flap is, in fact, a neuro-fasciocutaneous one based on the accompanying vessels of the posterior femoral cutaneous nerve. Its axial artery is the cutaneous branch of inferior gluteal artery. It might be transferred posteriorly outwards to repair a pressure sore on the greater trochanter or medially to repair the perineal region.

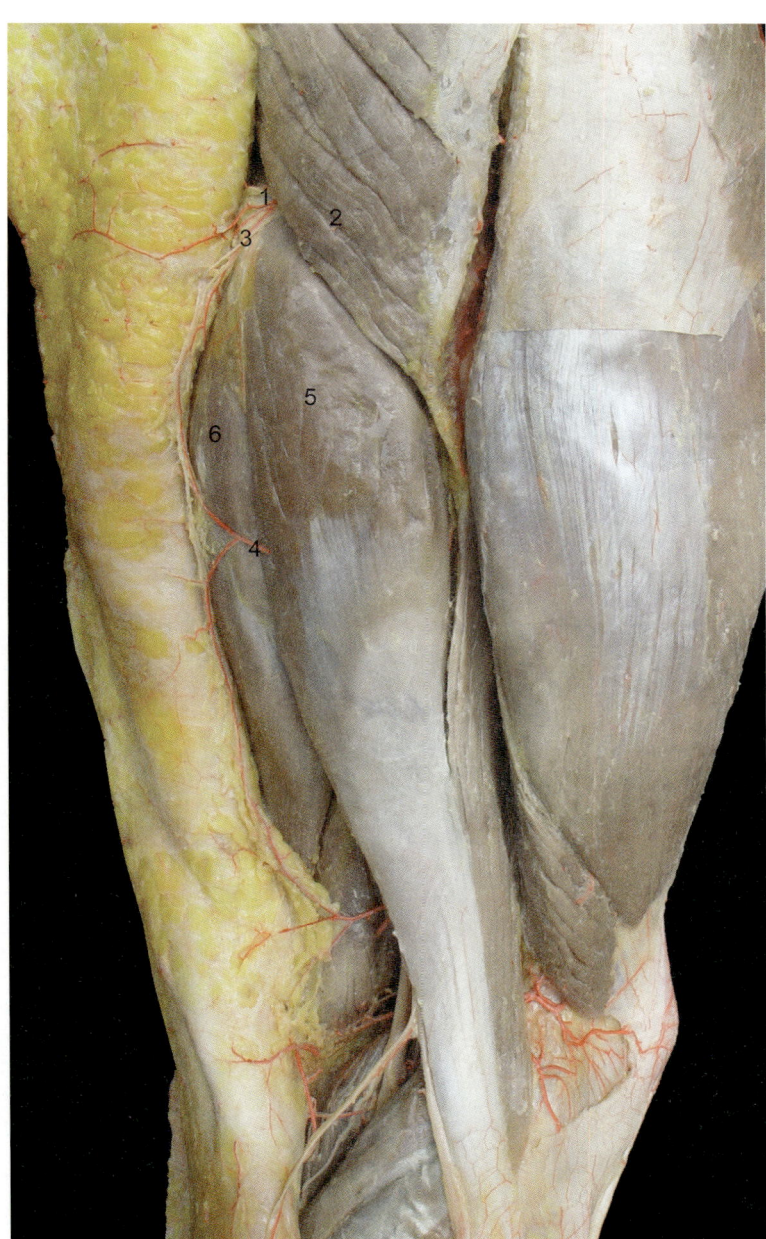

1. Cutaneous branch of inferior gluteal artery
2. Gluteus maximus muscle
3. Posterior femoral cutaneous nerve
4. Cutaneous branch of perforating artery
5. Biceps femoris muscle
6. Semitendinous muscle

Figure 1-128	Applied anatomy

The cutaneous branch of the inferior gluteal artery is the axis of the inferior gluteal posterior thigh flap. It extends through the spatium under the gluteus maximus muscle and sends cutaneous branches, usually 1-4 branches, to accompany the posterior femoral cutaneous nerve over the posterior leg. These cutaneous arteries are about 0.4-0.8 mm in diameter, and generally have 2 accompanying veins in the same diameter.

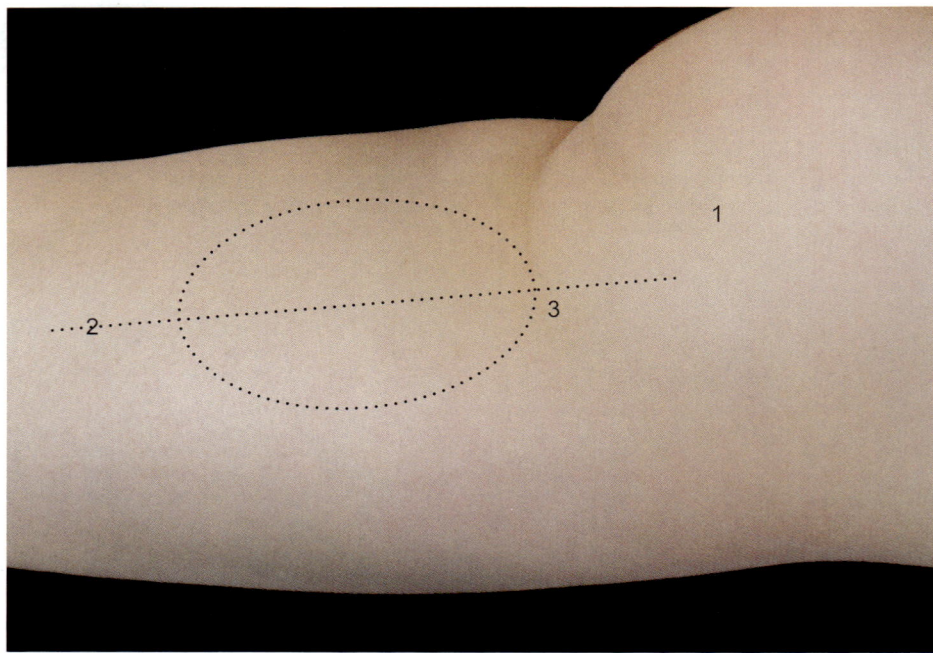

1. Gluteus maximus muscle
2. Posterior median line of upper leg
3. Pivot point of flap

Figure 1-129   Design of the flap

The flap should be designed on the posterior upper thigh with its bilateral borders extending to 5cm from the posterior midline, its distal border extending to 10cm above the popliteal fossa and its pivot point located at the inferior margin of the gluteus maximus muscle.

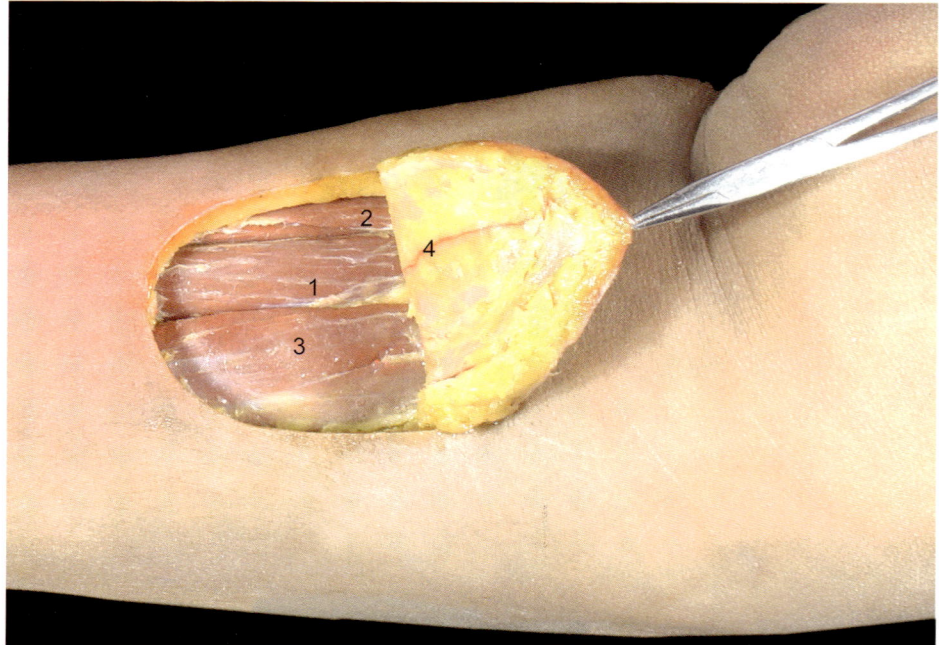

1. Semitendinous muscle
2. Semimembranous muscle
3. Biceps femoris muscle
4. Cutaneous branch of inferior gluteal artery

Figure 1-130   Dissection of the flap

The flap should be incised at its distal border and dissected from distal to proximal under the deep fascia. Along the course, the small branches that perforate through the posterior femoral muscular septum should be ligated. Care should be taken to preserve the proximal cutaneous vessels that enter the flap.

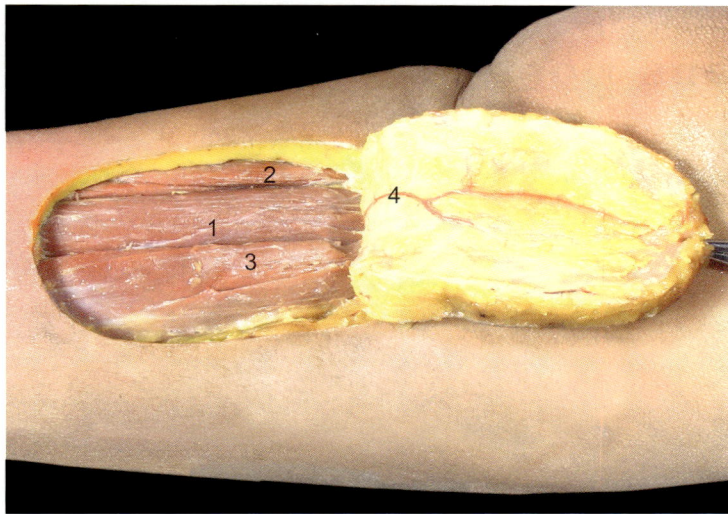

1. Semitendinous muscle
2. Semimembranous muscle
3. Biceps femoris muscle
4. Cutaneous branch of inferior gluteal artery

Figure 1-131   Elevation of the flap

The dissection of the flap should continue to the inferior border of the gluteus maximus muscle to expose the posterior thigh cutaneous branch of the inferior gluteal artery, which should be given great attention to avoid damages. Then, an island flap should be separated with a pedicle of the cutaneous branch of the inferior gluteal artery.

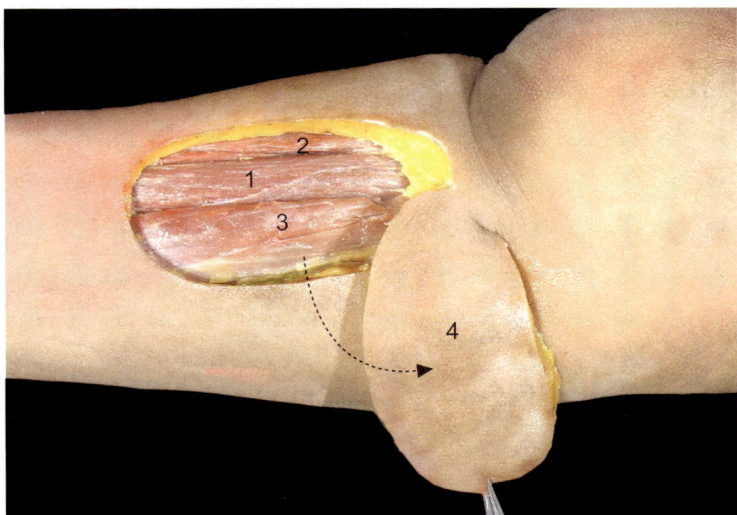

1. Semitendinous muscle
2. Semimembranous muscle
3. Biceps femoris muscle
4. Flap

Figure 1-132   Transposition of the flap

The island flap might be transferred laterally to restore a pressure sore on the greater trochanter.

Key points in applied anatomy

The flap might have a size with its superior margin at the inferior 1/3 of the buttock, and its inferior margin at the proximal 2/3 of the posterior thigh. Secondly, the inferior edge of the gluteus maximus muscle should be elevated at the intermuscular septum to expose the inferior gluteal artery and the posterior femoral cutaneous nerve that enter the subcutaneous tissue. Thirdly, since the inferior gluteus maximus muscle extends obliquely from mediosuperior to lateroinferior, the gluteal skin crease should not be mistaken for the inferior edge of the gluteus maximus muscle. Actually, they are not in the same layer. Fourthly, as the cutaneous artery is small in diameter, it would be preferable to trace the artery superiorly to the trunk of the inferior gluteal artery to obtain a longer and larger vessel (1.2-1.5 mm in diameter).

24

Popliteus-posterior Thigh Flap

The popliteus-posterior thigh flap is a fasciocutaneous flap that obtains its nutrition from the direct popliteal cutaneous artery of the popliteal artery. The flap should be raised with a distal pedicle and transferred to restore a skin and soft tissue defect on the medial or lateral knee or to relieve the scar contracture of the popliteal fossa.

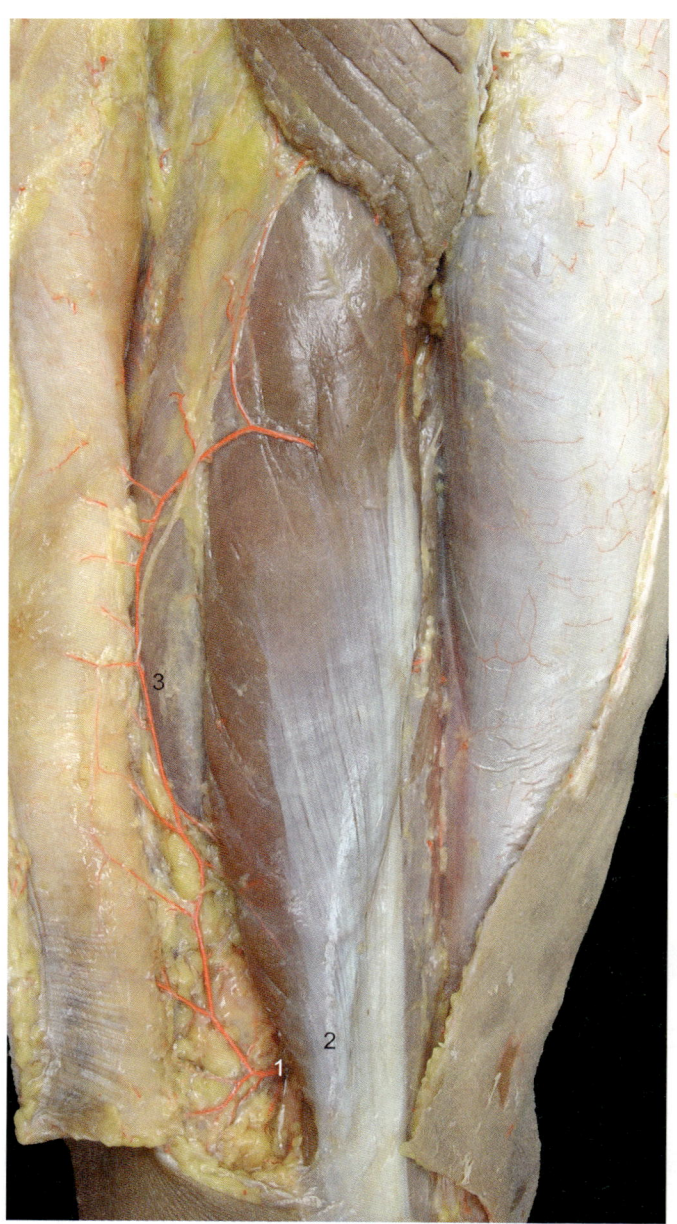

1. Direct popliteal cutaneous artery
2. Biceps femoris muscle
3. Semitendinous muscle

Figure 1-133	**Applied anatomy**

The superior popliteal artery gives a constant direct popliteal cutaneous artery at 7-11 cm above the joint level. The direct cutaneous artery extends superficially in the spatium intermusculare between the biceps muscle and the semitendinous muscle. It is 2.0 (1.5-2.5) mm in diameter and 8 (6-12) cm in length. It extends over the middle-inferior segment of the thigh, and anastomoses with the communicating branches of the vessels that accompany the posterior femoral cutaneous nerve. There are the concomitant veins, the posterior femoral cutaneous nerve running through the donor site.

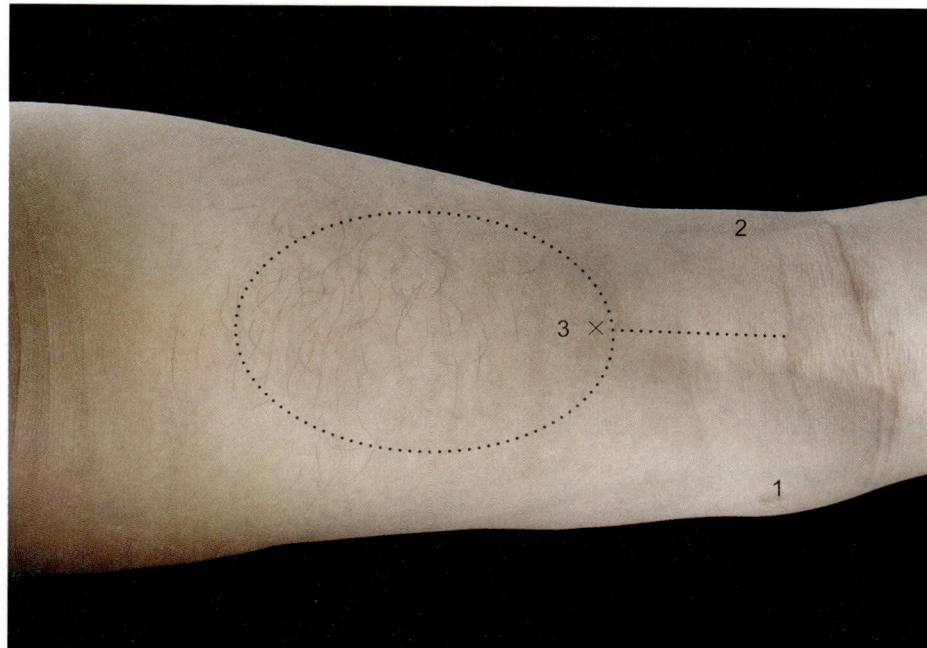

1. Semitendinous muscle
2. Biceps femoris muscle
3. Cutaneous branch of
   3rd perforating artery

Figure 1-134   **Design of the flap**

The flap should be designed with its pivot point located at 10cm above the connecting line between the internal and the external epicondyles of the posterior femur. This is the point where the 3rd perforating artery passes through the deep fascia. It should be confirmed with the Doppler.

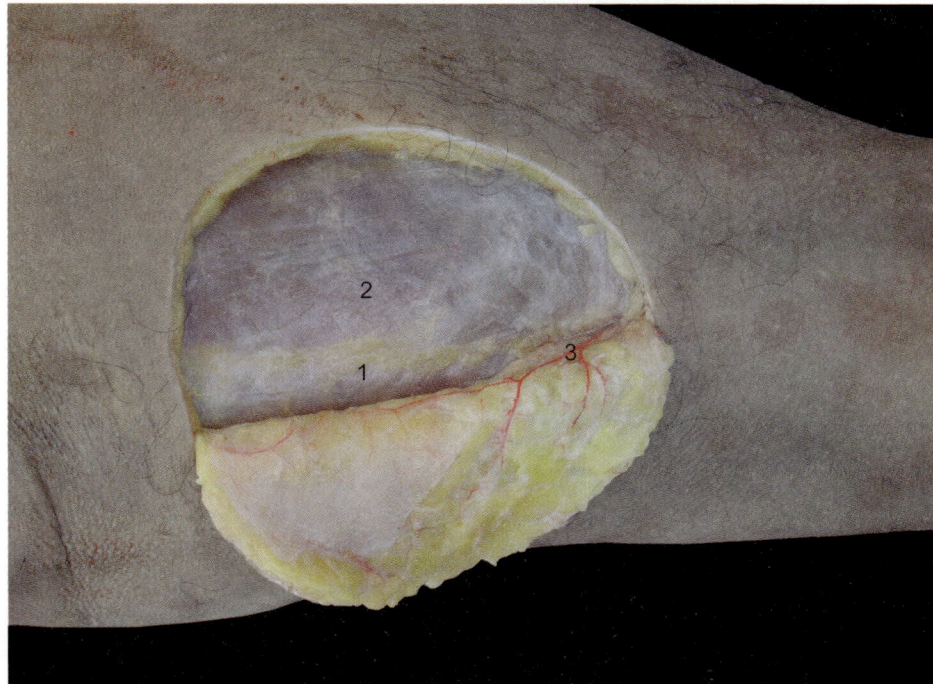

1. Semitendinous muscle
2. Biceps femoris muscle
3. Cutaneous branch of
   3rd perforating artery

Figure 1-135   **Dissection of the flap**

The flap should be incised down to the deep fascia from medial or lateral, and elevated from under the deep fascia to make it a fasciocutaneous one. The dissection should continue until it reaches the spetum intermusculare among the semitendinous muscle, the semimembranous muscle and the biceps muscle to ensure that the cutaneous artery has been included in the flap.

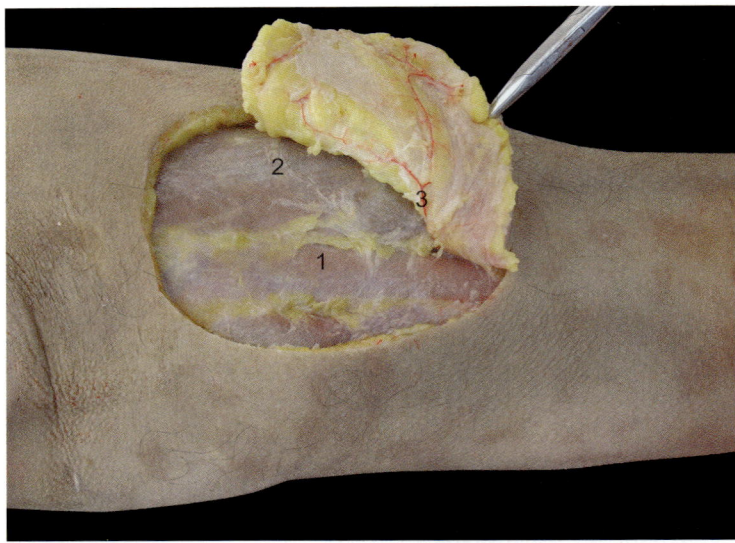

1. Semitendinous muscle
2. Biceps femoris muscle
3. Cutaneous branch from 3rd perforating artery

Figure 1-136   Elevation of the flap

The dissection of the flap should continue and the small branches of the arteries on its superior part ligated to make it an island based on a pedicle of the cutaneous branch from the 3rd perforating artery.

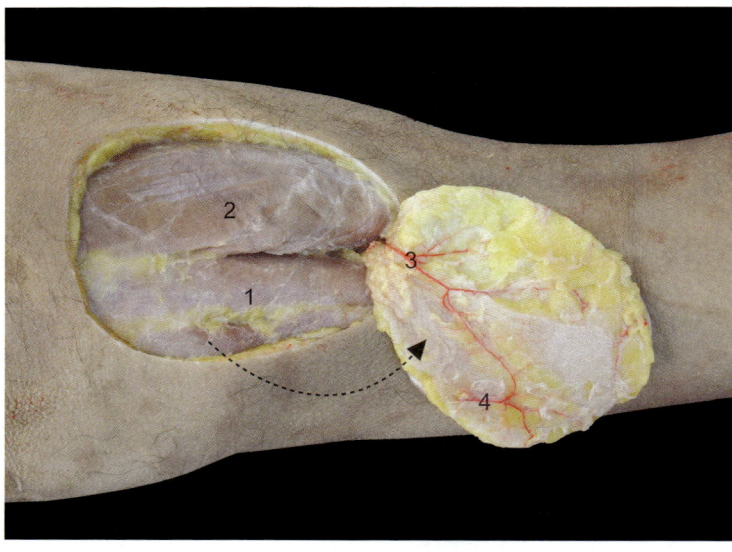

1. Semitendinous muscle
2. Biceps femoris muscle
3. Cutaneous branch from 3rd perforating artery
4. Cutaneous branch from 2nd perforating artery

Figure 1-137   Transposition of the flap

The flap might be transferred distally by rotation to repair a wound in the popliteal fossa.

Key points in applied anatomy

Firstly, the flap should be designed along the posterior midline of the thigh to make it a fasciocutaneous one. Its pivot point should be located at 10 cm above the knee joint level. Its superior margin extends to the gluteal skin transverse crease and its inferior to the popliteal transverse crease. Secondly, the vascular pedicle should not get twisted while the flap is being rotated. The pedicle should be longer enough to guarantee a smooth transposition. If necessary, the loose fat tissue of the popliteal fossa should be dissected to get a longer pedicle. Thirdly, the donor region is relatively hidden, and it might be directly sutured under the condition that it is less than 10 cm wide.

Medial Genicular Flap

25

The flap should be located in the medial side of the knee. The medial genicular flap might obtain its supplies from the saphenous branch of the descending genicular artery. The type of the flap has such advantages as fine soft skin, long vascular pedicle, large size, concealed donor region and good sensory innervation. It might be transferred locally to restore a tissue defect around the popliteal fossa or the knee. It might also be transferred crossover to repair a wound on the opposite lower leg or on the foot.

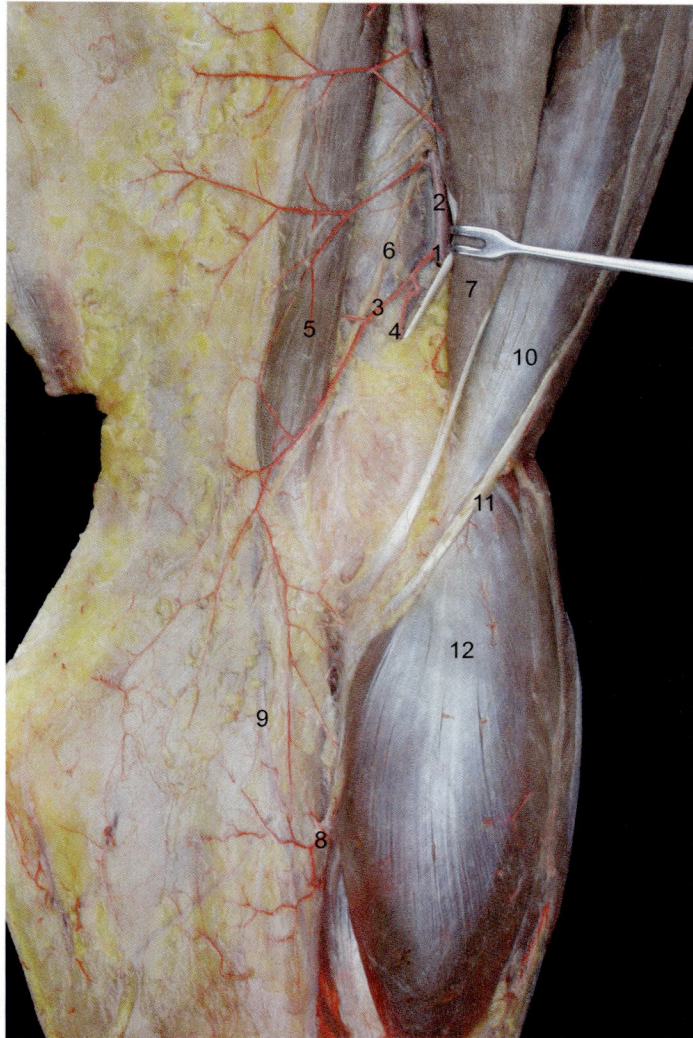

1. Descending branch of genicular artery
2. Femoral artery
3. Saphenous branch
4. Articular branch
5. Sartorius muscle
6. Saphenous nerve
7. Gracilis muscle
8. Intermuscular branches of posterior tibial artery
9. Greater saphenous vein
10. Semimembranous muscle
11. Semitendinous muscle
12. Gastrocnemius muscle

Figure 1-138	Applied anatomy

The descending branch of the genicular artery emerges from the femoral artery above the hiatus of the abductor magnus muscle. It then bifurcates into a cutaneous branch called the saphenous branch and a genicular articular branch. The saphenous branch perforates through the tendon abductor muscle in the deep layer of the sartorius muscle at the middle-inferior segment of the leg and extends distally with the saphenous nerve for about 10cm in the septum between the gracilis muscle and the sartorius muscle. It then courses superficially to the subcutaneous tissue to fan out over the medial skin of the knee and the proximal lower leg. Along the course, it anastomoses with the medial inferior genicular artery and the intermuscular branches of the posterior tibial artery. The saphenous artery has its accompanying nerve above and the saphenous nerve beneath the knee. The venous blood returns of the flap depend on the saphenous vein and the greater saphenous vein.

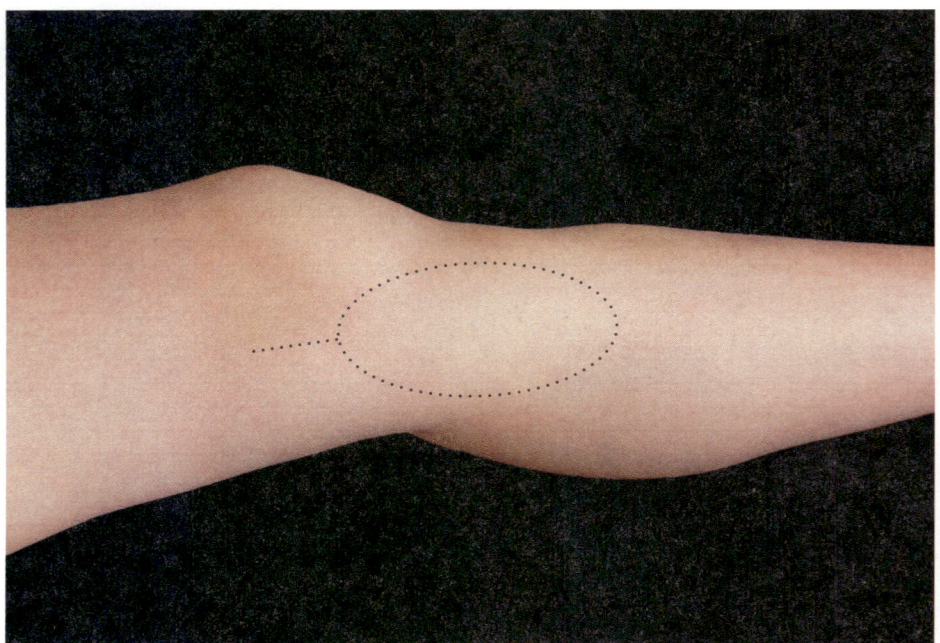

| **Figure 1-139** | **Design of the flap** |

The flap should be designed along the medial lower limb, ranging from 10cm above and 20cm beneath the genicular joint line.

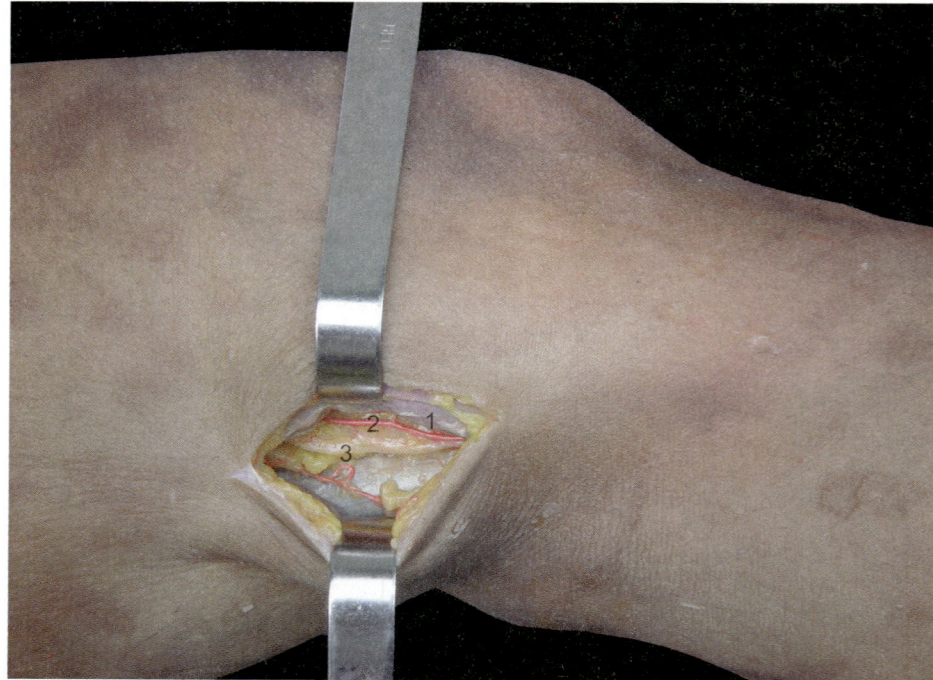

1. Sartorius muscle
2. Descending genicular artery
3. Saphenous nerve

| **Figure 1-140** | **Exposure of the flap** |

The proximal border of the flap should be incised to expose the adductor canal and the femoral artery at the lateral aspect of the sartorius muscle. The adductor canal should then be opened, and the sartorius muscle pulled laterally to expose the descending genicular artery, its concomitant vein and the saphenous nerve.

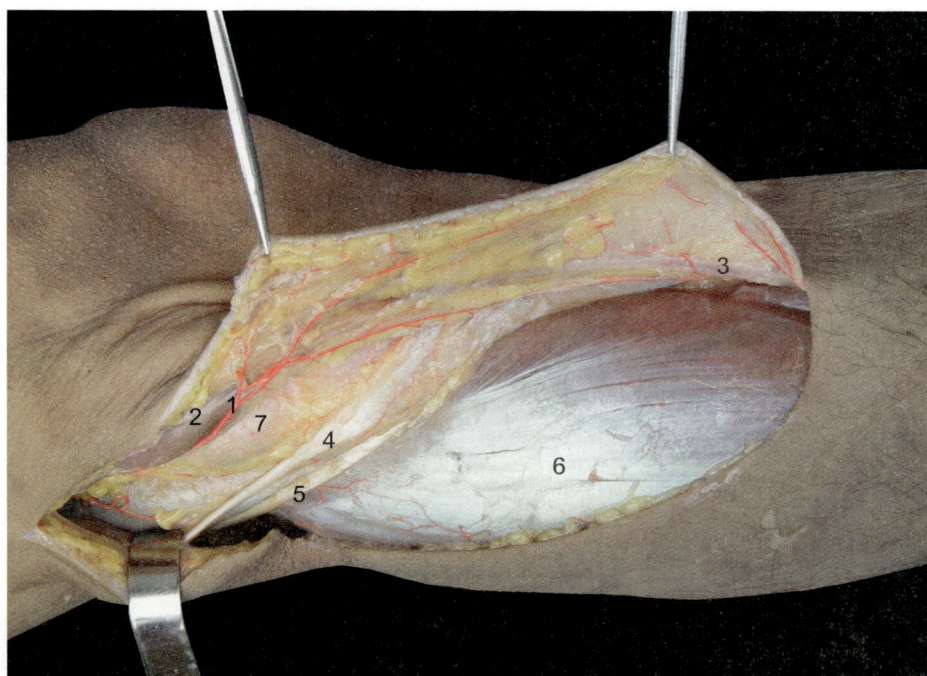

1. Neurovascular plexus
2. Sartorius muscle
3. Greater saphenous vein
4. Gracilis muscle
5. Semitendinosus muscle
6. Medial head of
   gastrocnemius muscle
7. Medial epicondyle

Figure 1-141   Dissection of the flap

The flap should be incised along its posterior border and elevated anteriorly under the deep fascia. The dissection should continue distally along the neurovascular bundle. If necessary, the sartorius muscle should be separated to keep the vessel intact. The saphenous artery and the saphenous vein should be ligated and cut at the distal end of the flap to search for the greater saphenous vein in the subcutaneous region and get it ligated at the distal end of the flap.

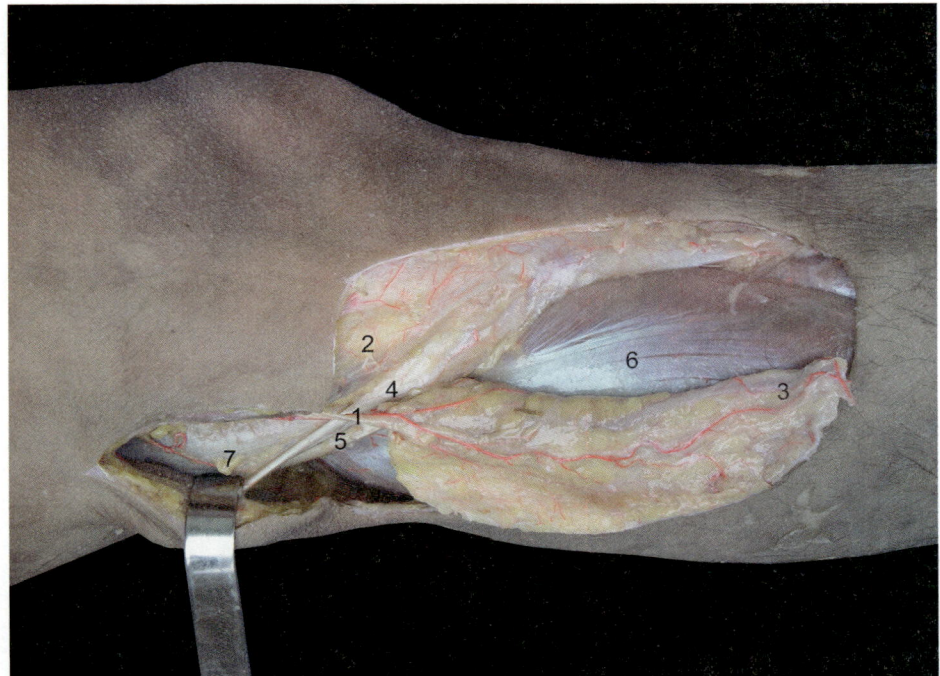

1. Neurovascular plexus
2. Sartorius muscle
3. Greater saphenous vein
4. Gracilis muscle
5. Semitendinosus muscle
6. Medial head of
   gastrocnemius muscle
7. Medial epicondyle

Figure 1-142   Elevation of the flap

As is designed, the flap should be incised at its distal-anterior borders, and elevated completely to make it an island, with a pedicle of the proximal saphenous neurovascular bundle.

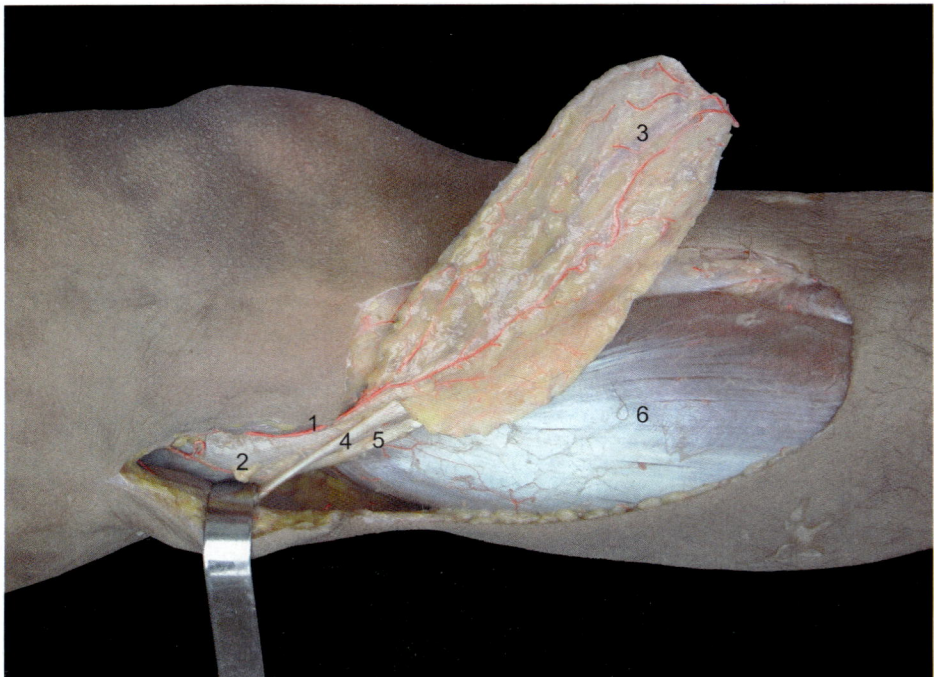

Figure 1-143   **Transposition of the flap**

The island flap might be transferred proximally to repair a wound on the recipient region.

1. Neurovascular plexus
2. Sartorius muscle
3. Greater saphenous vein
4. Gracilis muscle
5. Semitendinosus muscle
6. Medial head of gastrocnemius muscle

Key points in applied anatomy

Firstly, the conditions of the vessels should be confirmed preoperatively with the Doppler. The courses of the descending genicular artery and its saphenous branch should be marked to indicate the range of the flap. Secondly, a longitudinal incision (about 10 cm long) should be made proximally on the anterior medial knee. Here, the greater saphenous vein in the superficial subcutaneous tissue should be given great attention to avoid getting it damaged. Thirdly, the flap should be raised under the deep fascia, and some sutures should be put to avoid disconnection of the skin and the deep fascia. Fourthly, when the neurovascular pedicle is being dissected, the medial femoral cutaneous nerves should be protected from damages. Fifthly, the vessels should be traced backwards to their origins to obtain a large pedicle and guarantee an easy anastomosis. The genicular articular branches from the descending genicular artery should be ligated carefully. Sixthly, if the flap donor is situated in the medial aspect of the genicular joint, a split-skin graft is preferred to cover the defect to avoid genicular dysfunction.

Medial Inferior Genicular Flap

26

The medial inferior geniculate flap is based on the medial inferior genicular artery of the medial superior lower leg. The flap has such advantages as a concealed position, soft skin and a constant sensory nerve. It might be transferred anterogradely to the knee, or retrogradely to the middle-lower leg. It might also be designed as a compound one with a piece of bone.

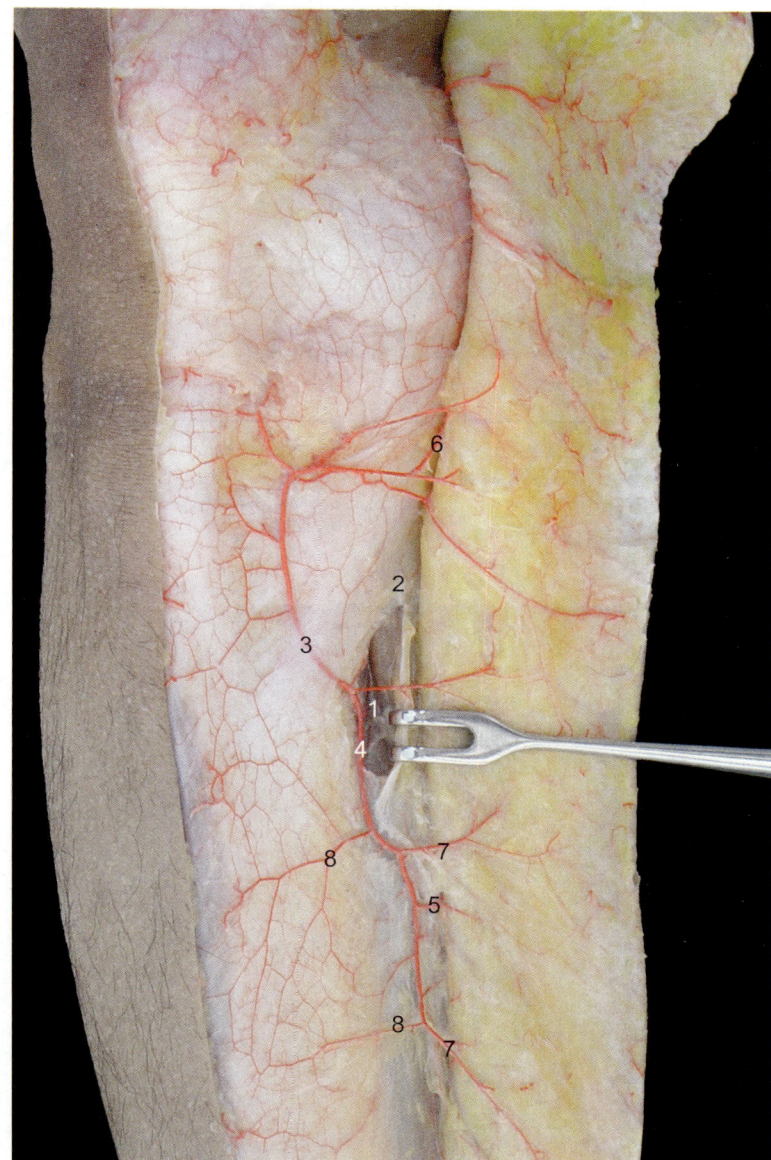

1. Medial inferior genicular artery
2. Popliteal muscle
3. Articular branch
4. Periost-fasciae-cutaneous branches
5. Intermuscular artery
6. Saphenous artery
7. Cutaneous branch
8. Periost branch

Figure 1-144   **Applied anatomy**

The medial inferior genicular artery emerges constantly from the popliteal artery and extends anteriorly between the medial tibial border and the popliteal muscle. It then bifurcates into the articular branch and the periost-fasciae-cutaneous branch at the medial antero-inferior popliteal aspect. The periost-fasciae-cutaneous branch extends along the popliteal muscle until it reaches the tibial insertion. It then descends vertically to anastomose with the intermuscular perforator of the posterior tibial artery, and sends ascending branches to anastomose with the saphenous artery and distribute over the proximal skin and the periosteum of the medial lower leg.

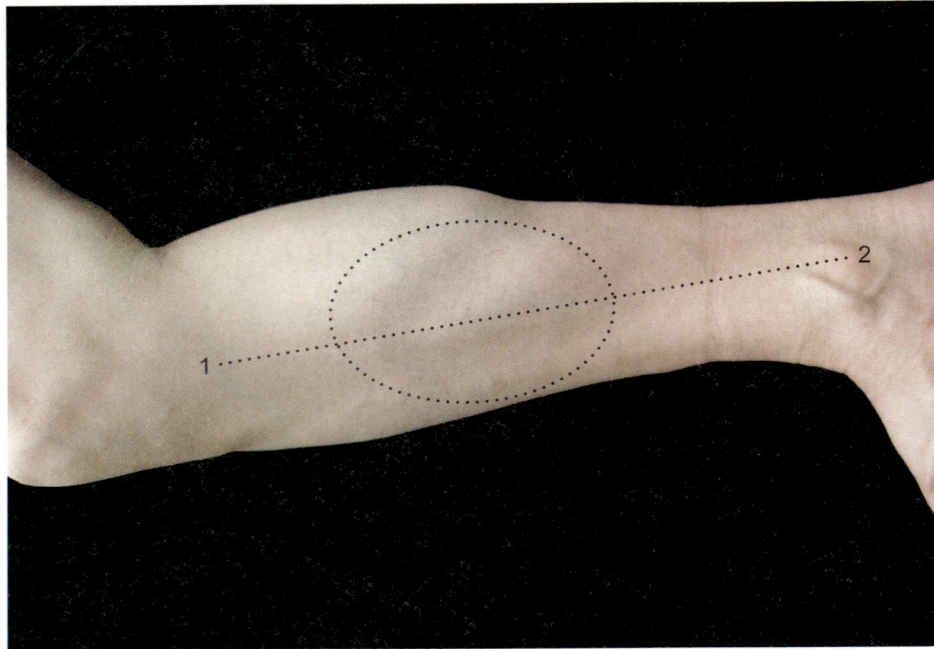

1. Medial condyle of tibia
2. Medial malleolus

Figure 1-145   Design of the flap

The flap should be designed with its vertical axis falling on the connecting line between the medial condyle of the tibia and the medial malleolus. It could be drawn on the medial lower leg, with its superior border to the medial condyle of tibia, its inferior to 10 cm below the tibial tuberosity, its anterior to the spine of the tibia and its posterior to the posterior midline.

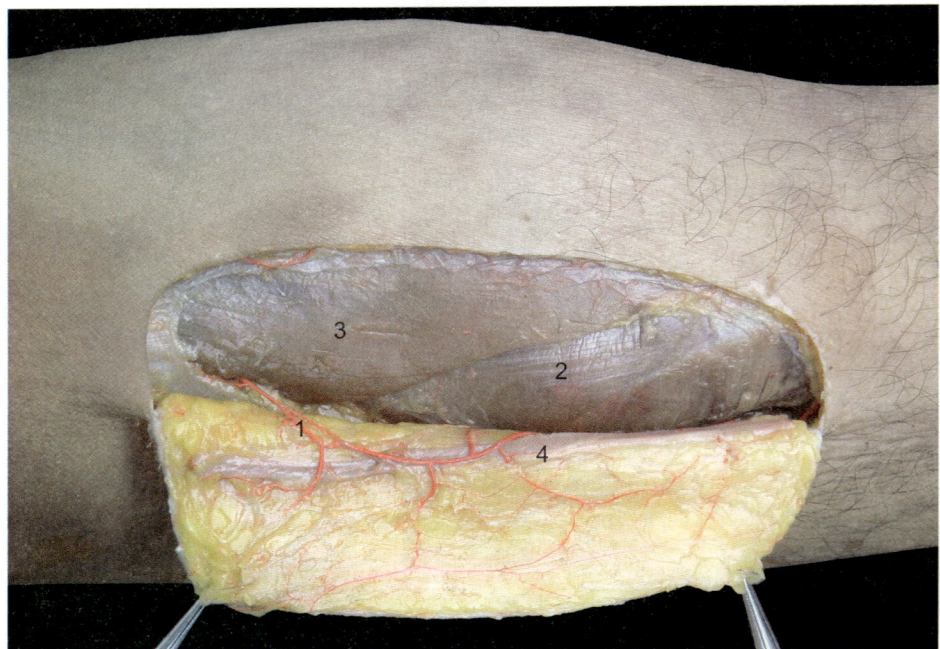

1. Cutaneous branch of medial inferior genicular artery
2. Soleus muscle
3. Gastrocnemius muscle
4. Greater saphenous vein

Figure 1-146   Exposure of the vessels

The skin should be cut open along the posterior border of the flap and then the flap turned forward from under the deep fascia to the medial tibia. Care should be taken to protect the cutaneous branch of the medial inferior genicular artery that enters the skin. The proximal and the distal ends of the flap might be adjusted to the distribution of the cutaneous branches of the artery.

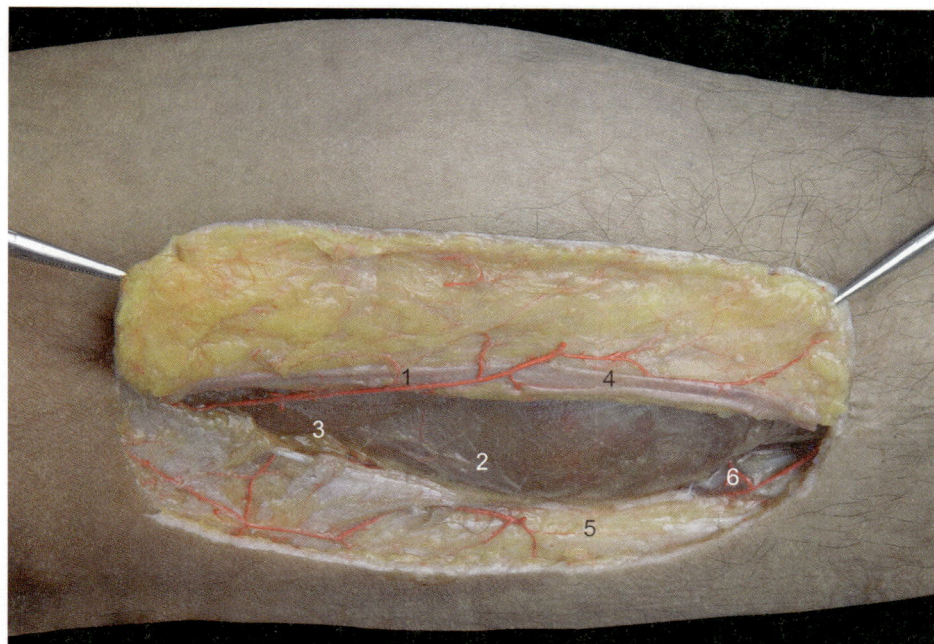

1. Cutaneous branch of
   medial inferior genicular
   artery
2. Soleus muscle
3. Gastrocnemius muscle
4. Greater saphenous vein
5. Tibia
6. Intermuscular branch

Figure 1-147   Elevation of the flap

The flap should first be incised at its anterior border and then dissected from under the deep fascia.
The dissection should continue posteriorly to the posterior tibia.

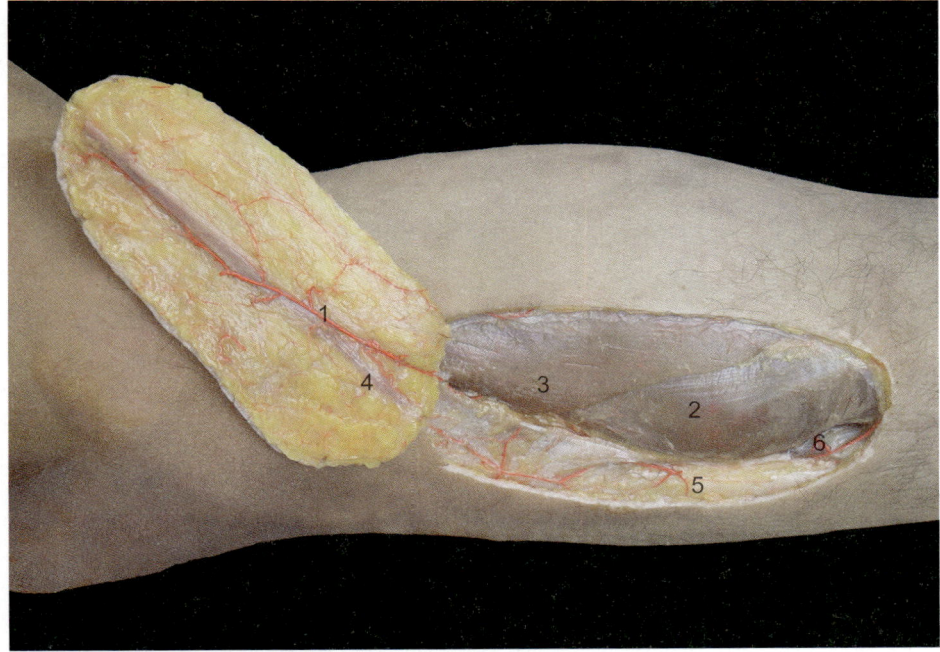

1. Cutaneous branch of
   medial inferior genicular
   artery
2. Soleus muscle
3. Gastrocnemius muscle
4. Greater saphenous vein
5. Tibia
6. Intermuscular branch

Figure 1-148   Anterograde transposition of the flap

Once the flap is isolated, the intermuscular branches should be cut at the distal end of the flap and
the dissection continue proximally along the medial inferior genicular artery to its origin. The flap
might be transferred proximally to repair a wound on the knee.

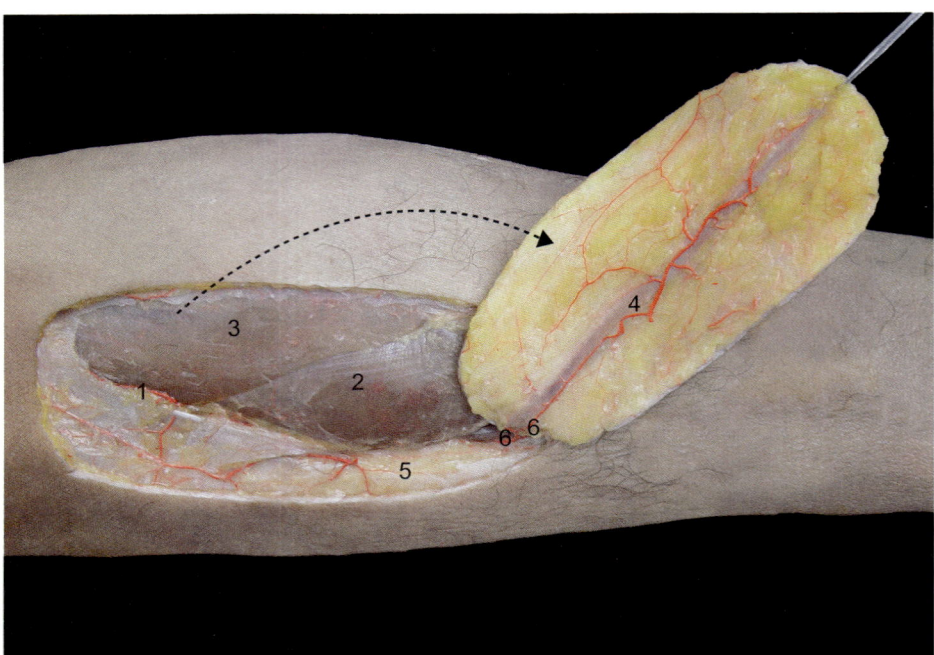

| **Figure 1-149** | **Retrograde transposition of the flap** |

The medial inferior genicular artery should be cut but the distal intermuscular branch retained. The medial inferior genicular artery should be separated downwards to the intermuscular branch. The distally based septum cutaneous perforator flap might be transferred distally to repair a wound on the middle lower leg.

1. Cutaneous branch of medial inferior genicular artery
2. Soleus muscle
3. Gastrocnemius muscle
4. Greater saphenous vein
5. Tibia
6. Intermuscular branch

Key points in applied anatomy

Firstly, the medial tibia should be explored preoperatively with the Doppler to confirm the position where the cutaneous branch of the medial inferior genicular artery perforates through. Secondly, when a distally based flap is designed, the arterial pedicle should be exposed first to visualize the conditions of the cutaneous branch and its anastomosis. The flap obtains its nutrition from the intermuscular branch of the posterior tibial artery. Its pivot point should be located at 7cm under the tibial tuberosity. Thirdly, when a periosteal flap is designed proximally based on the medial superior crural artery, the periosteum should be harvested at 8cm below the medial tibial plateau to protect the pes anserinus tendon. Fourthly, the rotation arch of the flap, with the pedicle of the saphenous artery, might reach as far as the middle lower leg. As the superior saphenous artery is covered under the sartorius muscle and the cutaneous brach is very small, it is preferable that the distal end of the flap should be restricted to 10 cm above the knee. The descending genicular artery and the saphenous branch should be separated from the septum between the sartorius muscle and the gracilis muscle, and then the flap raised as a fasciocutaneous one.

Medial Lower Leg Flap

27

The flap located at the medial lower leg obtains its nutrition from the spatium intermusculare cutaneous branch of the posterior tibial artery. It has such advantages as a concealed donor site, thick skin and little subcutaneous fat. A large flap could obtain its nutrition from the posterior tibial artery and vein as well as some segmental intermuscular cutaneous branches. A small flap could obtain its nutrition from the spatium intermusculare cutaneous branch (large in diameter) or a 2cm posterior tibial artery segment that gives the cutaneous branch. There are the greater saphenous vein and the saphenous nerve in the donor region. The flap might be transferred as a free one, antegrade-flow island one to the knee, retrograde-flow island one to the foot and ankle, or a cross one to the opposite leg.

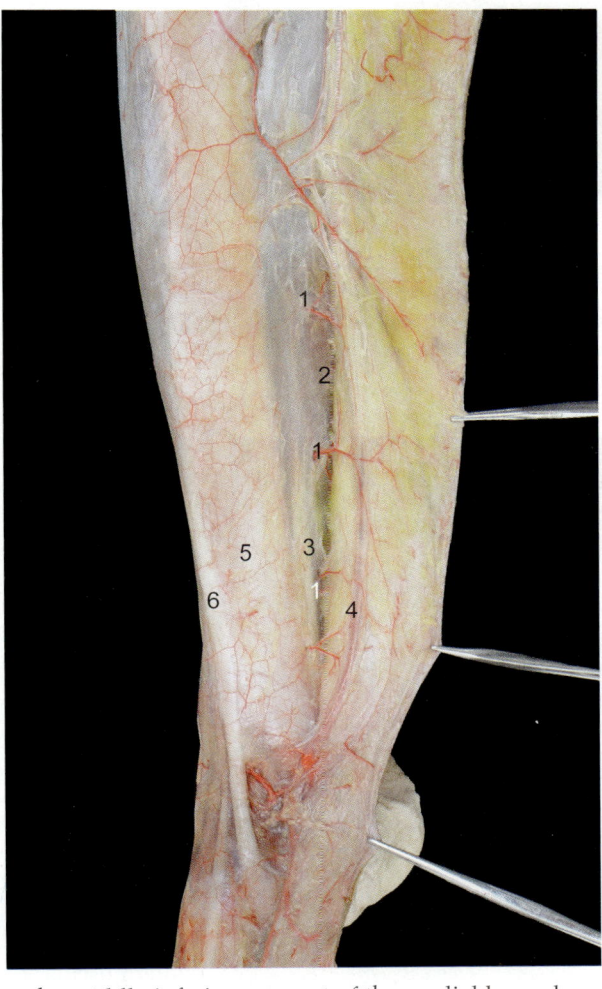

1. Intermuscular cutaneous artery
2. Soleus muscle
3. Flexor digitorum longus muscle
4. Greater saphenous vein
5. Tibia
6. Anterior tibial muscle

Figure 1-150	Applied anatomy

The flap based on the middle-inferior segment of the medial lower leg obtains its blood supply from the medial spatium intermusculare cutaneous branch of the posterior tibial artery. The vessel perforates through the spatium intermusculare between the soleus muscle and the flexor digitorum longus muscle and extends superficially along the deep fascia of the medial lower leg. The posterior tibial artery gives 2-7 cutaneous arteries at the middle-inferior segment of the medial lower leg, among which 2-4 branches (about 75% cases) emerge from the middle-superior segment of the middle lower leg. These septum cutaneous arteries are distributed along an axial line between the midpoint of the medial tibia and the midpoint of the medial malleolus and the Achilles tendon. The cutaneous artery is generally about 1.0 mm in diameter. The septum cutaneous perforators are 2.5-5.0 cm long in the proximal part of the lower leg since the posterior tibial artery is situated deep in the soleus muscle, and 0.2-1.1 cm long in the distal part of the lower leg since the posterior tibial artery is situated in the groove between the gastrocnemius muscle and the flexor digitorum longus muscle. The tibial artery of the middle-distal segment is easy to expose since it is situated under the deep fascia of the medial lower leg. The posterior tibial artery is 2.4 mm in diameter in the middle segment of the lower leg.

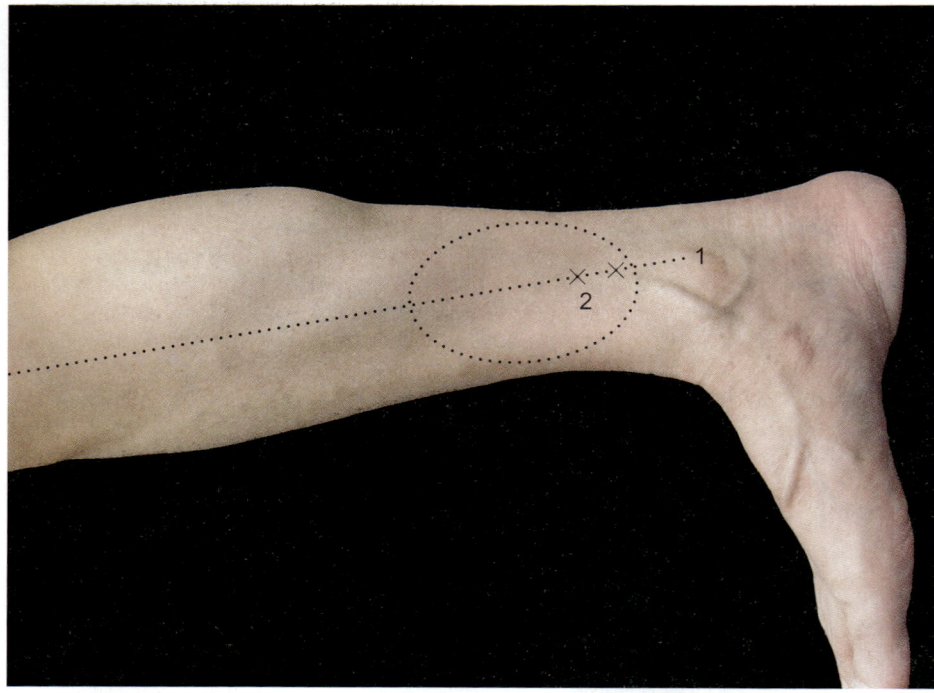

1. Internal malleolus
2. Point through which the cutaneous branch perforates

Figure 1-151   **Design of the flap**

The positions of the two septum cutaneous branches of the posterior tibial artery above the medial malleolus should be first confirmed with the Doppler. The flap should be designed with the two arteries as its pedicle and its distal margin might reach as far as 10 cm beneath the knee.

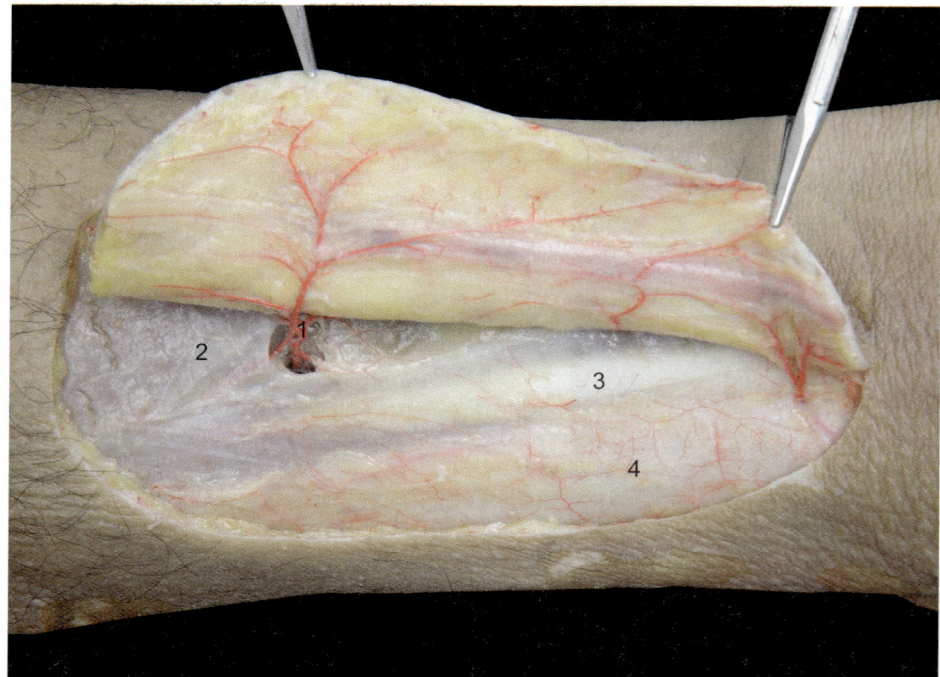

1. Intermuscular cutaneous artery
2. Soleus muscle
3. Flexor digitorum longus muscle
4. Tibia

Figure 1-152   **Dissection of the flap**

The skin of the flap should be cut open from its anterior border and the flap raised posteriorly from under the deep fascia to the medial tibia.

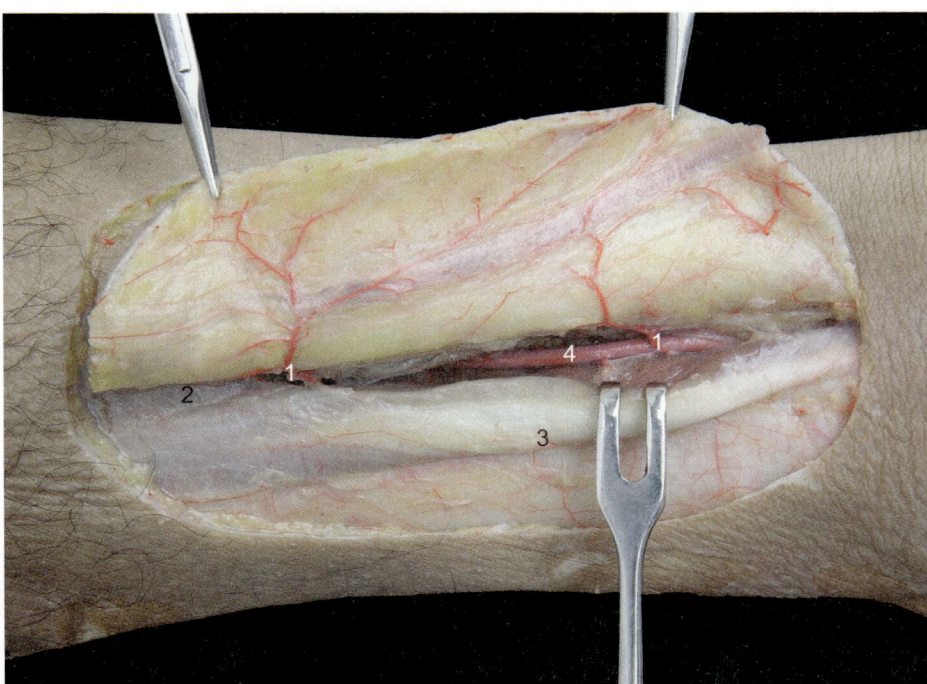

1. Intermuscular cutaneous artery
2. Soleus muscle
3. Flexor digitorum longus muscle
4. Posterior tibial artery

Figure 1-153   Exposure of the vessels

The deep fascia at the medial tibia should be incised with great care to expose the posterior tibial artery and its cutaneous branches in the space between the calcaneal tendon and the tibia. Since the cutaneous branches of the posterior tibial artery enter the subcutaneous tissue via the spatium intermusculare, the perforator vessels should be given great attention to avoid damages.

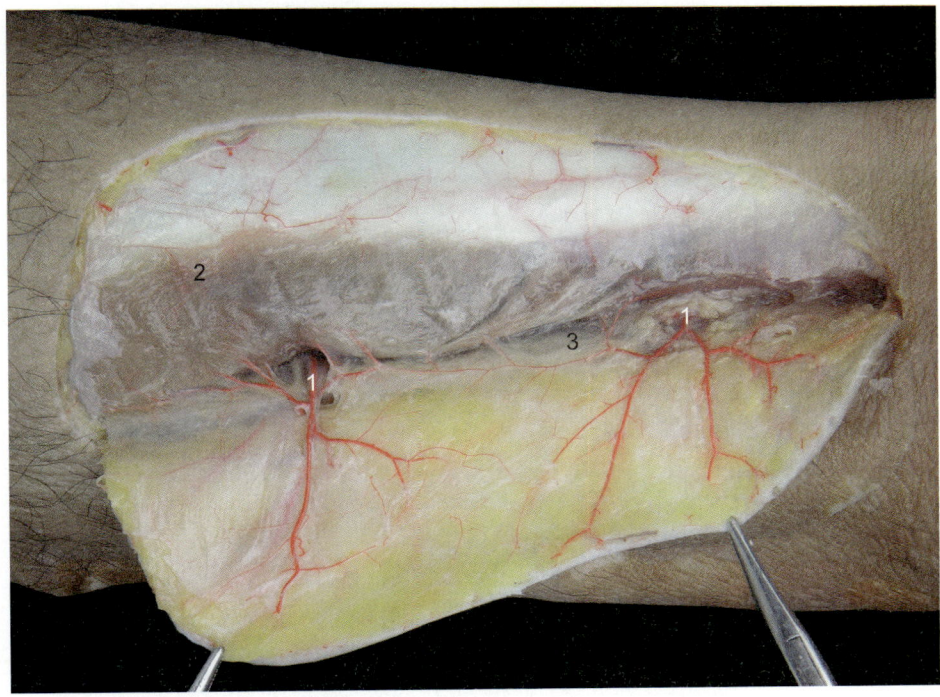

1. Intermuscular cutaneous artery
2. Soleus muscle
3. Flexor digitorum longus muscle

Figure 1-154   Elevation of the flap

The posterior border of the flap should be incised, the flap raised forward from under the deep fascia to the deep layer of the spatium intermusculare, and the cutaneous branches of the posterior tibial artery included in the flap.

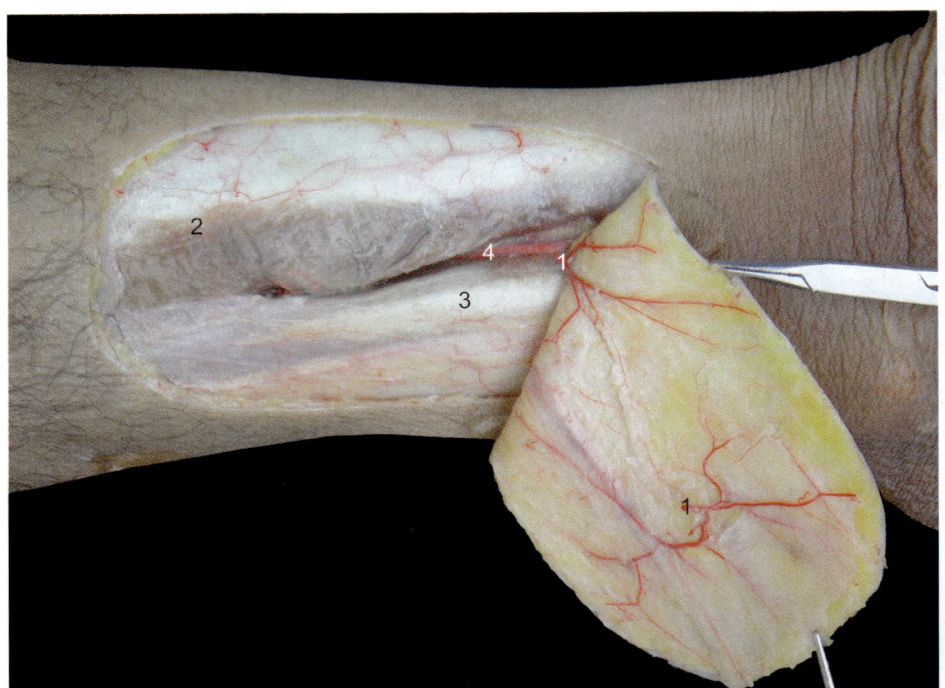

| **Figure 1-155** | **Transposition of the flap** |

Once the flap is isolated completely, it might be transferred to repair a wound on the heel region. The wound of the donor could be repaired with a split-thickness skin graft.

1. Intermuscular cutaneous artery
2. Soleus muscle
3. Flexor digitorum longus muscle
4. Posterior tibial artery

Key points in applied anatomy

Firstly, the conditions of the vessels should be confirmed preoperatively with the Doppler. The size of the flap should be marked according to the body surface projection of the posterior tibial artery and the intermuscular cutaneous artery. Secondly, in cases with abnormal posterior tibial artery (4.7%), the medial leg flap should include the peroneal artery other than the posterior tibial artery. In cases with small posterior tibial artery whose inferior segment is replaced by the communicating branch of the peroneal artery, medial leg flap should be given up. Thirdly, since the anatomical plane of the flap is under the deep fascia, the deep fascia should be sutured with the skin border interruptedly to avoid a disconnection of the two and an affect on the blood supply. Fourthly, when the elevation of the flap continues along the spatium intermusculare, the positions of the cutaneous arteries should be given great attention to avoid damages. Fifthly, when the flap is being dissected, the tibial nerve as well as its muscular branches should be given great attention to avoid damages. Sixthly, since the proximal segment of the posterior tibial artery is situated deep whereas its distal situated superficial, it is preferable that elevation of the flap be carried out in the upward direction.

Anterolateral Flap of the Lower Leg

28

The anterior lateral flap of the lower leg obtains its supply from an axial pedicle of the superficial peroneal artery. It is a sepocutaneous flap, and located at the middle-superior segment of the anterior lateral lower leg. It might be transferred anterogradely with the vascular pedicle to the proximal lower leg or the knee or retrogradely to the heel or the foot. It might also be transferred as a free flap to the hand.

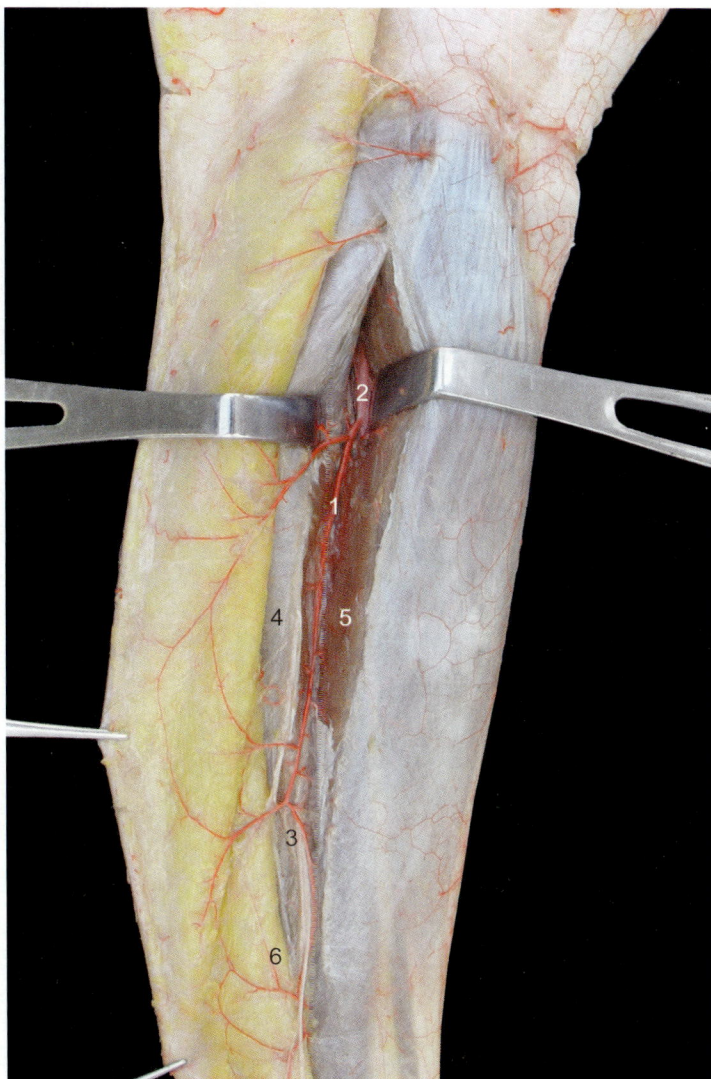

1. Superficial peroneal artery
2. Anterior tibial artery
3. Superficial peroneal nerve
4. Musculus peroneus longus
5. Extensor digitorum longus
6. Intermuscular cutaneous artery

Figure 1-156	Applied anatomy

The superficial peroneal artery emerges from the anterior tibial artery at 6cm distal to the fibular head. It extends distally with the superficial peroneal nerve in the spatium intermusculare between the musculus peroneus longus and the extensor digitorum longus. At about 14 cm distal to the fibular head, the vessel passes through the septum and distributes under the deep fascia (subfascial portion) for a distance. It then passes through the deep fascia at about 22 cm distal to the fibular head and distributes in the subcutaneous tissue (superior fascial portion). The superficial peroneal artery anastomoses with the intermuscular cutaneous arteries of the anterior tibial artery and the anterior perforating branch of the peroneal artery at the inferior spatium intermusculare. It is 1.0 mm in diameter at the origin. It has two accompanying veins, about 1.9 mm and 1.6 mm in diameter, respectively. The vascular pedicle is 9.8 cm in length.

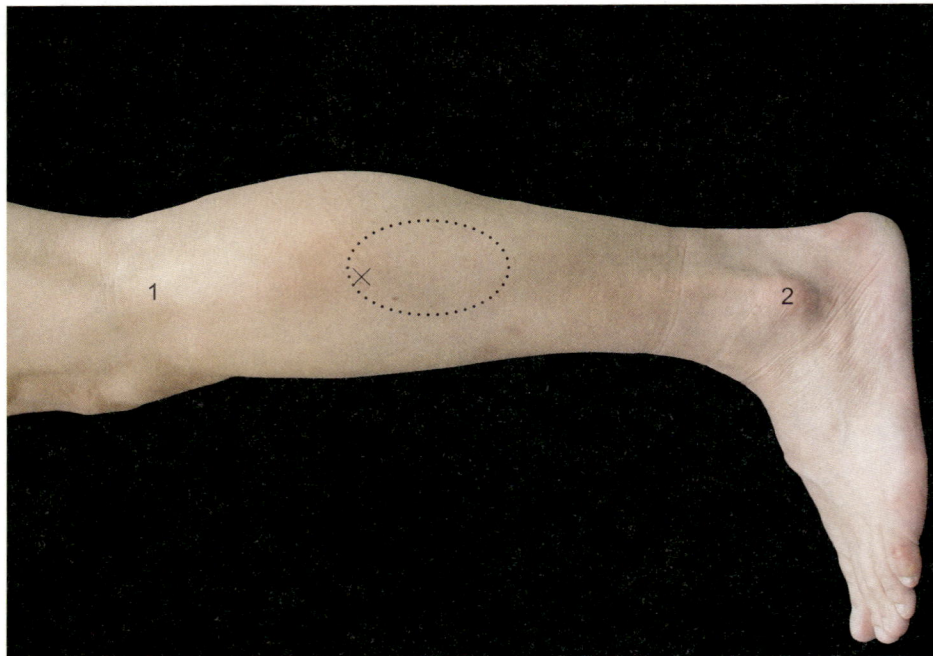

1. Capitulum fibulae
2. External malleolus

| **Figure 1-157** | **Design of the flap** |

The superficial peroneal artery extends superficially to perforate through the deep fascia at 22cm below the fibular head at the lateral anterior spatium intermusculare of the lower leg. The point should be confirmed preoperatively with the Doppler. The flap should be adjusted to the requirement of the recipient region.

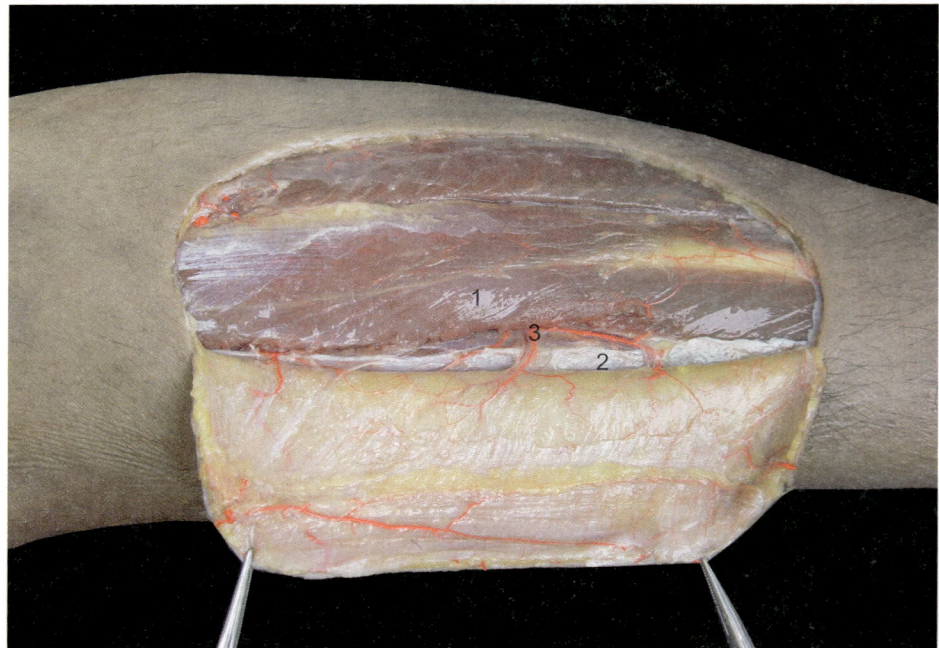

1. Musculus peroneus longus
2. Extensor digitorum longus
3. Superficial peroneal artery

| **Figure 1-158** | **Dissection of the flap** |

The flap should be incised from its posterior border and elevated from under the deep fascia. The dissection should continue to the spatium intermusculare between the musculus peroneus longus and the extensor digitorum longus to expose the superficial peroneal artery.

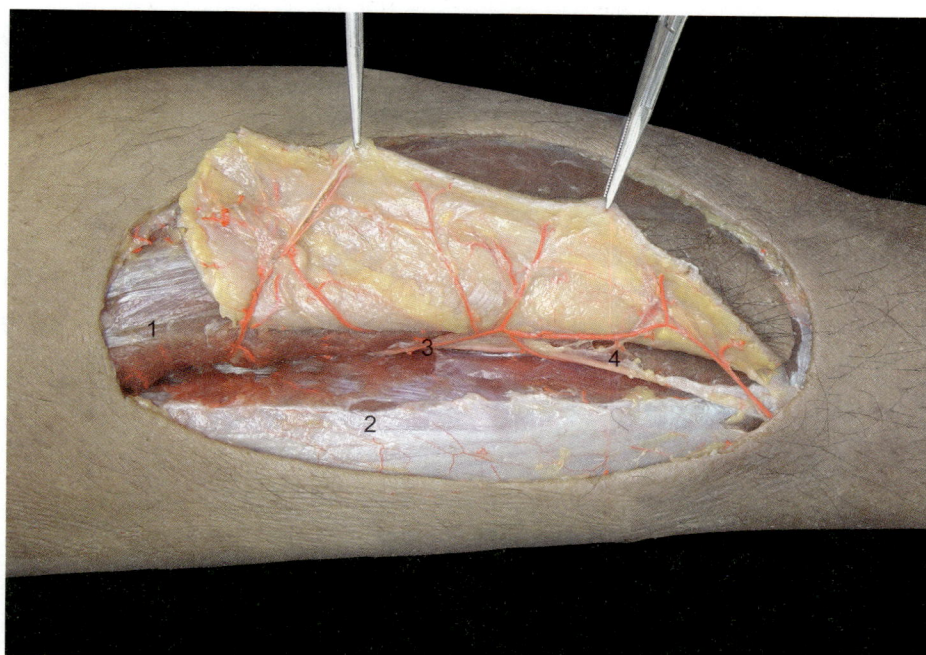

1. Musculus peroneus longus
2. Extensor digitorum longus
3. Superficial peroneal artery
4. Superficial peroneal nerve

Figure 1-159   Elevation of the flap

The anterior border of the flap should be incised. The separation should be done under the deep fascia and continue posteriorly to the spatium intermusculare between the extensor digitorum longus and the musculus peroneus longus.

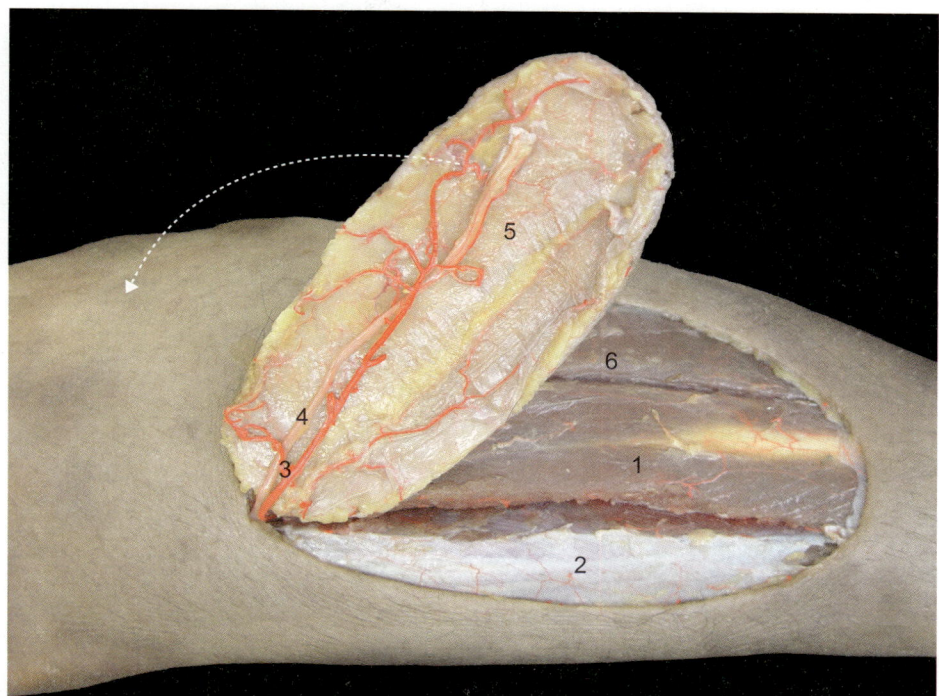

1. Musculus peroneus longus
2. Extensor digitorum longus
3. Superficial peroneal artery
4. Superficial peroneal nerve
5. Flap
6. Soleus muscle

Figure 1-160   Anterograde transposition of the flap

The superficial peroneal artery should be cut at the distal end and the flap dissected toward the proximal vascular base. Once the flap is elevated completely, it might be transferred to restore a wound on the proximal recipient region.

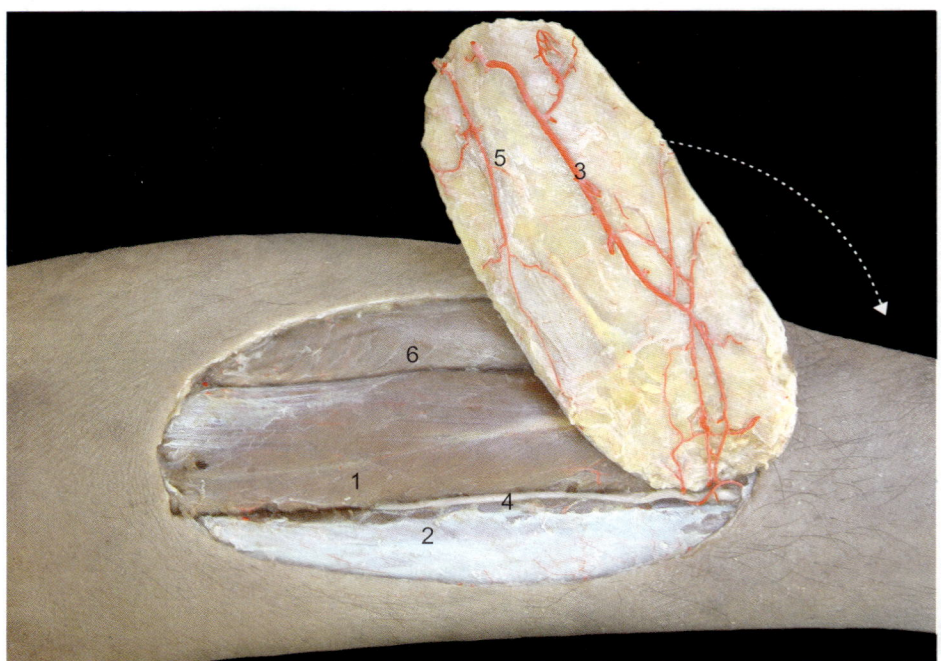

| Figure 1-161 | Retrograde transposition of the flap |

The superficial peroneal artery should be ligated at the proximal end of the flap to make it a retrograde island with a pedicle of the distal vessel and the perivascular fascia. Flaps of this type might be transferred distally to repair a wound on the middle or the inferior lower leg.

1. Musculus peroneus longus
2. Extensor digitorum longus
3. Superficial peroneal artery
4. Superficial peroneal nerve
5. Flap
6. Soleus muscle

Key points in applied anatomy

Firstly, when the anterior lateral spatium intermusculare is separated, the superficial peroneal artery should be given great attention, for it is the main artery that supplies the flap with blood. Secondly, the flap should be made as an antegrade-flow island, with its distal end of superficial peroneal artery ligated so that it could be transferred for the knee reconstruction. Thirdly, the perivascular fascia (0.5-1.0cm wide) should be dissected sharply with care to avoid damages. Fourthly, if a retrograde island flap is designed, the pedicle should be raised with a fascia cuff to protect and enrich its vascularity.

Lateral Flap of the Lower Leg

29

The lateral flap of the lower leg is based on the cutaneous branch of the peroneal artery. It could be incorporate part of the muscle or the bone. It might be transferred antegradely to restore a wound on the knee, or retrogradely to restore a wound on the foot and the ankle. The advantage of the flap is that it sacrifices only one non-dominant artery to the foot or makes it useful even if one of the anterior or the posterior tibial artery is damaged.

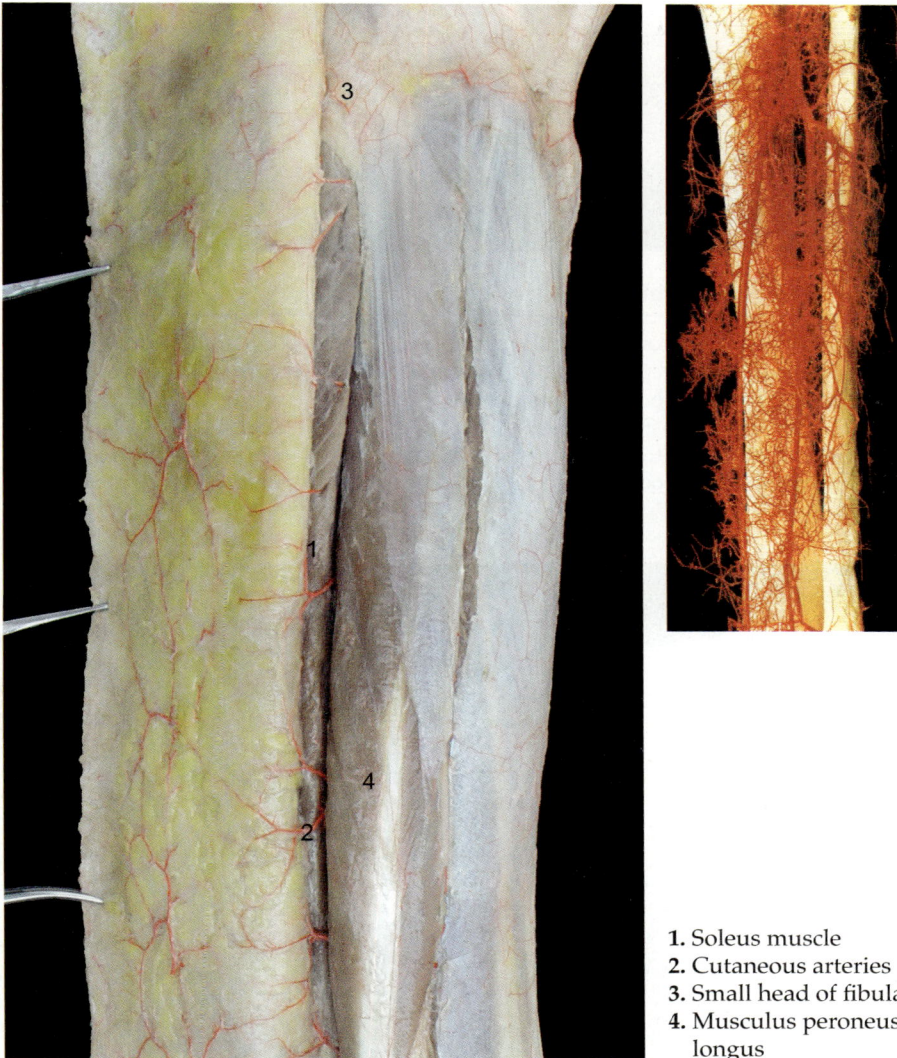

1. Soleus muscle
2. Cutaneous arteries
3. Small head of fibula
4. Musculus peroneus longus

Figure 1-162   **Applied anatomy**

The peroneal artery emerges from the posterior tibial artery, extends laterally downwards along the deep layer of the soleus muscle to the middle lower leg and then continues distally in the space between the fibula and the flexor hallucis longus muscle. Along the course, it gives several septum cutaneous and musculocutaneous arteries, among which 2-3 are larger than the others. The two larger musculocutaneous branches are situated at 9-20 cm below the fibular head. The peroneal artery gives 2 terminal branches at 8 cm above the lateral malleolus. One communicates with the posterior medial malleolar artery of the posterior tibial artery, and the other with the branch of the anterior lateral malleolar artery from the anterior tibial artery. Via these communicating branches, the anterior and the posterior tibial arteries supply the flap with blood on the condition that the flap is being retrogradely transferred. The size of the flap might account for 30cm×16cm.

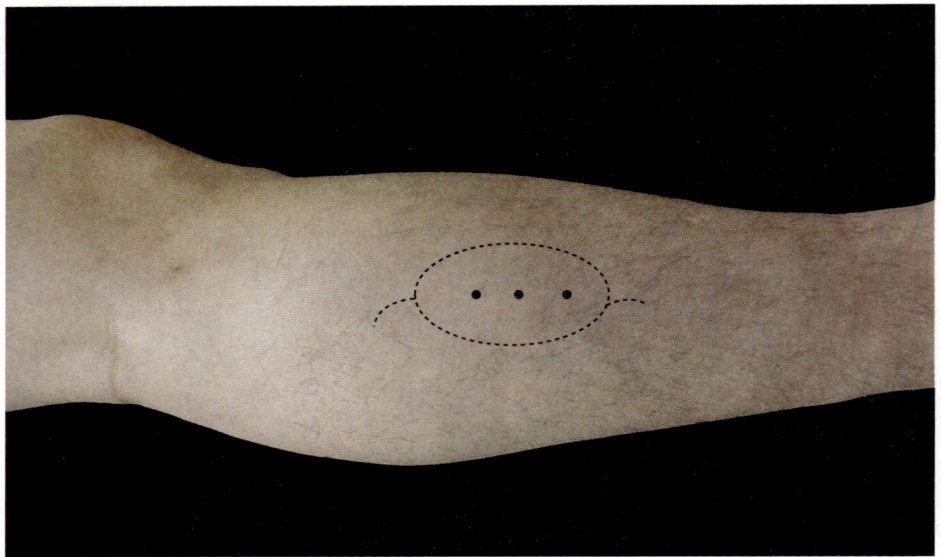

| **Figure 1-163** | **Design of the flap** |

Firstly, The perforating site should be confirmed preoperatively with the Doppler. The flap should be designed with its longitudinal axial line falling along the posterolateral septum of the lower leg, 1/3 of its size located anteriorly and 2/3 located posteriorly. The vascular pedicles should be designed long enough that the flap could be transferred freely. As for an antegradely pedicled flap, it should be designed near the distal end; as for a retrogradely pedicled flap, it should be near the proximal one. In both cases, the point at which the cutaneous artery enters the skin should be included in the flap.

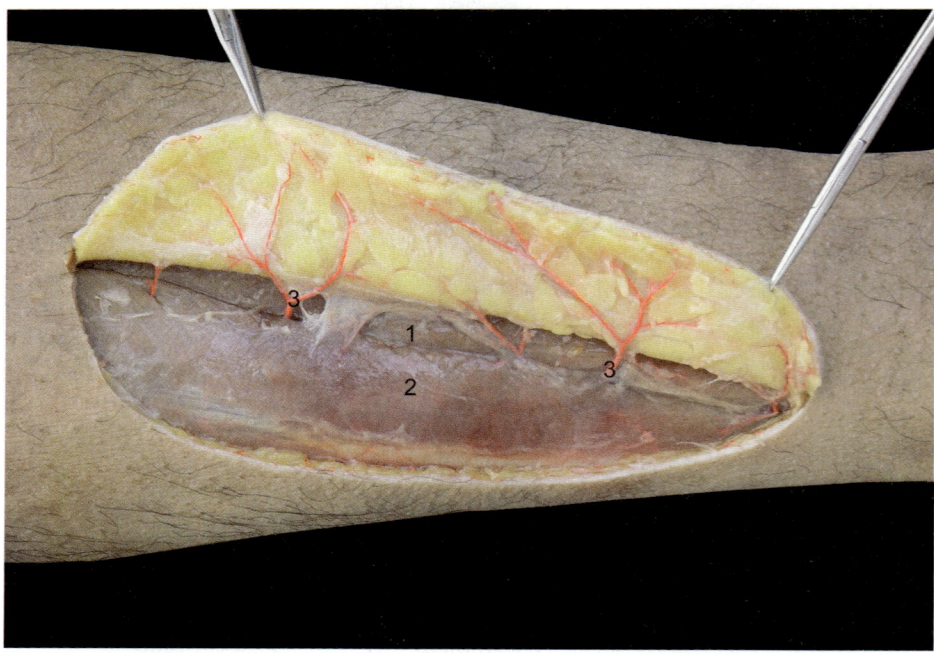

1. Musculus peroneus longus
2. Soleus muscle
3. Cutaneous branches of peroneal artery

| **Figure 1-164** | **Dissection of the flap** |

The skin of the posterior flap should be incised down to the deep fascia, and then the flap dissected anteriorly from under the deep fascia to the posterior border of the fibula to expose the spatium intermusculare between the musculus peroneus longus and the soleus muscle, where the cutaneous branch of the peroneal artery perforates through. The distal and the proximal ends of the flap should be adjusted to the location of the cutaneous branches.

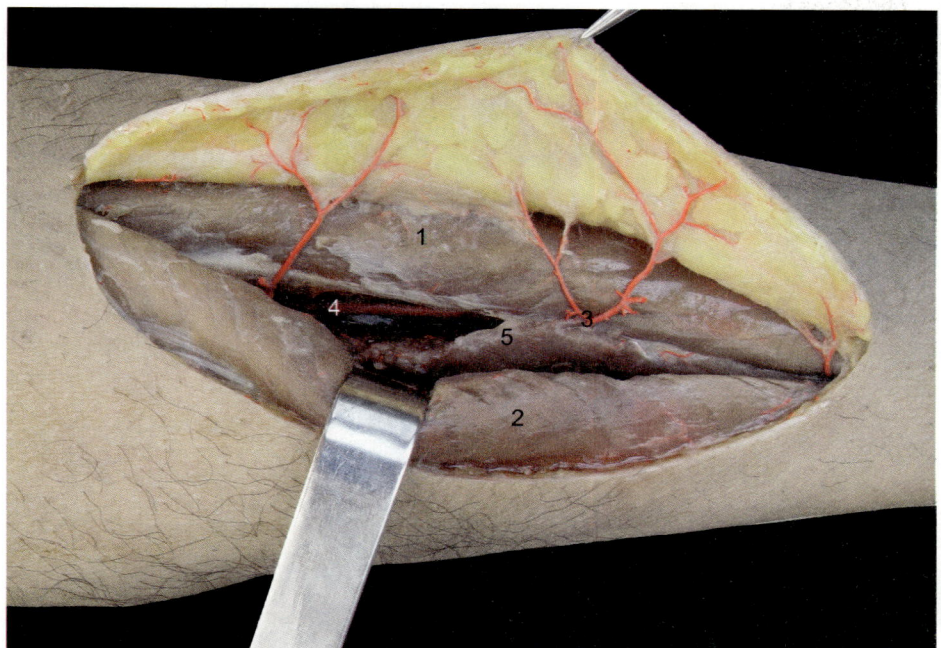

1. Musculus peroneus longus
2. Soleus muscle
3. Cutaneous branches of peroneal artery
4. Peroneal artery
5. Flexor hallucis longus muscle

Figure 1-165   Exposure of the peroneal artery

The septum between the musculus peroneus longus and the soleus muscle should be incised, and the incision trace along the cutaneous branches to the deep tissue to expose the peroneal artery that is situated at the posterior fibula. The peroneal artery in the distal lower leg is situated deep and covered under the flexor hallucis longus muscle.

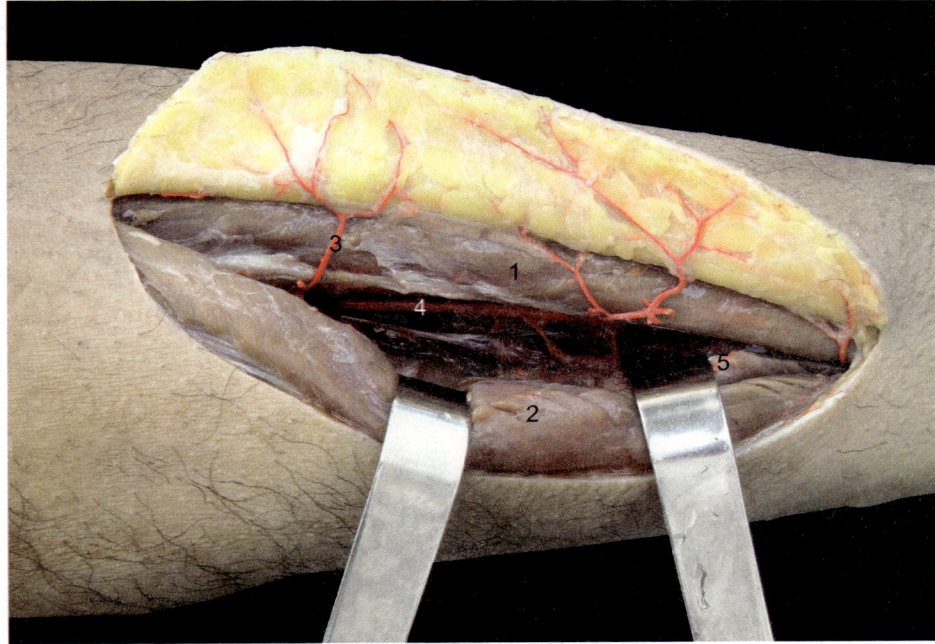

1. Musculus peroneus longus
2. Soleus muscle
3. Cutaneous branches of peroneal artery
4. Peroneal artery
5. Flexor hallucis longus muscle

Figure 1-166   Separation of the artery

The flexor hallucis longus muscle should be separated along the vessel to expose the distal peroneal artery.

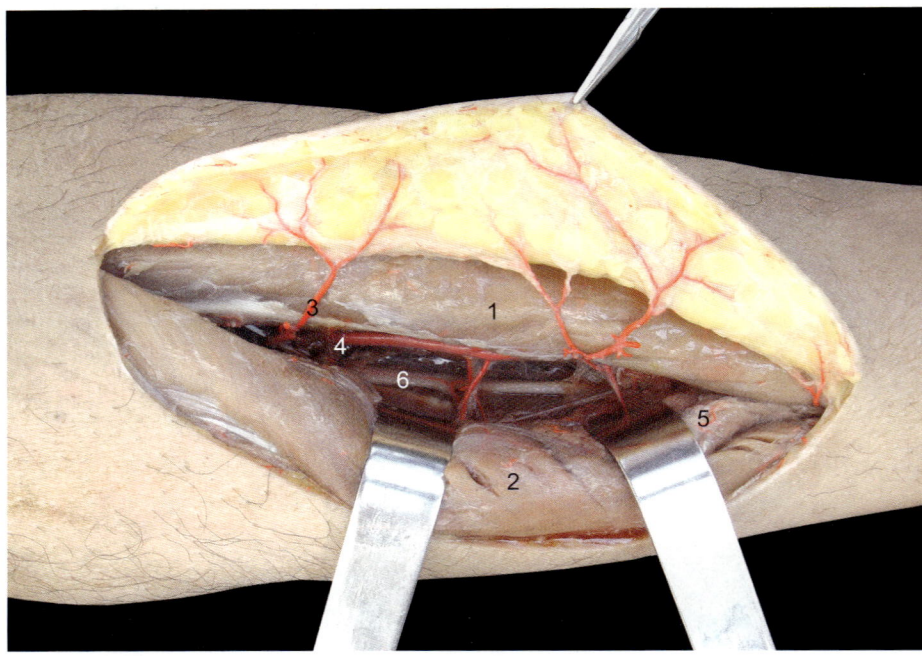

1. Musculus peroneus longus
2. Soleus muscle
3. Cutaneous branches of peroneal artery
4. Peroneal artery
5. Flexor hallucis longus muscle
6. Tibial nerve

| **Figure 1-167** | **Separation of the nerve** |

The tibial nerve adjacent to the peroneal artery should be separated and properly protected. The peroneal artery as well as the cutaneous branches should be included in the flap and kept intact.

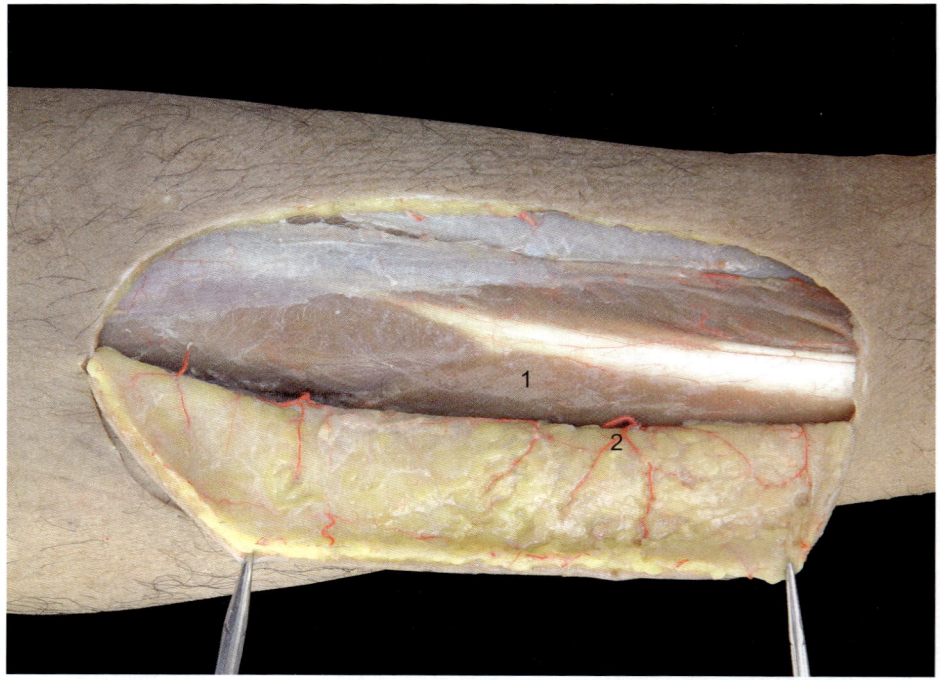

| **Figure 1-168** | **Dissection of the flap** |

The anterior border of the flap should be incised and separated under the deep fascia and the dissection continue to the lateral spatium intermusculare.
1. Musculus peroneus longus
2. Cutaneous branches of peroneal artery

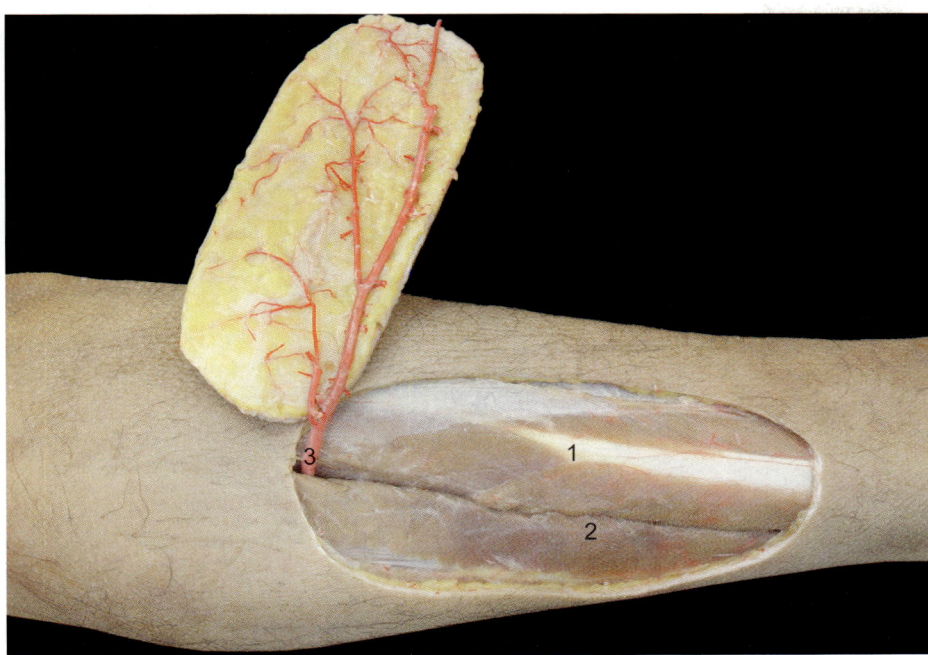

1. Musculus peroneus
   longus
2. Soleus muscle
3. Peroneal artery

Figure 1-169   **Anterograde transposition of the flap**

Once the flap is isolated, it might be transferred proximally with an antegrade flow to restore a wound on the knee. The artery should be cut at the distal end of the flap and elevated toward its origin.

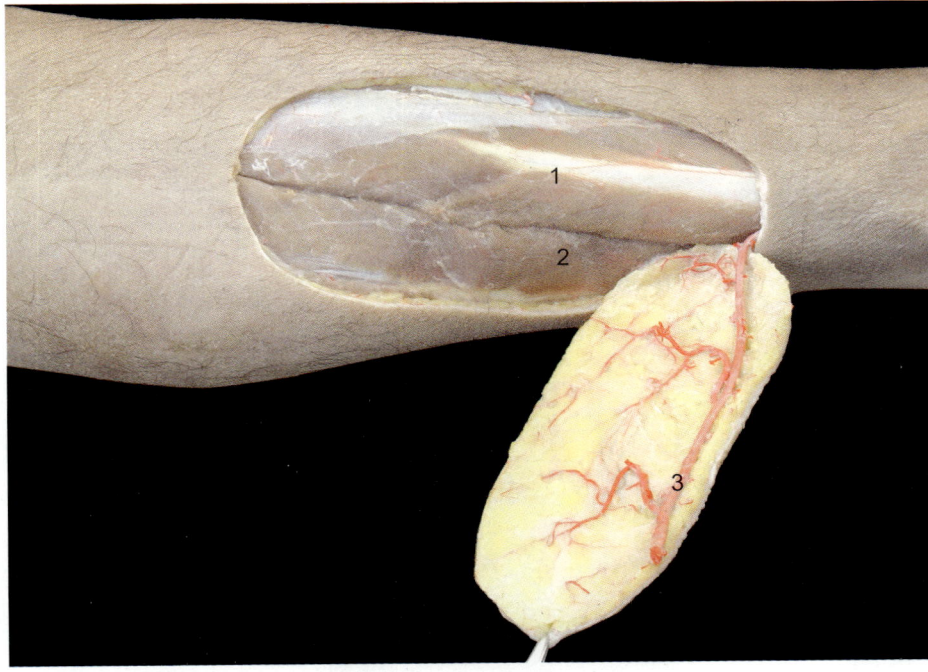

1. Musculus peroneus
   longus
2. Soleus muscle
3. Peroneal artery

Figure 1-170   **Retrograde transposition of the flap**

The peroneal artery should be separated towards the distal end until it is long enough for a retrograde transfer. The distal dissection should be restricted to the level of the lateral malleolus, to avoid damaging the communicating branches. Then the proximal peroneal artery should be interrupted for 10 minutes with a soft clamp to monitor the blood supply of the foot and the flap. If both are normal, the proximal vessel should be cut and ligated, and the flap transferred retrogradely to the foot or the ankle.

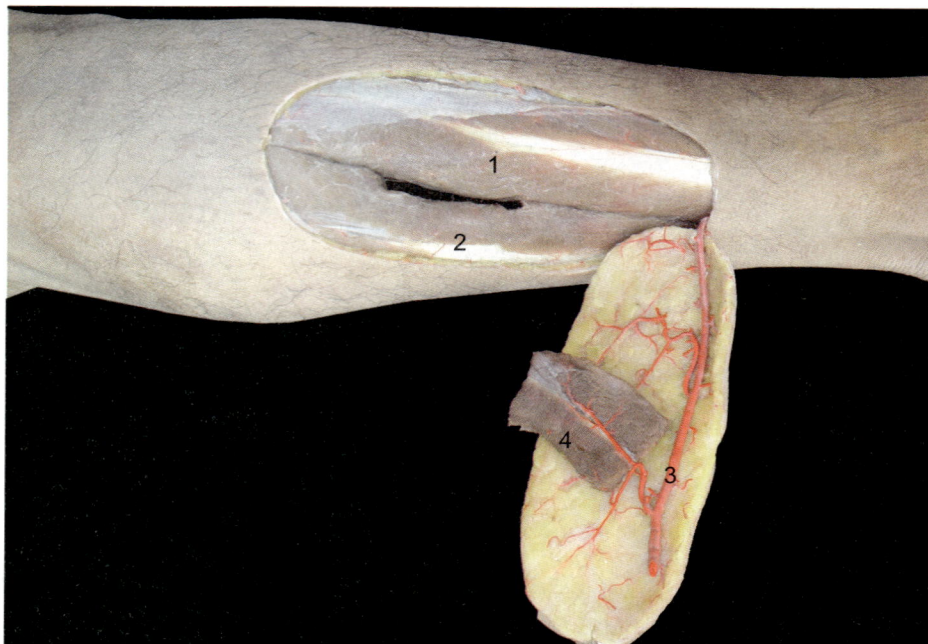

1. Musculus peroneus longus
2. Soleus muscle
3. Peroneal artery
4. Flexor hallucis longus
   muscle

| Figure 1-171 | Formation of the musculocutaneous flap |

The lateral lower leg flap could carry a slip of the flexor hallucis longus muscle or the gastrocnemius muscle to form a musculocutaneous flap. The composite flap might be transferred to treat the chronic osteomyelitis, whose muscular part is used to fill up the wound cavity and whose skin to cover the wound.

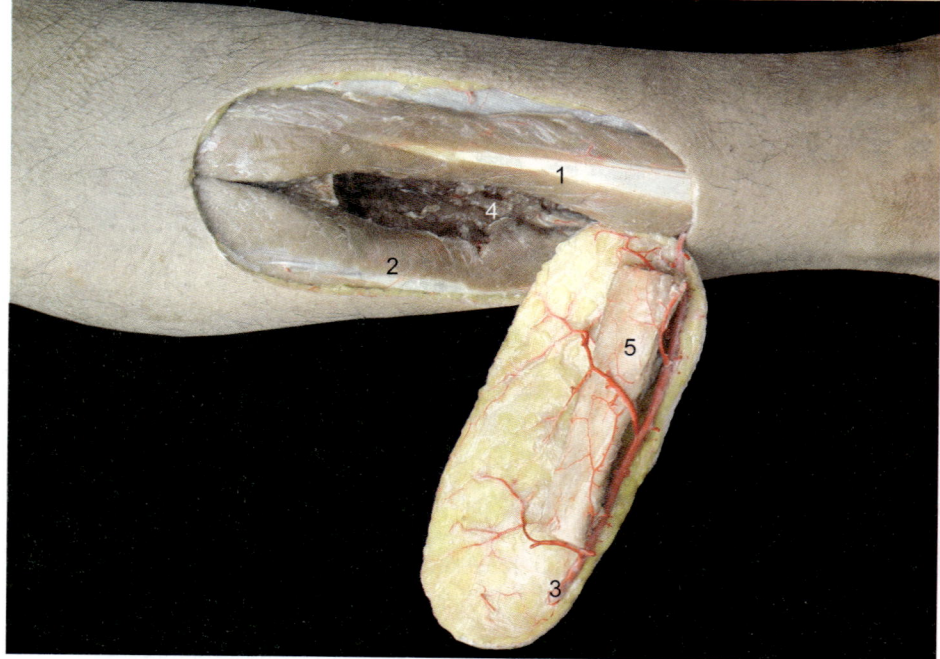

1. Musculus peroneus longus
2. Soleus muscle
3. Peroneal artery
4. Flexor hallucis longus
   muscle
5. Part of the fibula

| Figure 1-172 | Formation of the osseous cutaneous flap |

The peroneal artery pedicle could also supply an osseous cutaneous flap by carrying a peace or a segment of the fibular bone. A flap based on it might be transferred to restore a titial defect with a soft tissue wound.

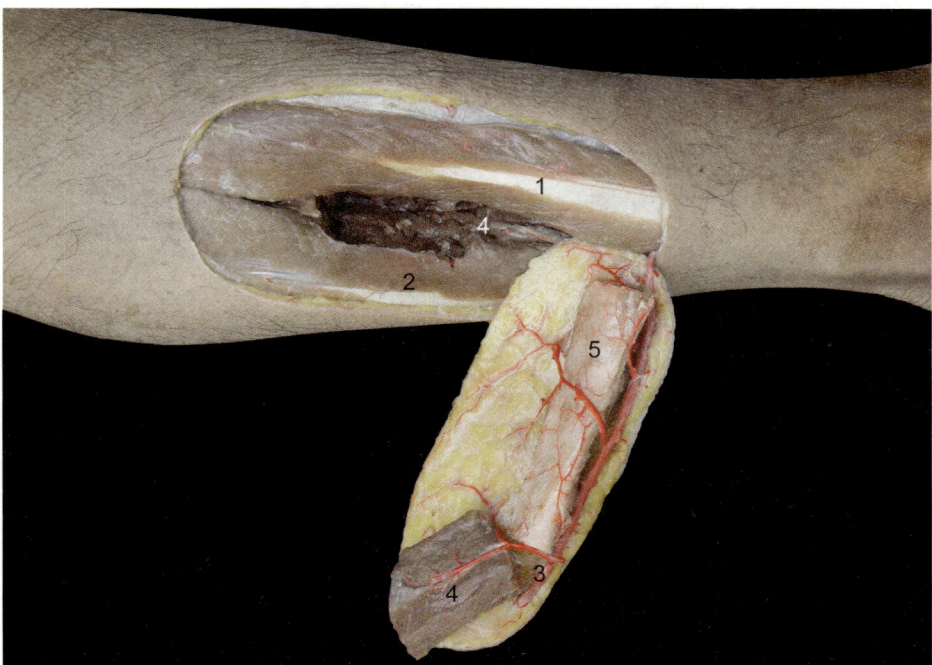

| **Figure 1-173** | **Formation of the osseous muscular flap** |

A compound osseous muscular flap could be made with a pedicle of the peroneal artery. It might be transferred to restore a tibial wound and soft tissue defects.

1. Musculus peroneus longus
2. Soleus muscle
3. Peroneal artery
4. Flexor hallucis longus muscle
5. Part of the fibula

Key points in applied anatomy

Firstly, the body surface projection of the axial line of the flap should fall on the connecting line between the fibula head and the lateral malleolus. The 2nd, 3rd, and 4th septum cutaneous arteries are the larger ones that perforate through at 9-20 cm below the fibula head. The size of the flap should be determined with its anterior about 5-6cm and its posterior about 8-10 cm to the axial line. Secondly, the flap should be elevated from under the deep fascia to the posterolateral spatium intermusculare to expose the proper septum cutaneous perforator. The muscular fibers should be separated along the perforating cutaneous artery and traced to the deep fascia. Parts of the perivascular muscular cuff should be retained to protect the vessels from injury. Thirdly, when the posterior border of the flap is being incised, the lesser saphenous vein and its branches, as well as the sural nerve, should be separated and marked to make ready for anastomosis. Fourthly, since the vascular pedicles of the flap are situated very deep, they should be given great attention in operation to avoid vascular injuries.

30

Lateral Supramalleolar (fascia) Flap

The lateral supramalleolar flap obtains its supply through the perforating peroneal artery. It has such advantages as a long vascular pedicle, a long rotating arch, easy dissection under the deep fascia, and no sacrifice of any main arteries. It might be transferred to restore a wound on the distal 1/3 segment of the lower leg, or transferred retrogradely to restore a wound on the 5th metatarsal bone, under the condition that the vascular pedicles should be separated to the horizontal tarsal sinus.

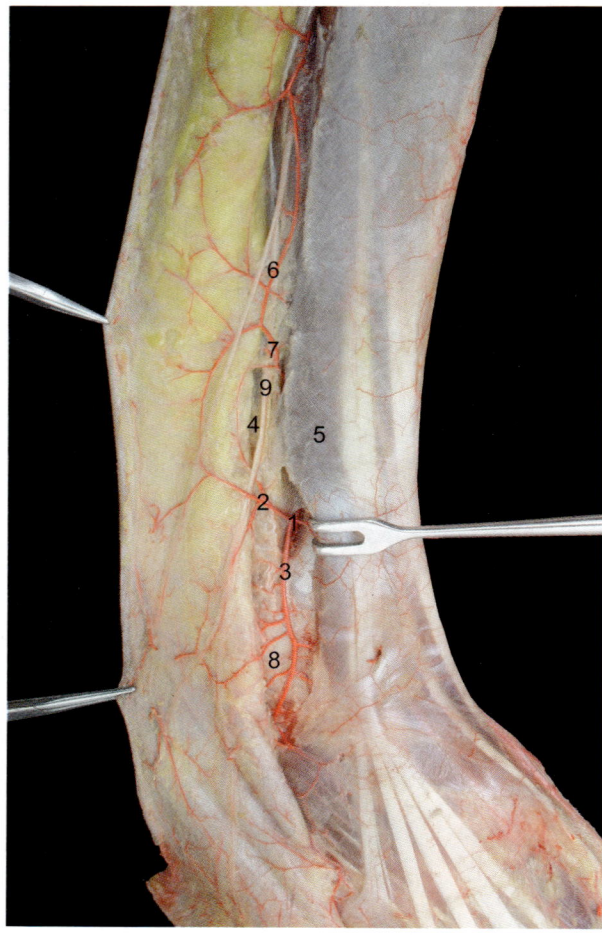

1. Perforating peroneal artery
2. Ascending branch
3. Descending branch
4. Peroneal brevis muscle
5. Extensor digitorum longus
6. Superficial peroneal artery
7. Intermuscular facial cutaneous branches of peroneal artery
8. External malleolus
9. Superficial peroneal nerve

Figure 1-174   Applied anatomy

The peroneal artery perforates through the interosseous membrane at 5.7-7.0 cm above the lateral malleolus, and there it is termed as the perforating peroneal artery. The artery gives constant ascending and descending branches. The ascending branch extends in the anterolateral spatium intermusculare between the peroneal brevis muscle and the extensor digitorum longus, and perforates through the spatium intermusculare and the deep fascia to enter the subcutaneous tissue. It then ascends vertically in the superficial fascia and anastomoses with the superficial peroneal artery or the intermuscular fascial cutaneous branches of the anterior tibial artery to form a longitudinal anastomotic net adjacent to the superficial peroneal nerve. Meanwhile, it anastomoses extensively with the intermuscular fascial cutaneous branches of the peroneal artery to nourish the skin of the lateral half of the lower leg. The descending branch extends inferiorly in the loose connective tissue under the deep fascia and enters the space between the lateral malleolus and the talus tuberosity to anastomose with the anterior lateral artery in the talus groove. The anastomotic artery descends anteriorly outwards to the tuberosity of the 5th metatarsal bone. The perforating peroneal artery is 0.4-1.0 cm in length and 1.5-2.0 mm in diameter. The descending branch is 4.5-6.9 cm in length and 0.6-1.2 mm in diameter.

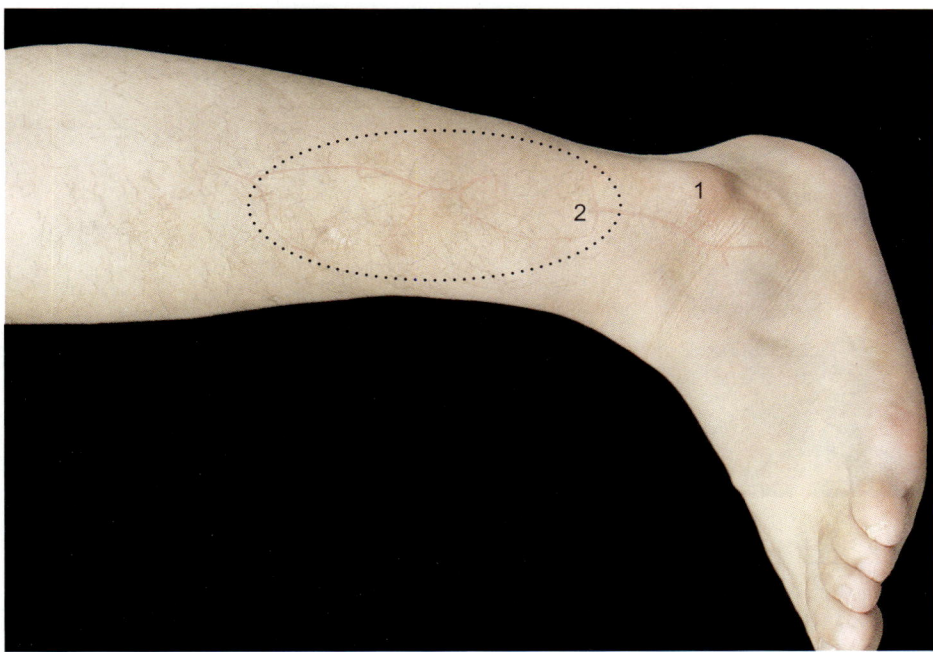

1. External malleolus
2. Perforating peroneal artery

| **Figure 1-175** | **Design of the flap** |

The pivot point at which the perforating peroneal artery perforates through the interosseous membrane is generally located at 5cm above the lateral malleolus. It should be confirmed with the Doppler. A flap of this type should be designed anteriorly to the crest of the tibia, posteriorly to the fibula and proximally to the middle lower leg. It might account for about 18×9 cm in size.

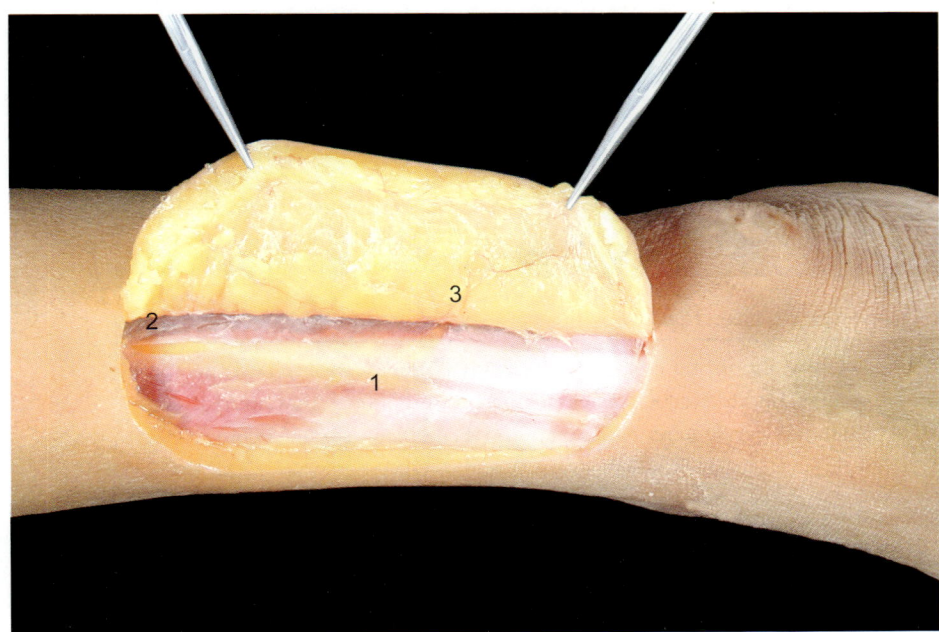

1. Extensor digitorum muscle
2. Peroneal muscle
3. Perforating cutaneous branch

| **Figure 1-176** | **Dissection of the flap** |

The flap should first be incised at its anterior border and elevated posteriorly from under the deep fascia to the spatium intermusculare between the extensor digitorum muscle and the peroneal muscle to expose the perforating peroneal artery that perforates through the spatium. The superficial peroneal nerve could be seen to extend obliquely along the medial side of the artery and should be kept intact.

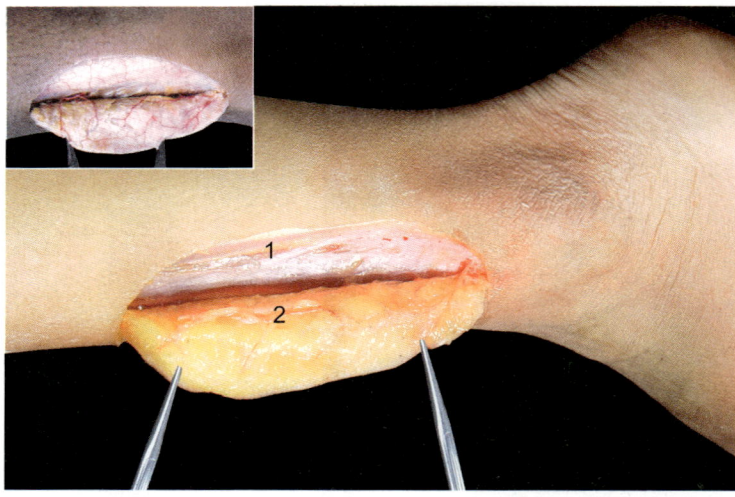

1. Peroneal muscle
2. Perforating cutaneous branch

Figure 1-177   Elevation of the flap

With the ascending branch of the perforating peroneal artery included, the flap should be incised from its posterior border and separated under the deep fascia.

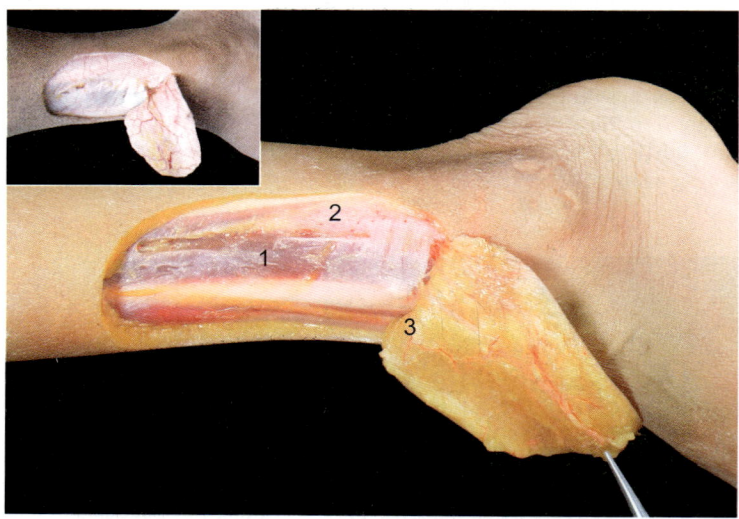

1. Extensor digitorum muscle
2. Peroneal muscle
3. Ascending branch of perforating artery

Figure 1-178   Transposition of the flap

The trunk of the perforating peroneal artery should be ligated before it gives the ascending and the descending branches and then the dissection continue distally along the descending branch that nourish the flap. A flap of this type might be transferred locally to repair a wound on the malleolus or the heel.

Key points in applied anatomy

Firstly, since the perforating branch of the peroneal artery has its anatomical variants, the point through which the cutaneous branch of the terminal branch of the peroneal artery perforates should be confirmed preoperatively with the Doppler. Secondly, the flap should be incised first from its anterior border and dissected under the deep fascia. Its posterior border should not be incised before the perforating peroneal artery is included in the flap. Thirdly, since the venous blood returns via the small accompanying vein to the final perforating branch of the peroneal artery, the conditions of the pedicles should be checked to avoid getting them twisted and compressed. Fourthly, the superficial peroneal nerve should be kept intact during the operation. Fifthly, it is preferable that the flap should take parts of perivascular fascia and subcutaneous tissue (2-3 cm wide) to protect the vessel and to increase blood return in it.

Sural Flap

31

The popliteal artery that supplies the skin of the posterior lower leg gives three direct cutaneous branches into the popliteal fossa: the lateral, the intermediate and the medial popliteal cutaneous arteries. Since it has its accompanying nerve, it could be harvested as a sensate flap for the sensory restoration. A sural flap with such a pedicle might be transferred to the knee, the distal thigh or the proximal leg. It might also be used for the hand or the forearm reconstruction.

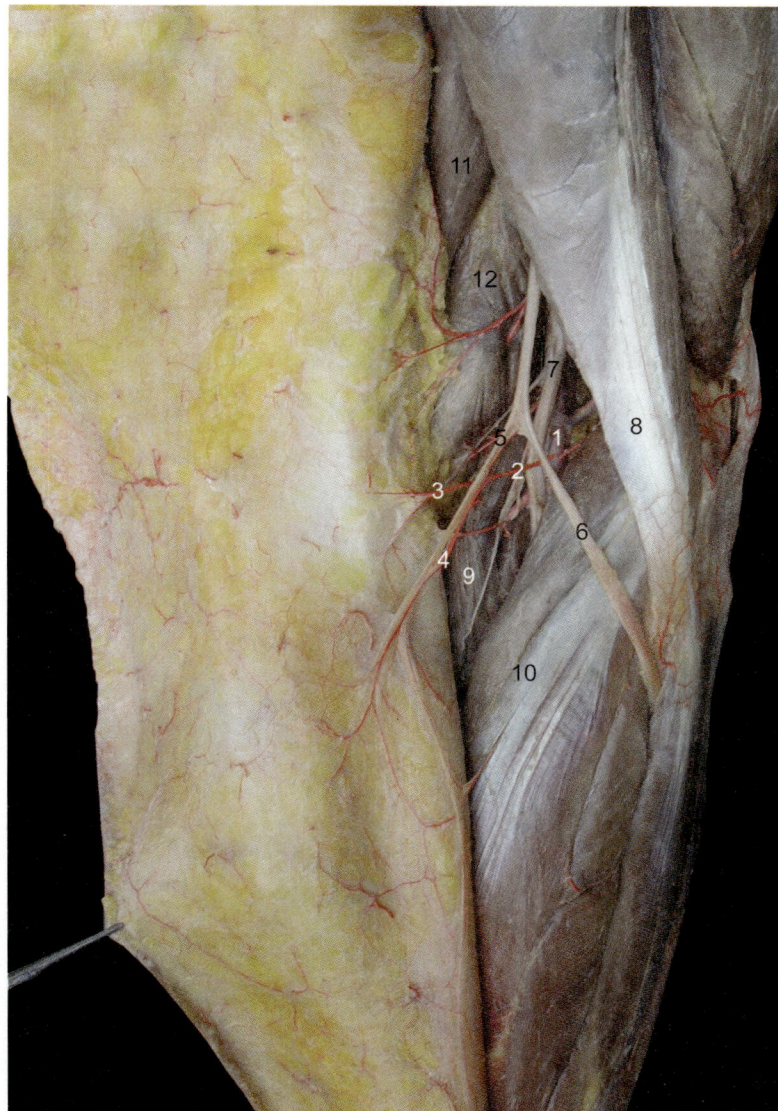

1. Popliteal artery
2. Lateral popliteal cutaneous artery
3. Collateral branch
4. Descending branch
5. Lateral sural cutaneous nerve
6. Common peroneal nerve
7. Tibial nerve
8. Biceps femoris muscle
9. Medial head of gastrocnemius muscle
10. Lateral head of gastrocnemius muscle
11. Semitendinous muscle
12. Semimembranous muscle

Figure 1-179	Applied anatomy

In most cases, the popliteal artery (the sural artery in a few cases) sends three direct cutaneous branches: the lateral, the intermediate and the medial popliteal cutaneous arteries. These cutaneous branches perforate through the deep fascia at the midline of the leg (18 mm, 13 mm and 16 mm, respectively) to enter the subcutaneous tissue. Along the course, they give the ascending the, collateral branches and the descending branches to form an extensive vascular net. The descending branch extends for 14 cm below the medial and the lateral femoral condyles. After perforating through the deep fascia, it courses with the lateral sural cutaneous nerve and sends smaller branches to fan out over the skin. The flap could be harvested for size of 30×15cm.

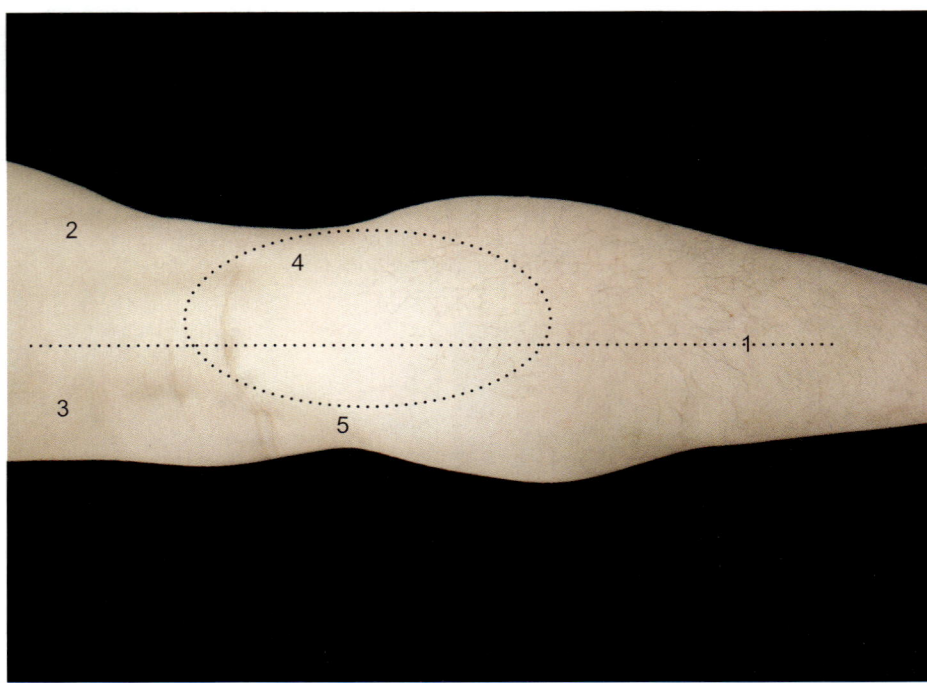

1. Posterior median line of the lower leg
2. Biceps femoris muscle
3. Semitendinous muscle, semimembranous muscle
4. Lateral head of gastrocnemius muscle
5. Medial head of gastrocnemius muscle

Figure 1-180   Design of the flap

Take the flap based on the lateral popliteal cutaneous artery. Its pivot point should be located at the popliteal fossa and its axis 2cm lateral to the posterior midline of the lower leg.

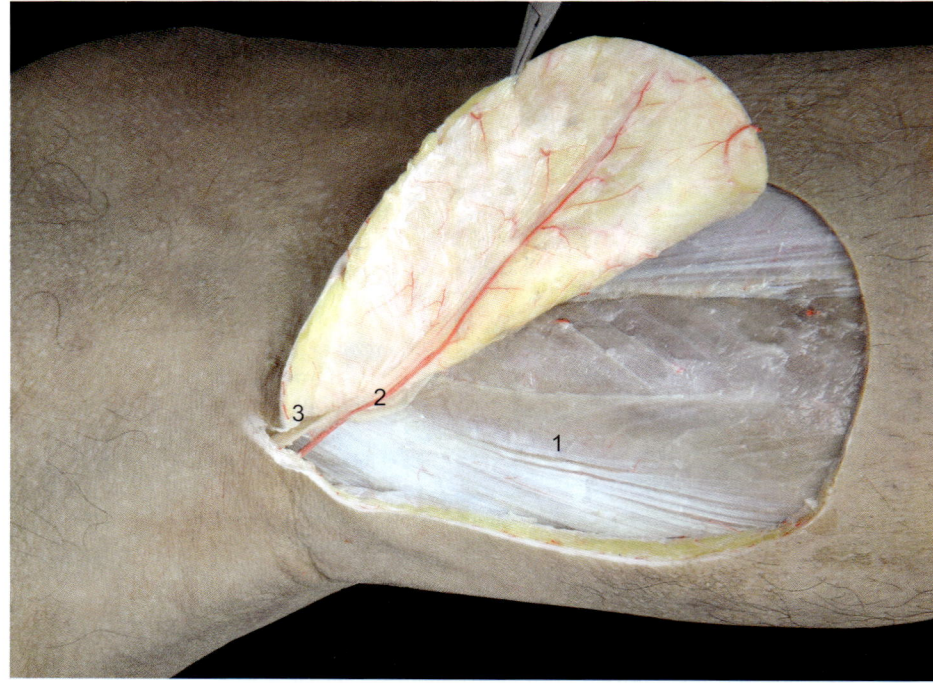

1. Lateral head of gastrocnemius muscle
2. Cutaneous artery of lateral popliteal fossa
3. Sural nerve

Figure 1-181   Dissection of the flap

The flap should be incised from the distal border and dissected retrogradely under the deep fascia, and the dissection should continue to the proximal base. The sural nerve at the posterior midline of the lower leg should be given great attention, and so should the vessel that perforates through the deep fascia to enter the flap to avoid getting it damaged.

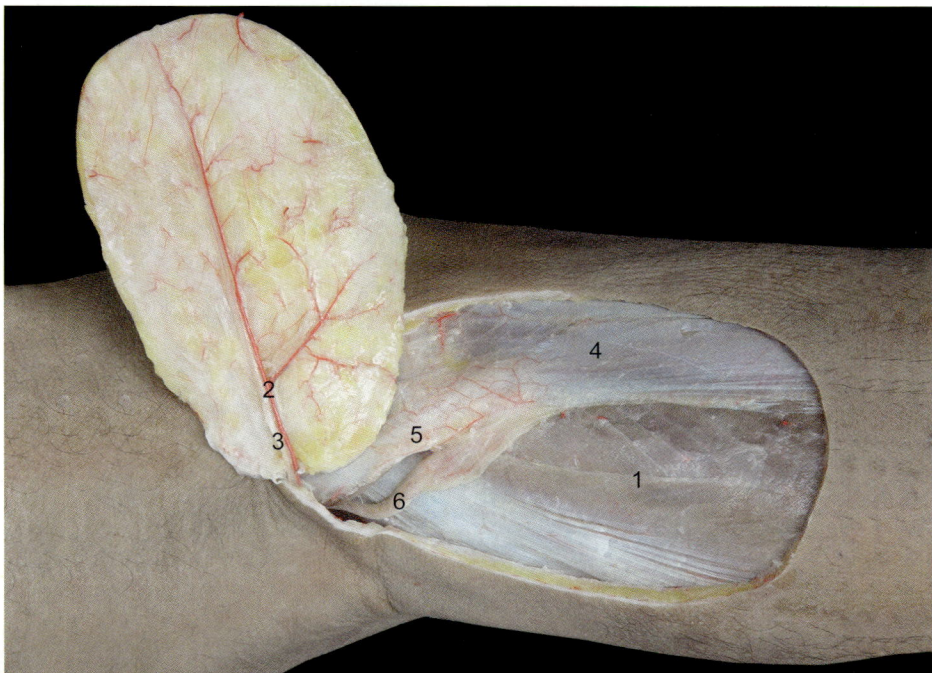

Figure 1-182   Transposition of the flap

Once the flap is isolated, it might be transferred locally to repair a wound on the middle-superior segmeat of the lower leg or on the knee. The donor region could be covered with a split-thickness skin.

1. Lateral head of gastrocnemius muscle
2. Lateral popliteal cutaneous artery
3. Sural nerve
4. Peroneal muscle
5. Biceps femoris muscle
6. Common peroneal nerve

Key points in applied anatomy

Firstly, a large flap should be harvested, with its superior margin to the connecting line between the medial and the lateral epicondyles of the femur, its inferior to 5cm above the medial and the lateral malleolus, its lateral to the lateral femur epicondyle and the lateral malleolus line, and its medial to the medial femur epicondyle and the medial malleolus line. The flap might account for about 30×15cm in size. Secondly, either the lateral or the medial popliteal cutaneous artery could serve as the pedicle of the flap. The flap should be dissected on the anatomic plane to avoid damaging the common fibular nerve. Thirdly, the superior margin of the flap should be located below the connecting line between the medial and the lateral femoral condyles, to avoid the formation of a cicatrix scar in the popliteal fossa, which might in turn affect the knee flexion and extension. Fourthly, the perivascular fascia of the pedicle should be cut off to form an island flap, so that it could be transferred upwards to the knee. When the flap is intended for the tibial coverage, the vascular pedicle should not be exposed, and nor should the base of the skin be cut off.

32

Medial Pedis Flap

The medial pedis flap is located in the region between the medial plantar and the medial dorsal pedis. It has such advantages as a concealed location, a non-weight-bearing part, a good-quality skin and a multiple blood supply. It has many arteries that could be chosen as its pedicles, the deep branch of the medial plantar artery, the superficial branch of the medial plantar artery, the medial anterior malleolar artery or the medial tarsal artery, for example. The pedicled medial pedis flap might be transferred to the adjacent recipient site on the medial malleolus, the calcaneal tendon, the dorsal pedis or the plantar. Microsurgical free medial pedis flap is suitable for the hand repair and reconstruction.

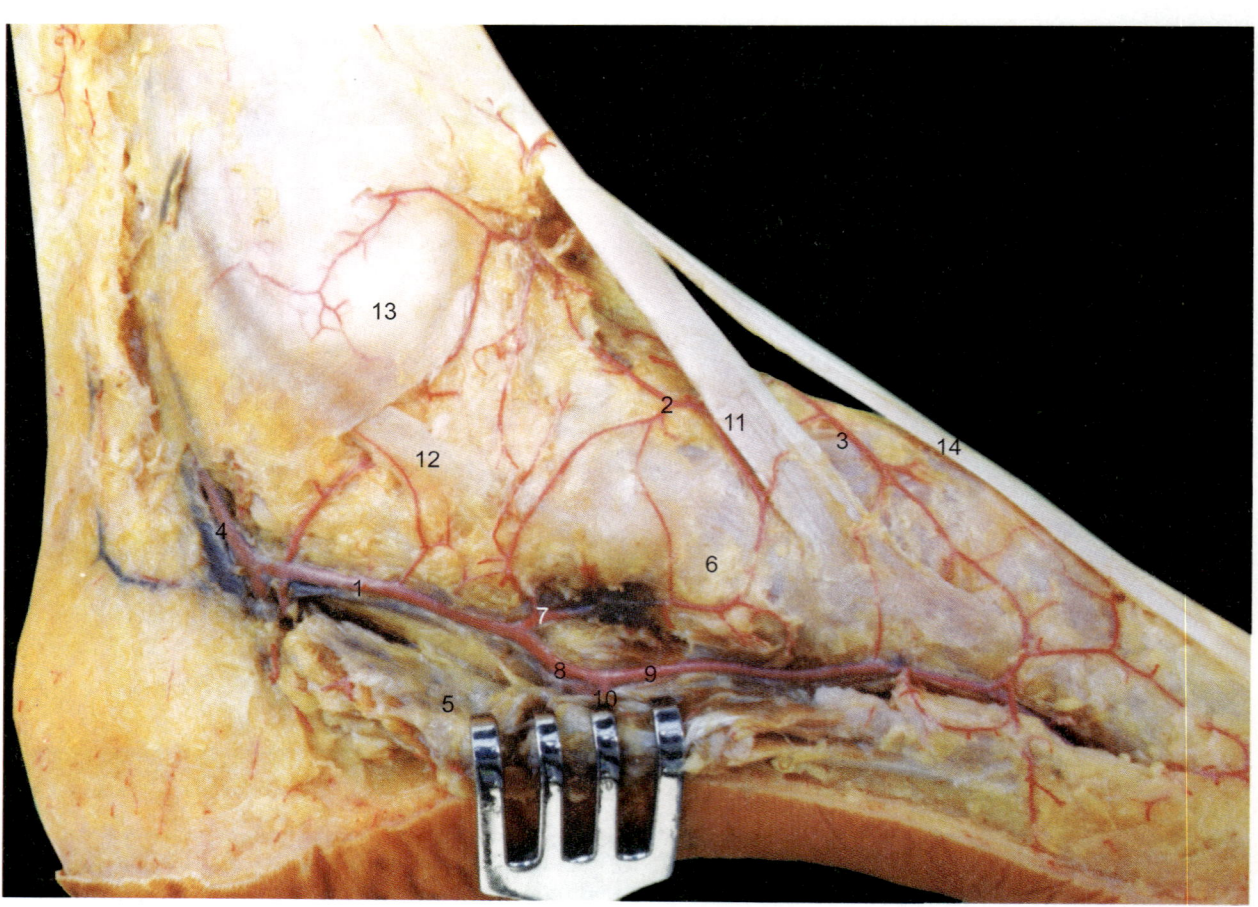

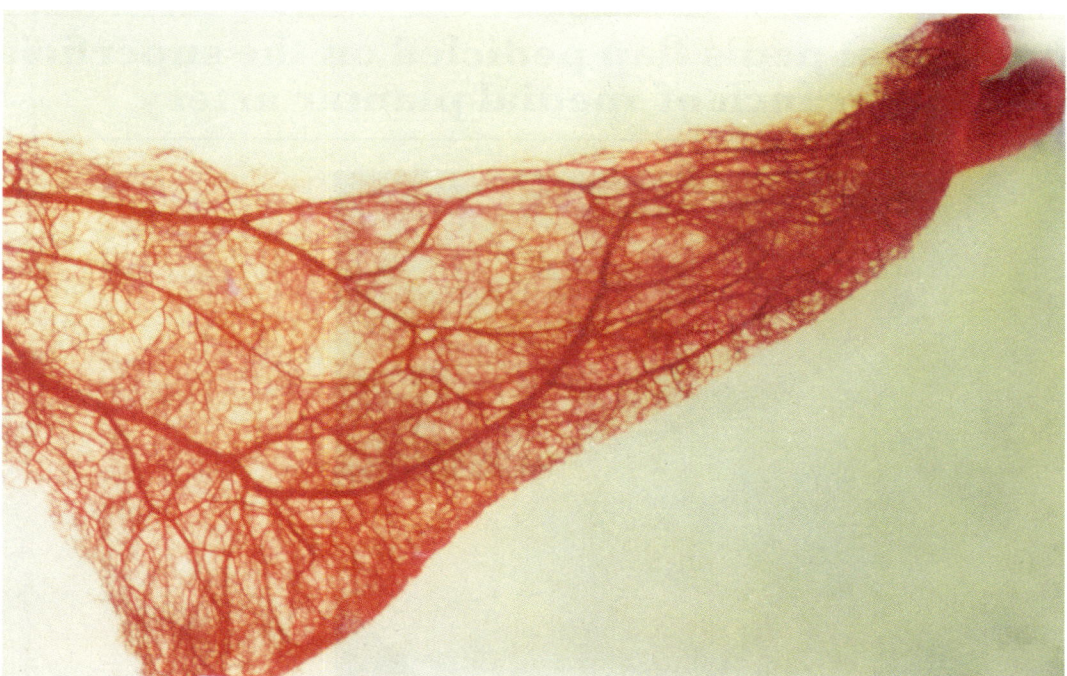

Figure 1-183	Applied anatomy

The medial pedis skin gets its blood supply from multiple sources: the superficial branches of the medial plantar artery, the medial anterior malleolar artery and the medial tarsal artery. Firstly, the medial plantar artery emerges from the posterior tibial artery in the tarsal tunnel, passes through the deep surface of the abductor hallucis muscle and bifurcates into superficial and deep branches behind the tuberositas ossis navicularis. The superficial branch courses anteriorly in the interosseous fascia between the abductor hallucis muscle and the tarsal bone. The deep branch subdivides into medial and lateral deep branches. The medial deep branch extends along the deep surface of the abductor hallucis muscle and runs superficial at the tuberositas ossis navicularis. Secondly, the medial anterior malleolar artery emerges from the anterior tibial artery and extends anteriorly, close to the medial side of the neighboring anterior tibial tendon in the medial region of the foot. The medial anterior malleolar artery is 5.2 cm in length and 1.6 mm in diameter. Thirdly, the medial tarsal artery emerges from the dorsal pedis arterial trunk and extends anteriorly, close to the lateral side of the neighboring anterior tibial tendon. It is 1.4 cm in length and 1.3 mm in diameter. All of these arteries anastomose with one another at the superficial or the deep layers of the anterior tibial tendon and give many cutaneous branches to nourish the medial skin of the foot.

1. Medial plantar artery
2. Medial anterior malleolar artery
3. Medial tarsal artery
4. Posterior tibial artery
5. Abductor hallucis muscle
6. Tuberositas ossis navicularis
7. Superficial branch
8. Deep branch
9. Medial deep branch
10. Lateral deep branch
11. Anterior tibial tendon
12. Posterior tibial tendon
13. Medial malleolus
14. Extensor hallucis longus muscle

A. The medial pedis flap pedicled on the superficial (or deep) branch of medial plantar artery

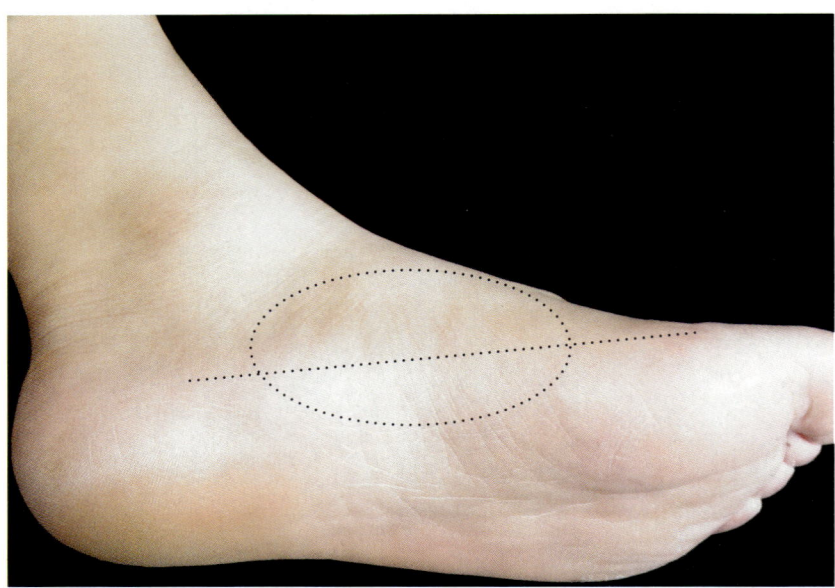

Figure 1-184   **Design of the flap**

The flap should be designed with its axial line falling on the connecting line between the tuberositas ossis navicularis and the medial 1st metatarsal bone. The flap might account for 3-5 cm in width. Its anterior border might extend to the middle segment of the 1st metatarsal bone, its lateral to the extensor pollicis longus muscle tendon, its medial to the medial plantar and its posterior to the vertical line at the medial malleolus. The flap might account for 9×6cm to 10×8 cm in size.

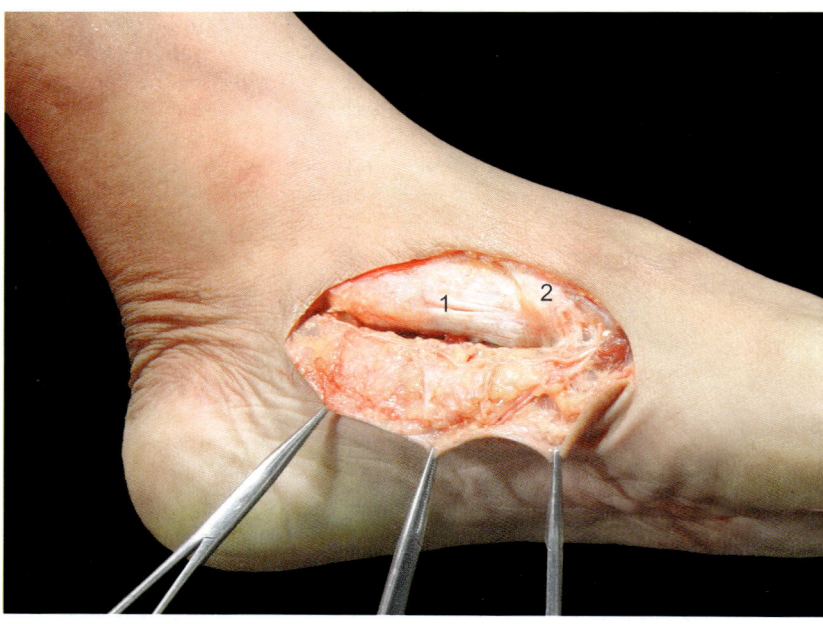

1. Abductor hallucis muscle
2. Anterior tibial tendon

Figure 1-185   **Exposure of the vessels**

The flap should be incised from its dorsal border and then elevated from under the deep fascia. The dissection should continue along the anterior medial artery and the medial tarsal artery to the abductor hallucis muscle and the tarsal bones to expose the medial plantar artery.

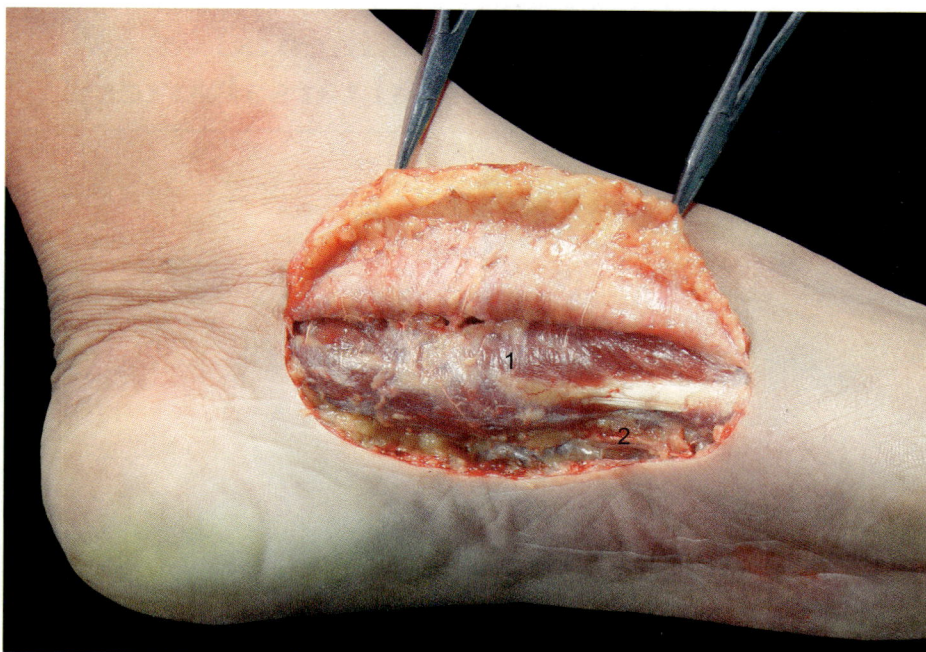

1. Abductor hallucis muscle
2. Medial plantar artery

Figure 1-186   **Dissection of the flap**

The dissection of the flap should begin with its plantar border and continue dorsally from the superficial layer of the abductor hallucis muscle to the posterior part of its anterior border. Then the superficial branch of the medial plantar artery should be separated along the superficial layer of the periosteum until it is included in the flap.

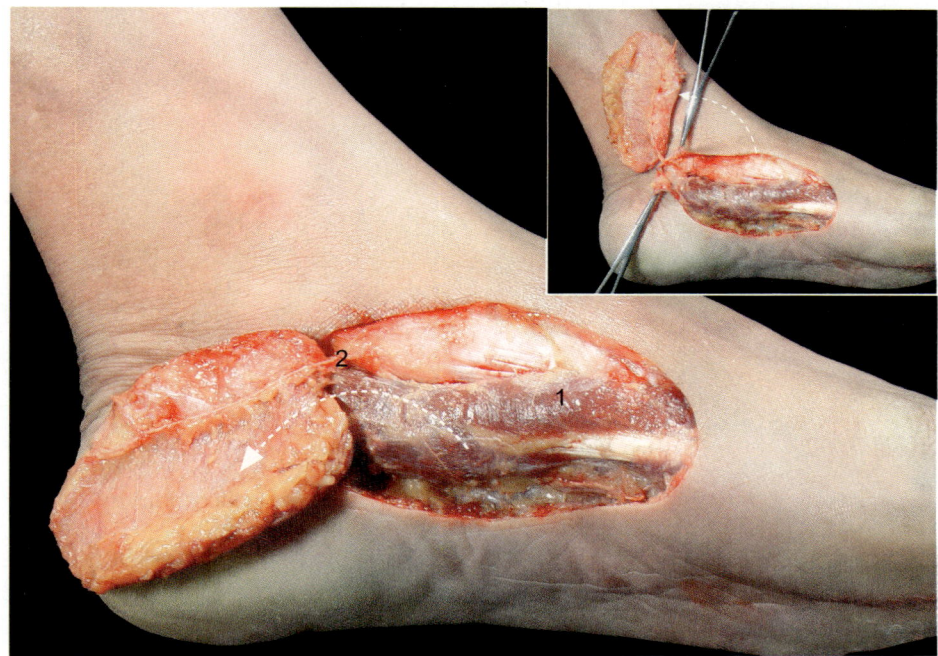

1. Abductor hallucis muscle
2. Superficial branch of medial plantar artery

Figure 1-187   **Elevation of the flap**

The distal end of the flap should be incised, and the abductor hallucis muscle drawn laterally. The pedicle should be separated towards the proximal end until it is long enough for a tension-free posterior transfer to the medial malleolus, the calcaneal tendon, or the heel.

B. The medial pedis flap based on the medial anterior malleolar artery or medial tarsal artery

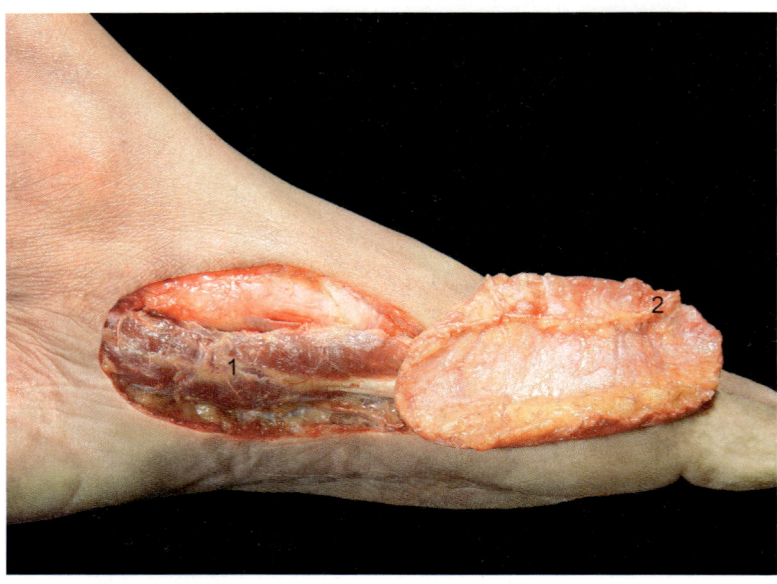

1. Abductor hallucis muscle
2. Superficial branch of medial plantar artery

| **Figure 1-188** | **A retrograde transposition of the flap** |

The design, incision, exposure and dissection of a retrograde flap are similar to those of an anterograde one. But its pivot point should be located at the middle segment of the 1ˢᵗ metatarsal bone.

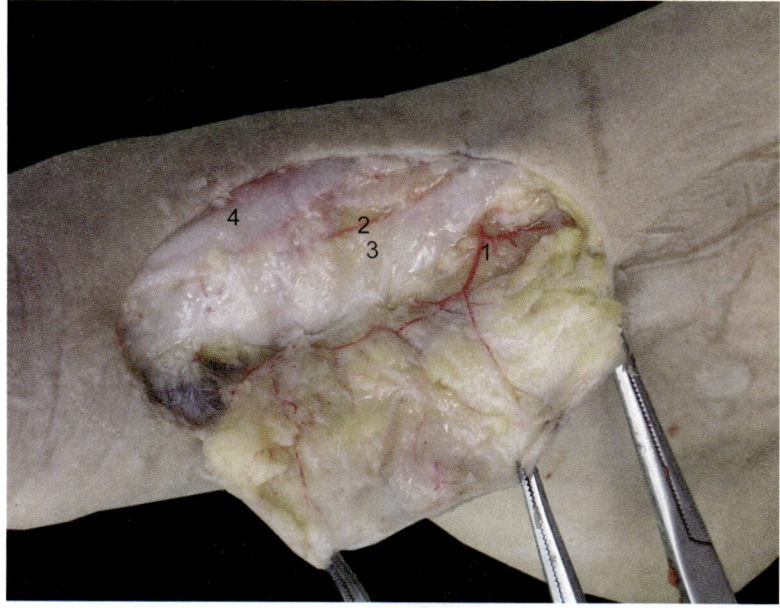

1. Medial anterior malleolar artery
2. Medial tarsal artery
3. Anterior tibial tendon
4. Extensor pollicis longus muscle tendon

| **Figure 1-189** | **Exposure of the vessels** |

The flap could be designed in the same way as the medial plantar one with a pedicle of the superficial (deep) branch of the medial plantar artery. It should be incised from its lateral border to expose the medial anterior malleolar artery and vein as well as the medial tarsal artery and vein. Among these vessels, the larger artery and vein should be selected as the pedicle of the flap. The vascular pedicle should be harvested with part of the perivascular fascia (0.5-1.0 cm wide) to keep them intact.

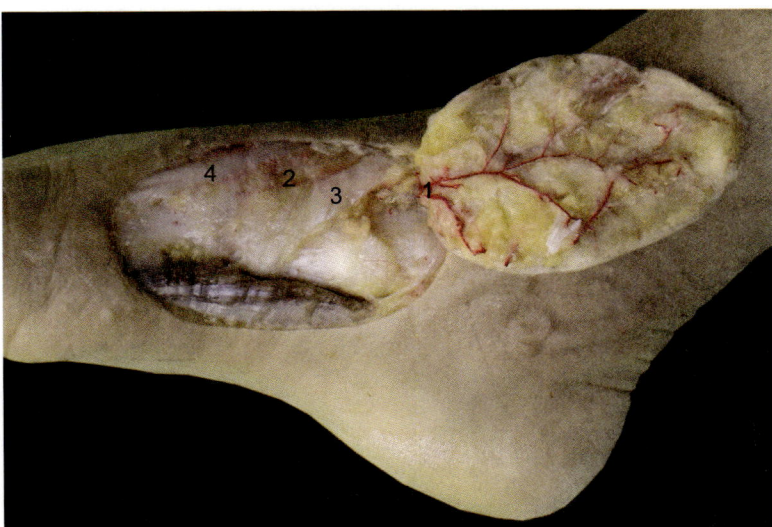

1. Medial anterior malleolar artery
2. Medial tarsal artery
3. Anterior tibial tendon
4. Extensor pollicis longus muscle tendon

Figure 1-190   **Dissection of the flap**

The lateral border of the flap should be incised, and the extensor pollicis longus muscle tendon drawn laterally. If necessary, the anterior tibial tendon should be incised in Z-plasty to facilitate the dissection of the vascular pedicle. The pedicle should be separated closely along the superficial surface of the periosteum and raised carefully. Then the circumference of the flap should be incised. The flap could be made a sensate one with the saphenous nerve or medial dorsal pedis cutaneous nerve included in it.

Key points in applied anatomy

Firstly, the pedicle of the superficial branch of the medial plantar artery has many advantages. The artery is located superficial and so it could be found and harvested easily. It gives many cutaneous branches. And its pedicle could be extended to the medial plantar artery or even the posterior tibial artery. The medial pedis flap based on the superficial branch of the medial plantar artery might be transferred anterogradely to the medial malleolus, the calcaneal tendon or the heel. Secondly, the pedicle of the deep branch of the medial plantar artery extends relatively deep and gives medial deep and superficial branches to anastomose with the medial anterior malleolar artery and the medial tarsal artery. Its final branch generally anastomoses with the plantar metatarsal artery, which is large enough to serve as the vascular pedicle of a medial flap that might be transferred retrogradely to restore a defect on the dorsal foot or on the distal plantar foot. Thirdly, the pedicle of the medial anterior malleolar artery is situated in the deep layer of the extensor hallucis tendon and could not be dissected easily because of the overlying tendons. However, this pedicle is suitable for a flap that might be transferred to the medial malleolus or the calcaneal tendon. Fourthly, the pedicle of the medial tarsal artery varies in length from case to case. The flap might be transferred only to the dorsal pedis or the distal plantar. Fifthly, the vascular direction and anastomotic position should be confirmed preoperatively with the Doppler. Sixthly, the medial pedis flap, whether it is transferred anterogradely, retrogradely, or freely, should be harvested under the deep fascia and be dissect include the arteries and the perivascular deep fascia to guarantee an adequate blood supply. Seventhly, when the medial plantar artery is being harvested as its pedicle, the flap should first be incised from the posterior inferior border. Then the abductor hallucis muscle should be dissected to expose the medial pedis artery and its branches, and sequentially, the other borders be dissected. Eighthly, the flap donor site should be restricted excluding the weight-bearing area, especially the 1st metatarsal head. Ninthly, as for a free flap with a pedicle of the medial anterior malleolar artery or the medial tarsal artery, the vascular pedicle should be harvested from the proximal to the dorsal pedis artery to ensure that it is long and large enough. Tenthly, a retrograde medial pedis flap should be based on the anastomotic branch of the medial pedis artery and the plantar metatarsal artery, with its pivot point located at the middle segment of the 1st metatarsal bone. When the flap is being transferred with its distal base, the perivascular fascia should be retained so that the pedicle could be wide enough (1.5-2.0 cm) to include the anastomotic branch.

33   Lateral Pedis Flap

The lateral pedis flap is located at the lateral dorsal pedis. It depends on the lateral tarsal artery for its blood supply. It might be transferred to repair a wound on the lateral malleolus, the calcaneal tendon, the dorsal pedis or the plantar. It might also be transferred retrogradely to restore a skin defect on the forefoot.

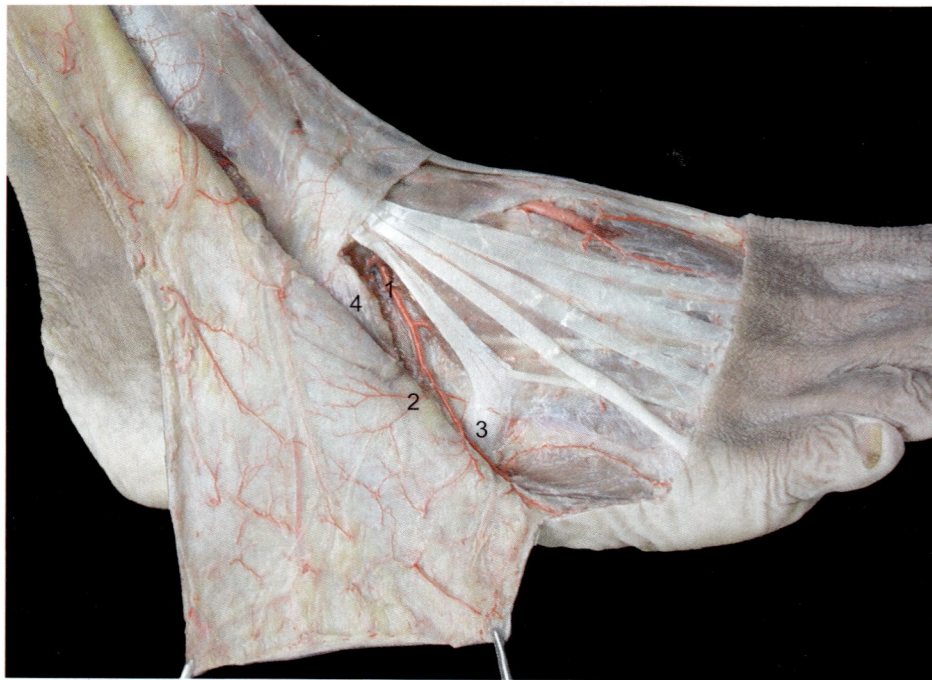

1. Lateral tarsal artery
2. Lateral tarsal cutaneous branch
3. Tuberosity of 5th metatarsal bone
4. Extensor digitorum brevis

Figure 1-191	Applied anatomy

The lateral tarsal artery emerges from the dorsal pedis artery and courses laterally along the navicular bone. It extends in the deep layer of the extensor digitorum brevis, close to the dorsal cuboid bone until it reaches the base of the 5th metatarsal bone. It sends two final branches: the anterior and the posterior branches. Its body surface projection might fall on the connection between the pulsatile point of the dorsal artery and the 5th metatarsal base. The lateral tarsal artery gives muscular branch (0.2-0.7 mm in diameter), osseous branch, direct cutaneous branch and perforating musculocutaneous branch. The direct cutaneous artery enters the deep fascia and extends superficially to the subcutaneous tissue. The perforating musculocutaneous artery passes vertically through the extensor digitorum brevis to the deep fascia and then extends superficially to the subcutaneous tissue. It is 0.3-0.7 mm in diameter and 0.8-1.2 cm in length.

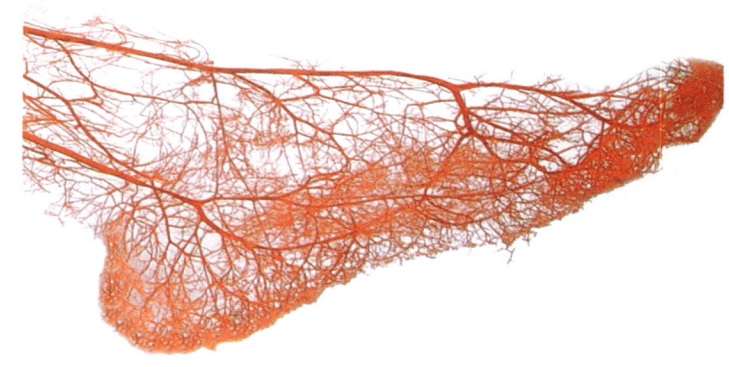

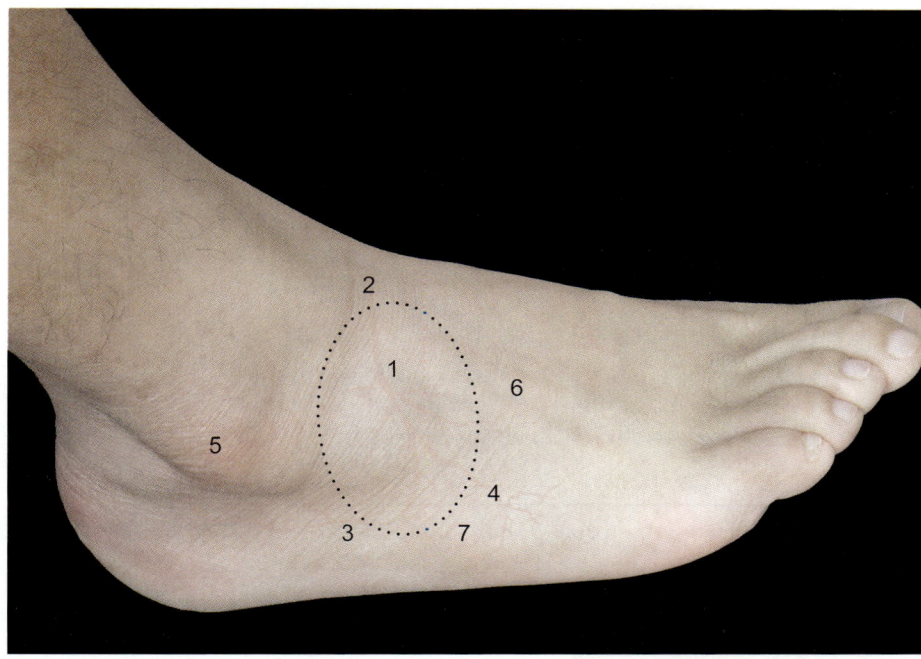

1. Body surface projection of lateral tarsal artery
2. Pivot point of the pedicle of lateral tarsal artery
3. Pivot point of the posterior branch of final branch
4. Pivot point of the anterior branch of final branch
5. Lateral malleolus
6. Extensor digitorum longus tendon
7. Plantar 5st metatarsal bone

Figure 1-192   Design of the flap

The flap should be designed with the lateral tarsal artery as its axis line, its pivot point located on the pulsating point of the dorsal pedis artery, which is at the level of the connecting line between the medial malleolus and the lateral malleolus. If it is based on the posterior branch of the lateral tarsal artery, its pivot point should be located at 2cm behind the 5th metatarsal base. If it is based on the anterior branch of lateral tarsal artery, its pivot point should be located at 2.0 cm in front of the 5th metatarsal base. The flap might account for a size of 6.0cm×4.0cm.

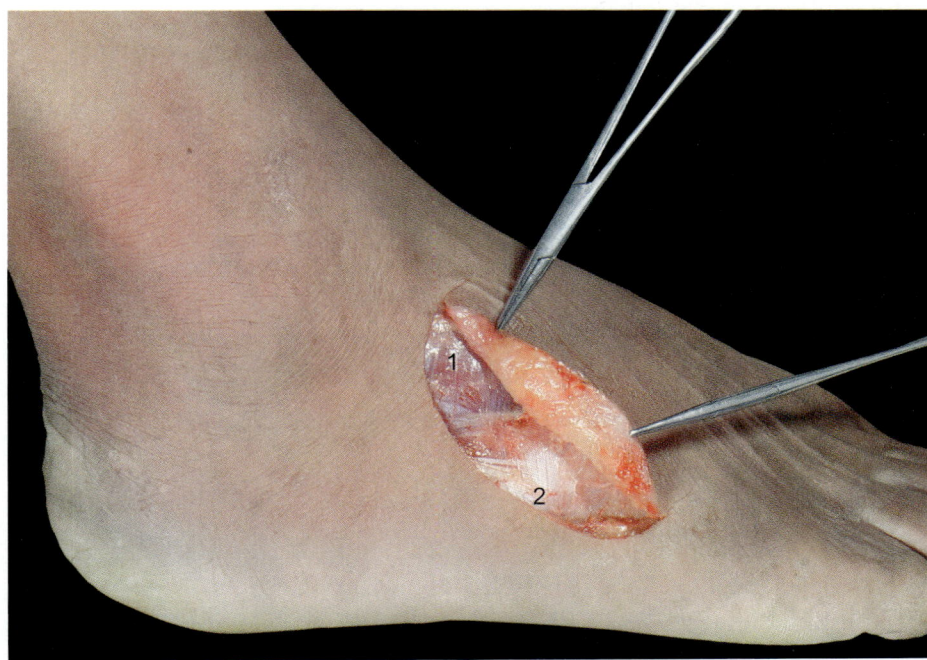

1. Extensor digitorum brevis
2. Tuberosity of 5th metatarsal bone

Figure 1-193   Dissection of the flap

The flap should be first incised from its posterior border and then elevated from under the deep fascia to expose the extensor digitorum brevis.

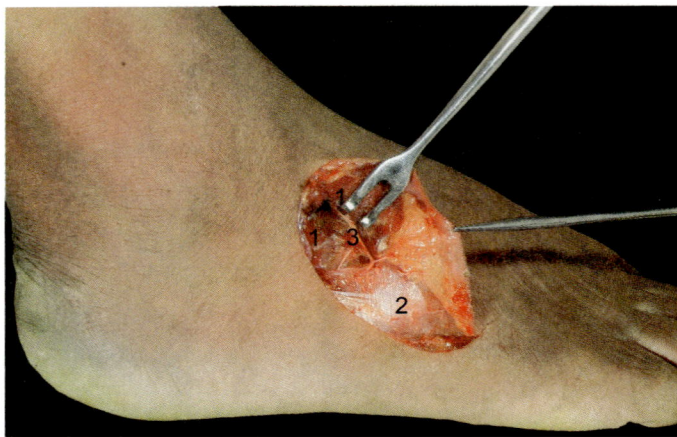

1. Extensor digitorum brevis
2. Tuberosity of 5th metatarsal bone
3. Lateral tarsal artery

Figure 1-194 **Exposure of the vessels**

The extensor hallucis brevis muscle and the extensor digitorum brevis should be cut and turned distally to expose the lateral tarsal artery.

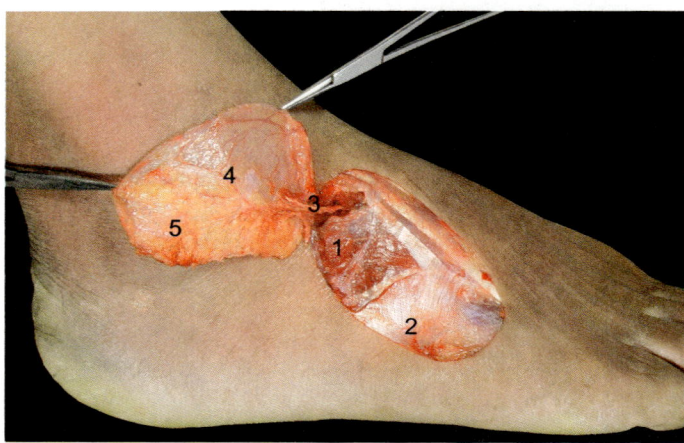

1. Extensor digitorum brevis
2. Tuberosity of 5th metatarsal bone
3. Lateral tarsal artery
4. Cutaneous branch of lateral tarsal artery
5. Flap

Figure 1-195 **Elevation of the flap**

Once the branch of the lateral tarsal artery is confirmed to have been included in, the other borders should be incised, and the flap elevated with the pedicle. If a retrograde one is needed, the separation of the pedicle should be done along the lateral tarsal artery in the medial extensor digitorum brevis and trace to the plantar 5th metatarsal bone onto the pivot point. The flap could be harvested pedicled with either the anterior or the posterior branch of the lateral tarsal artery.

Key points in applied anatomy

The flap based on the lateral pedis artery might be transferred to the heel, the lateral malleolus, the dorsal foot, or the distal plantar foot. A free flap might be transferred to the hand. Firstly, the flap for the restoration of the heel or the lateral malleolus should be designed with its axial line falling on the body surface projection of the lateral tarsal artery and its pivot point located at 2 cm behind the 5th plantar metatarsal bone. The flap for the restoration of the dorsal foot or the distal plantar foot should be designed with its pivot point at 2 cm in front of the 5th plantar metatarsal bone. Secondly, the courses and branches of the vessels should be confirmed preoperatively with the Doppler. Thirdly, from the hemodynamic viewpoint of retrogration, a stally-based flap might have a relatively poor blood supply compared with an anterograde one and so it should be restricted in size. Fourthly, the vessel and the skin should be properly sutured together to prevent a pull-off. Fifthly, the vascular pedicle should be long enough to reach the recipient region without tension, twist or sharp angulation. If the pedicle vessel is too small in certain cases, it should be harvested with part of the perivascular muscle and fascia (2 cm wide) to guarantee its blood supply.

Lateral Calcaneal Flap

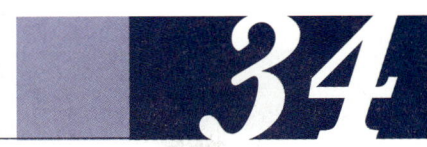

The lateral calcaneal flap is based on the lateral calcaneal artery and vein, the lesser saphenous vein and sural nerve. It is situated at the lateral side of the calcaneus and has such advantages as an adequate blood circulation, a concealed location, a dense tissue and a sensory function. It might be transferred anterogradely to restore a defect on the calcaneus, the plantar or the lateral malleolus, or transferred retrogradely to restore a defect on the forefoot, or transferred freely to repair a wound on the palm, the first web space, or the wrist. This type of flaps might also be designed as a musculocutaneous one with part of the extensor digitorum brevis to reconstruct hand intrinsic muscular function.

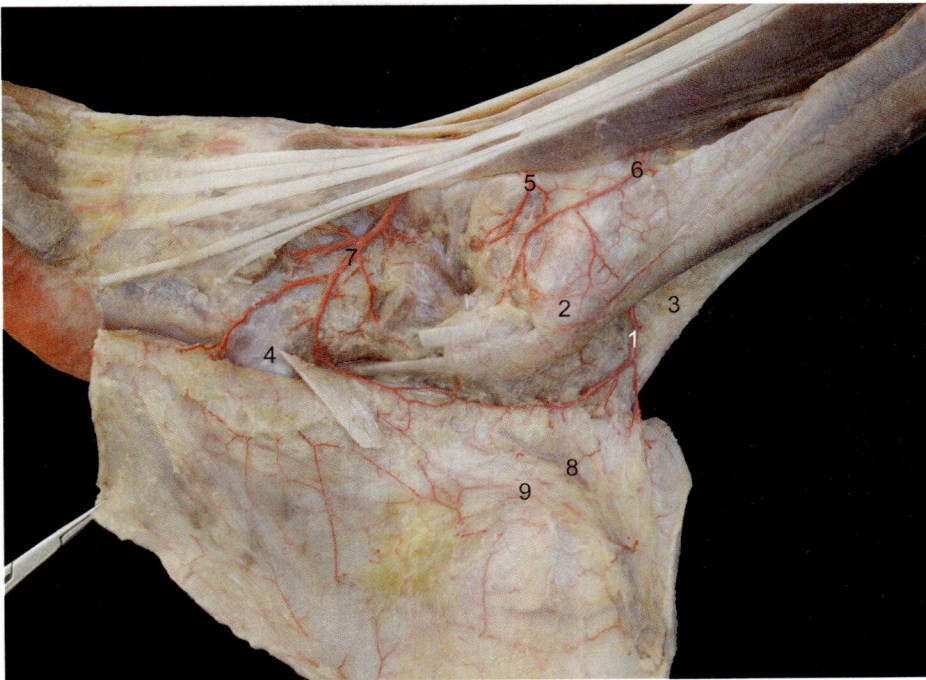

1. Lateral calcaneal artery
2. Lateral malleolus
3. Calcaneal tendon
4. Tuberosity of 5th metatarsal bone
5. Anterior lateral malleolus artery
6. Descending branch of peroneal perforating artery
7. Lateral tarsal artery
8. Lesser saphenous vein
9. Sural nerve

Figure 1-196	Applied anatomy

The lateral calcaneal artery, the axial artery of the flap, is an anastomotic branch of the terminal branch of peroneal artery and the posterior tibial artery. It extends distally and covers 5-8mm in front of the calcaneal tendon at the lateral malleolus level. It continues inferiorly in an arch to 3cm below the lateral malleolus, and then horizontally to the base of the 5th metatarsal bone. The lateral calcaneal artery anastomoses extensively with the anterior lateral malleolus artery, the descending branch of the peroneal perforating artery and the lateral tarsal artery. The lesser saphenous vein extends through the superficial layer of the flap. The sural nerve extends from the posterolateral of the lower leg to the dorsal pedis and there it is termed as the lateral dorsal cutaneous nerve of the foot. The nerve divides into two final branches under the lateral malleolus: the medial and the lateral branches. The medial branch fans out over the lateral calcaneal skin.

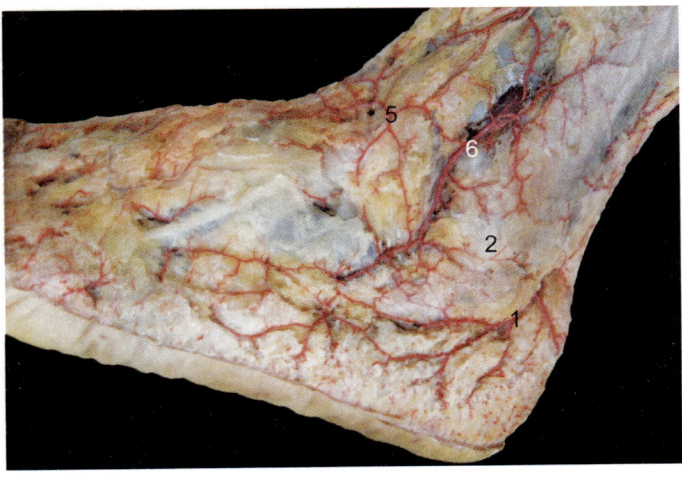

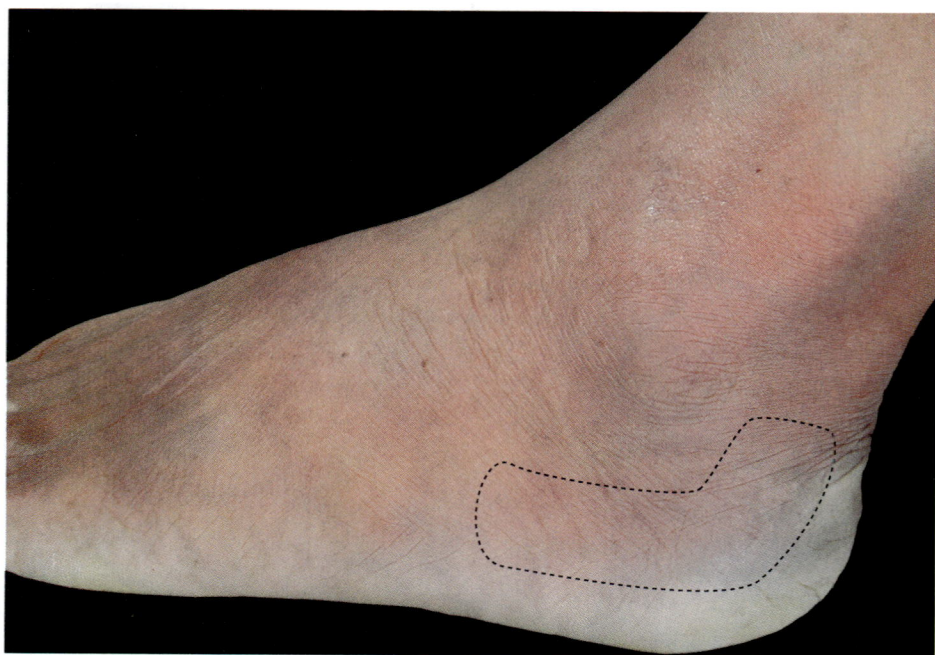

Figure 1-197	**Design of the flap**

The flap should be designed in L-shape with the lateral calcaneal artery or the midline between the lateral malleolus and the calcaneal tendon as its axial line. Its posterior margin should be the connecting line between the lateral malleolus and the calcaneal tendon, its anterior extending to the tuberosity of the 5th metatarsal bone, its medial to about 1/3 lateral dorsal pedis and its lateral to the lateral pedis

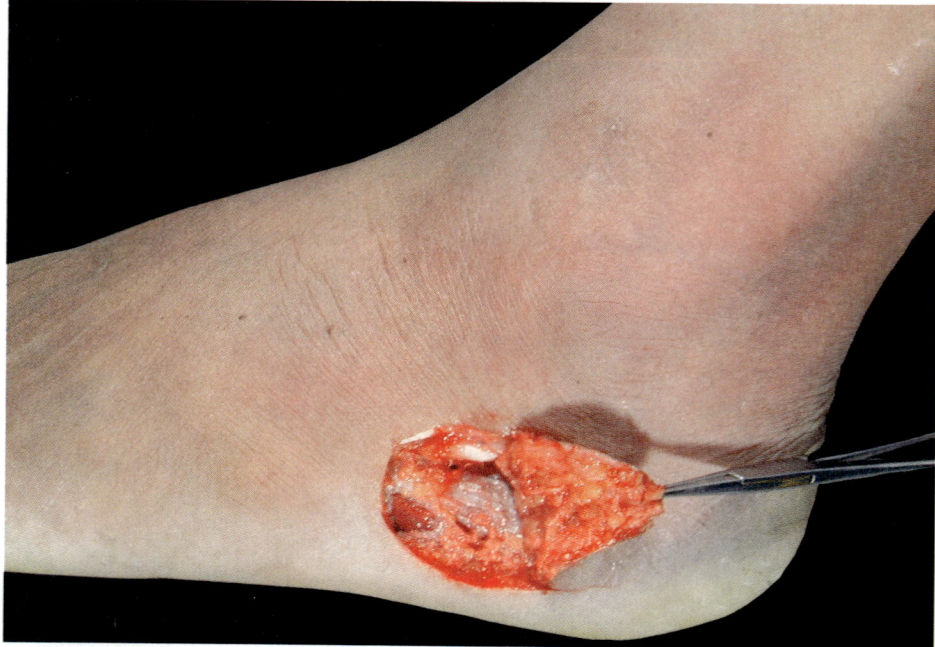

Figure 1-198	**Dissection of the flap**

The flap should be incised from its distal border and then its bilateral ones down to the deep fascia. It should then be elevated from distal to proximal, attaching closely to the periosteum, the abductor digiti minimi, the musculus peroneus longusi and the musculus peroneus brevis. The dissection should extend to its pivot point in the space of the calcaneal tendon and the lateral malleolus. The lateral calcaneal artery should be given great attention to avoid damages.

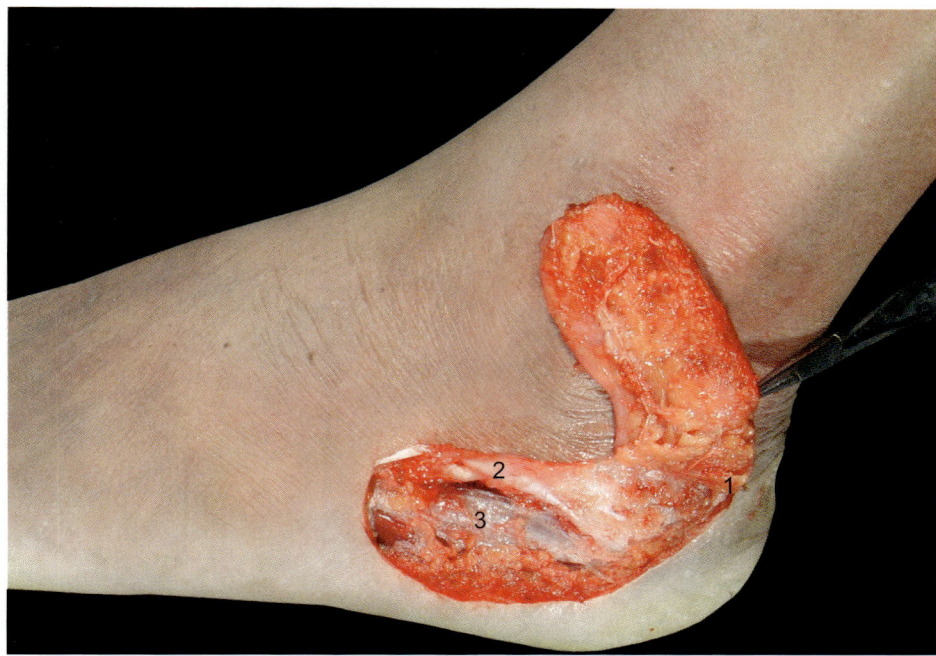

1. Lateral calcaneal artery
2. Musculus peroneus longus /brevis
3. Muscular branch of abductor digiti minimi

Figure 1-199   **Elevation of the flap**

There are communicating branches that enter the plantar metatarsal region. These branches should be ligated in the operation. The lateral calcaneal vessels should be identified and included before the flap is isolated.

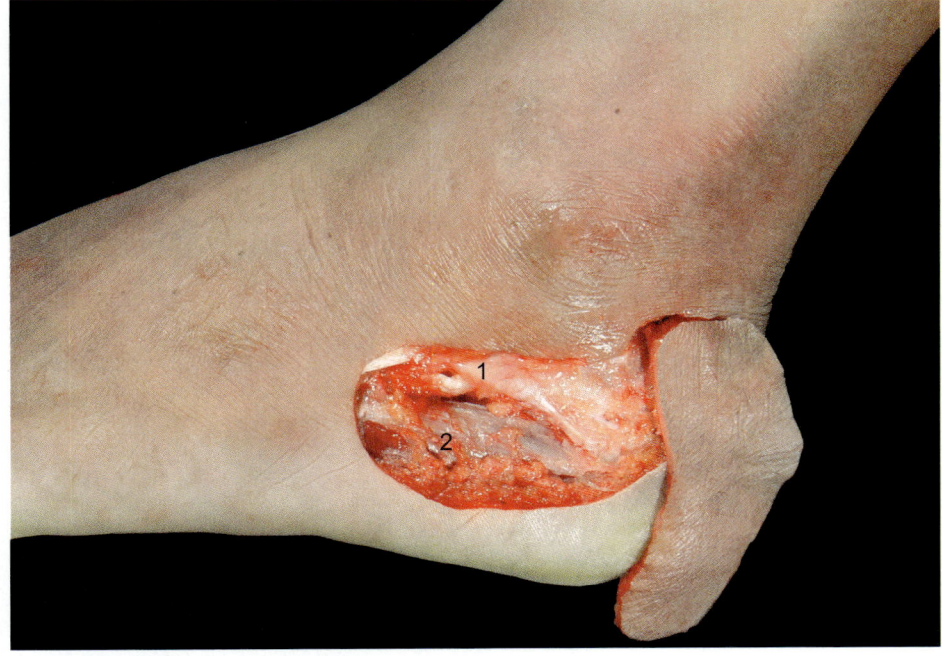

1. Musculus peroneus longus/brevis
2. Abductor muscle of little finger

Figure 1-200   **Transposition of the flap**

Once the flap is elevated completely, it might be transferred posteriorly to repair a wound on the calcaneus. The donor region might be repaired with a split-thickness skin graft.

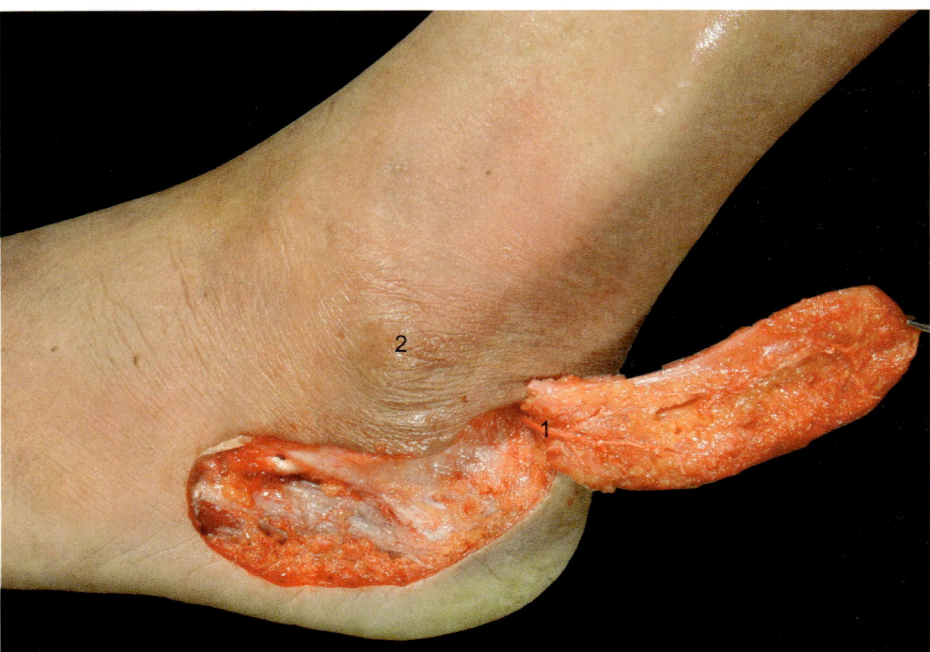

| **Figure 1-201** | **Transposition of the flap** |

The pedicled lateral calcaneal flap might be rotated through the subcutaneous tunnel or the direct skin opening to the recipient region.

1. Lateral calcaneal artery
2. Lateral malleolus

Key points in applied anatomy

Firstly, the course and the branches of the lateral calcaneal artery should be confirmed preoperatively with the Doppler. Secondly, there are generally 4 groups of arteries from different sources in the donor region. Anyone of them might be chosen as the pedicle of the lateral calcaneal flap. In a few cases (9.1-15.0%), the terminal branches of the perforating peroneal artery are smaller than 0.5mm in diameter, or there may be no terminal branches at all. In some other cases (5%), the perforating peroneal artery is large and extends as the dorsal pedis artery, one of the major arteries for foot circulation. Therefore, in either of the two variations, it is preferable that other artery be chosen as the flap pedicle. Thirdly, according to the relation between the vascular pedicle and the osseous blood supply in the flap, different osseous cutaneous flaps might be designed. The lateral calcaneal artery might serve as the main vascular pedicle of a osseous cutaneous flap carrying a bloc of the posterior lateral calcaneal bone; the descending branch of peroneal artery, the main vascular pedicle of the osseous cutaneous flap carrying a bloc of the anterior lateral calcaneal bone; the lateral tarsal artery, the main vascular pedicle of the osseous cutaneous flap carrying a bloc of the cuboid bone. In an operation, attention should be given to avoid a disconnection of the skin and the bone. Fourthly, once the lateral tarsal artery in a distally based flap is ligated proximally, its end should be sutured with the skin to avoid damaging the cutaneous branch due to a directly pull. Fifthly, the pedicle should be separated laterally to make it long enough for a tension-free transplantation. If the artery is small in diameter, the perivascular muscular tissue and fascia (2cm wide) should be retained so that the pedicle could be wide enough to guarantee a sufficient blood supply. Sixthly, the lateral dorsal cutaneous nerve of the foot gives the medial and the lateral branches at 2.7cm below the lateral malleolus. The medial branch should be included in the flap for the sensory function. It should be separated proximally until it is long enough for the recipient suture. The lateral branch should be retained in situ to guarantee the sensory function of the 4th and 5th digital regions. Seventhly, the proximal portion of the flap should be restricted to keep intact the skin overlying the lateral malleolus and the calcaneal tendon and to avoid the scar formation.

Chapter II
Muscle and Musculocutaneous Flaps

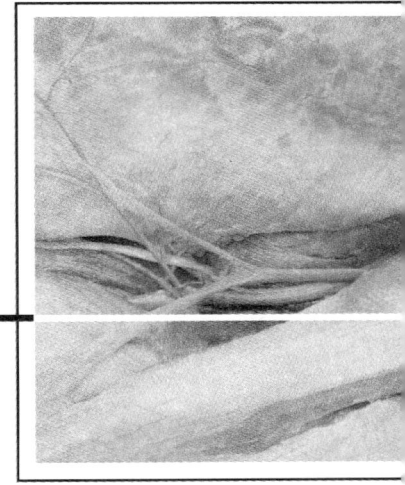

Types of Blood Supply for Muscles

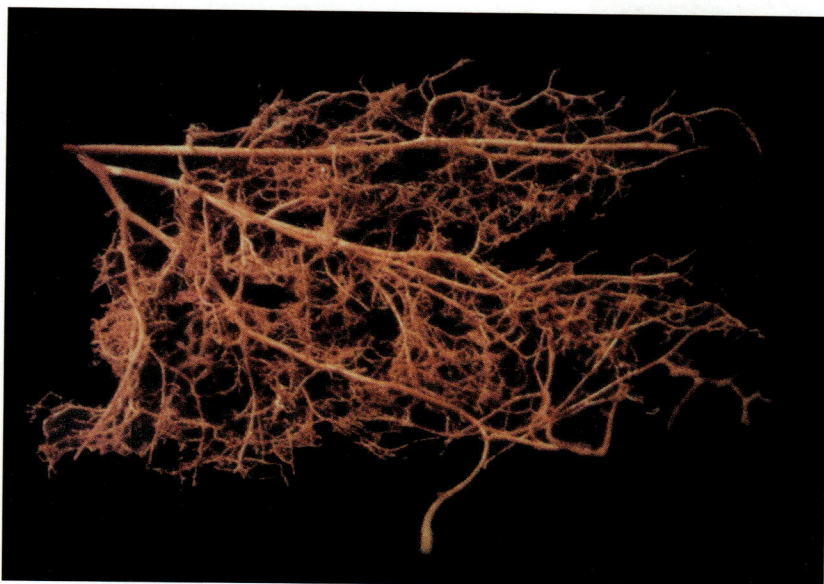

| Figure 2-1 | A single arterial-trunk flaps |

There is only one arterial trunk in the muscle that extends along the long muscular axis and gives main branches to nourish the whole muscle. Along the course, these branches send many smaller sub-branches to fan out over the muscle belly, such as the tensor fasciae latae muscle, the medial head of the gastrocnemius muscle, and the lateral head of the gastrocnemius muscle.

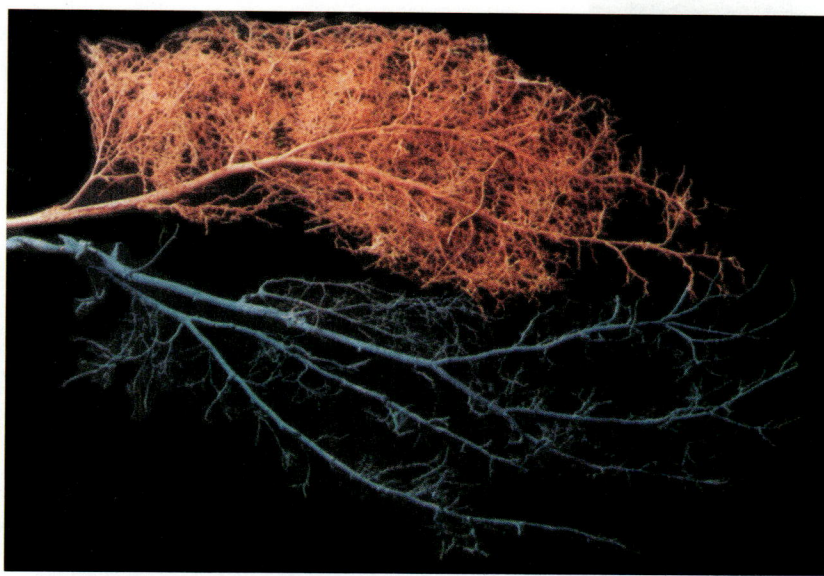

| Figure 2-2 | Double arterial-trunks flaps |

There are two arterial trunks that enter the muscle at different positions and extend in different regions. It is not necessary that the two are equal in vascular diameter and supplied area. Cases in point are the gluteus maximus muscle (upper and lower part), the rectus femoris muscle and the gastrocnemius muscle (medial and lateral head).

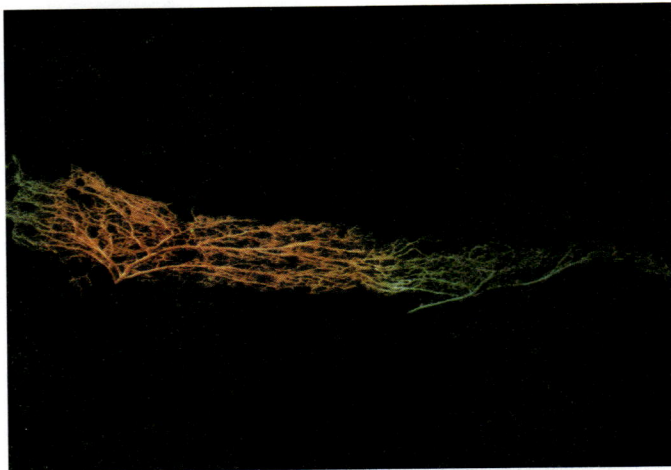

| Figure 2-3 | Segmental-arterial flaps |

There are several arteries that enter the muscle at different positions, extend in different regions and anastomose with one another rather extensively. Cases in point are the sartorius muscle, the gracilis muscle and the sternocleidomastoid muscle.

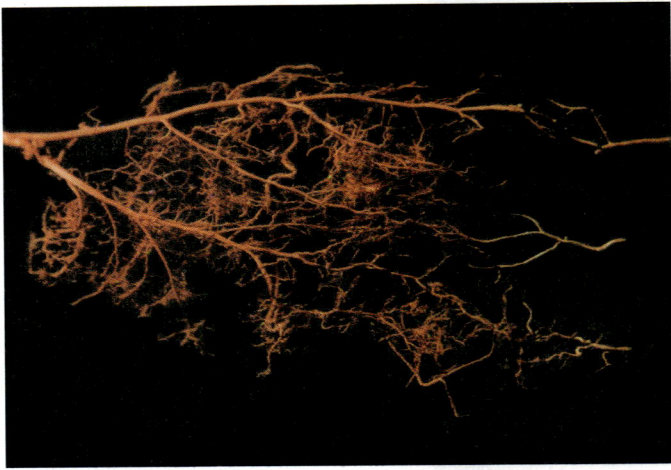

| Figure 2-4 | Combined-arterial flaps |

There are many arteries to nourish the muscle, among which, the largest one enters the muscle through the muscular portal to fan out over most part of the muscle belly. Other small arteries enter the muscle peripherally to fan out over the peripheral part of the muscle. Cases in point are the latissimus dorsi muscle and the trapezius muscle.

Key points in applied anatomy

Firstly, as for the single trunk type and the double-trunk type, the myoplasm is concentrated to form a visible muscle belly. The arteries are constant in diameter and enter the muscle at constant places, accompanied by the motor nerves and the lymphatic vessels to form a clear muscular portal. Therefore, muscle flaps of these types might be harvested with long neurovascular pedicles. And it is possible that muscular or musculocutaneous flaps be designed for free grafting. Secondly, as for the segmental arterial type, it is possible that a muscular flap be designed for transplantation under the condition that one vessel is retained as a pedicle. Thirdly, as for the combined vascular type, it is possible that a whole muscle or musculocutaneous flap be designed based on the main arterial trunk. It is also possible that a partial muscle flap be designed nourished by several arterial branches but still pedicled with the main arterial trunk.

Deltoid Muscle Flap

2

The deltoid flap depends on the posterior circumflex humeral artery for its blood supply and on the superior lateral brachial cutaneous nerve for its innervation. A flap of this type might be transferred locally to restore a soft tissue defect on the ipsilateral shoulder, on the superior back or in the axillary fossa.

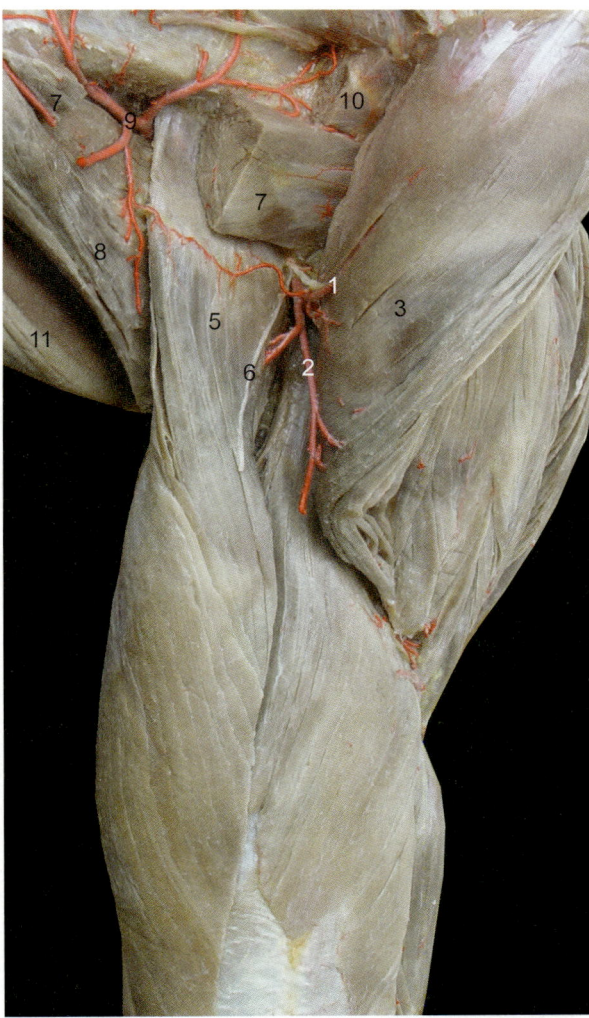

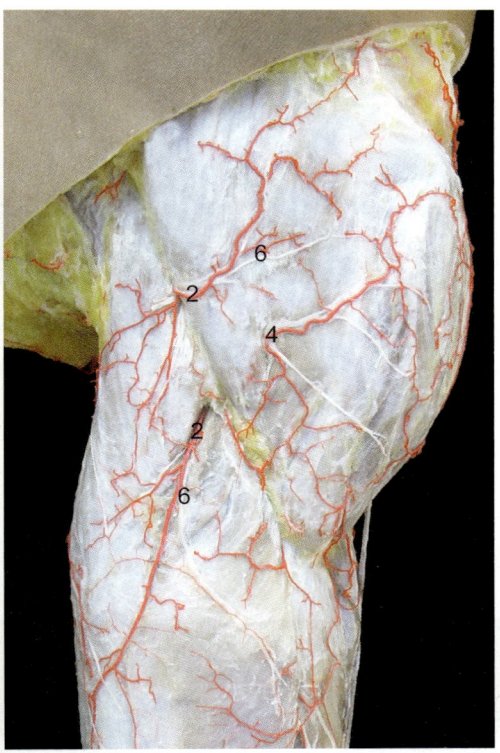

Figure 2-5	Applied anatomy

The posterior circumflex humeral artery passes through the quadrilateral space, and turns around the posterior lateral side of the surgical neck of the humerus to give the deltoid muscular and the posterior marginal branches. The former nourishes the deltoid muscle, and is 2.0-2.5 mm in diameter. In addition, some smaller perforating branches perforate through the deltoid muscle to fan out over the superficial skin. The latter (1-2 in general) is 0.8mm in diameter and 5cm in length. It extends inferiorly outwards and perforates through the septum of the deltoid muscle and the triceps brachii muscle via the mid portion of the posterior margin of the deltoid muscle to enter directly the subcutaneous tissue. It accompanies the superior lateral brachial cutaneous nerve.

1. Muscular branches of deltoid muscle
2. Posterior marginal branch
3. Deltoid muscle
4. Perforating branches
5. Triceps brachii muscle
6. Superior lateral brachial cutaneous nerve
7. Teres minor muscle
8. Teres major muscle
9. Circumflex scapular artery
10. Infraspinous muscle
11. Latissimus dorsi muscle

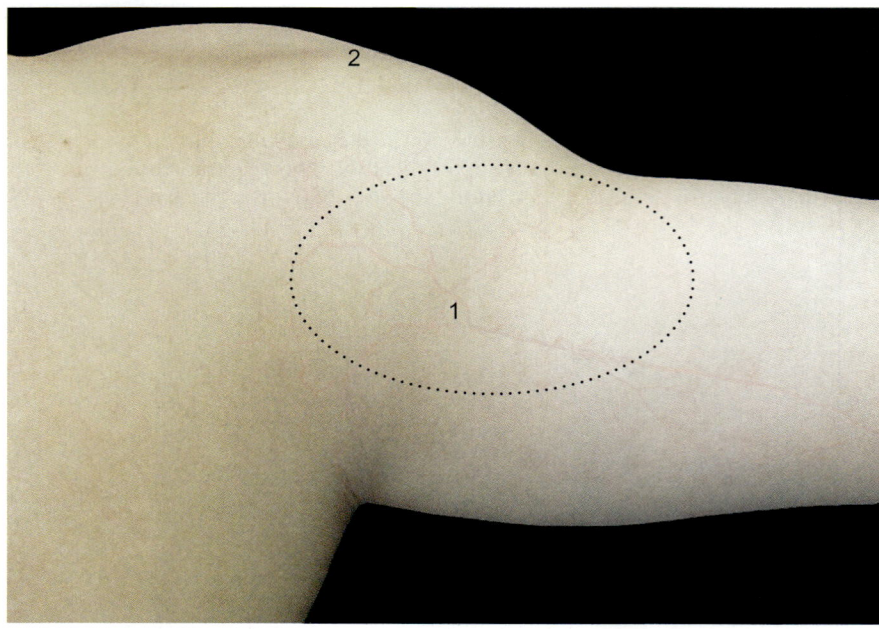

1. Point through which the posterior marginal branch perforates
2. Acromial angle

| Figure 2-6 | Design of the musculocutaneous flap |

The point through which the posterior marginal branch perforates the middle portion of the deltoid muscle should be confirmed with the Doppler. Based on it, the flap might be designed with its pivot point located at the quadrangular space or at 7cm below the acromial angle correspondingly and its distal end reaching 5cm above the olecranon.

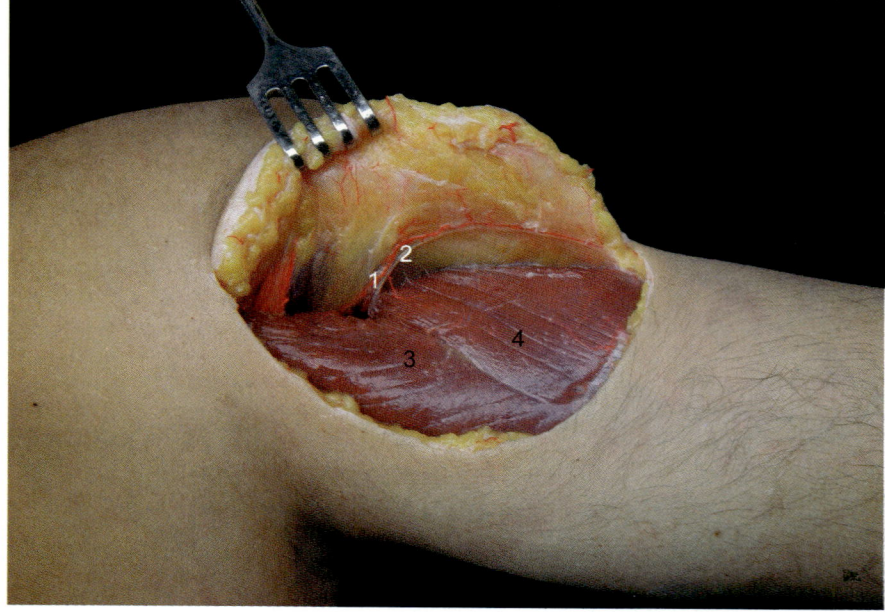

1. Cutaneous branch of posterior circumflex humeral artery
2. Superior lateral brachial cutaneous nerve
3. long head of triceps brachii muscle
4. lateral head of triceps brachii muscle

| Figure 2-7 | Dissection of the musculocutaneous flap |

As has been designed, the flap should be incised from its posterior border and elevated anteriorly along the plane beneath the deep fascia to the posterior margin of deltoid muscle. The perforating cutaneous branches at this region should be given great attention to avoid getting them damaged.

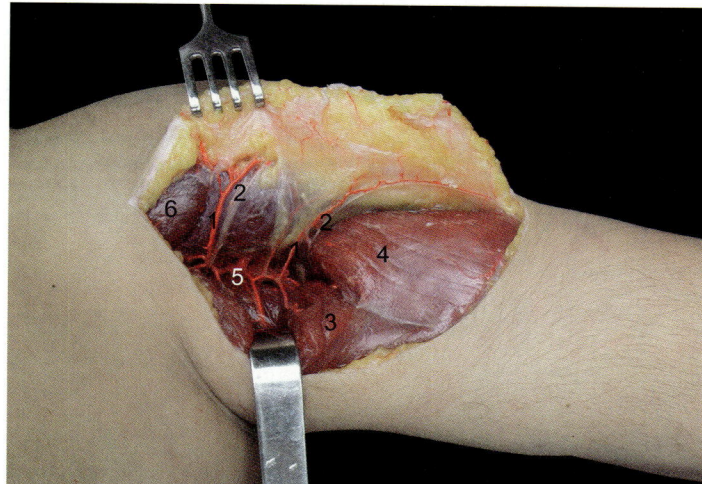

Figure 2-8   Exposure of the vessels

The incision of the flap should begin with its proximal border and continue retrogradely along the cutaneous branch to the quadrangular space to expose the trunk of the posterior circumflex humeral artery.

1. Cutaneous branch of posterior circumflex humeral artery
2. Superior lateral brachial cutaneous nerve
3. Long head of triceps brachii muscle
4. Lateral head of triceps brachii muscle
5. Trunk of posterior circumflex humeral artery
6. Deltoid muscle

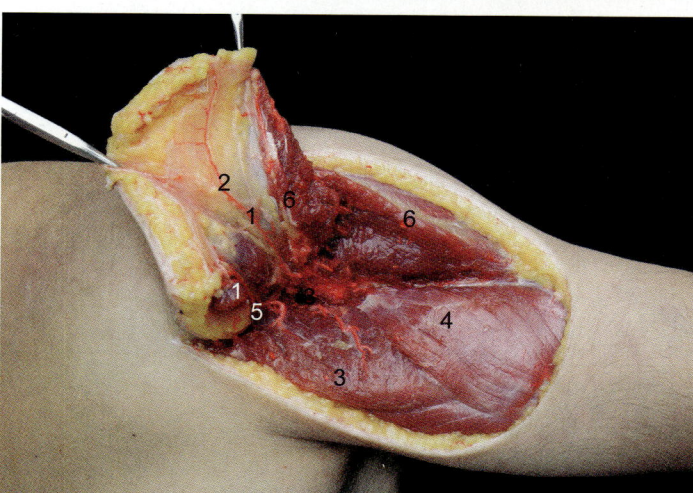

1. Cutaneous branch of posterior circumflex humeral artery
2. Superior lateral brachial cutaneous nerve
3. Long head of triceps brachii muscle
4. Lateral head of triceps brachii muscle
5. Trunk of posterior circumflex humeral artery
6. Deltoid muscle

Figure 2-9   Elevation of the musculocutaneous flap

The posterior portion of the deltoid muscle should be separated bluntly. After the vascular direction in the deep muscle is identified, part of the deltoid muscle and the overlying skin should be cut to make a compound flap with a pedicle of the posterior circumflex humeral artery. A flap of this type might be transferred locally to repair an adjacent trauma.

Key points in applied anatomy

Firstly, the flap should be dissected including only the posterior part of the deltoid muscle and the overlying skin. Secondly, since the posterior marginal branch of the posterior circumflex humeral artery and its accompanying nerves perforate through the lower portion of the posterior deltoid muscle (equal to the quadrangular space which is 7cm below the acromion) to enter the skin, the incision of the flap should begin from the medial portion to the posterior portion of the deltoid muscle. Thirdly, in some cases the ascending branch of the deep brachial artery might take the place of the posterior circumflex humeral artery, it should not be mistaken for a common branch nor should it be ligated. In other cases no arterial trunk could be found in the quadrangular space. Fourthly, the motor branches of the superior lateral brachial cutaneous nerve to the deltoid muscle and teres minor muscle should be retained and untouched when a sensitive flap is expected. The superior lateral brachial cutaneous nerve should be dissected bluntly from distal to proximal in the procedure. Fifthly, since the deltoid muscle is closely integrated with the fascia and subcutaneous tissue, there is little mobility between the different layers. A deltoid flap might be transferred to restore the weight-bearing area on the heel or the planta with satisfactory result.

Brachioradialis Muscular Flap

The brachioradial muscle is situated superficial. It depends on the radial collateral artery and the radial recurrent artery for its blood supply. Its motor innervation comes from the radial nerve. Its function is to supplement the elbow flexion and the forearm pronation. The muscle might be used as a dynamic muscle to replace the paralyzed biceps brachii muscle.

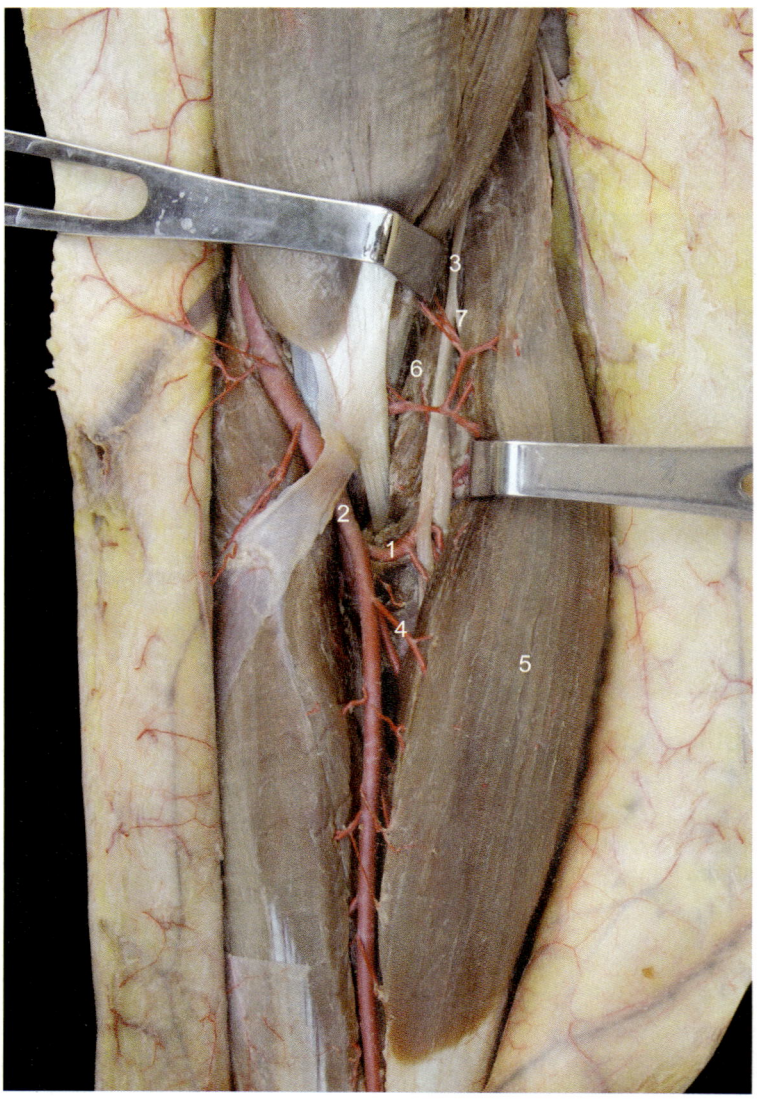

Figure 2-10   Applied anatomy

The radial recurrent artery emerges from the radial artery and extends laterall upwards across the radial nerve to anastomose with the radial collateral artery. Along the course, it gives branches to nourish the middle-superior segment of the brachioradial muscle. The radial collateral artery is the terminal branch of the deep brachial artery, whose anterior branch accompanies the radial nerve, perforates through the lateral brachial intermuscular septum to extend in the septum between the brachialis muscle and the brachioradial muscle and gives branches to nourish the superior segment of the brachioradial muscle. The motor innervation of the brachioradial muscle comes from the branches of the radial nerve, which enters the muscle at the superior one-third.

1. Radial recurrent artery
2. Radial artery
3. Radial nerve
4. Muscular branch
5. Brachioradial muscle
6. Brachial muscle
7. Branches of radial nerve

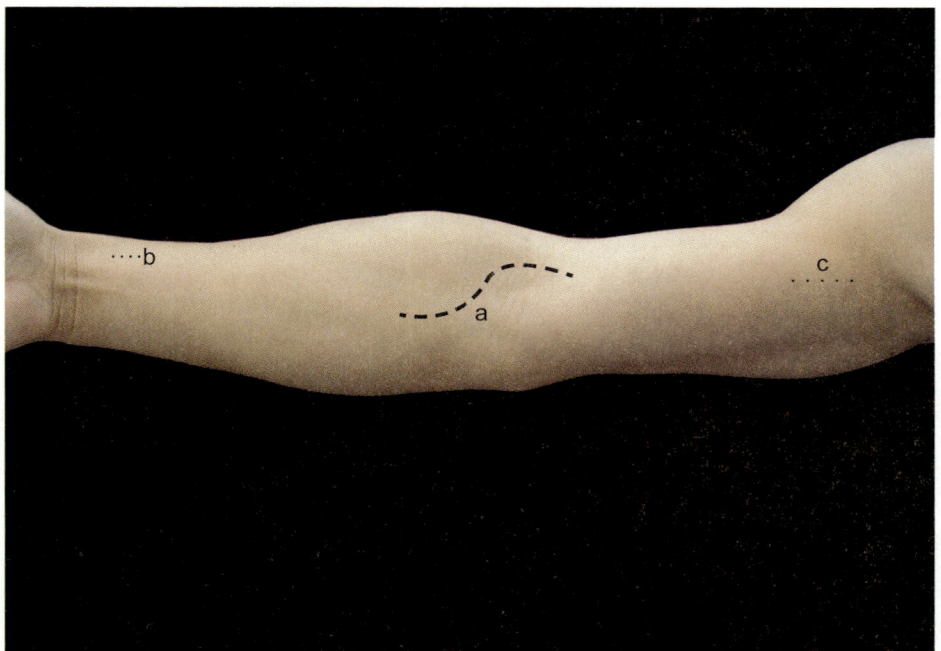

Figure 2-11   Design of the incision

The patient should be placed in supine position, and three incisions designed: 'S'-shaped incision A should be designed at the anterior elbow, its superior extends to 9cm above the external epicondyle of humerus, its inferior extends along the anterior margin of the brachioradial muscle to 2cm under the cubital transverse crease; incision B extends at 1cm above the styloid process of the radius on the anterior surface for 2cm long; incision C under the insertion of the pectoralis major muscle for 4cm long.

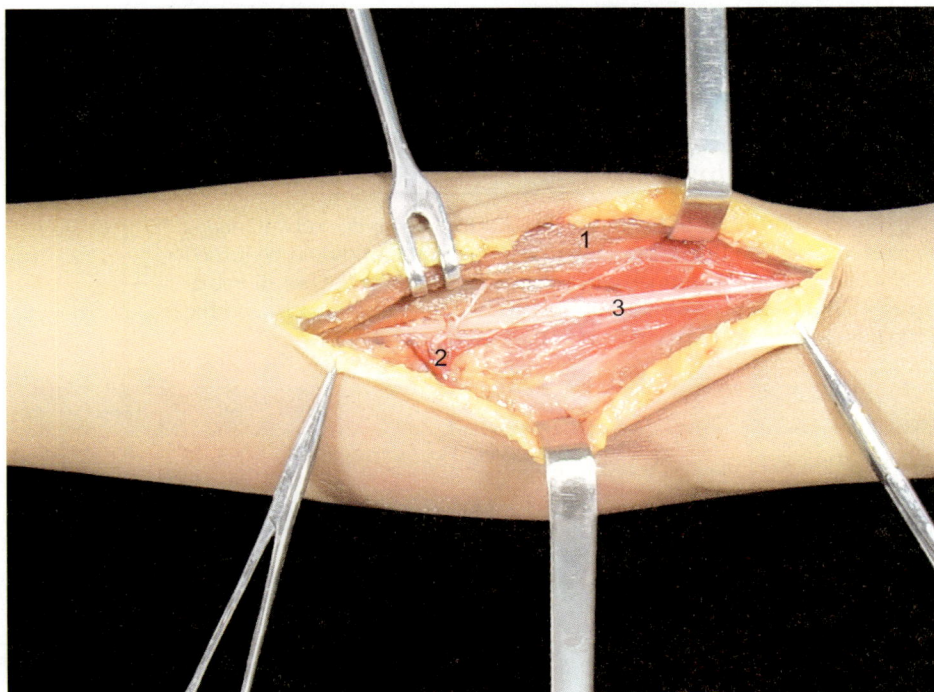

1. Brachioradial muscle
2. Radial recurrent artery
3. Radial nerve

Figure 2-12   Exposure of the vessels

Incision A should be made to expose the brachioradial muscle, from whose medial surface enter the arterial and nerval branches.

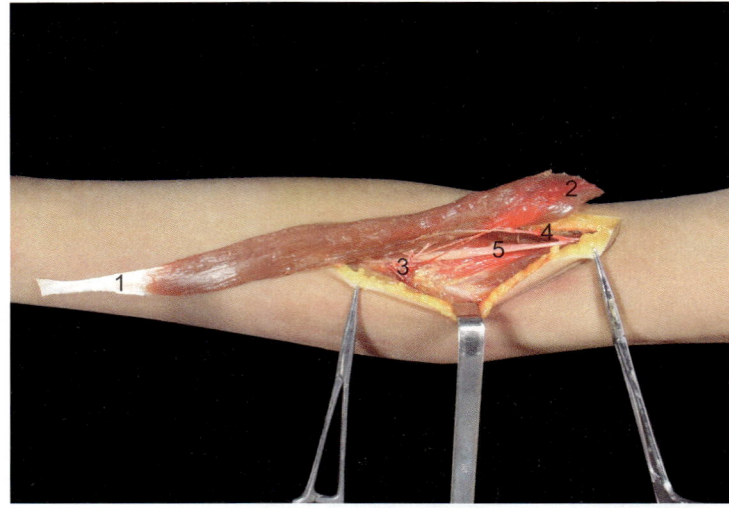

Figure 2-13   Elevation of the flap

The insertion of the brachioradial muscle should be cut at incision B, and its origin cut at incision A. The radial collateral artery should be ligated, and the neurovascular pedicle of the flap separated until it is long enough to guarantee a smooth transfer of the brachioradial muscle through the subcutaneous tunnel.

1. Insertion of brachioradial muscle
2. Origin of brachioradial muscle
3. Vascular pedicle
4. Nerval pedicle
5. Radial nerve

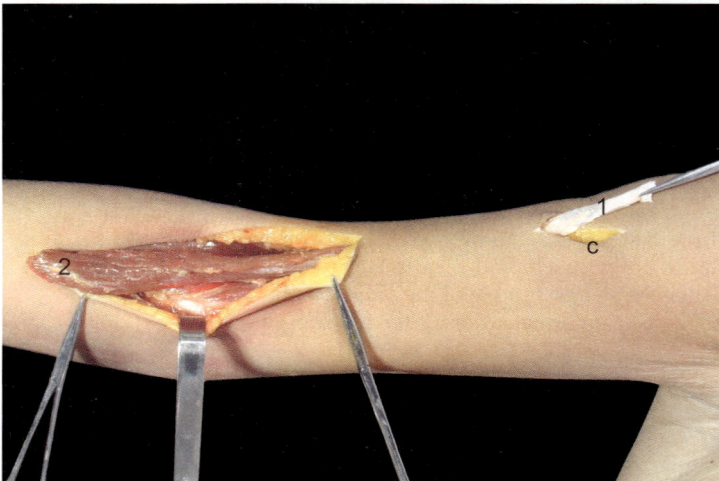

1. Insertion of brachioradial muscle
2. Origin of brachioradial muscle

Figure 2-14   Transposition of the muscular flap

Incision C should be made to expose the short head of the biceps brachii muscle, and a subcutaneous tunnel made along the muscle to reach the incision B. The brachioradialis muscular flap should be turned over 180 degree and pulled through the subcutaneous tunnel to incision C. The origin of the brachioradial muscle should be sutured and fixed with the aponeurosis insertion of the biceps brachii muscle, and the insertion of the muscular flap fixed with the origin of the short head of the biceps brachii muscle.

Key points in applied anatomy

Firstly, the tendon of the brachioradial muscle should be about 10cm long, which might be adjusted to the need of the recipient area when the flap is being dissected. Secondly, the origin of the brachioradial muscle is not a tendinous structure, but there is strong fascia attached on its surface, which is connected with the lateral brachial intermuscular septum. In the procedure, the fascia together with the septum should be included in the flap to guarantee a safe suture after the flap is transferred. Thirdly, the two groups of the neurovascular pedicles to the brachioradial muscle are both constant in origins and courses. The radial collateral artery is easy to find in the deep surface of the lateral head of the triceps brachii muscle under the insertion of the deltoid muscle; and since the radial recurrent artery is relatively short, its source vessel of the radial artery might be partially harvested as a pedicle if necessary. Fourthly, both groups of vessels give branches to nourish the adjacent muscle of the brachioradialis and the extensor carpi radialis longus, the two muscles might be cut together to make a compound muscular or musculocutaneous flap so that the muscular power and the flap area could be increase for a dynamic reconstruction.

Pronator Quadratus
Muscular Flap

4

The pronator quadratus muscle is situated in the deepest layer of the distal forearm and depends on the anterior interosseous artery for its blood supply. The flap should not be designed a musculocutaneous one but a deeply located muscular one that could be used to restore an adjacent soft tissue defect.

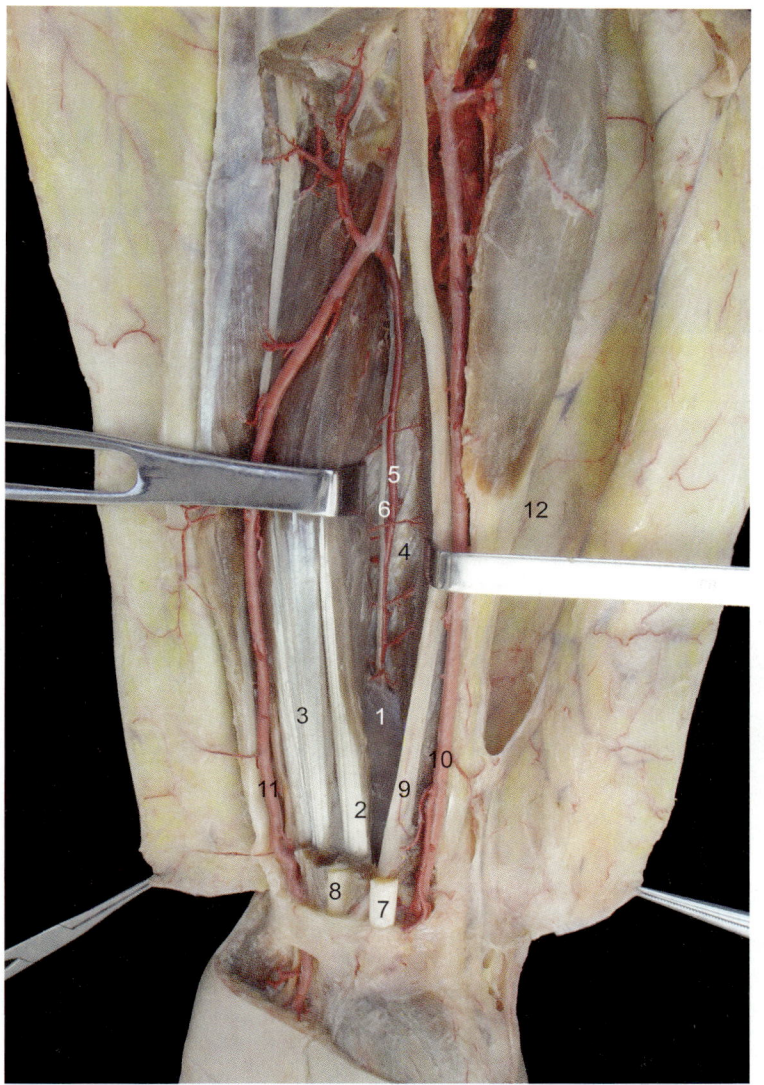

Figure 2-15   **Applied anatomy**

The pronator quadratus muscle is situated under the deep surface of the flexor pollicis longus muscle and the flexor digitorum profundus muscle at the distal anterior region of the forearm. It attaches closely to the radius, the ulna and the anterior interosseous membrane. The muscle looks like a quadrate with each limb about 4.5cm in length. The anterior interosseous artery descends just closely to the anterior interosseous membrane. It is 1.6 mm in diameter at the superior margin of the pronator quadratus muscle. It continues its way in the deep surface of the muscle and gives 3-7 branches to nourish the latter. These branches are 0.3-0.8mm in diameter. The anterior interosseous nerve accompanies the homonymous vessels.

1. Pronator quadratus muscle
2. Flexor pollicis longus muscle
3. Flexor digitorum profundus muscle
4. Interosseous membrane
5. Anterior interosseous artery
6. Anterior interosseous nerve
7. Flexor carpi radialis muscle
8. Flexor digitorum superficialis muscle
9. Median nerve
10. Radial artery
11. Ulnar artery
12. Brachioradial muscle

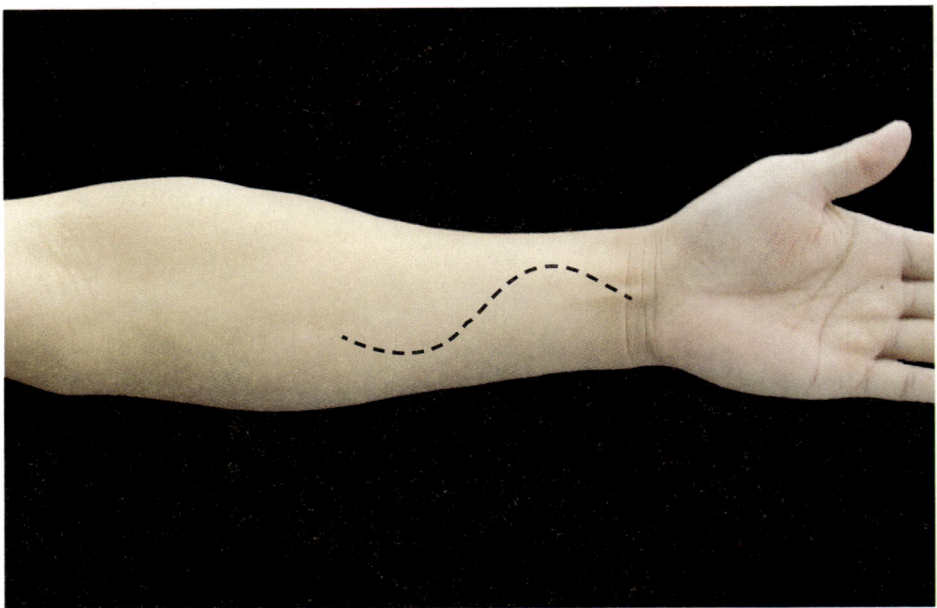

Figure 2-16   Design of the incision

A lazy "S"-shaped incision should be designed at the anterior forearm region proximally to the wrist crease.

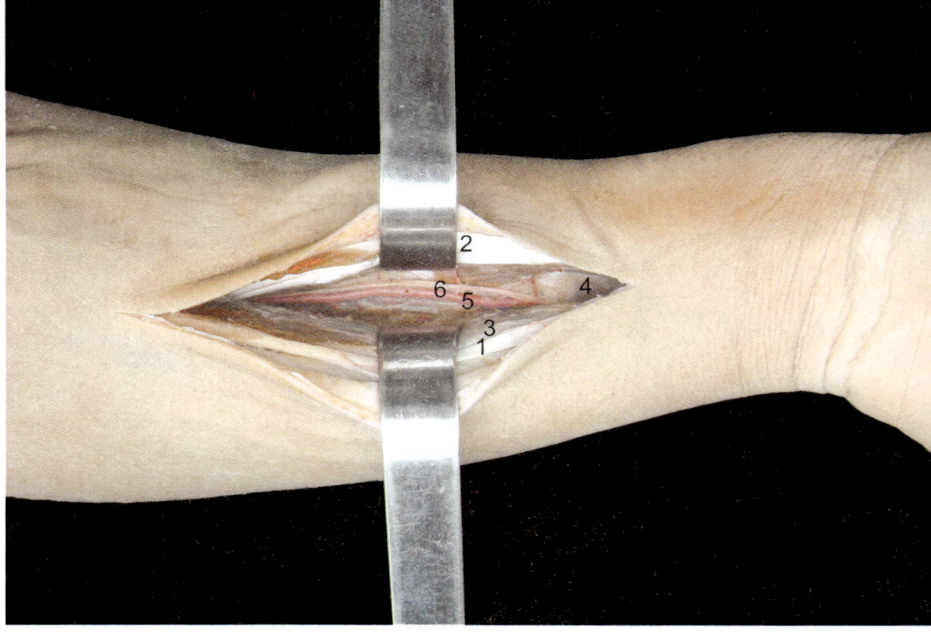

1. Palmaris longus muscle
2. Flexor pollicis longus muscle
3. Flexor digitorum profundus muscle
4. Pronator quadratus muscle
5. Anterior interosseous artery
6. Anterior interosseous nerve

Figure 2-17   Exposure of the muscle

The skin, the subcutaneous tissue and the deep fascia should be incised to expose the median nerve and keep it intact. The palmaris longus muscle and the flexor pollicis longus muscle should be drawn bilaterally to expose the pronator quadratus muscle at the deep layer between the flexor pollicis longus muscle and the flexor digitorum profundus muscle. The anterior interosseous artery and nerve descend closely to the anterior interosseous membrane to enter the muscle.

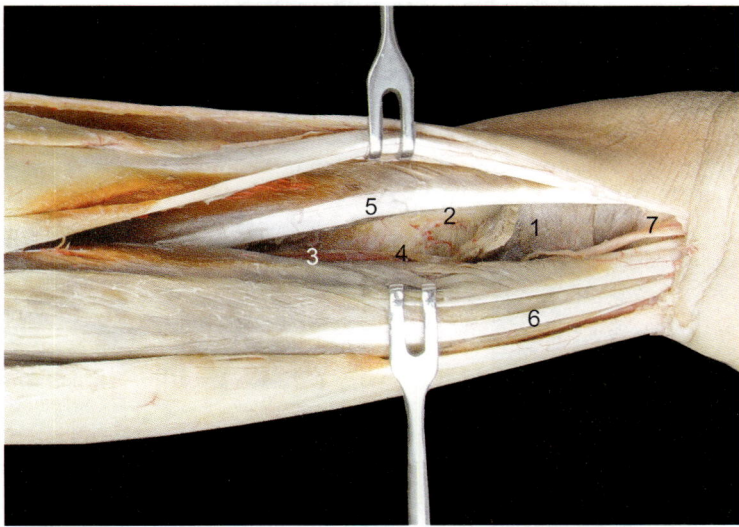

1. Pronator quadratus muscle
2. Radius
3. Anterior interosseous artery
4. Anterior interosseous nerve
5. Flexor pollicis longus muscle
6. Flexor digitorum superficialis muscle
7. Median nerve

Figure 2-18   **Dissection of the muscular flap**

The deep layer of the pronator quadratus muscle should be separated carefully, and then the muscle cut off from its attachment to the ulna and the radius.

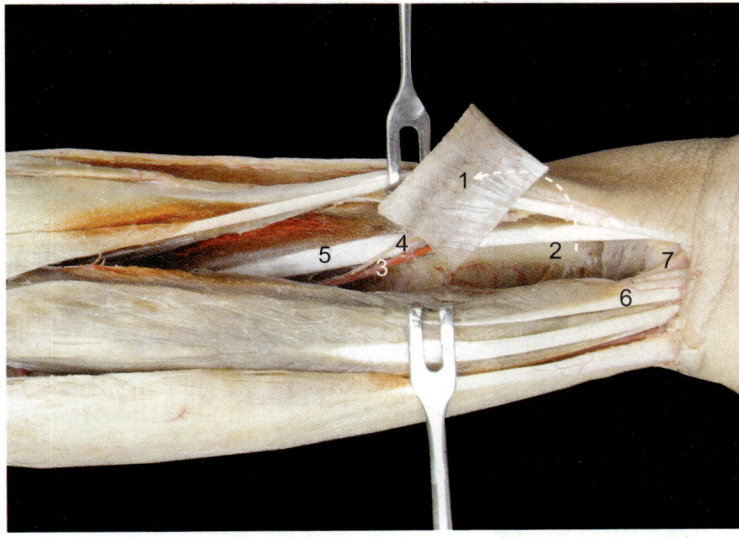

1. Muscular flap
2. Ulna
3. Anterior interosseous artery
4. Anterior interosseous nerve
5. Flexor pollicis longus muscle
6. Flexor digitorum superficialis muscle
7. Median nerve

Figure 2-19   **Transposition of the muscular flap**

Once the flap is completely dissected, the pedicle of the anterior interosseous vessels should be traced retrogradely to get enough length. The dissected flap might be used to restore a defect on the proximal area.

Key points in applied anatomy

Firstly, the median nerve should be kept intact in the procedure. Secondly, the flexor pollicis longus muscle and the flexor digitorum profundus muscle should be drawn bilaterally to expose adequately the pronator quadratus muscle and the vascular plexus. Thirdly, the vascular branches that enter the muscle should be protected when the flap is being elevated. Fourthly, the anterior interosseous nerve should be kept intact during the operation.

5

Abductor Digiti Minimi Musculocutaneous Flap

The abductor digiti minimi is situated in the hypothenar region. Based on it, a dynamic muscular flap might be designed and transferred to restore the opposition and abduction of the thumb at the cost of the abducent function of the digitus minimus.

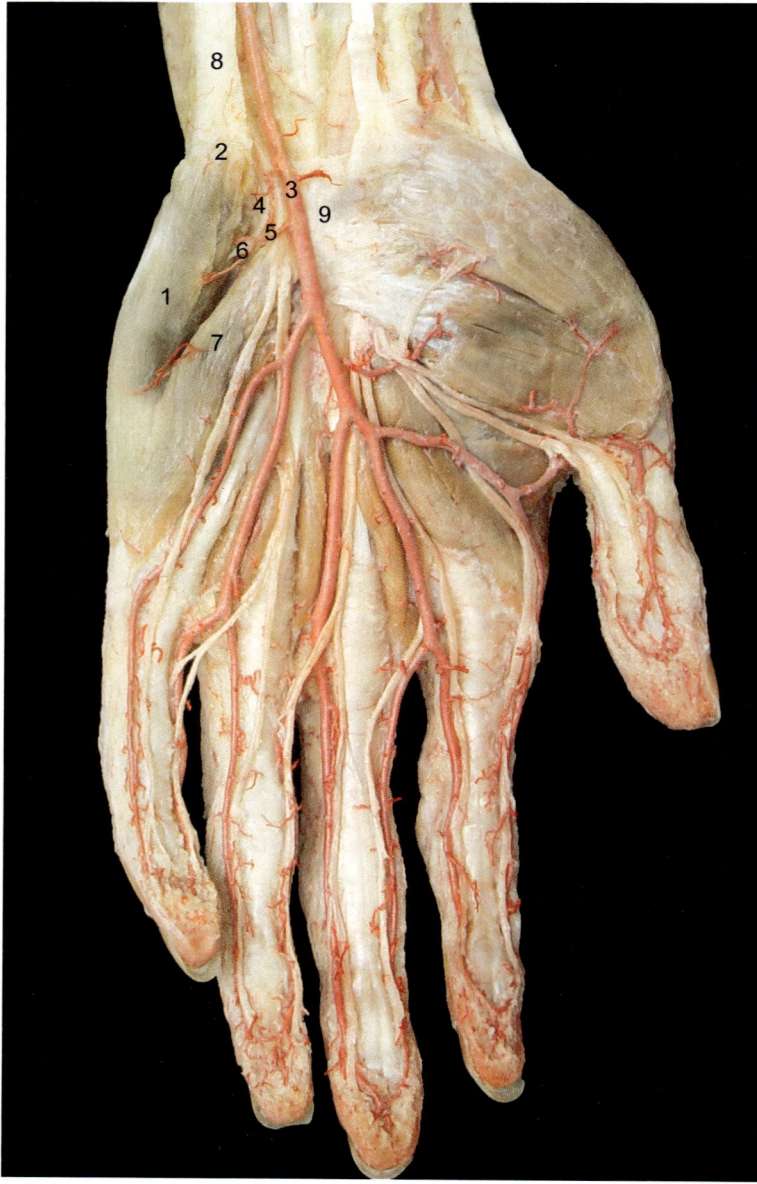

Figure 2-20	Applied anatomy

The abductor digiti minimi originates from the pisiform bone and the piso-hamate ligament and terminates at the ulnar condyle of the base of proximal phalanx base of the digitus minimus. The artery in the muscle emerges from the ulnar artery and the nerve from the deep branch of the ulnar nerve. At the hamate bone level, the ulnar artery is situated lateral to the ulnar nerve. It sends one muscular branch into the muscle at 1cm below the hamate bone and is accompanied by the muscular branch of the ulnar nerve. The musculocutaneous perforators and the direct cutaneous branches from the ulnar artery nourish the superficial layer of the hypothenar skin.

1. Abductor digiti minimi
2. Pisiform bone
3. Ulnar artery
4. Deep branch of ulnar nerve
5. Abductor digiti minimi muscular branch of ulnar artery
6. Abductor digiti minimi muscular branch of ulnar nerve
7. Flexor digiti minimi brevis muscle
8. Flexor carpi ulnaris muscle
9. Flexor retinaculum

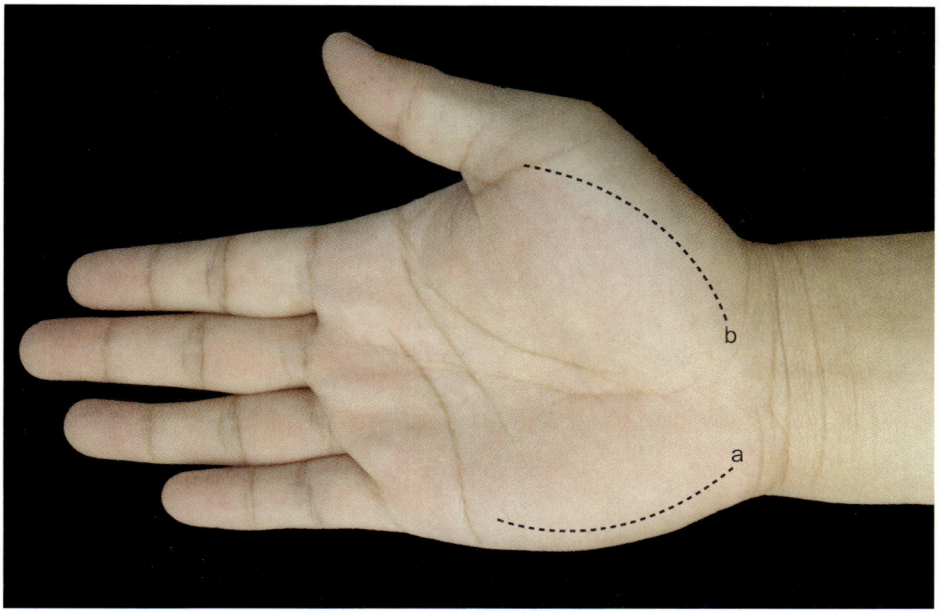

| Figure 2-21 | Design of the incision |

Take the functional reconstruction of opposition and abduction of the thumb for example. Incision A and incision B should be designed at the ulnar and the radial palm, respectively.
a. Ulnar palmar incision
b. Radial palmar incision

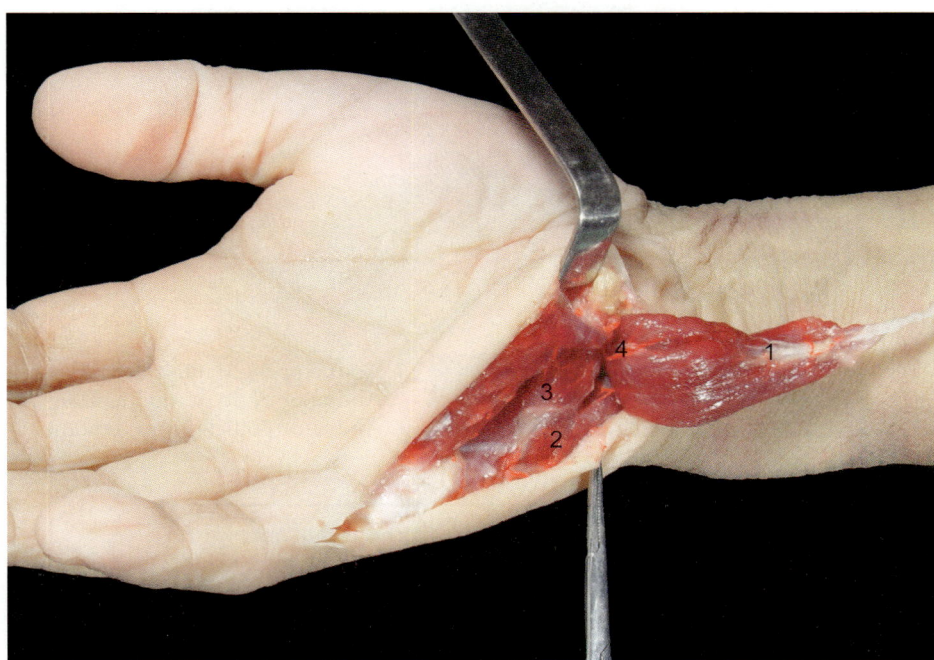

1. Abductor digiti minimi
2. Flexor digiti minimi brevis
3. Opponens digiti minimi
4. Neurovascular pedicle

| Figure 2-22 | Dissection of the muscular flap |

The incision A should be made to expose the abductor digiti minimi, and the muscular tendon cut at the distal. The flap should be elevated at the superficial layer of the flexor digiti minimi brevis and the opponens digiti minimi from distal to proximal. The neurovascular pedicle that enters the muscle around the hamate bone should be carefully protected.

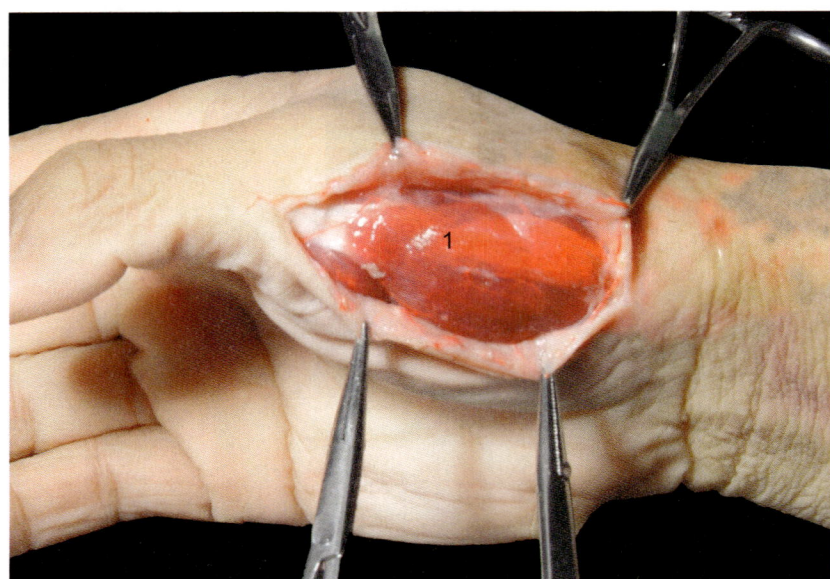

1. Abductor pollicis brevis

| **Figure 2-23** | **Separation of the abductor pollicis brevis muscle** |

The radial palmar incision should be made to expose and separate the abductor pollicis brevis.

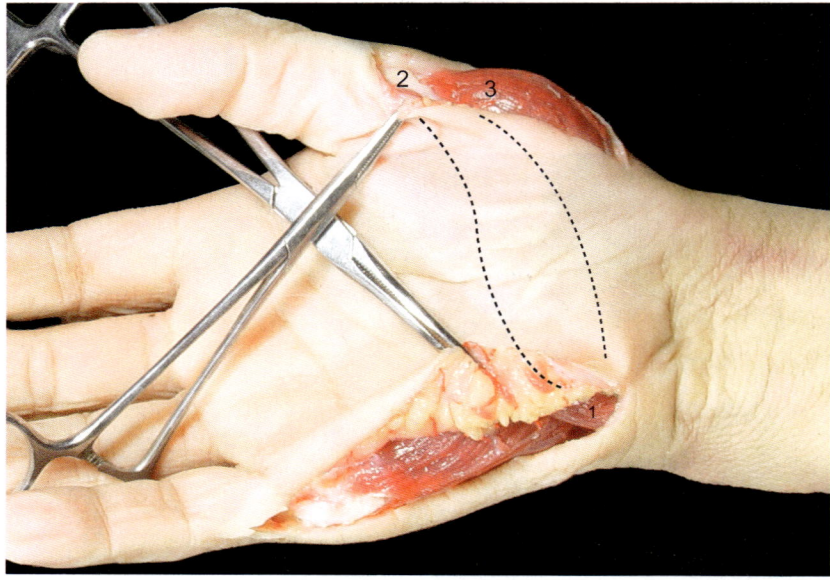

1. Abductor digiti minimi
2. Abductor digiti minimi tendon
3. Abductor pollicis brevis tendon

| **Figure 2-24** | **Transposition of the muscular flap** |

A wide subcutaneous tunnel should be made from the radial incision to the ulnar one, and the isolated abductor digiti minimi pulled out through the tunnel to the radial incision. The abductor digiti minimi tendon should be sutured with the abductor pollicis brevis tendon at the abduction-opposition position of the thumb, and the thumb fixed with a plaster cast for 4 weeks postoperatively.

Key points in applied anatomy

Firstly, the neurovascular pedicle of the muscle flap is constant. Its original position, which is around the hamate bone, might serve as the axis of the flap. Secondly, the neurovascular pedicles that enter the muscle should be kept intact around the hamate bone. Thirdly, the subcutaneous tunnel should be wide enough to guarantee a spacious pass for the muscular flap.

Gluteus Maximus Musculocutaneous Flaps

6

The gluteus maximus is the largest rhomboid muscles in the gluteal region. Since there are two main nutrient arteries (the superior gluteal artery and the inferior gluteal artery) in the muscle, double-arterial-trunk flaps might be designed in various shapes. A flap of this type might be mainly used in the treatment of decubitus pressure ulcer in the sacro-gluteal region. In nonparalytic patients, only part of the superior or the inferior gluteus maximus muscle should be included in the flap so that the hip-stretching function of the muscle could be preserved and the stability of the hip retained.

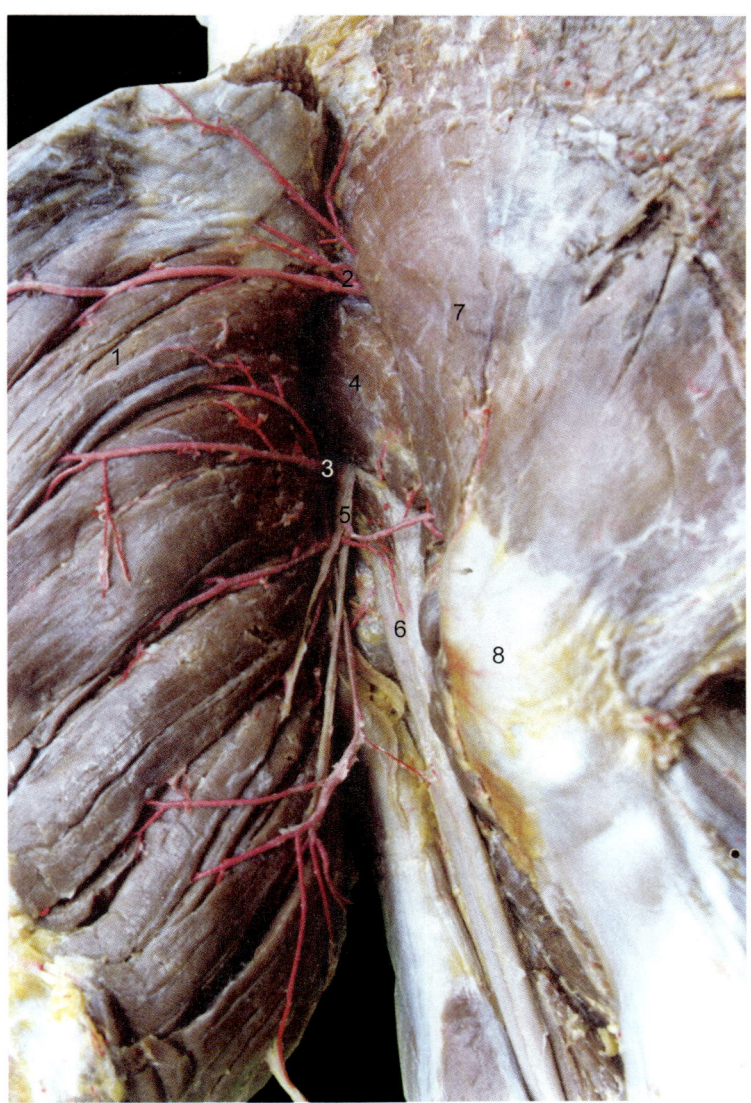

Figure 2-25	Applied anatomy

The superior gluteal artery and the inferior gluteal artery nourish the gluteus maximus muscle. The superior gluteal artery emerges from the superior margin of the piriformis muscle and immediately divides into the deep and the superficial branches. The deep branch runs deep with the superior gluteal nerve in the deep surface of the gluteus medius muscle. The superficial branch perforates superficially through the spatium between the piriformis muscle and the gluteus medius muscle and sends branches to fan out over the superior half of the gluteus maximus muscle. The inferior gluteal artery together with the inferior gluteal nerve runs out of the inferior margin of the piriformis muscle and gives muscular branches to the inferior half of the gluteus maximus muscle. It also gives cutaneous branches that extend superficially along the inferior margin of the gluteus maximus muscle to nourish the posterior thigh. Both the superior and the inferior gluteal arteries anastomose extensively with each other in the muscle.

1. Gluteus maximus muscle
2. Superior gluteal artery
3. Inferior gluteal artery
4. Piriformis muscle
5. Inferior gluteal nerve
6. Sciatic nerve
7. Gluteus medius muscle
8. Greater trochanter

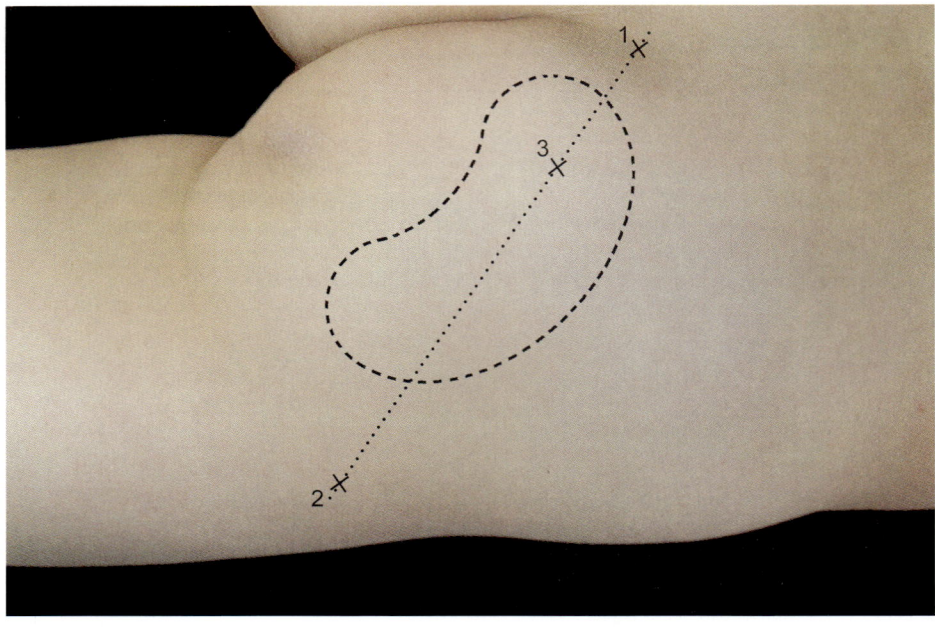

1. Posterior superior iliac
   spine
2. Greater trochanter of
   femur
3. The rotation point

Figure 2-26   **Design of the flap**

The patient in prone position, the flap should be designed along the line between the posterior superior iliac spine and the tip of greater trochanter of femur. Its pivot point should fall on the proximal 1/3 intersection of the line, where the superior gluteal artery perforates through the superior margin of the piriformis muscle.

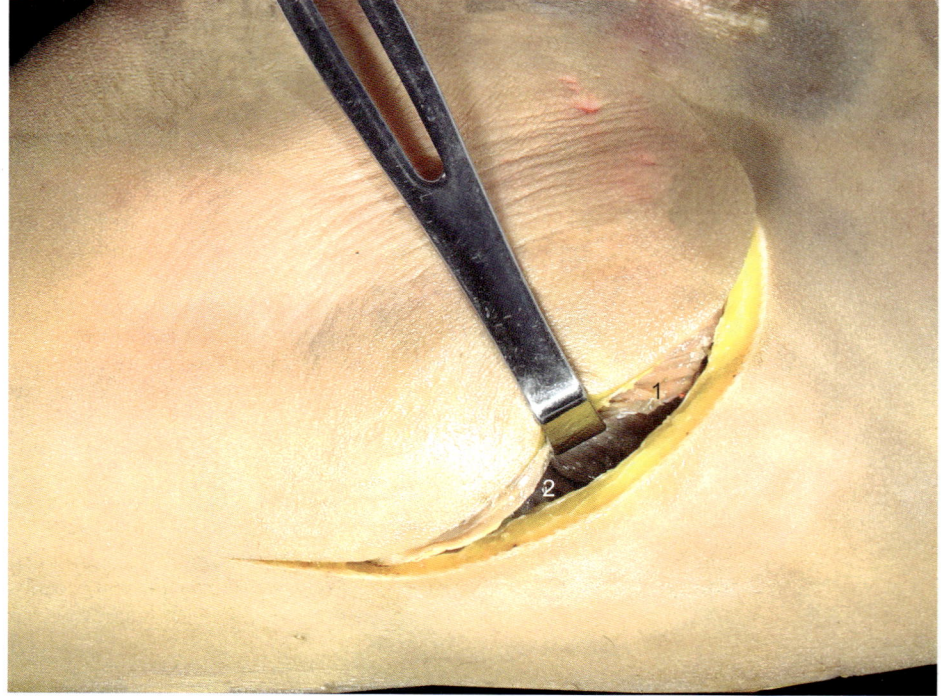

1. Gluteus maximus muscle
2. Gluteus medius muscle

Figure 2-27   **Exposure of the superior margin of gluteus maximus muscle**

As has been designed, an arch incision of the posterolateral hip approach should be made along the connecting line between the posterior superior iliac spine and the greater trochanter to identify the septum between the gluteus maximus muscle and the gluteus medius muscle.

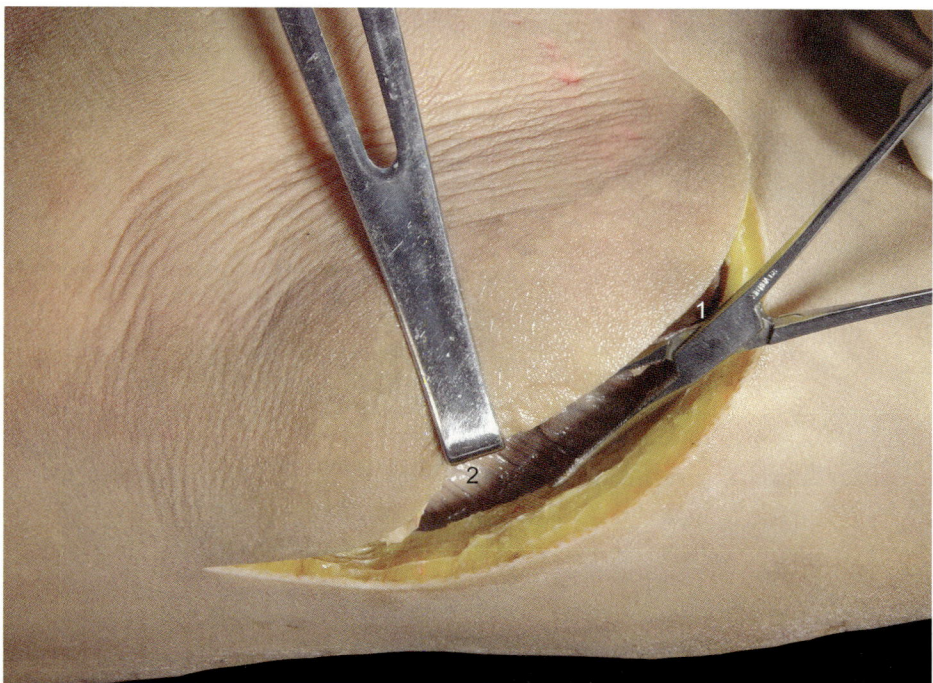

1. Gluteus maximus muscle
2. Gluteus medius muscle

Figure 2-28   **Separation of the gluteus maximus muscle**

The septum of the two muscles should be bluntly separated.

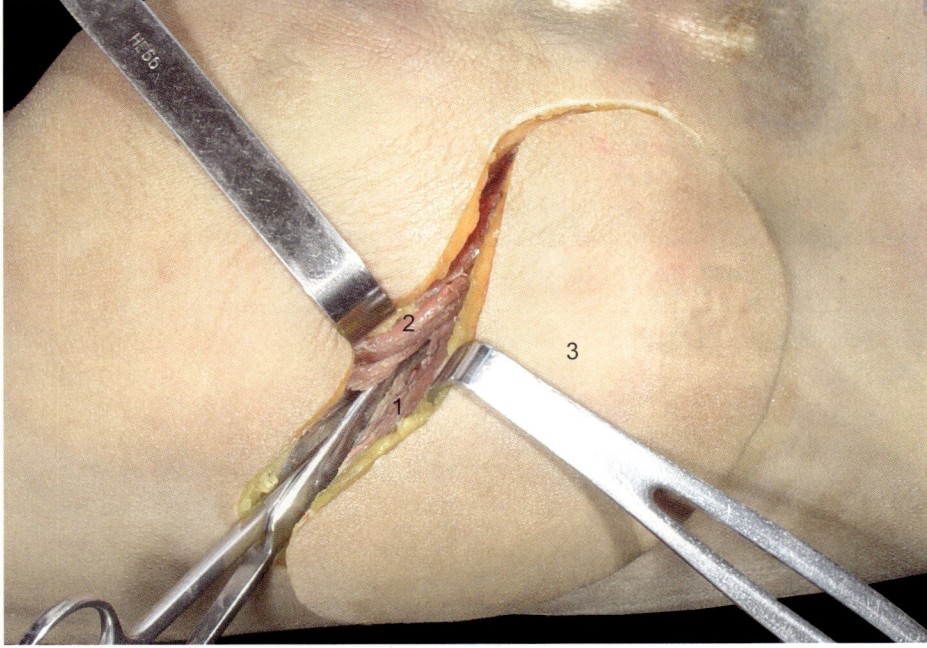

1. Superior portion of the gluteus maximus muscle
2. Inferior portion of the gluteus maximus muscle
3. Musculocutaneous flap

Figure 2-29   **Dissection of the muscular flap**

The separation should extend distally under the deep surface of the gluteus maximus muscle with the surgeon's finger, and then the gluteus maximus muscle should be elevated to expose the superficial branches (3-4 branches) of the superior gluteal artery in the deep surface. According to the distribution of these superficial branches, the inferior border of the flap should be incised, and the gluteus maximus muscular fibers split along the incision.

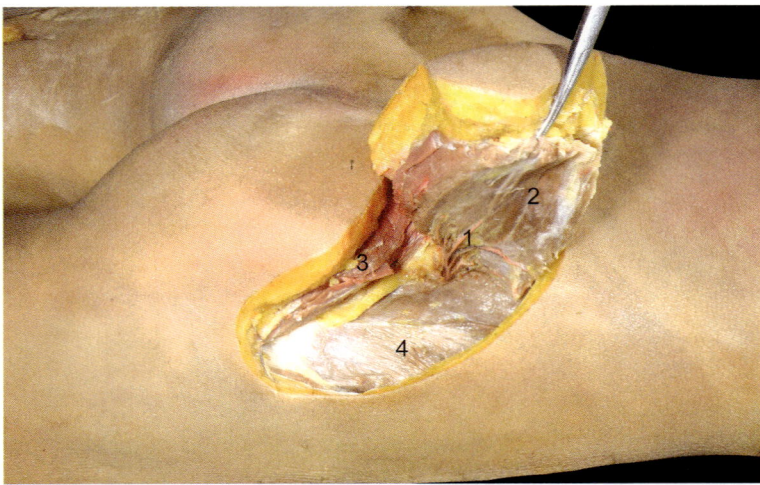

Figure 2-30   Elevation of the flap

The separation should trace toward the vessels in the deep surface until reaching the base of the superficial branch of the superior gluteal artery. The complete separation of the flap might not finish until the medial incision is made. In this way, an island flap could be made with a pedicle of the superficial branch of superior gluteal artery.
1. Superficial branch of superior gluteal artery
2. Superior portion of gluteus maximus muscle
3. Inferior portion of gluteus maximus muscle
4. Gluteus medius muscle

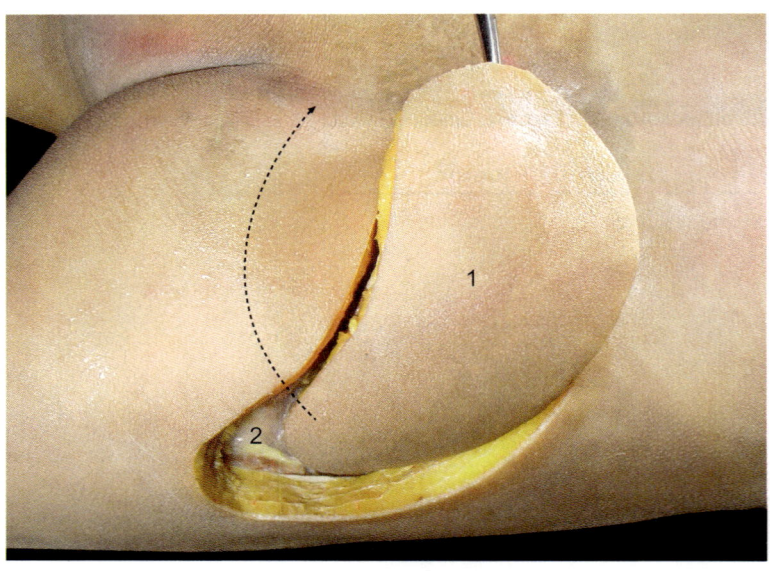

1. Gluteus maximus musculocutaneous flap.
2. Gluteus medius muscle

Figure 2-31   **Transposition of the flap**

The flap might be rotated about 150 degree to repair a wound on the sacral region.

Key points in applied anatomy

Firstly, the size and shape of the flap should be adjusted to that of the sacral wound, and the distance from the pivot point to the distal end of the flap should be longer than that from the pivot point to the distal end of the wound. Secondly, the fibers of the gluteus maximus muscle extend from the mediosuperior to the lateroinferior obliquely while those of the gluteus medius muscle extend vertically. The different directions of the two muscles might serve as an indication to identify the septum between them. Thirdly, when the pedicle is being isolated, it is preferable that part of the perivascular muscle be retained to keep the vessels intact and make the flap easy to transfer. Fourthly, since there are two groups of large and regular neurovascular plexuses in the gluteus maximus muscle, it is possible that a muscular or musculocutaneous flap be harvested based on the superior portion or the inferior portion of the gluteus maximus muscle to repair a large defect or reconstruct the breast.

Sartorius Musculocutaneous Flap

The sartorius muscle, a long thin ribbon muscle, gets its blood supply from the segmental vessels. A superior sartorius flap based on the proximal nutrient vessels might be transferred to repair a wound on the greater trochanter or on the pubic region. An inferior sartorius flap based on the distal vessels might be transferred to repair a wound on the knee, the popliteal fossa or the superior extremity of the tibia.

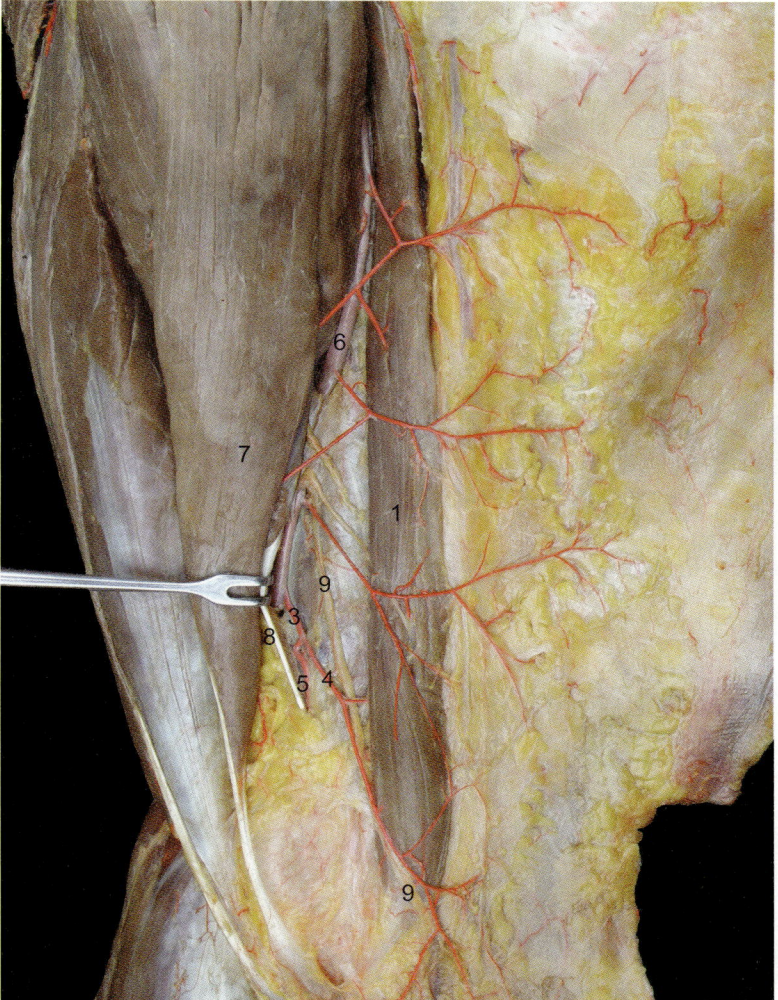

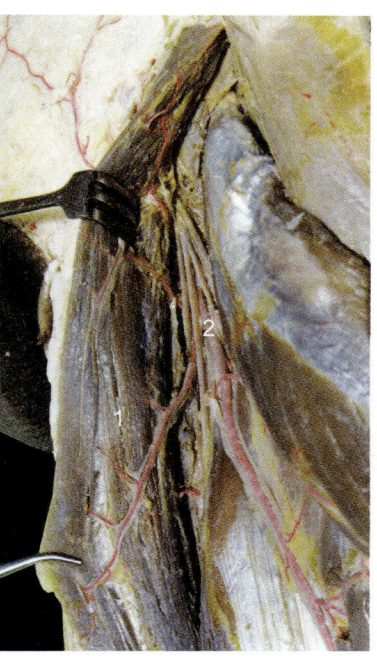

| **Figure 2-32** | **Applied anatomy** |

The sartorius muscle begins at the anterior superior iliac spine, goes medially downwards and stops at the medial area of the proximal tibia. The arteries that nourish the muscle are distributed segmentally: they originate from the deep femoral artery, the lateral circumflex femoral artery or the femoral artery in the superior half of the muscle. Among them, there is a dominant one at 8 cm below the inguinal ligament that could nourish the proximal muscle for 15 cm long. There are other branches of the descending genicular artery and the saphenous artery in the inferior half of the muscle.

1. Sartorius muscle
3. Descending genicular artery
5. Articular branch
7. Gracilis muscle
9. Saphenous nerve

2. Lateral circumflex femoral artery
4. Saphenous artery
6. Femoral artery
8. Great adductor muscle

A. Superior sartorius musculocutaneous flap

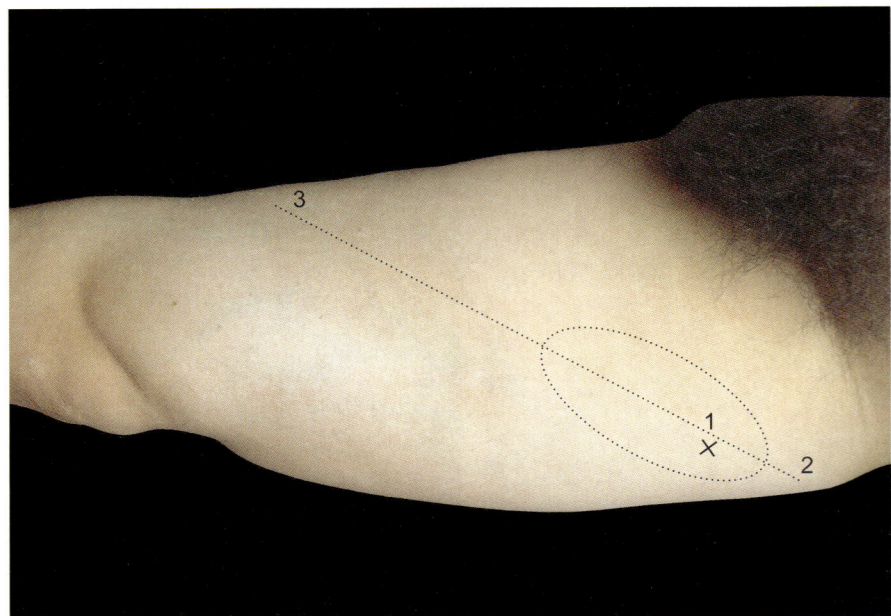

1. Pivot point of the flap
2. Anterior superior iliac spine
3. Adductor tubercle

| **Figure 2-33** | **Design of the musculocutaneous flap** |

Take the pressure sore on the greater trochanter for example. The flap might be designed with its axial line falling on the connecting line between the anterior superior iliac spine and the adductor tubercle, and with its pivot point located at 8 cm below the inguinal ligament.

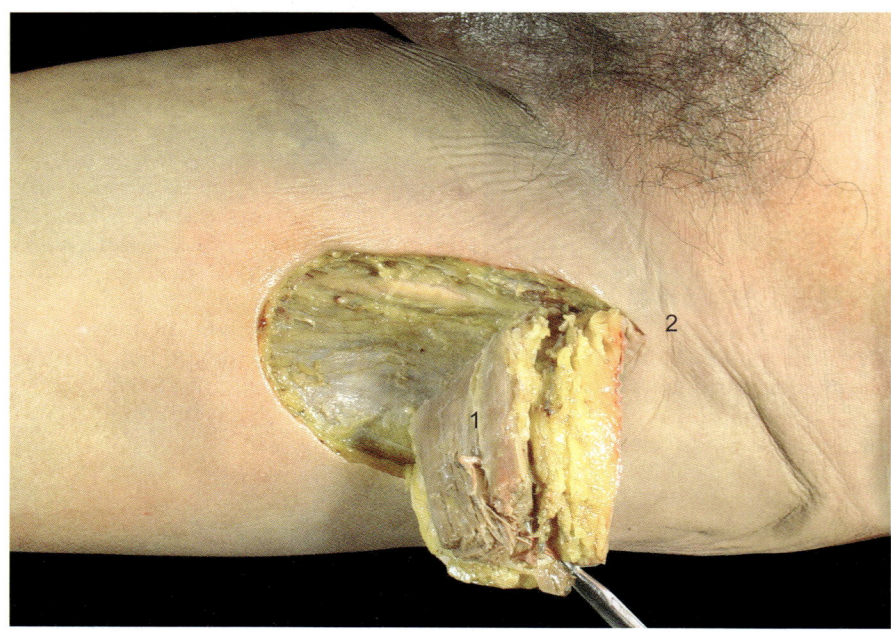

1. Sartorius muscle
2. Inguinal ligament

| **Figure 2-34** | **Exposure of the vessels** |

The flap should be incised from the lateral border to the deep fascia and the sartorius muscle exposed and cut at its distal end.

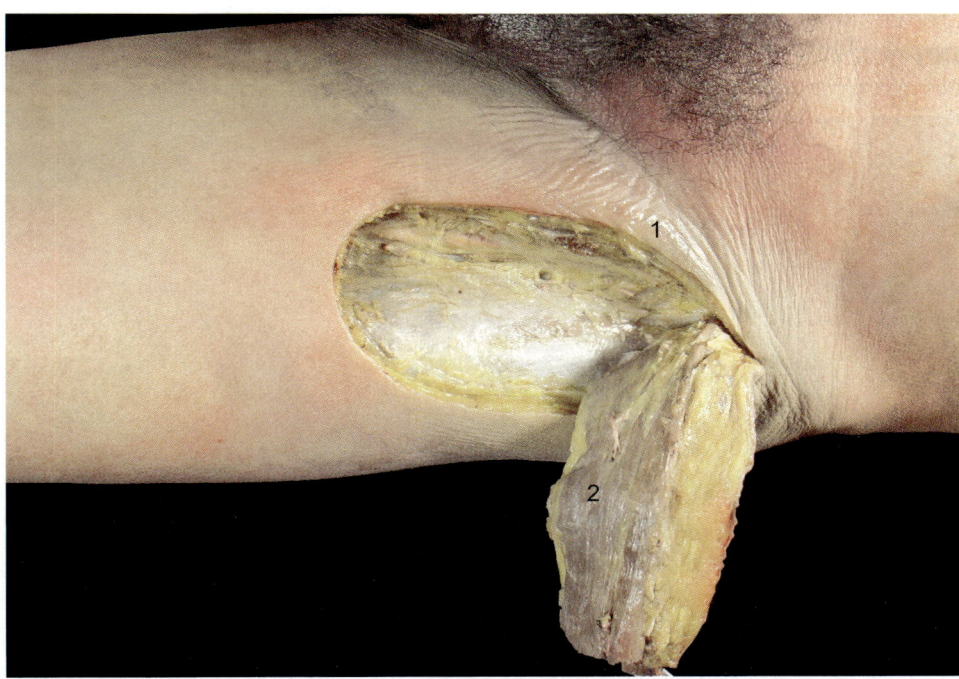

1. Inguinal ligament
2. Sartorius muscle

Figure 2-35   Elevation of the flap

The deep layer of the muscle should be separated upwards from the inferior to the superior to expose the dominant artery, which is usually situated at 8cm below the inguinal ligament. The artery should be carefully protected, and other non-main arteries ligated for a smooth transposition.

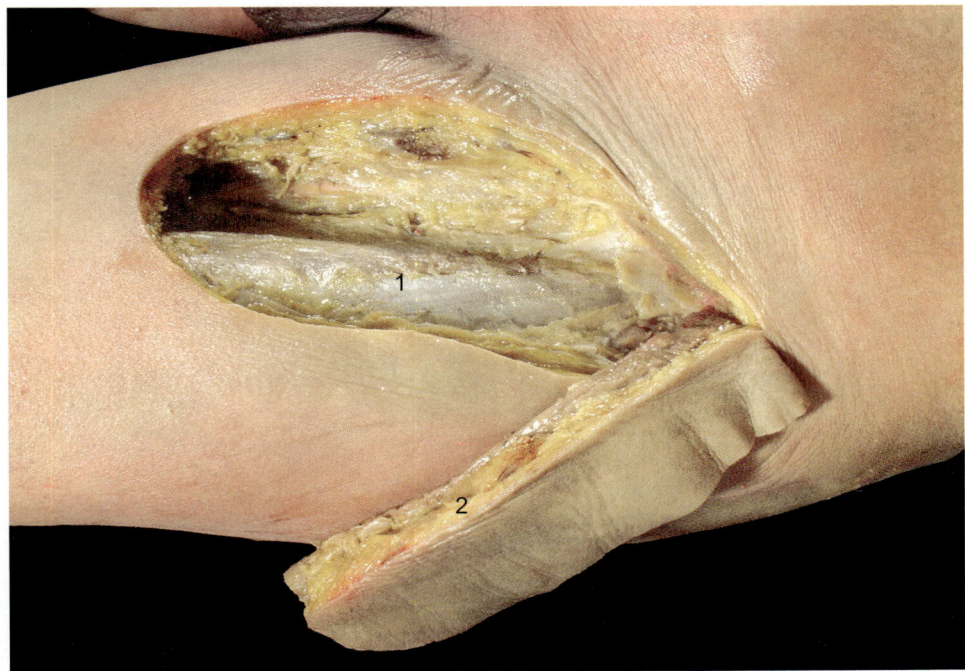

1. Donor site
2. Musculocutaneous flap

Figure 2-36   Transposition of the musculocutaneous flap

After the decubital necrosis on the greater trochanter has been debrided, the skin between the recipient and the donor sites should be incised and the flap transferred to the recipient region. If necessary, the proximal end of the skin and the muscle in the donor site might be incised to make an island flap for a smooth transfer.

B.Inferior sartorius musculocutaneous flap

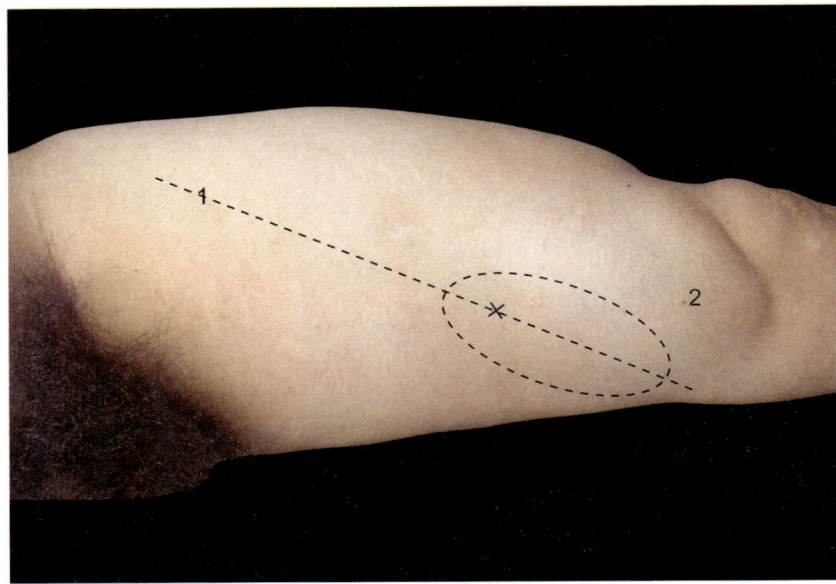

1. Pivot point of the flap
2. Patella

| **Figure 2-37** | **Design of the flap** |

Take the restoration of a wound on the anterior knee. The flap should be designed with its pivot point located at 10cm above the adductor tubercle along the body surface projection line of the sartorius muscle.

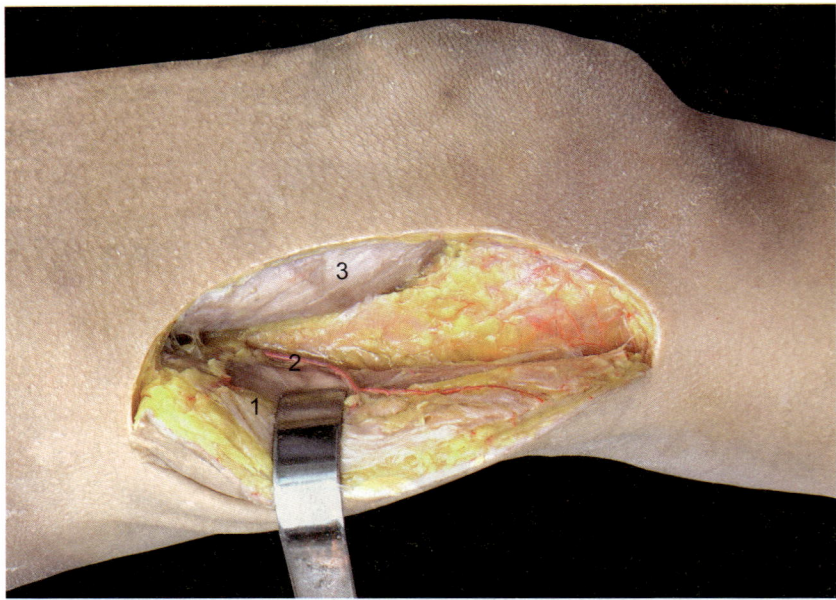

1. Sartorius muscle
2. Descending genicular artery
3. Medial vastus muscle

| **Figure 2-38** | **Exposure of the vessels** |

The flap should be incised from its anterolateral border and dissected backward under the deep fascia until reaching the anterior margin of sartorius muscle. Then it should be elevated from the deep surface of the muscle and the adductor canal cautiously opened to expose the femoral artery and the descending genicular artery. The incision should extend along theses vessels to the distal margin of the flap. Attention should be given to the arterial branches that enter the muscle or the branches that goes into the flap from bilateral sides of the muscle.

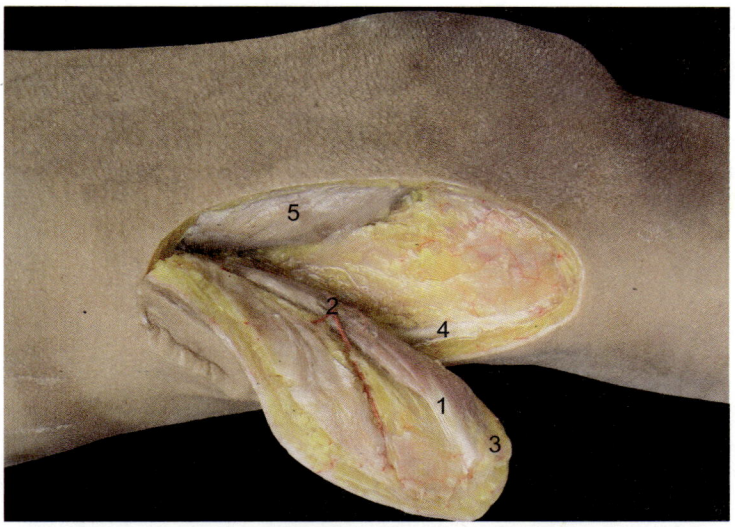

Figure 2-39 Elevation of the flap

The distal border of the flap should be incised before the sartorius muscle, the saphenous artery and the greater saphenous vein are dissected. Then its posterior border should be incised so that it could be elevated completely.

1. Sartorius muscle
2. Saphenous artery
3. Greater saphenous vein
4. Gracilis muscle
5. Medial vastus muscle

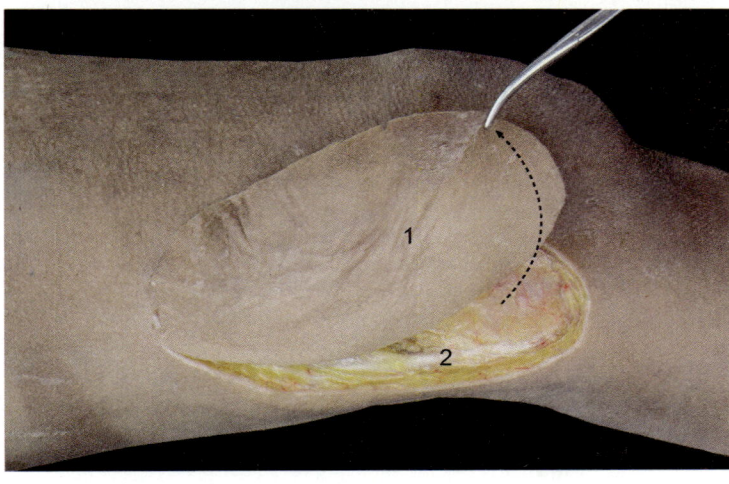

1. Musculocutaneous flap
2. Gracilis muscle

Figure 2-40 Transposition of the musculocutaneous flap

After the wound on the recipient site has been completely debrided, the flap might be transferred to the recipient site.

Key points in applied anatomy

Firstly, when the proximal portion of the muscle is being dissected, great attention should be given to the lateral femoral cutaneous nerve that runs across the muscle from medial to lateral at 7cm under the anterosuperior iliac spine. When the distal portion of the muscle is being dissected, great attention should be given to the saphenous nerve at the plane of the patellar apex, where it extends in the septum between the sartorius muscle and the gracilis muscle. Secondly, the two groups of constant vessels in the muscle could serve as pedicles of the flap. The proximal group comprises the deep femoral artery and the lateral circumflex femoral arteries. A transpositional or free flap based on this pedicle might be designed about 15cm long with its medial extending to the anterior midline of the thigh and its lateral to the anterior margin of tensor fasciae latae muscle. The distal group comprises the descending genicular arteries. A flap based on it might reach 20cm in length. Thirdly, since the sartorius muscle has a large skin contact surface, and many musculocutaneous perforators and direct cutaneous arteries run superficially along its deep layer to nourish the adjacent skin, a relatively long and wide flap could be harvested. Fourthly, there is sometimes a transverse muscular branch from the popliteal artery (1.2mm in diameter) in the inferior portion of sartorius muscle. The branch should be ligated when the inferior sartorius musculocutaneous flap is harvested.

8 Vastus Lateralis Musculocutaneous Flap

The vastus lateralis muscle is situated at the anterolateral region of the thigh. The muscle is thick and rich in blood supply. Its main nutrient artery is the lateral circumflex femoral artery. An island flap including the muscle and the distal overlying skin could be harvested to fill in the cavity on the greater trochanter after the decubital necrosis is debrided. Harvesting the flap does no damage to the function of the lower leg.

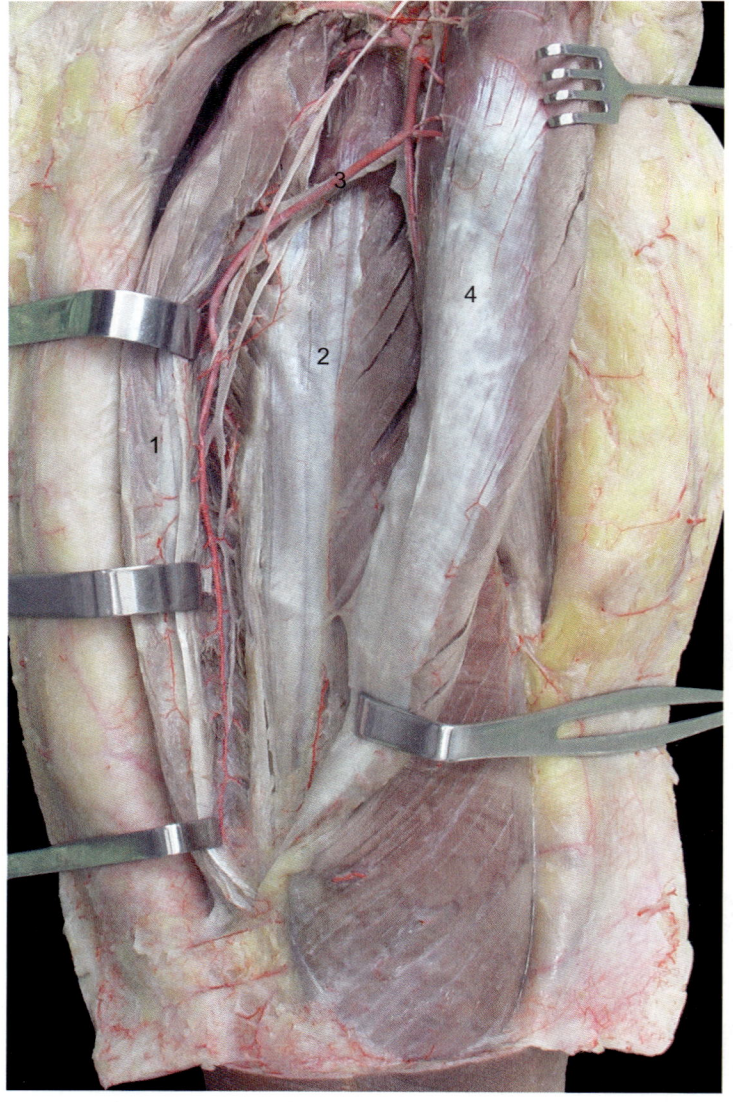

| Figure 2-41 | Applied anatomy |

The vastus lateralis muscle is part of the quadriceps femoris muscle. Its superior 2/3 segment is clearly separate from the vastus intermedius muscle but its inferior 1/3 is closely stick to the muscle. The blood supply of the vastus lateralis comes from the descending branch of the lateral circumflex femoral artery, which descends first in the deep layer of the rectus femoris and then along the anterior border of the vastus lateralis muscle. The artery enters the muscle at 10cm under the greater trochanter (equal to the place above middle-superior intersection of the vastus lateralis muscle). The vascular pedicle is about 6cm long. Its superficial layer is covered with the rectus femoris and the tensor fasciae latae muscle. There are no direct muscular cutaneous branches that perforate through the skin from the upper segment of the vastus lateralis, and so it is impossible that a musculocutaneous flap be made. But there are musculocutaneous branches at its inferior segment that enter the subcutaneous tissue and the skin to anastomose extensively with those branches from the rectus femoris and the tensor fasciae latae muscle, and so it is possible that an musculocutaneous island flap could be based on the distal segment of the vastus lateralis.

1. Vastus lateralis muscle
2. Vastus intermedius muscle
3. Descending branch of lateral circumflex femoral artery
4. Rectus femoris muscle

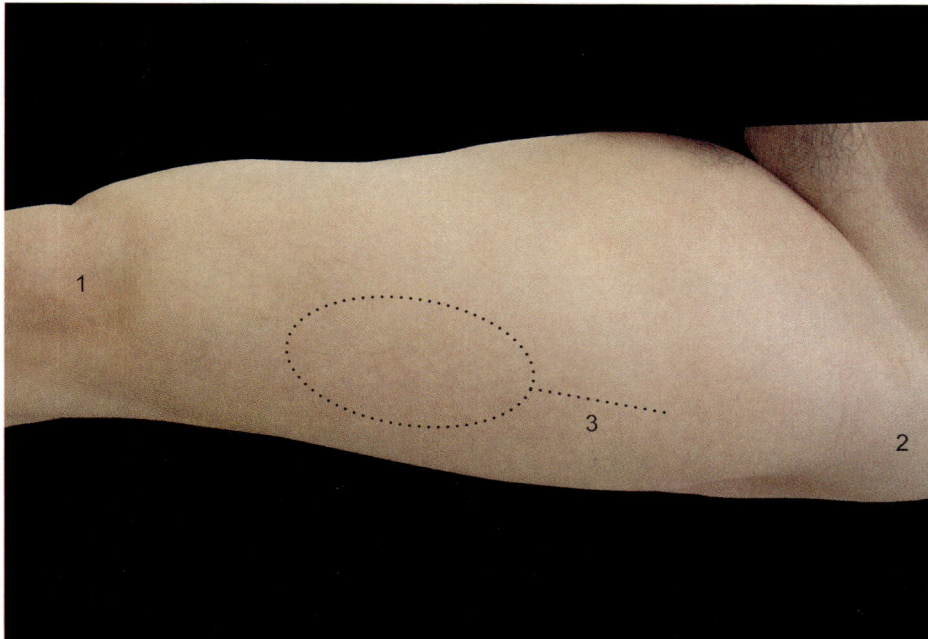

1. Patella
2. Anterior superior iliac spine
3. Incision line

Figure 2-42   **Design of the musculocutaneous flap**

The flap should be designed on the lateral thigh and its anterior border located within the connecting line between the anterior superior iliac spine and the superolateral point of the patella. The distal flap might extend to 4cm above the patella. The largest one might amount to 10×7cm in size. The proximal incision line between the wound on the greater trochanter and the superior border of the flap should be clearly marked.

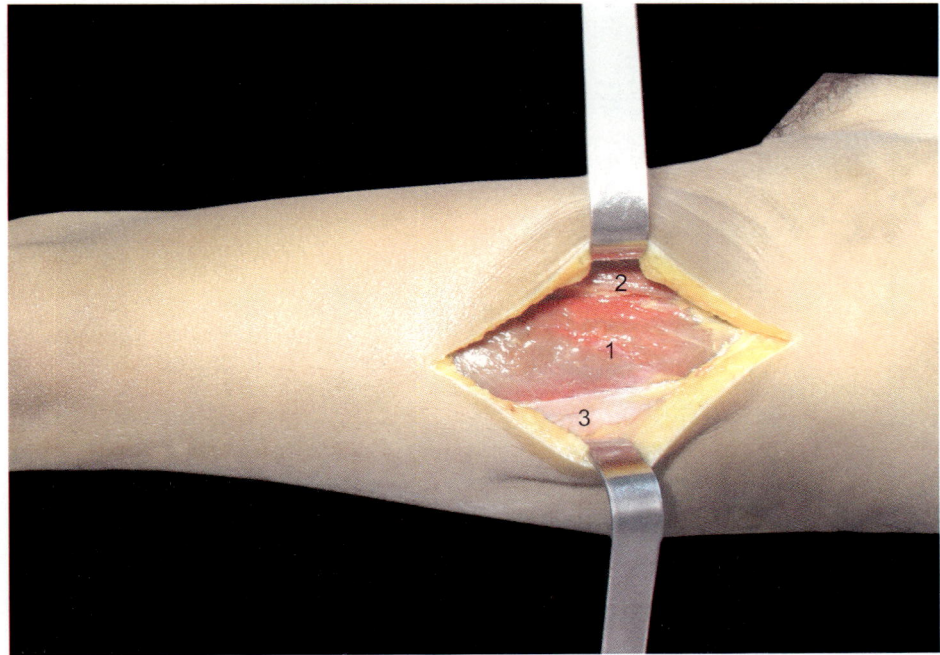

1. Vastus lateralis muscle
2. Rectus femoris muscle
3. Tractus iliotibialis

Figure 2-43   **Exposure of the vastus lateralis muscle**

The incision should begin with the proximal line to expose the vastus lateralis muscle to determine its relation with the rectus femoris muscle and the tensor fasciae latae muscle.

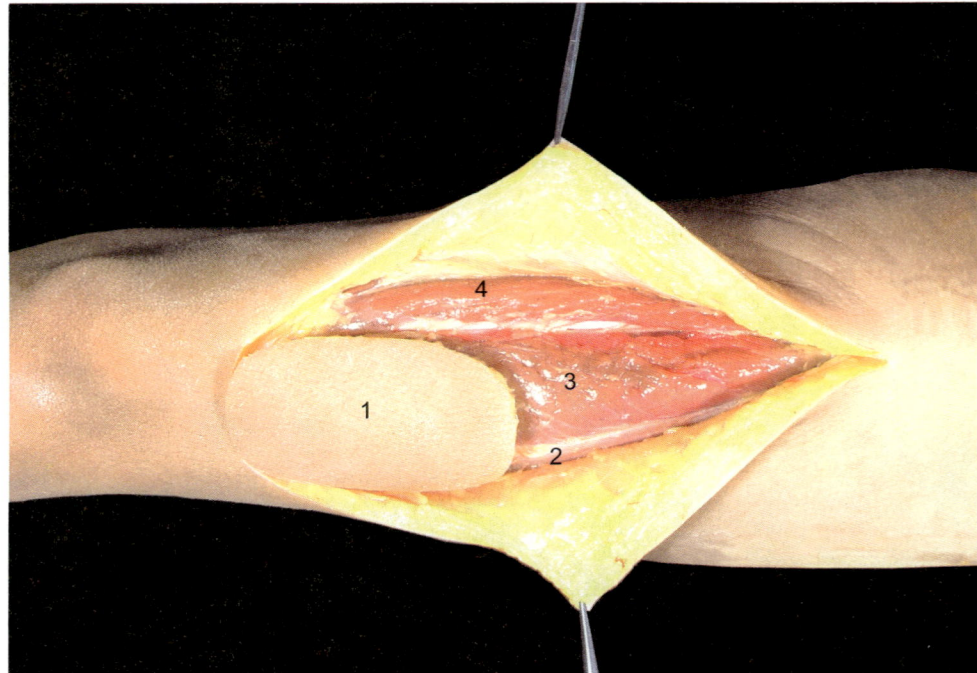

| **Figure 2-44** | **Dissection of the flap** |

1. Flap
2. Tractus iliotibialis
3. Vastus lateralis muscle
4. Rectus femoris muscle

As has been designed, the flap should be incised circumsferentially. The tractus iliotibialis should be opened at its proximal end to separate the vastus lateralis muscle from the rectus femoris muscle and the vastus intermedius muscle.

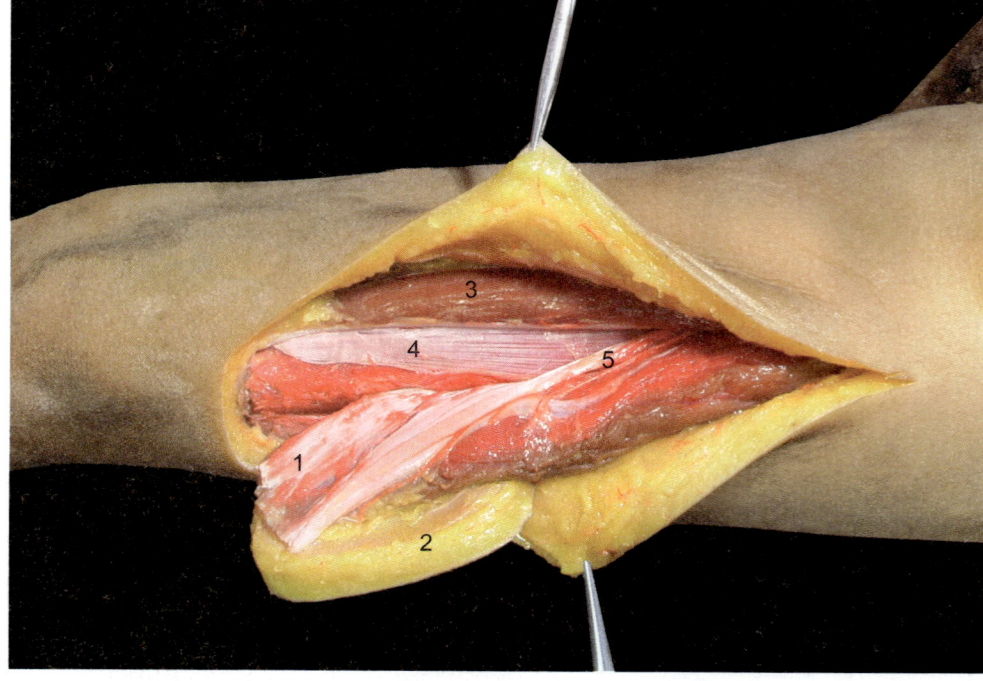

| **Figure 2-45** | **Elevation of the flap** |

1. Vastus lateralis muscle
2. Flap
3. Rectus femoris muscle
4. Vastus intermedius muscle
5. Descending branch of lateral circumflex femoral artery

The vastus lateralis muscle should be separated at 5cm above the patella (intersection of the muscle belly and the tendon). Then the flap should be elevated and dissected superiorly until the neurovascular pedicle extends as long as is expected (about 5cm long).

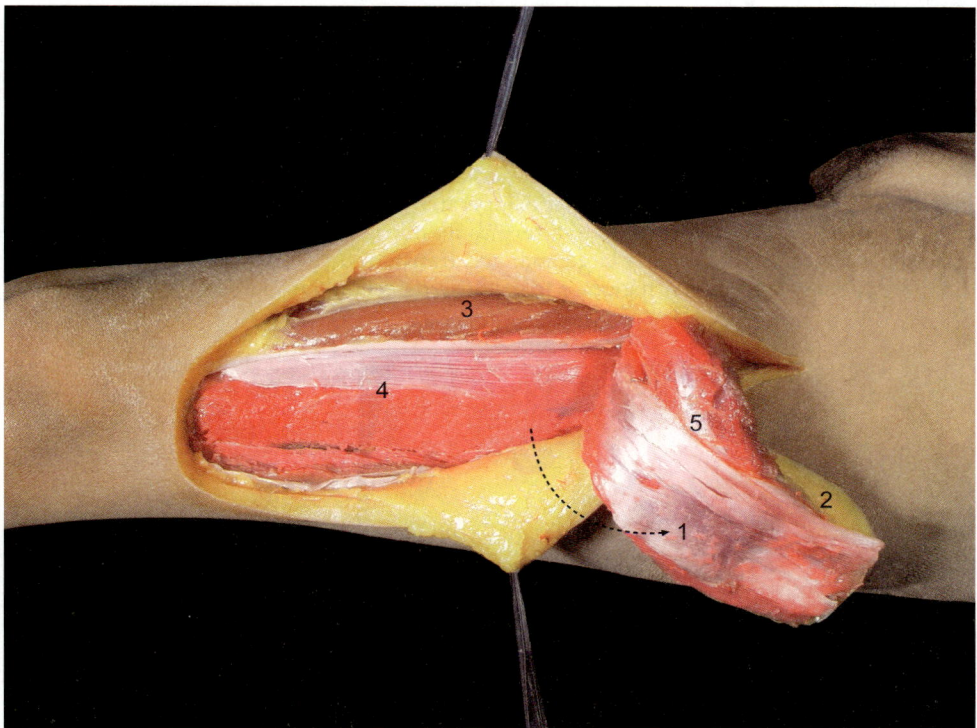

Figure 2-46   **Transposition of the flap**

The flap might be transferred upwards to repair a decubital ulcer on the greater trochanter. Its muscle belly could fill in the cavity and the skin cover up the wound surface.

1. Vastus lateralis muscle
2. Flap
3. Rectus femoris muscle
4. Vastus intermedius muscle
5. Descending branch of lateral circumflex femoral artery

Key points in applied anatomy

Firstly, since the superior 2/3 segment of the vastus lateralis is clearly separate from the vastus intermedius muscle but its inferior 1/3 closely stick to the muscle, the flap should be dissected from proximal to distal to get the muscle separated from the rectus femoris and the vastus intermedius. Secondly, the tractus iliotibialis should be incised at the proximal edge of the flap, and it together with the vastus lateralis muscle, fixed temporarily with the skin in the flap dissection to avoid disconnection of the layers. Thirdly, no damage should be done to the suprapatellar bursa. Fourthly, if the recipient site is located at a superior position, the flap should be elevated upwards until the neurovascular pedicle is as long as has been expected (about 5cm long). Fifthly, a median-thick skin graft is needed to cover the donor surface.

Rectus Femoris Musculocutaneous Flap

The rectus femoris muscle is part of the quadriceps femoris muscle. The flap should be situated superficially and connected loosely with the medial, lateral and intermediate vastus muscles, so that it could be easily harvested with little postoperative harm to the leg function. It has constant branches of the lateral circumflex femoral artery as its nutrient vessels. A flap based on the rectus femoris muscle might be rotated in a large arch and transferred to repair a wound on the perineal, the pubic or the greater trochanter region or to restore a defect on the abdomen.

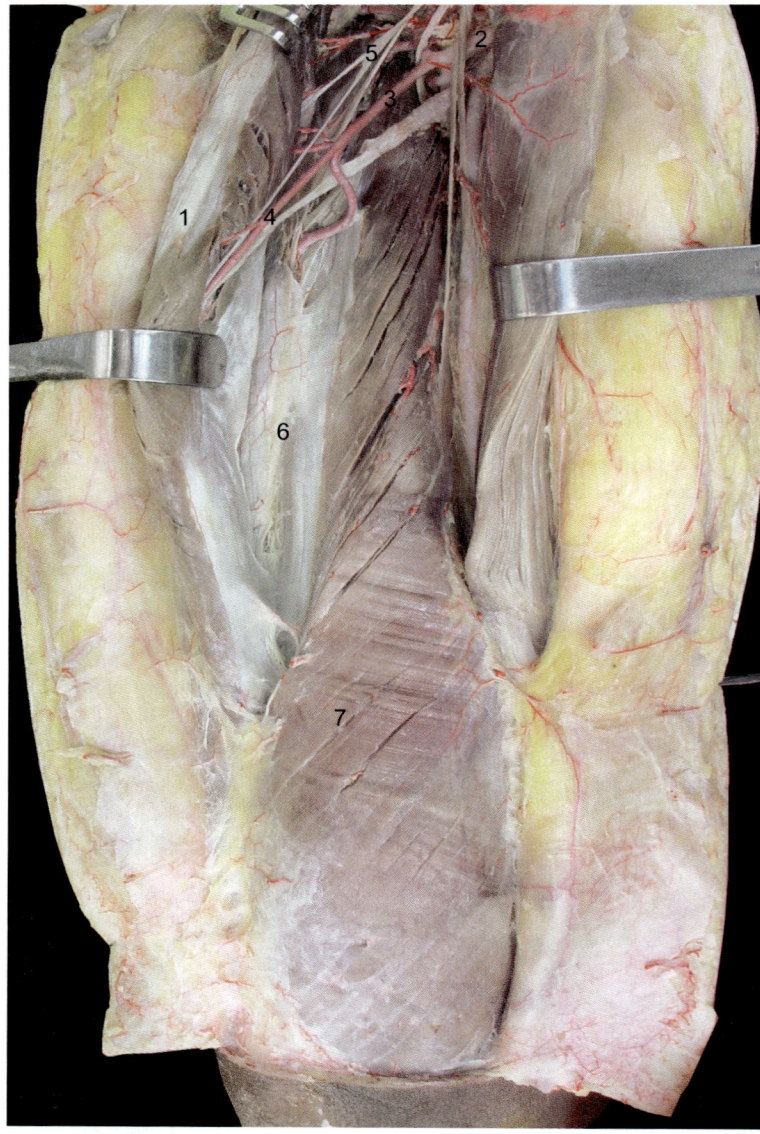

1. Rectus femoris muscle
2. Lateral circumflex femoral artery
3. Descending branch of lateral circumflex femoral artery
4. Muscular branch of rectus femoris muscle
5. Nerve of rectus femoris muscle
6. Vastus intermedius muscle
7. Vastus medialis muscle

Figure 2-47   Applied anatomy

The rectus femoris muscle originates from the supersulcus between the anterior inferior iliac spine and the superior edge of the acetabulum. It has the muscular branches of the descending vessel of the lateral circumflex femoral artery as its main nutrient vessels. The muscular branches extend inferiorly along the medial border of the muscle to 8cm below the central point of the inguinal ligament, where they accompany the motor branches of the femoral nerve and enter the middle-superior segment of the muscle. The pedicle is about 4cm long.

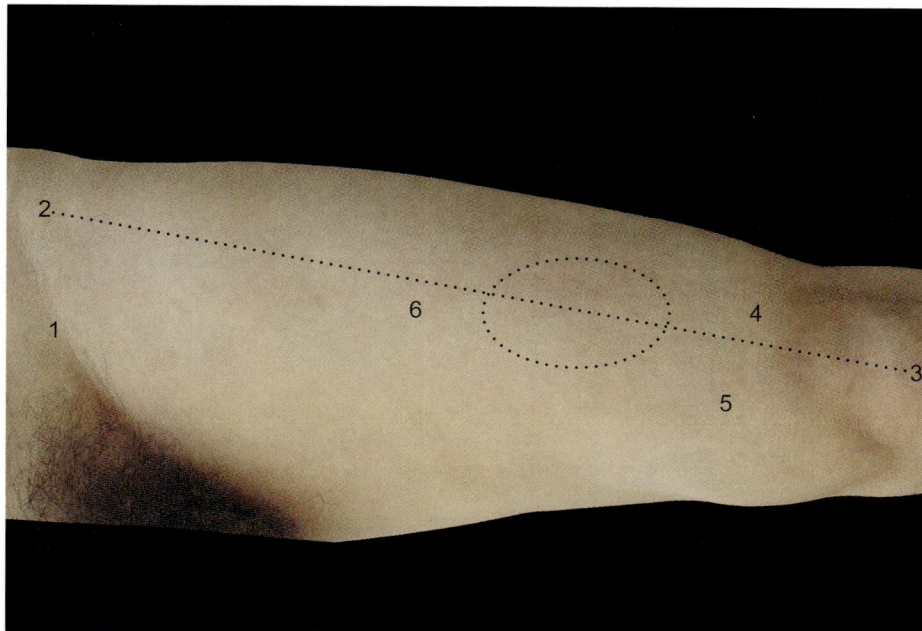

1. Inguinal ligament
2. Anterior superior iliac spine
3. Patella
4. Vastus lateralis muscle
5. Vastus medialis muscle
6. Rectus femoris muscle

Figure 2-48   Design of the flap

The flap should be designed with its pivot point located at about 8cm below the central point of the inguinal ligament and its axis falling on the connecting line between the anterior superior iliac spine and the midpoint of the patella. The lateral margin of the flap should be located on the medial edge of the vastus lateralis muscle, and its medial margin on the lateral edge of the vastus medialis muscle and the sartorius muscle. Its distal margin reaches the terminal of the muscle. The size of the flap depends on the needs of the recipient site.

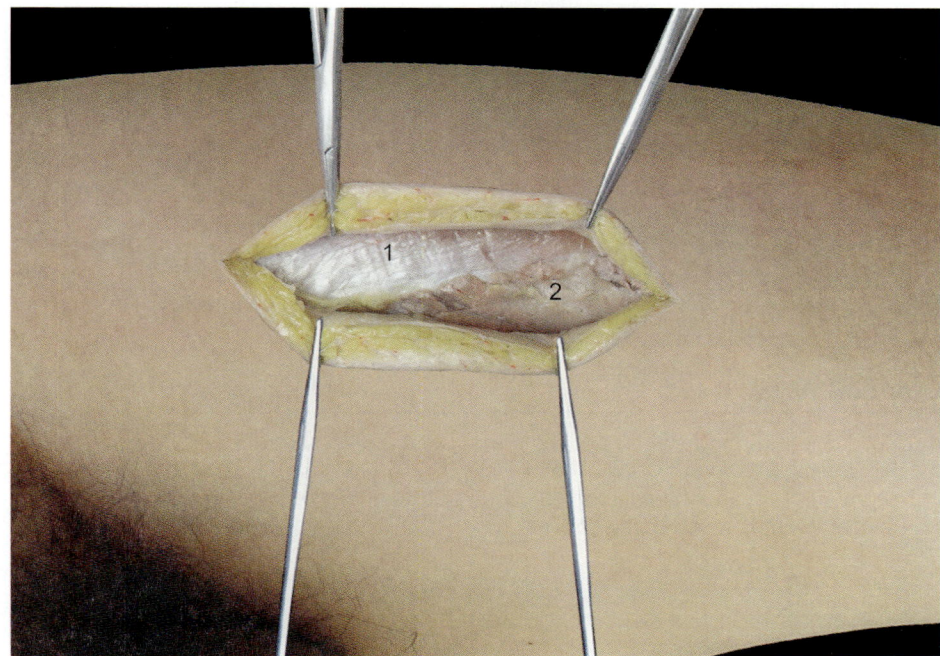

1. Vastus lateralis muscle
2. Rectus femoris muscle

Figure 2-49   Exposure of the rectus femoris muscle

The proximal border of the flap should be incised first to expose the rectus femoris muscle between the vastus lateralis muscle and the sartorius muscle.

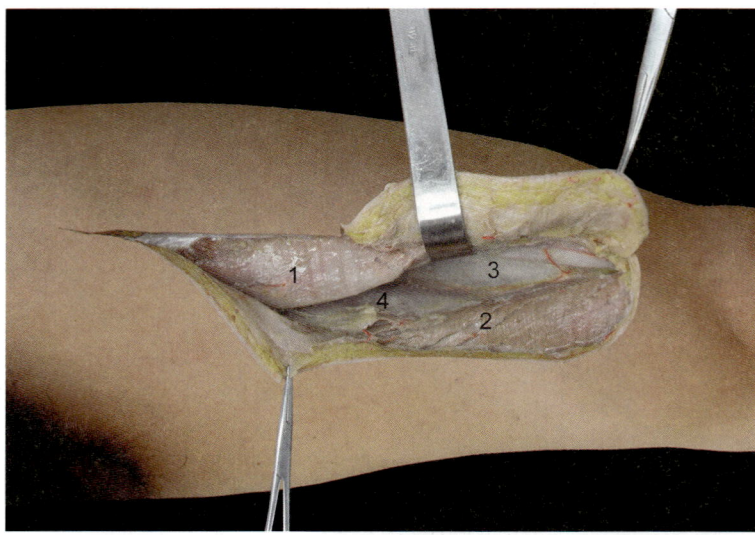

1. Rectus femoris muscle
2. Vastus medialis muscle
3. Vastus lateralis muscle
4. Vastus intermedius muscle

Figure 2-50   **Elevation of the flap**

The septum between the rectus femoris muscle and the vastus medialis/lateralis muscle should be determined clearly, and the septum and the deep surface of the muscle should be separated bluntly from the proximal to the distal.

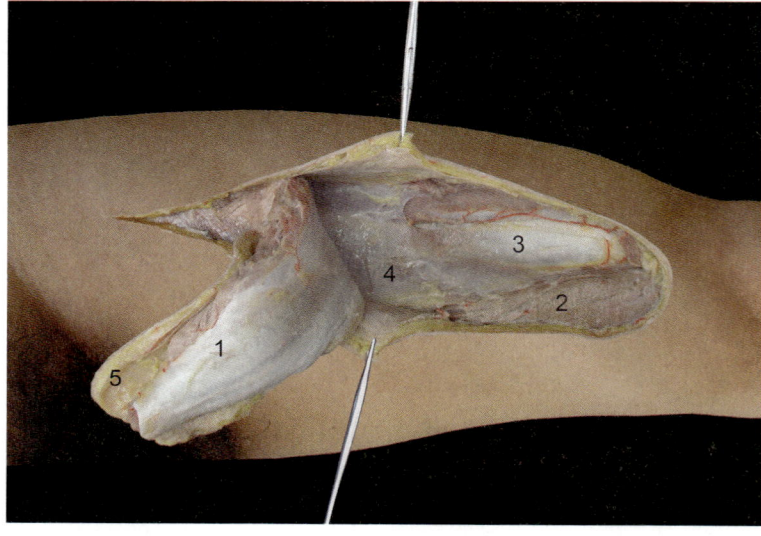

1. Rectus femoris muscle
2. Vastus medialis muscle
3. Vastus lateralis muscle
4. Vastus intermedius muscle
5. Flap

Figure 2-51   **Transposition of the flap**

The rectus femoris muscle should be cut off at the distal end of the flap. Then the flap should be elevated and separated upward from the deep surface of the muscle. The small vascular branches that enter the distal 2/3 segment of the muscle should be ligated and the main vessels and nerves, at 8cm below the inguinal ligament retained in the flap.

Key points in applied anatomy

Firstly, it is not uncommon that the nerve of the rectus femoris shares a common trunk with other anterior femoral muscular branches. Therefore, careful dissection was needed to avoid injuring other myoneural branches when the femoris flap is being harvested. Secondly, the skin and the muscle should be sutured and fixed temporarily during the operation. Thirdly, the subcutaneous tunnel should be wide enough to guarantee a smooth transfer of the muscular flap.

Medial Vastus Femoral Musculocutaneous Flap

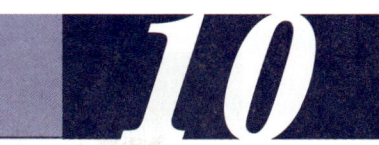

The vastus medialis muscle is situated at the anteromedial region of the thigh. Its blood supply is distributed segmentally. Based on the muscle, a musculocutaneous or a musculo-tendo-cutaneous flap might be designed. The flap might be transferred to repair a wound on the knee or to reconstruct the extending apparatus or the function of the knee.

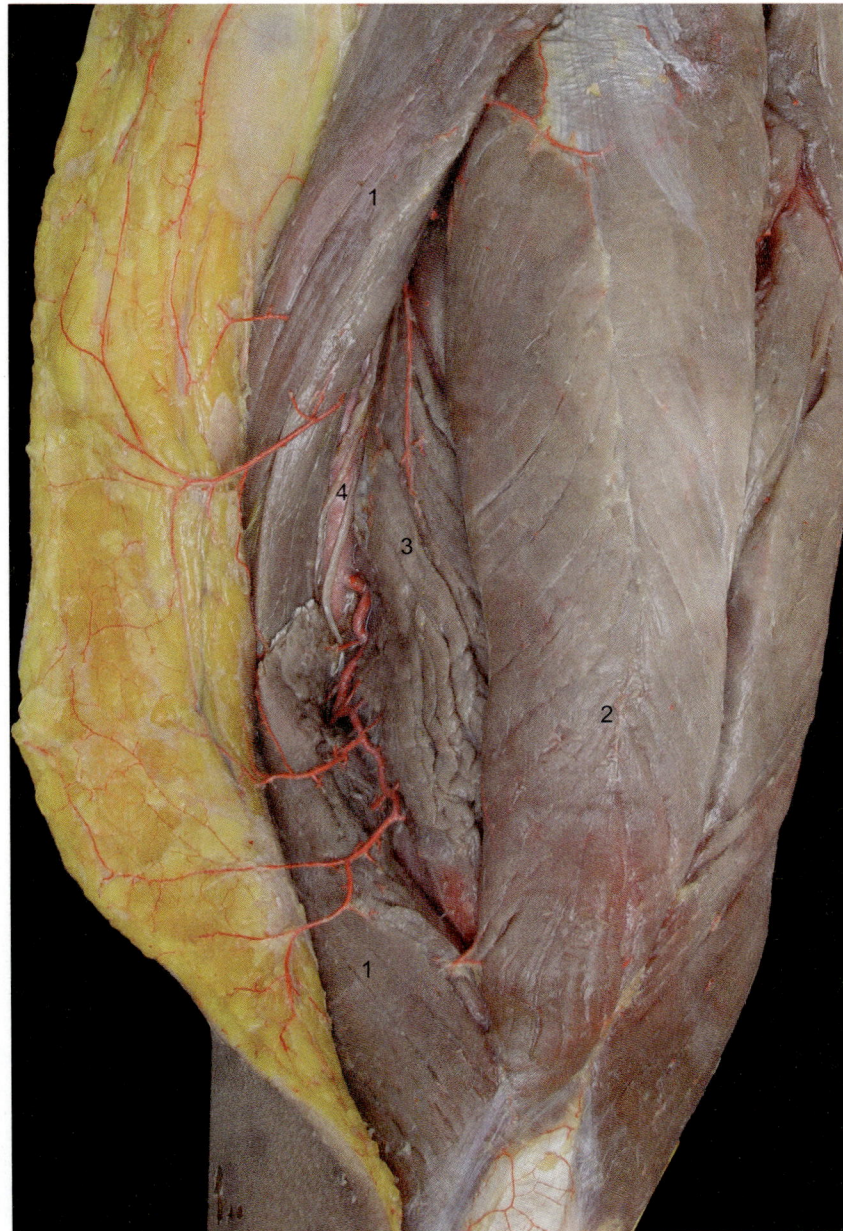

1. Vastus medialis muscle
2. Rectus femoris muscle
3. Vastus intermedius muscle
4. Femoral artery

Figure 2-52   **Applied anatomy**

The vastus medialis muscle gets its blood supply from the muscular branches of the femoral artery and the medial circumflex femoral artery. There are generally 4-6 muscular branches at the medial femoral side. These branches nourish the muscle and the overlying skin segmentally. The femoral nerve has 2 motor branches to innervate the muscle. One enters the proximal muscle through the neurovascular porta; the other enters it over the superficial venous surface at the central point of the medial muscle.

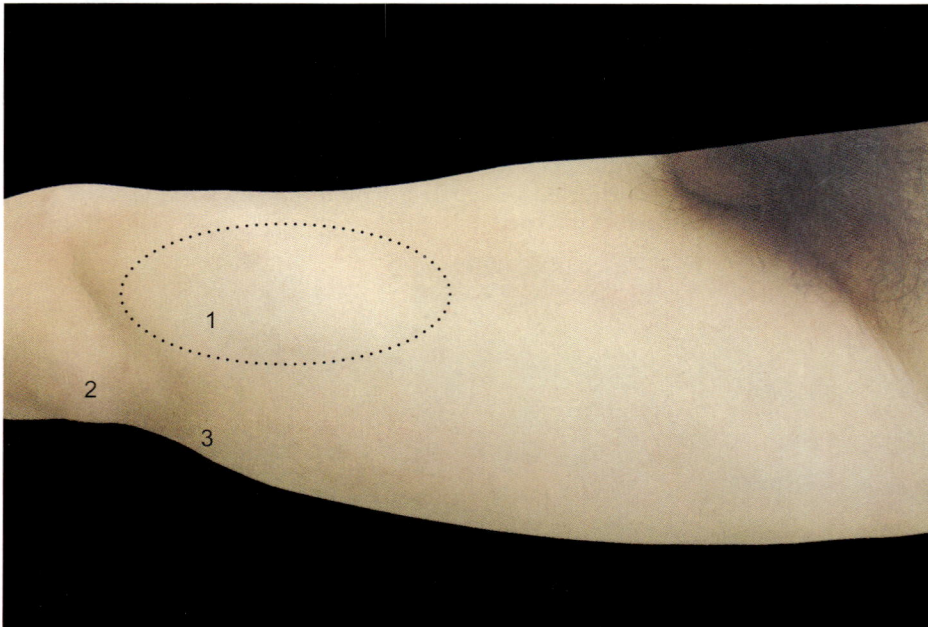

1. Vastus medialis muscle
2. Patella
3. Vastus lateralis muscle

| **Figure 2-53** | **Design of the flap** |

Take the restoration of the soft tissue defect on the anterior knee. The flap should be designed at the anteromedial region of the thigh. Its proximal edge might extend to the upper region of the medial thigh and its distal edge is connected with the border of the genicular wound. Its lateral edge might extend to the medial margin of the vastus lateralis muscle and its width is about one-third of the circumference of the inferior thigh.

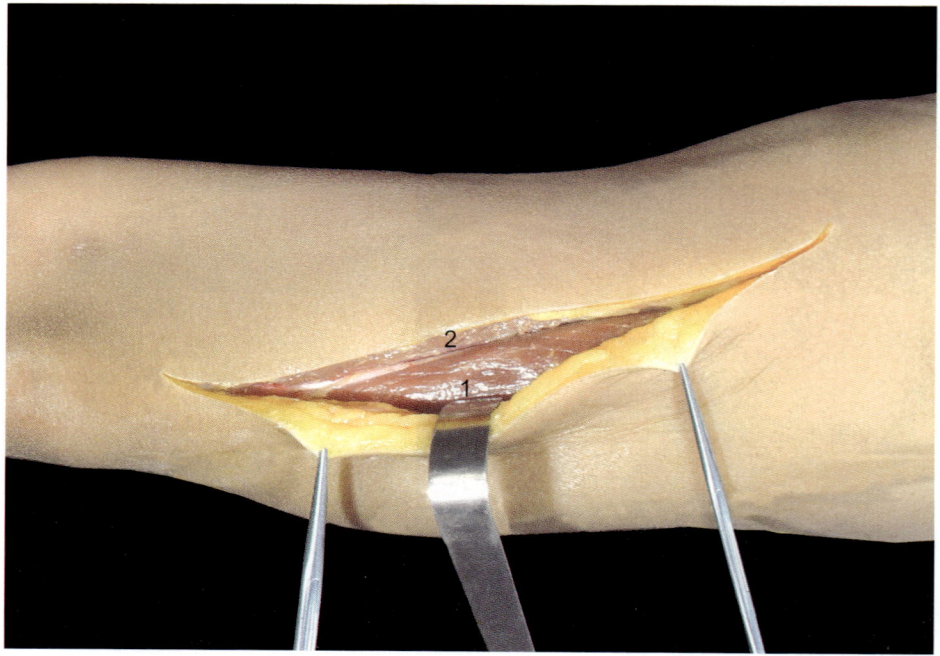

| **Figure 2-54** | **Exposure of the vastus medialis muscle** |

As has been designed, the flap should be first incised along its lateral border down to the deep fascia to expose the septum between the rectus femoris muscle and the vastus medialis muscle.

1. Rectus femoris muscle   **2.** Vastus medialis muscle

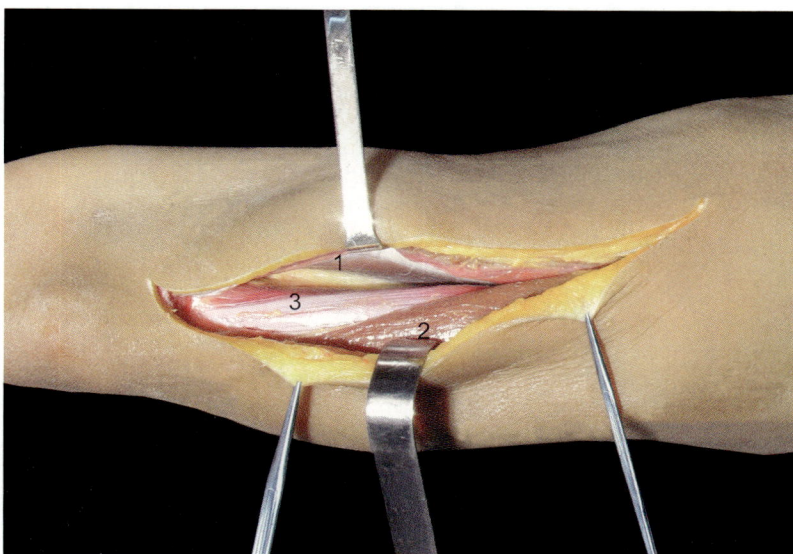

1. Vastus medialis muscle
2. Rectus femoris muscle
3. Vastus intermedius muscle

Figure 2-55   Separation of the muscle

The separation of the intermuscular septum should be done bluntly and continued along the deep surface of the vastus medialis onto the intermuscular septum between the vastus medialis muscle and the vastus intermedius muscle. The connection between the muscle and the skin should be preserved in the dissection.

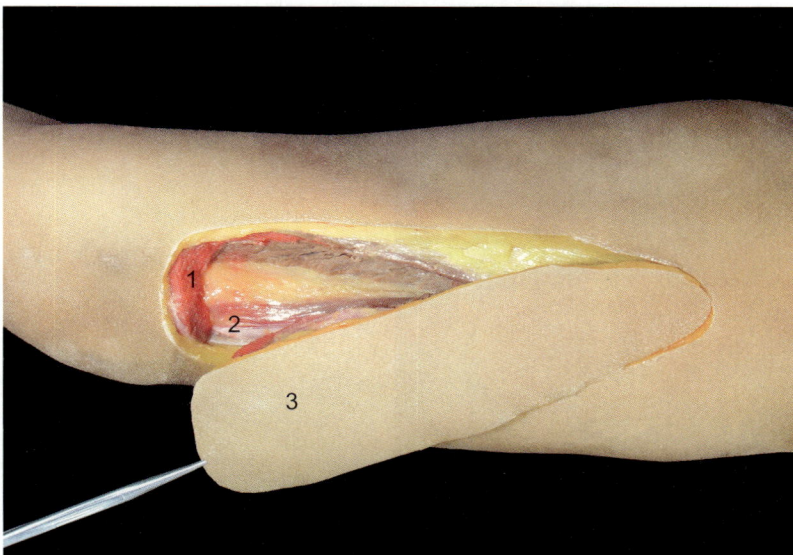

1. Rectus femoris muscle
2. Vastus intermedius muscle
3. Musculocutaneous flap

Figure 2-56   Elevation of the musculocutaneous flap

The medial border should then be incised to make an island flap. The nutrient vessels that enter the deep layer of the muscle should be kept intact. If necessary, the insertion of the muscle might be separated to enhance its mobility. Meanwhile, the neurovascular pedicle that is located around the insertion should be given further attention to avoid getting it damaged.

Key points in applied anatomy

Firstly, the skin and the muscle in the flap should be kept integrated by contemporary sutures during the operation. Secondly, the nutrient vessels that enter the muscle should be kept intact. Thirdly, if the insertion the vastus medialis muscle has to be cut to enhance its mobility, attention should be given to the adjacent neurovascular pedicle to avoid getting them damaged.

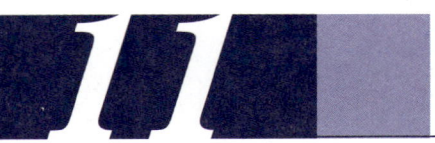

Gracilis Musculocutaneous Flap

The gracilis muscle is concealed at the medial portion of the thigh. The flap might be transferred locally to repair a wound on the medial thigh, the inguinal groove, the perineal region or the ischial tuberosity. The muscle is part of the medial group of the thigh and a dissection of it might not affect the leg function. The donor site might be closed primarily.

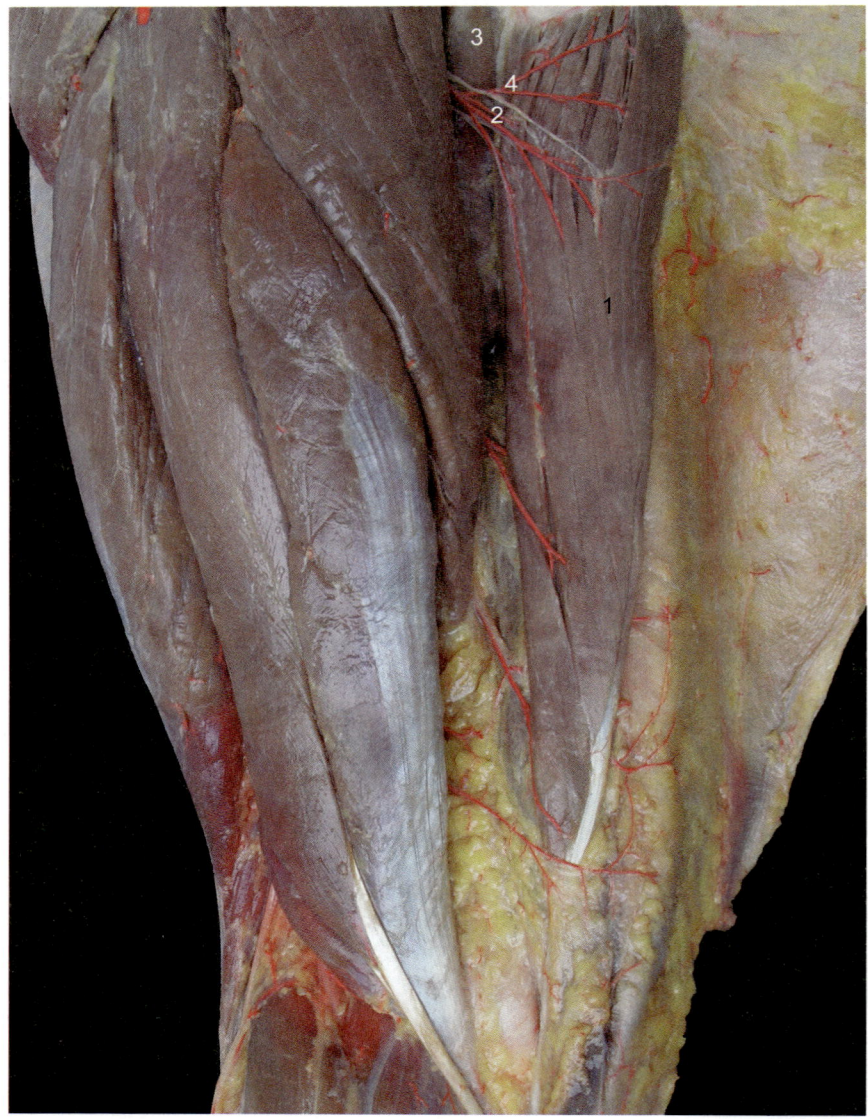

1. Gracilis muscle
2. Muscular branch of gracilis muscle
3. Adductor brevis muscle
4. Anterior branch of obturator nerve

| Figure 2-57 | Applied anatomy |

The gracilis muscle, a flat long ribbon muscle, is situated subcutaneous at the medial portion of the thigh. Its main nutrient vessel comes from the branches of the deep femoral artery. These branches extend medially downwards in the septum between the adductor longus and brevis muscles and enter the middle-superior segment of the gracilis muscle (8cm below the pubic tubercle) from its deep surface. The innervation of the muscle comes from the anterior branch of the obturator nerve. There is the sartorius muscle that crosses obliquely the distal segment of the gracilis muscle, but there are no musculocutaneous arteries that perforate through the muscle to the skin. That is why the gracilis musculocutaneous flap should be limited within the superior 2/3 segment of the muscle.

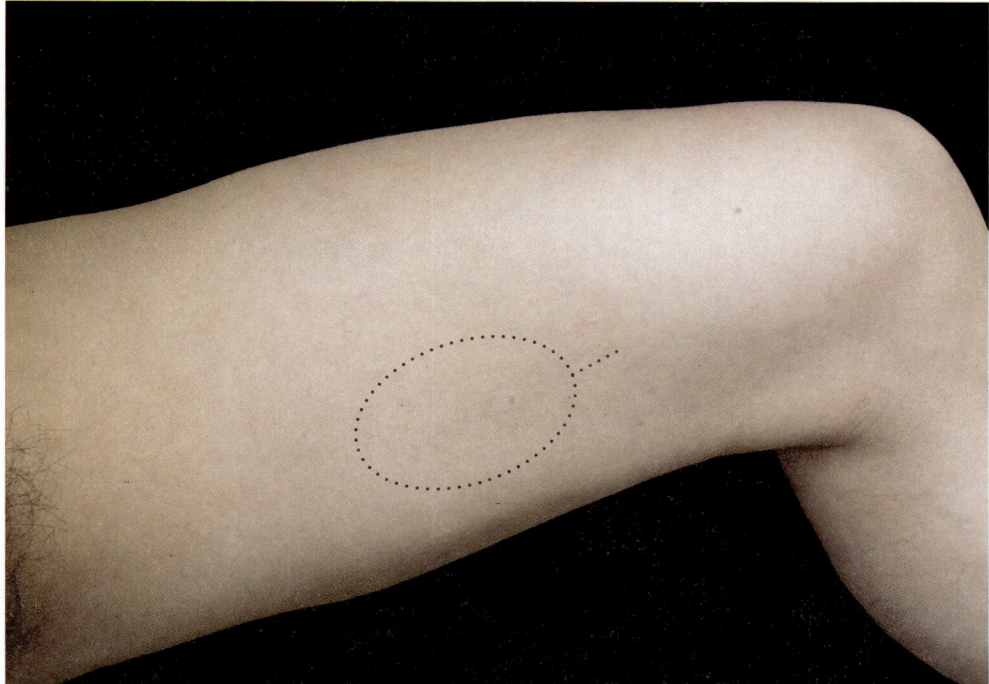

Figure 2-58   **Design of the musculocutaneous flap**

The flap should be located within 10cm behind the connecting line between the pubic tubercle and the tuberosity of tibia.

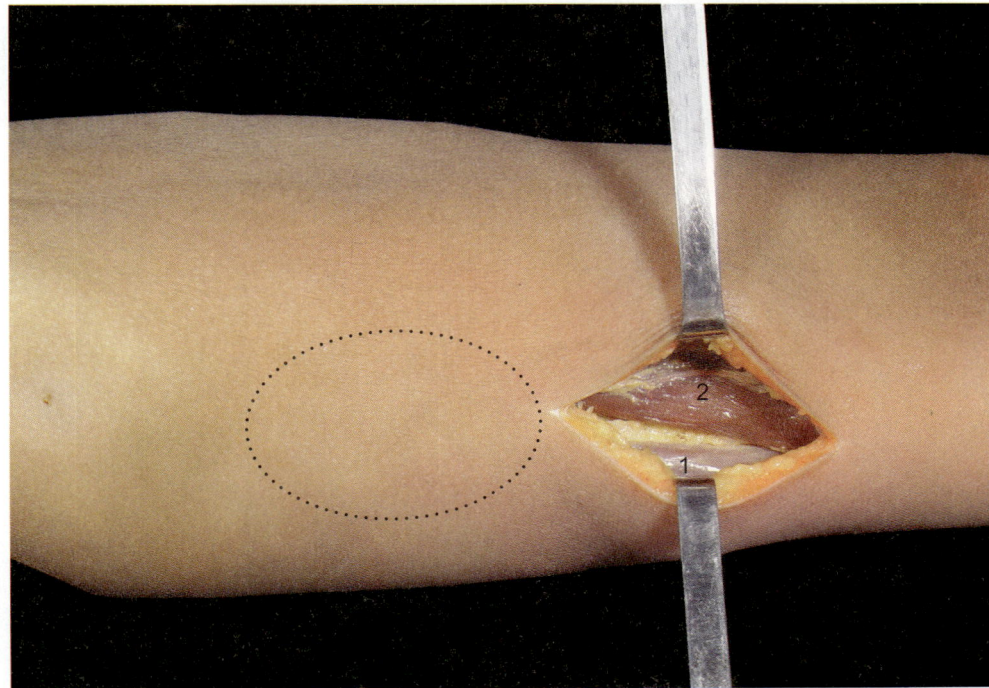

1. Gracilis muscle
2. Sartorius muscle

Figure 2-59   **Exposure of the muscle**

The flap should be firstly incised and traced distally to expose the gracilis muscle.

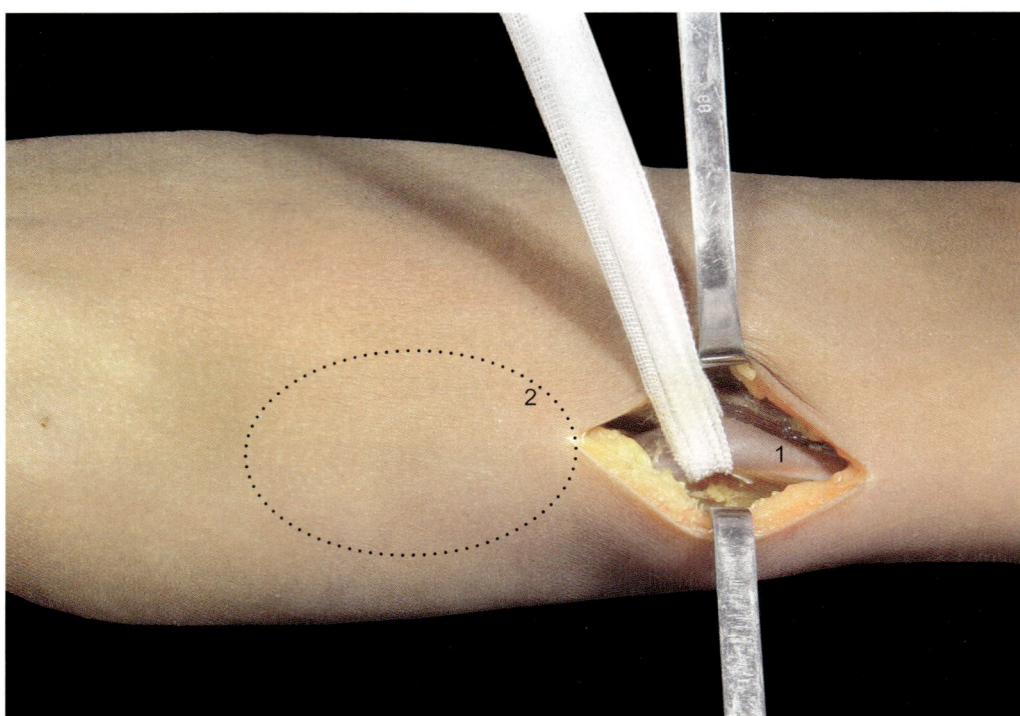

1. Gracilis muscle
2. Designing line

| **Figure 2-60** | **Separation of the muscle** |

The gracilis muscle should be separated and elevated to determine whether the muscle has been included in the flap. The design of the flap might be adjusted intraoperatively if necessary.

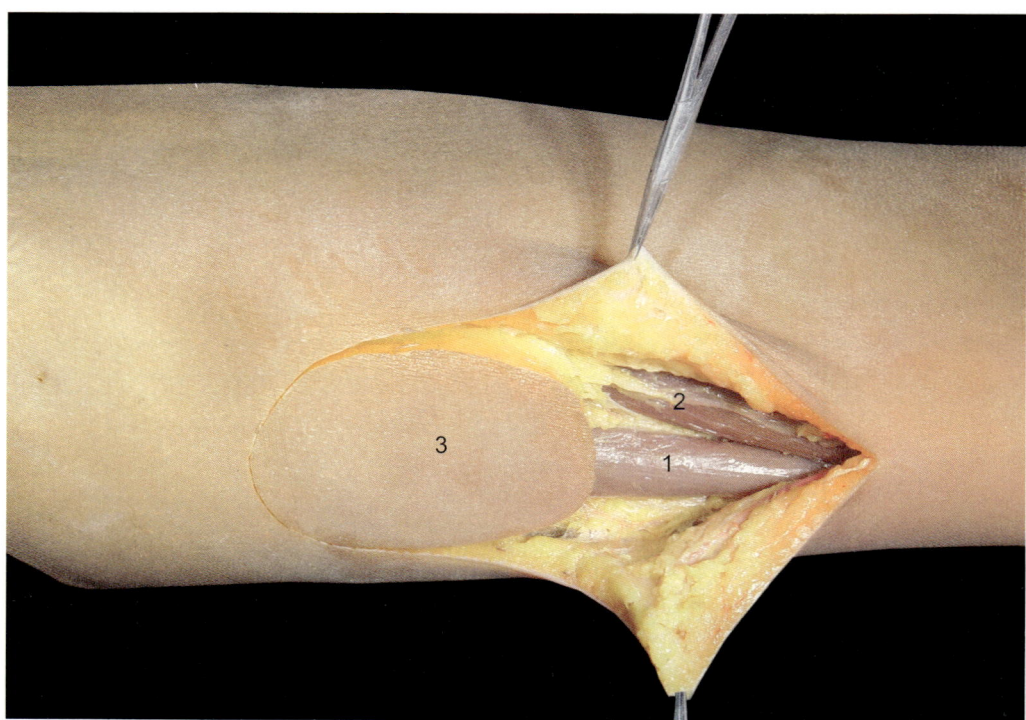

1. Gracilis muscle
2. Sartorius muscle
3. Flap

| **Figure 2-61** | **Dissection of the musculocutaneous flap** |

As has been designed, the flap should be incised one border after another along the designed line until it is completely dissected.

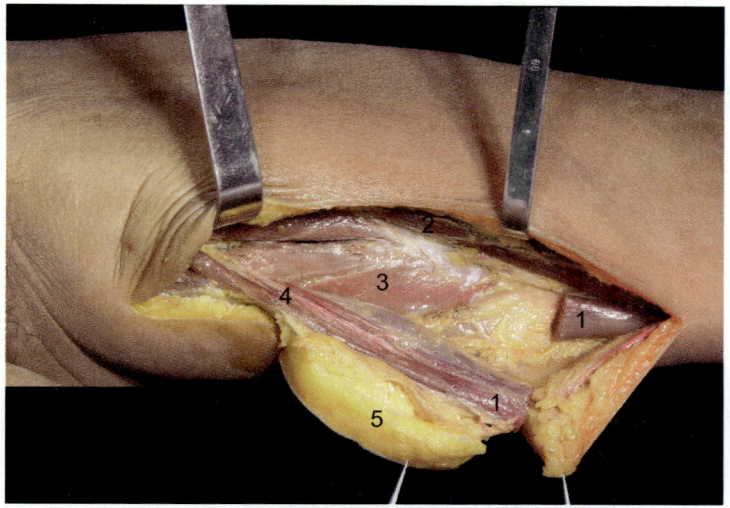

Figure 2-62 Elevation of the flap

The gracilis muscle should be cut off at the distal end of the flap. Then the flap should be elevated and separated towards its proximal end. The small nutrient vessels at the distal segment should be ligated and the main nutrient vessels that enter the superior 1/3 segment of the gracilis muscle kept intact.

1. Gracilis muscle
2. Sartorius muscle
3. Adductor magnus muscle
4. Nutrient vessels
5. Flap

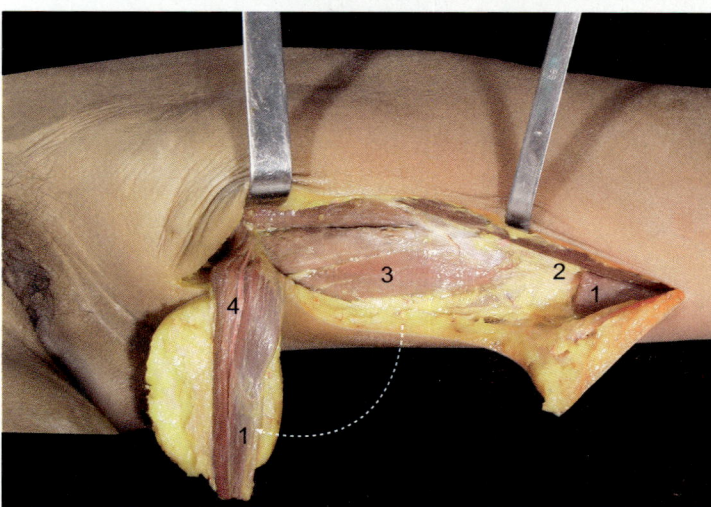

Figure 2-63 Transposition of the musculocutaneous flap

A broad subcutaneous tunnel should be made, through which the flap could be pulled to the recipient site. The muscle of the flap should be used to fill in the deep dead cavity and the skin to cover up the wound surface.

1. Gracilis muscle
3. Adductor magnus muscle

2. Sartorius muscle
4. Nutrient vessels

Key points in applied anatomy

Firstly, if it is difficult to locate the gracilis muscle, the distal incision might be extended downwards to expose the easily recognizable sartorius muscle and the gracilis muscle at its deep surface. It is not recommended to identify the gracilis muscle in the flap region in case any damages should occur to the perforating cutaneous arteries for the skin circulation. Secondly, since the gracilis muscle is connected loosely with the skin, it is necessary that the two be sutured temporarily to avoid disconnection of the layers. Thirdly, when the muscle is being separated, the small nutrient vessels at the distal segment should be ligated but the main nutrient vessels that enter the superior 1/3 segment of the muscle should be kept intact. Fourthly, since there exist the marginal branches, the skin island might extend to 2-3cm beyond the muscular edge so that it could be larger than the muscle island. Fifthly, if a large skin is needed, the superficial vein in the flap might be sutured in the recipient site to increase the blood reflow

12

Biceps Femoris
Musculocutaneous Flap

The posterior group femoral muscle consists of the biceps femoris muscle, the semitendinosus muscle and the semimembranosus muscle. These mucles are helpful for the hip extension and the knee flexion. They all originate from the ischial tuberosity, have a large muscle belly and are rich in blood circulation. These muscles should be cut off at their origins and transferred upward to repair a wound on the ischial tuberosity region.

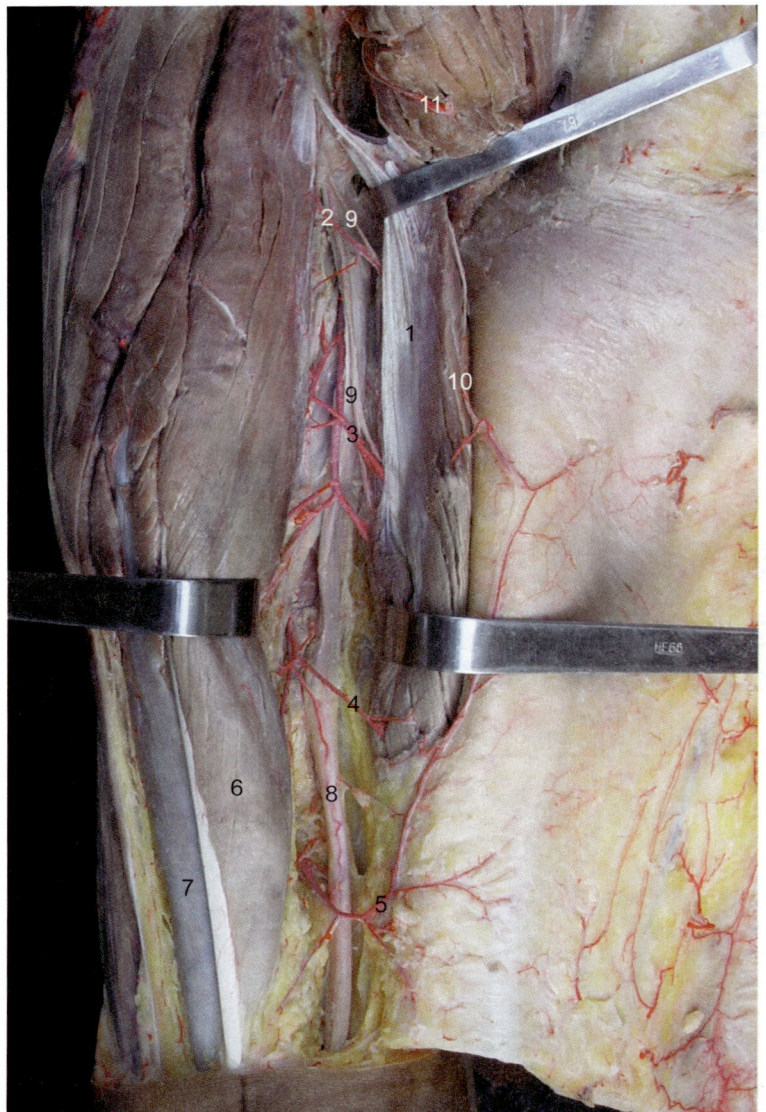

Figure 2-64   **Applied anatomy**

The biceps femoris muscle is situated at the posterior thigh. Most arteries of its long head emerge from the perforating artery, the medial circumflex femoral artery and the inferior gluteal artery. These arteries are about 1.3-1.7 mm in diameter. They enter the muscle at the middle-superior segment. The nerve of the biceps femoris muscle originates from the sciatic nerve, extends laterally downwards and enters the muscle with the vascular plexus.

1. Biceps femoris muscle (long head)
2. Muscular branch (from the 1st perforating artery)
3. Muscular branch (form the 2nd perforating artery)
4. Muscular branch (from the 3rd perforating artery)
5. Cutaneous branch (from the 4th perforating artery)
6. Semitendinosus muscle
7. Semimembranosus muscle
8. Sciatic nerve
9. Muscular branch (to the long head of biceps femoris muscle)
10. Posterior femoral cutaneous nerve
11. Inferior gluteal artery

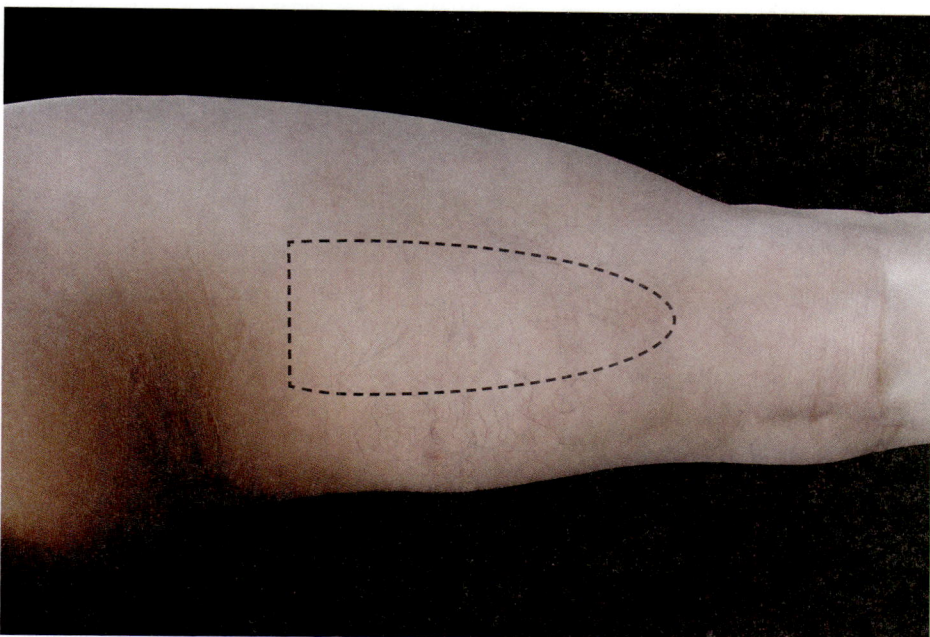

Figure 2-65   **Design of the musculocutaneous flap**

Take the repair of the decubital necrosis on the ischial tuberosity region. The patient in prone position, an inverted triangle flap should be designed at the posterior thigh. Its base should be proximally linked with the wound and as wide in transverse diameter as the wound; its tip should fall on the connecting line between the ischial tuberosity and the distal tendon of the biceps femoris muscle. If a composite flap based on either the semitendinous muscle or the semimembranous muscle is being made, its top tip should fall on the connecting line between the ischial tuberosity and the distal end of semitendinous muscle. If a composite flap includes the three muscles altogether, its top tip should fall on the line between the above two muscles.

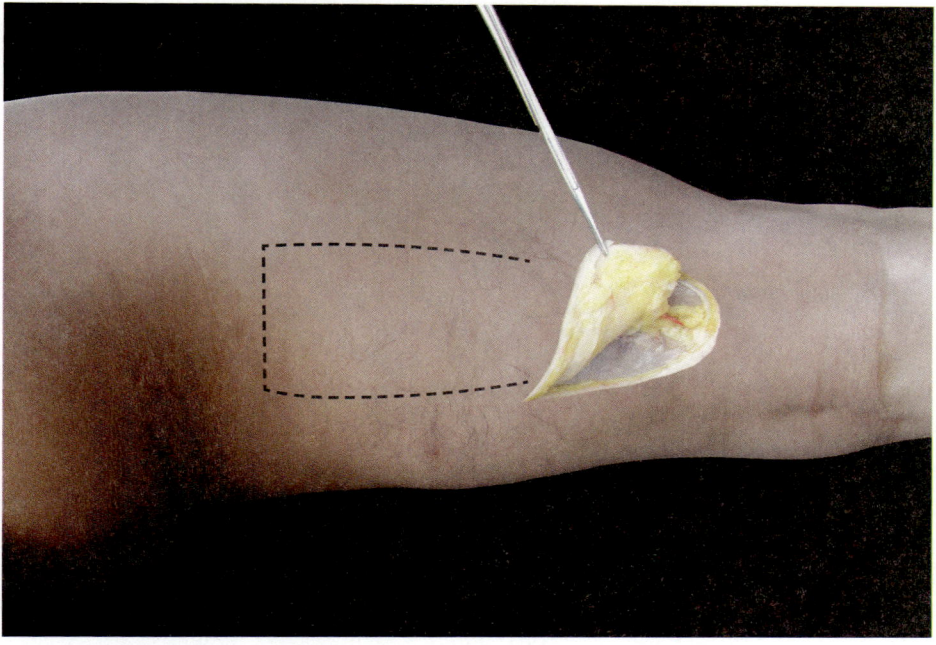

Figure 2-66   **Exposure of the muscle**

The tip of the flap should be incised down to the deep fascia to expose the long head of the biceps femoris muscle.

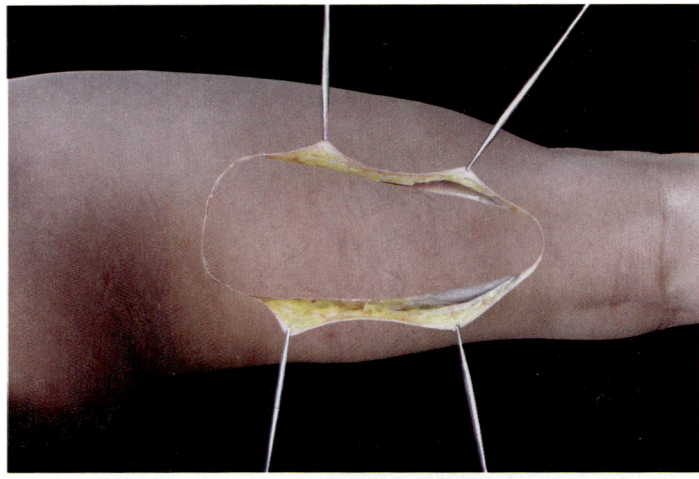

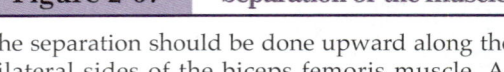

Figure 2-67   Separation of the muscle

The separation should be done upward along the bilateral sides of the biceps femoris muscle. At the lateral side the muscle should be freed from the short head of biceps femoris muscle and the vastus lateralis muscle, and at the medial side it freed from the semitendinosus muscle and the semimembranosus muscle.

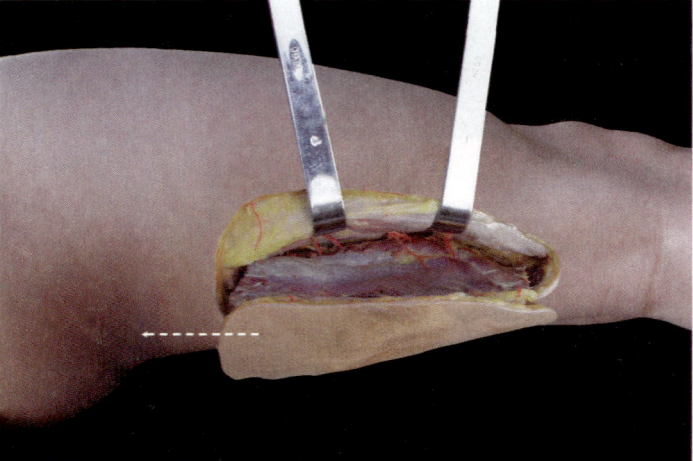

Figure 2-68   Transposition of the musculocutaneous flap

The flap then should be pushed proximally to repair a decubital necrosis on the ischial tuberosity region, its muscle used to fill in the deep cavity and its skin used to cover up the wound. If the recipient wound is large, the distal segment of the muscle could be separated to increase the flap mobility. Y-shaped closure should be presented after the flap is completely sutured.

Key points in applied anatomy

Firstly, the main muscular vessels that originate from the 1st perforating artery enter the deep surface of the long head of the biceps femoris muscle from its middle segment. From central incision in the posterior thigh, these vessels could be found just before the anterior margin of the muscle. Secondly, there is generally only one nerve in the long head of the biceps femoris muscle that enters the muscle at the same level as the main nutrient vessel. The nerve usually shares the trunk with the muscular branch of the semitendinosus muscle. The latter should be kept intact carefully in the procedure. Thirdly, it is preferable that the muscle and the skin be sutured and fixed with each other temporarily in the course of the operation, in case the blood circulation should be affected. Fourthly, the short head of the biceps femoris muscle attaches too long to the femur and the vascular pedicle is too short to be transferred. It is not suitable for muscular flap.

Gastrocnemius Musculocutaneous Flap

13

Gastrocnemius musculocutaneous flap is a composite flap pedicled with the sural vessel, which consists of two parts: the medial and the lateral ones. The medial gastrocnemius musculocutaneous flap is long and wide, and is one of most commonly used flaps in the restoration of the knee or the lower leg. The lateral gastrocnemius musculocutaneous flap is not as large as the medial one. Little harm might be done to the leg function when only part of the muscle is harvested, but the long scar left behind might affect the appearance of the leg.

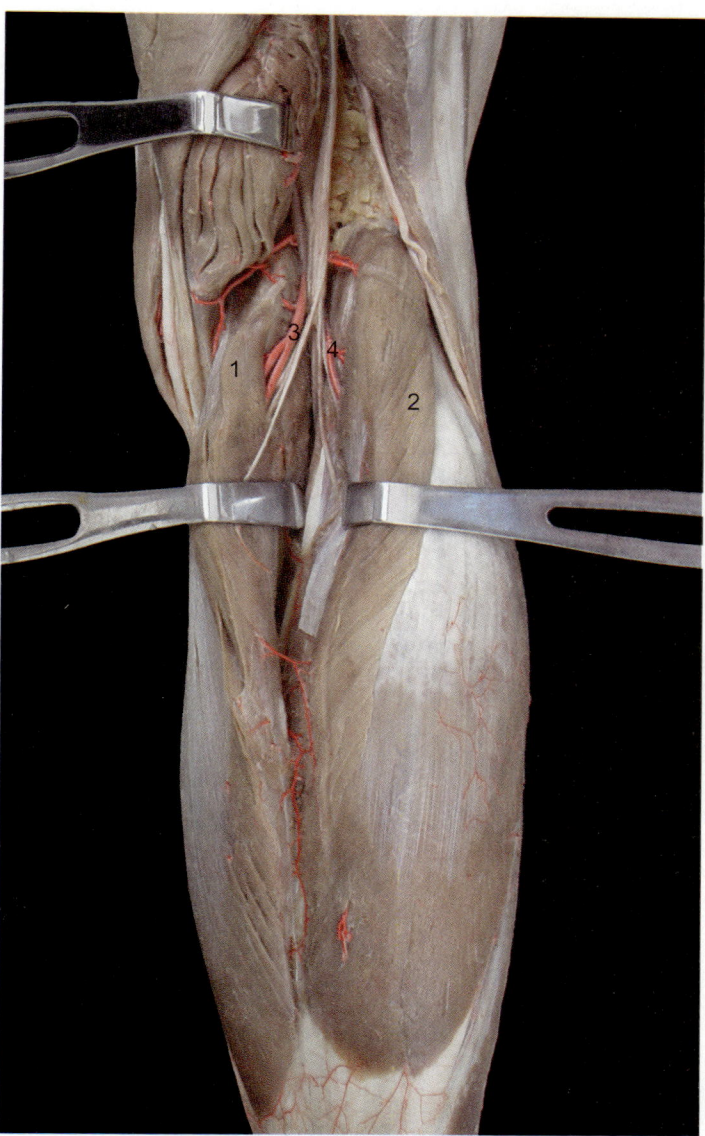

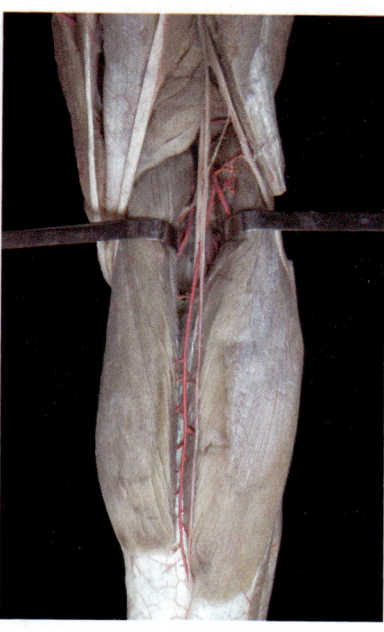

Figure 2-69	Applied anatomy

The medial and the lateral heads of the gastrocnemius muscle originate from the posterior region of the medial and the lateral condyles of the femur respectively. The muscle bellies of the two heads converge into each other and form a groove in which the lesser saphenous vein and the sural nerve run. The groove might serve as an anatomical mark in the operation. The nutrient arteries for the medial and the lateral heads originate medially and laterally from the popliteal arteries, respectively, and enter the muscle via its proximal deep surface and give many branches to form a vascular tree to nourish the muscle and the overlying skin. A flap based on the medial gastrocnemius muscle might be large in size, its superior to the mid popliteal fossa and its inferior to 5cm above the medial malleolus; its anterior to the medial margin of the tibia and its posterior to the posterior median line of the leg. A flap based on the lateral gastrocnemius muscle might be small in size, its lateral to the fibula and its distal to 10cm above the lateral malleolus.

1. Medial head of gastrocnemius muscle
2. Lateral head of gastrocnemius muscle
3. Medial sural artery
4. Lateral sural artery

A. Gastrocnemius muscular flap

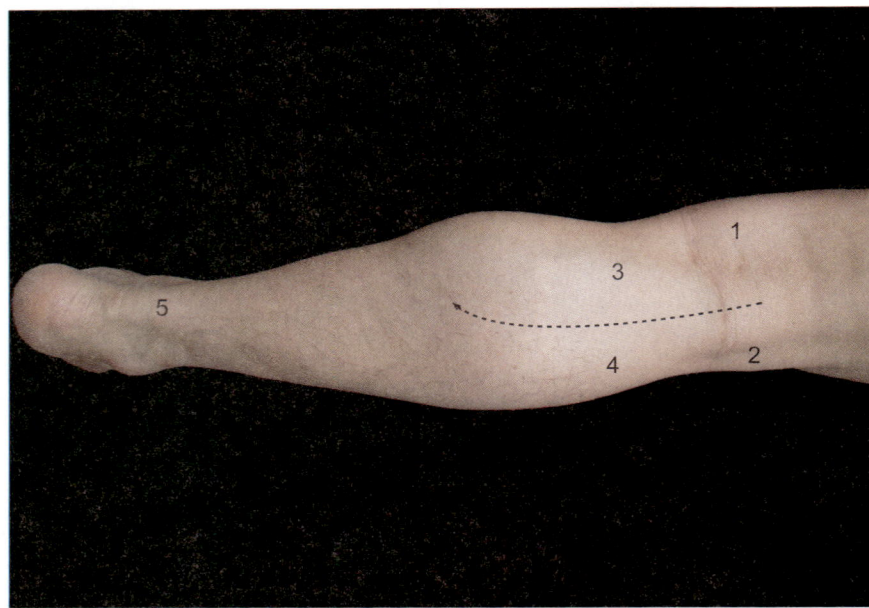

1. Semitendinosus muscle,
   Semimembranosus muscle
2. Biceps femoris muscle
3. Medial head of gastrocnemius
   muscle
4. Lateral head of gastrocnemius
   muscle
5. Calcaneal tendon

| **Figure 2-70** | **Design of the incision** |

Take the repair of a wound on the middle-superior segment of the leg. The incision of the flap should begin from the popliteal fossa, extend along the posterior midline of the leg, and curve medially at the intersection of the muscle and the tendon. The course of the incision should be presented in a J-shape. If the flap is based on the lateral head of gastrocnemius muscle, the distal of the incision should curve laterally.

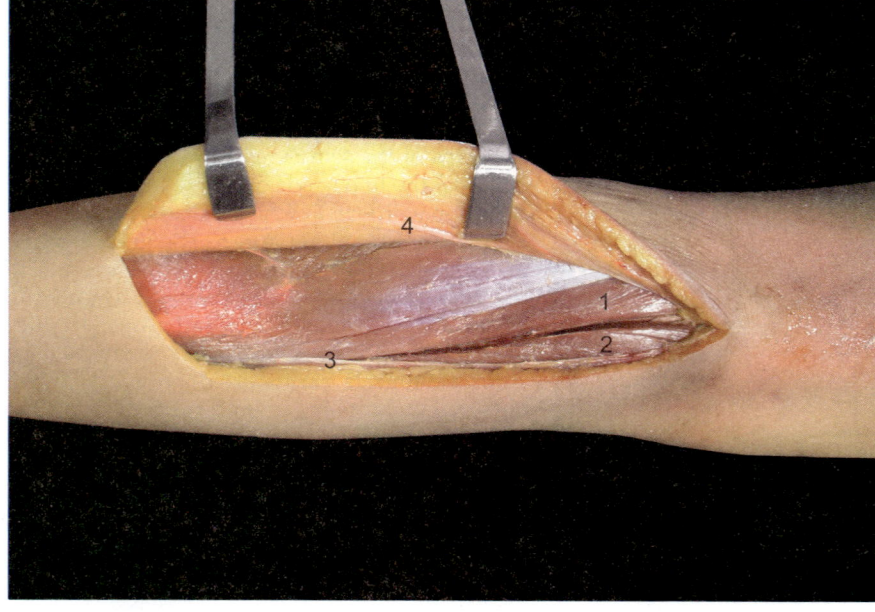

1. Medial head of
   gastrocnemius muscle
2. Lateral head of
   gastrocnemius muscle
3. Lesser saphenous vein
4. Sural nerve

| **Figure 2-71** | **Exposure of the muscle** |

The skin and the deep fascia should be incised and the flap elevated laterally to expose the medial and the lateral heads of the gastrocnemius muscle. The lesser saphenous vein and the sural nerve between the two heads should be kept intact.

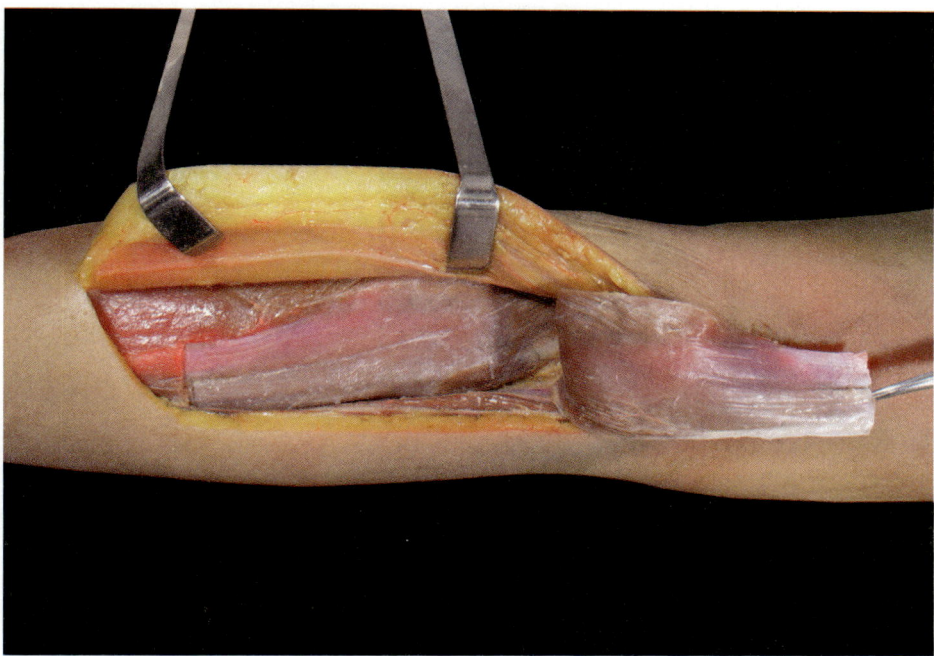

Figure 2-72   **Dissection of the flap**

The medial and the lateral heads of the gastrocnemius muscle should be separated bluntly under the superior incision to determine the spatium between the medial head and the soleus muscle. Then the two muscles should be separated with the doctor's fingers until the gastrocnemius is long enough to be transferred. A spacious tunnel should be made between the crural fascia and the deep fascia.

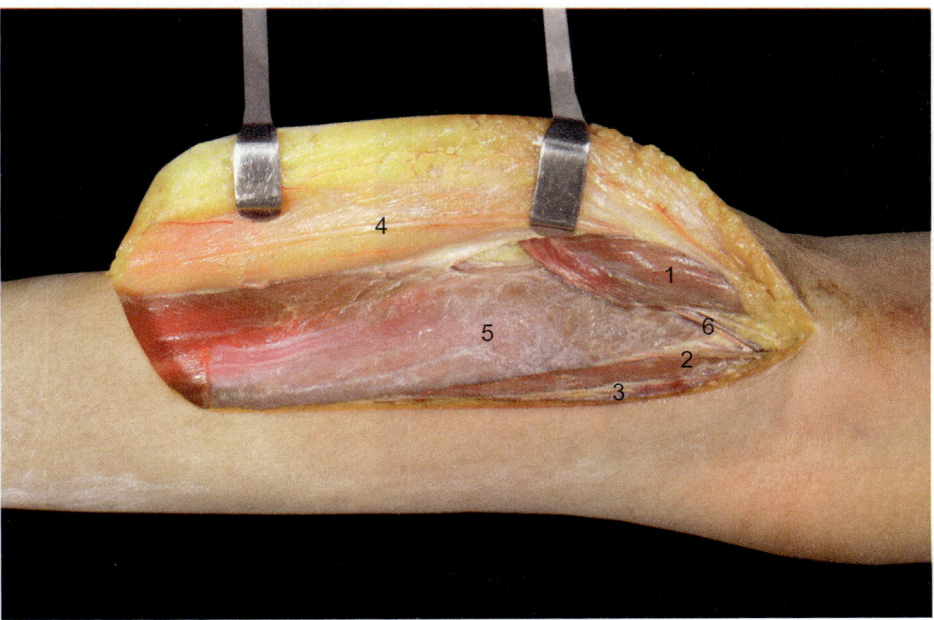

Figure 2-73   **Transposition of the muscle flap**

The muscular flap should be pulled through the tunnel to the recipient site.

1. Medial head of gastrocnemius muscle   2. Lateral head of gastrocnemius muscle
3. Lesser saphenous vein   4. Sural nerve
5. Soleus muscle   6. Medial sural artery

B. Retrograde gastrocnemius muscular flap

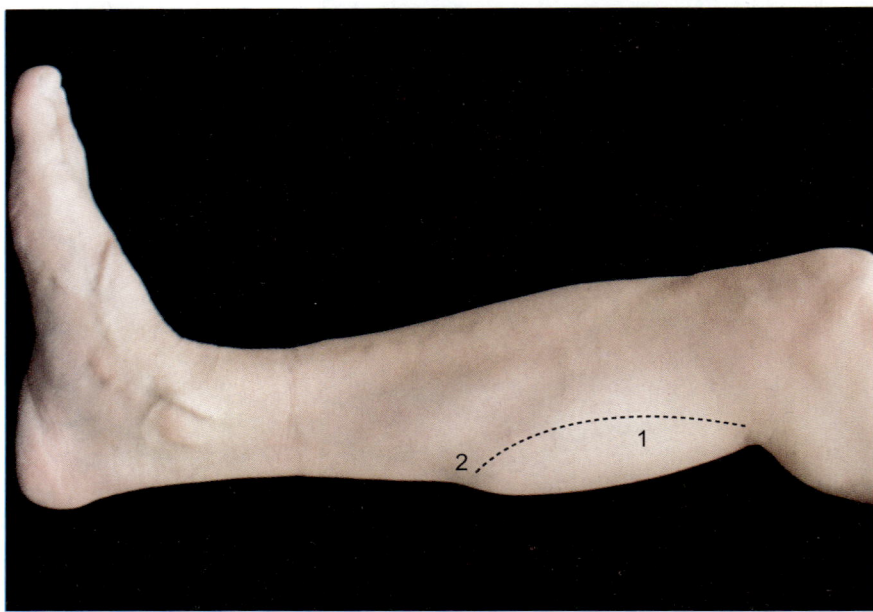

1. Gastrocnemius muscle
2. Soleus muscle

Figure 2-74   **Design of the incision**

Take the restoration of the infected osseous wound on the middle-inferior segment of the leg. A curved incision should be made from the popliteal fossa to the middle-inferior region of the leg.

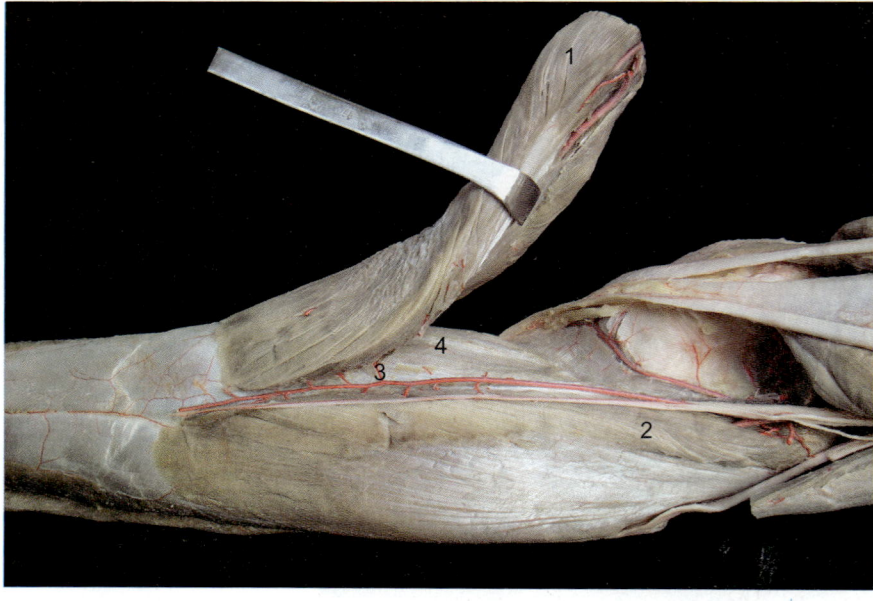

1. Medial head of gastrocnemius muscle
2. Lateral head of gastrocnemius muscle
3. Communicating branches
4. Soleus muscle

Figure 2-75   **Dissection of the muscle flap**

The skin should be incised to expose the gastrocnemius muscle and its medial head be cut off from the femoral attachment. The medial and the lateral heads of the muscle should be separated at the superior segment. The communicating arterial branches in the inferior segments of the two heads should be retained to guarantee a good blood supply for the flap. Finally the flap based on the medial head of the gastrocnemius muscle should be pulled through the tunnel to the recipient site and the dead cavity filled in with the muscle.

C. Gastrocnemius musculocutaneous flap

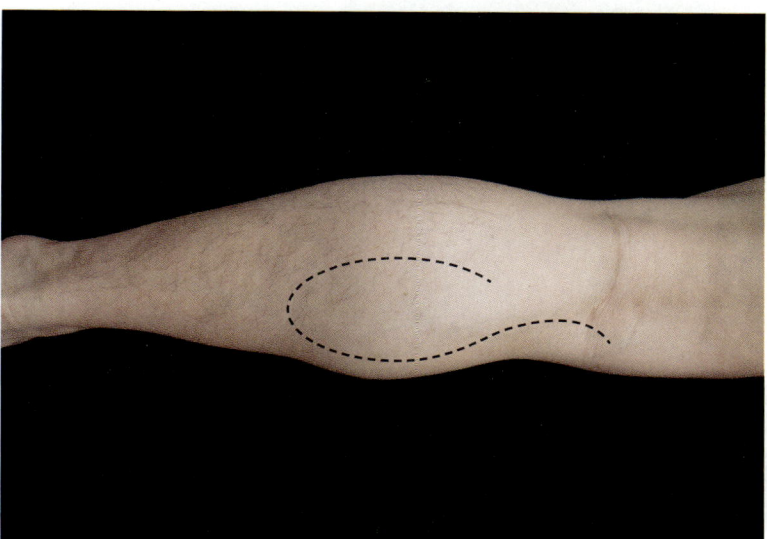

| Figure 2-76 | Design of the musculocutaneous flap |

Take the design of the musculocutaneous flap based on the medial gastrocnemius muscle. The patient lying on the operated side, the base of flap might be located at the posterosuperior portion of his leg, with its posterior margin to the posterior crural midline and its anterior connected with the wound edge with no normal tissue in between. Its distal end extends for 3-5cm over the level of the distal wound edge. The shape of the flap depends on that of the wound.

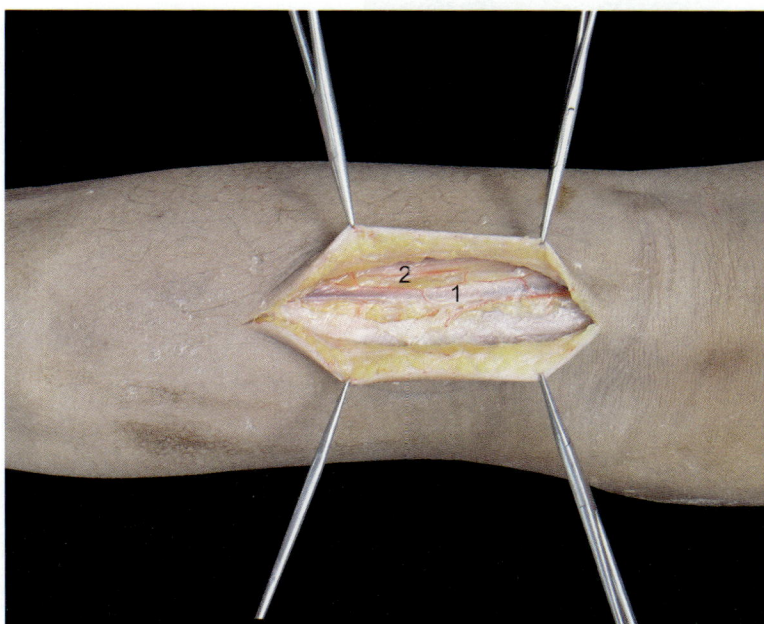

1. Lesser saphenous vein
2. Sural nerve

| Figure 2-77 | Exposure of the muscle |

The posterior superior incision of the flap should be made near the popliteal fossa. The deep fascia should be incised to expose the lesser saphenous vein and the sural nerve along the posterior crural midline. The two should be drawn laterally to keep them intact. The different directions of the muscle fibers of the medial and the lateral heads could serve as indications to determine the two heads and the spatium between them.

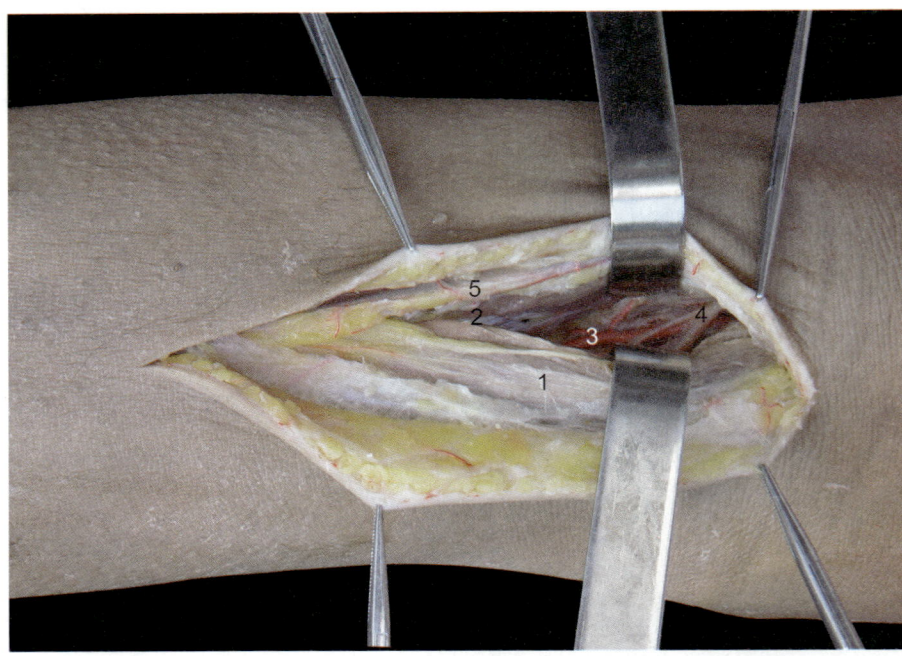

1. Medial head of gastrocnemius muscle
2. Lateral head of gastrocnemius muscle
3. Medial sural artery
4. Nerve of medial head of gastrocnemius muscle
5. Lesser saphenous vein

Figure 2-78	Separation of the intermuscular spatium

The intermuscular spatium between the medial and the lateral heads should be separated bluntly to expose a deep septum between the medial head of the gastrocnemius muscle and the soleus muscle, which is loosely connected and easy to be separated with the doctor's fingers. The medial sural artery enters the proximal deep surface of the gastrocnemius muscle, and it should be kept intact.

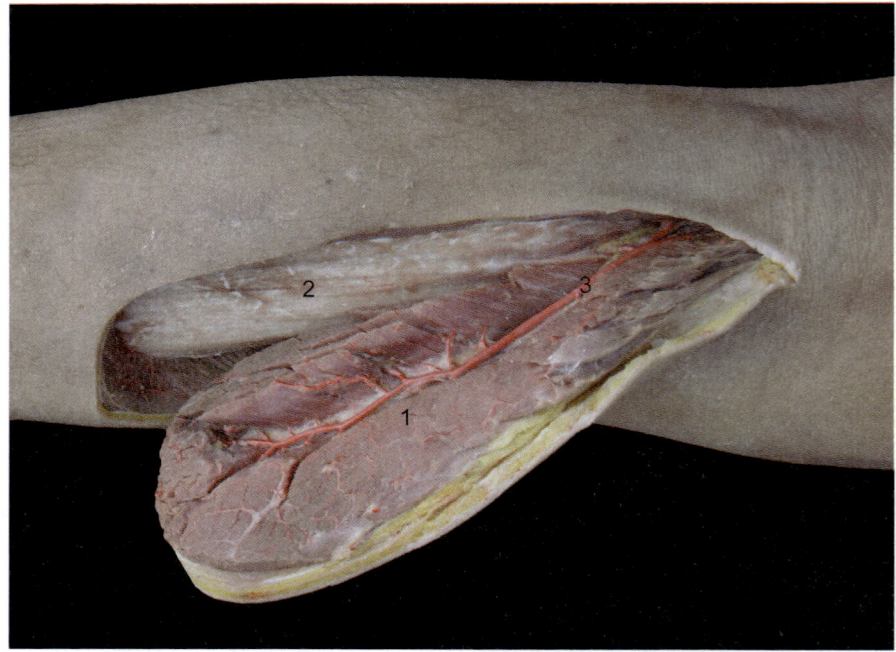

1. Medial head of gastrocnemius muscle
2. Soleus muscle
3. Medial sural artery

Figure 2-79	Dissection of the musculocutaneous flap

The spatium between the medial and the lateral heads together with the spatium of the medial head and the soleus muscle should be separated bluntly from proximal to distal with the doctor's fingers. The anterior and the distal borders of the flap should then be incised one by one so that the flap could be completely elevated. It is usually not necessary to separate the basal skin at the proximal pedicle.

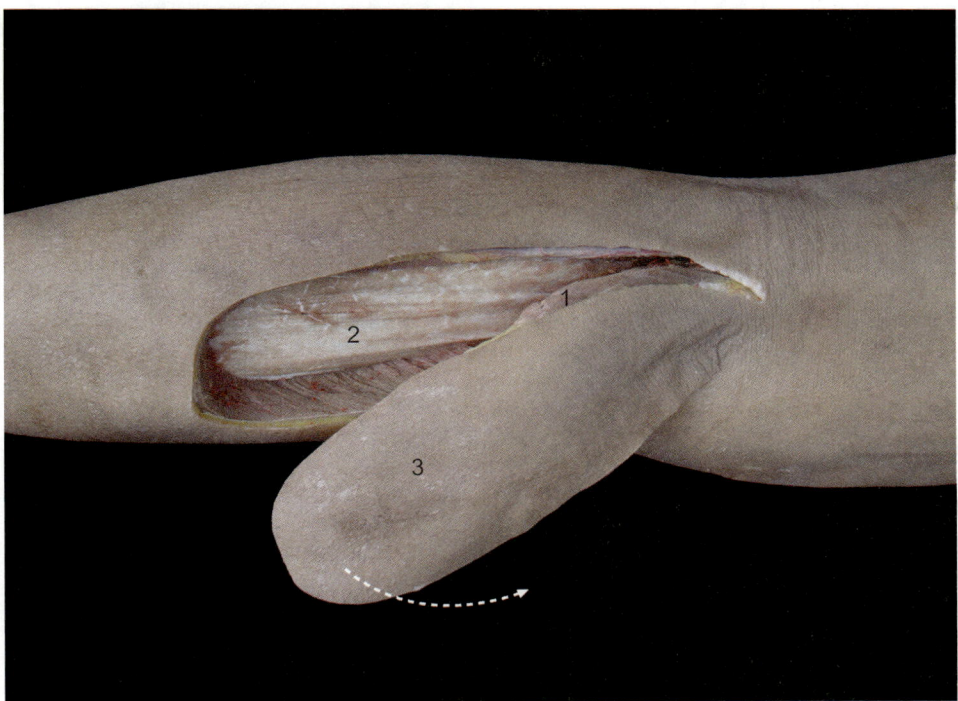

Figure 2-80   **Transposition of the musculocutaneous flap**

The made flap might be transferred anteriorly to repair a wound on the anterior tibia.

1. Medial head of gastrocnemius muscle
2. Soleus muscle
3. Musculocutaneous flap

Key points in applied anatomy

Firstly, when the recipient site is situated at the middle-superior segment of the tibia, it is not necessary that the vascular pedicle be exposed. Secondly, when the recipient site is situated at the inferior segment of the upper leg or on the knee, the flap should be made either as a musculofascial island flap with the medial head of the gastrocnemius muscle separated from the condylar attachment of the femur, or as a neurovascular island flap with the medial head cut off from its attachment. Both of them might augment the rotating arch of the flap. Thirdly, the distal portion of flap should be elevated from the deep surface of the fascia, and the loose connective tissue over the calcaneal tendon retained for skin grafting. When the distal portion of the medial head is cut off at the muscle-tendon intersection plane, care should be taken to avoid disconnection of the layers of the muscle and the subcutaneous tissue. Fourthly, if a free flap or a neurovascular pedicled flap is being made, the vessels in the pedicle should be kept intact. The arteries and the veins should not get disconnected from each other. Fifthly, the subcutaneous tunnel should be spacious enough to let the flap pass through to the recipient site and inset on the wound properly to guarantee a tension-free suture. Sixthly, the two skin edges of the donor site should be first subcutaneously sutured to reduce the size of wound surface. A split-thick skin graft should be then taken from the upper leg for a donor site closure. Seventhly, the two heads of the gastrocnemius muscle have constant nutrient arteries to anastomose with each other extensively over the superficial skin. The skin of the flap might be larger than the underlying muscle. Eighthly, the connective part of the medial and the lateral heads of the gastrocnemius muscle at the fibular head is the muscle portal through which the medial and the lateral sural arteries and nerves enter the gastrocnemius muscle.

Extensor Digitorum Brevis Musculocutaneous Flap

The extensor digitorum brevis musculocutaneous flap gets its blood supply from the dorsal pedal artery. It has such advantages as constant vascular situation and easy dissection. When the dorsal pedal artery is dissected proximally to the anterior tibial artery, the pedicle might be long enough to be transferred for a restoration of a soft tissue defect on the knee, the lower leg, the malleolus or the calcaneal region. The making of the flap might do little harm to the function of the foot but leave only the coverage of periosteum and epitendineum over the donor site, which might reduce the survival rate of a free skin graft. The scarred donor region might hardly resist wearing.

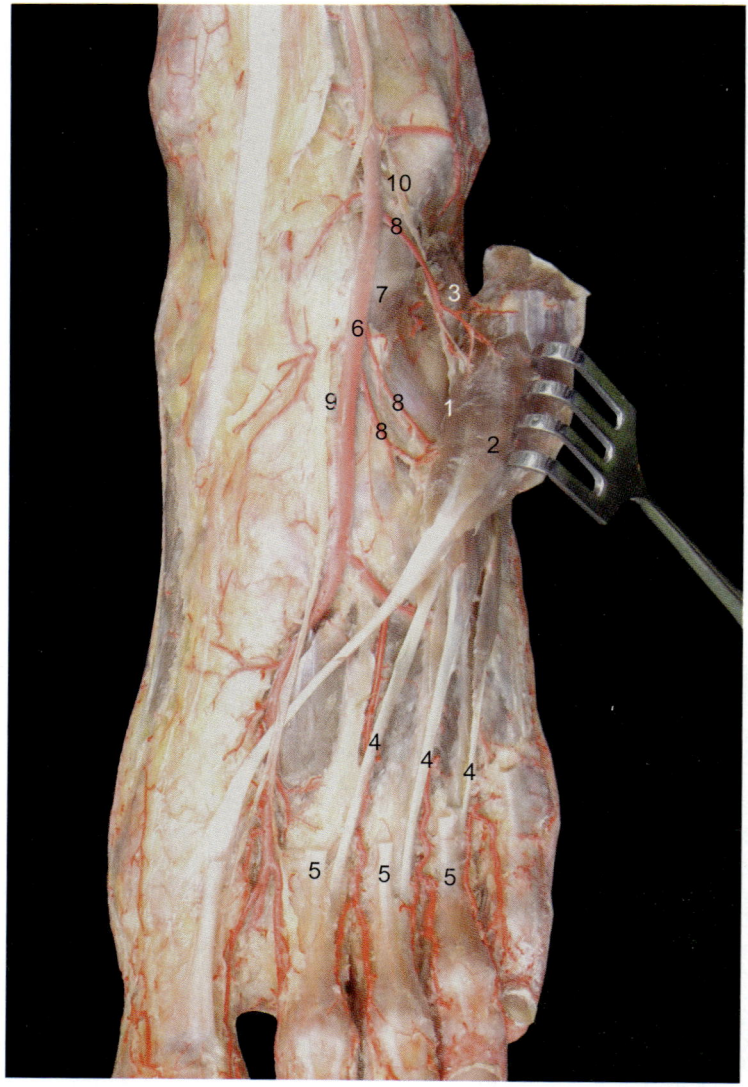

| **Figure 2-81** | **Applied anatomy** |

The extensor digitorum brevis originates from the anterior calcaneal bone before the tarsal sinus, together with the extensor hallucis brevis muscle. It divides into 3 small tendons that converge into the 2nd, the 3rd and the 4th extensor digitorum longus tendons to supplement extending the toes. The muscle has its blood supply from the lateral tarsal artery, which originates from the dorsal pedal artery around the talus head. The lateral tarsal artery runs anteriorly outwards along the deep surface of the muscle and sends branches to nourish it. The artery has 1-5 muscular branches, and in most cases (78%), it has 2. The proximal branch (about 1.8mm in diameter) accompanies the muscular branch of the deep peroneal nerve to enter the muscle. Besides, the extensor digitorum/hallucis brevis muscle also has branches from the anterior lateral malleolus artery.

1. Extensor digitorum brevis
2. Extensor hallucis brevis muscle
3. Calcaneal bone
4. Tendon of extensor digitorum brevis
5. Tendon of extensor digitorum longus
6. Dorsal pedal artery
7. Talus head
8. Lateral tarsal artery
9. Deep peroneal nerve
10. Nerve of extensor digitorum brevis

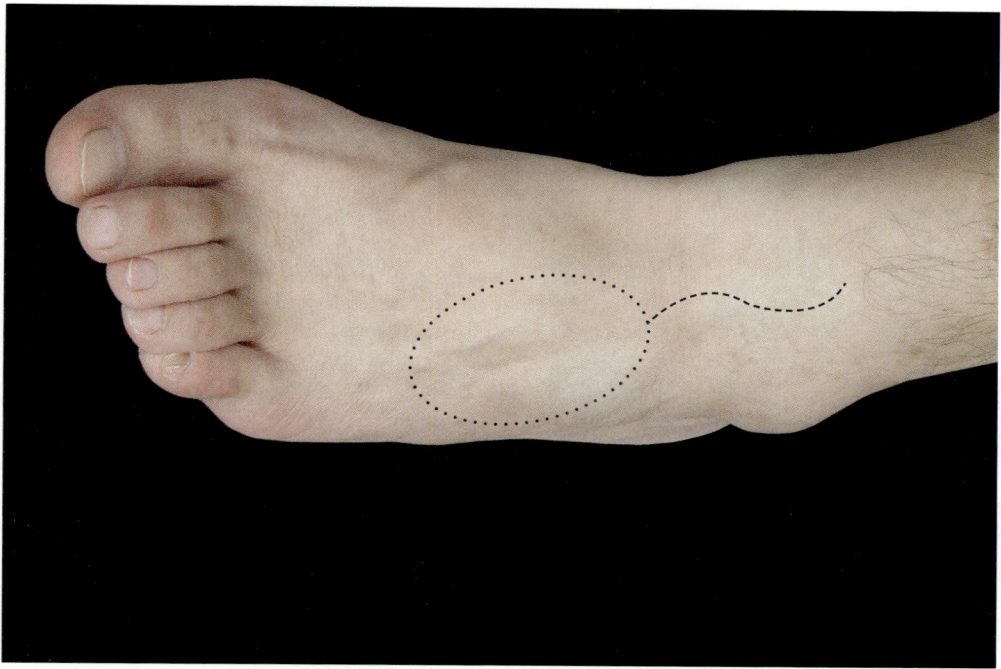

Figure 2-82   Design of the flap

According to the defect size of the recipient region, the flap should be designed along the outline of the extensor digitorum brevis, and its proximal incision extend in the direction of the artery.

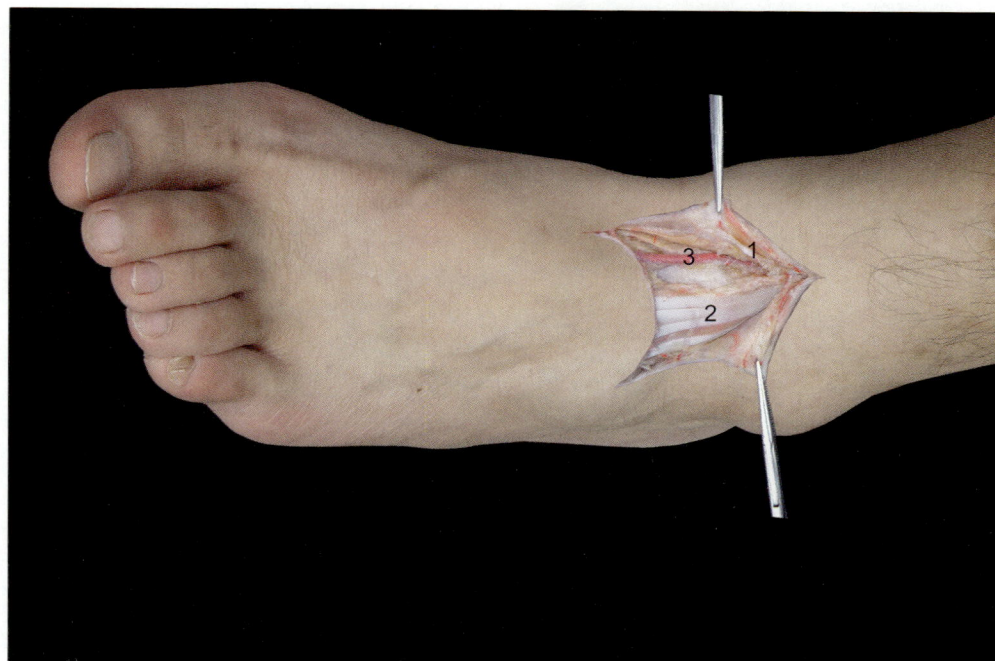

1. Extensor hallucis longus muscle
2. Extensor digitorum longus
3. Dorsal pedal artery

Figure 2-83   Exposure of the vessels

The flap should be incised first at its proximal portion. The incised tissue should be drawn bilaterally to expose the extensor hallucis and the digitorum longus muscle and the dorsal pedal artery and vein that are situated between the two muscles. Then the incision should continue along the dorsal pedal artery to the deep surface of the extensor digitorum brevis to find out the lateral tarsal artery.

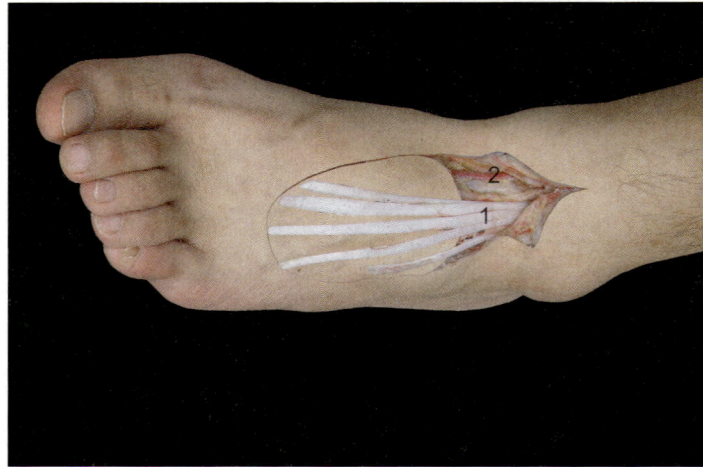

Figure 2-84   Dissection of the flap

As has been designed, the dorsal pedal skin should be incised. The tendon of the extensor digitorum longus and the extensor digitorum brevis should be cut off at the distal end of the flap, and the former pulled out through the proximal incision (the cut tendon might be sutured back to its normal position after the flap is dissected). The cut extensor digitorum brevis should be sutured with the skin edge to avoid disconnection of the two. The incision then should continue along the dorsal pedal artery to the 1st dorsal metatarsal artery, where the deep plantar branch could be found and ligated. The flap should then be elevated from the distal to the proximal at the superficial layer of the periosteum and the ligament. When the dissection continues to the lateral edge of the extensor digitorum brevis, the anastomotic branch between the lateral tarsal artery and the lateral calcaneal artery should be ligated and the origin of the extensor digitorum brevis separated near the tarsal sinus.

1. Extensor digitorum longus
2. Dorsal pedal artery

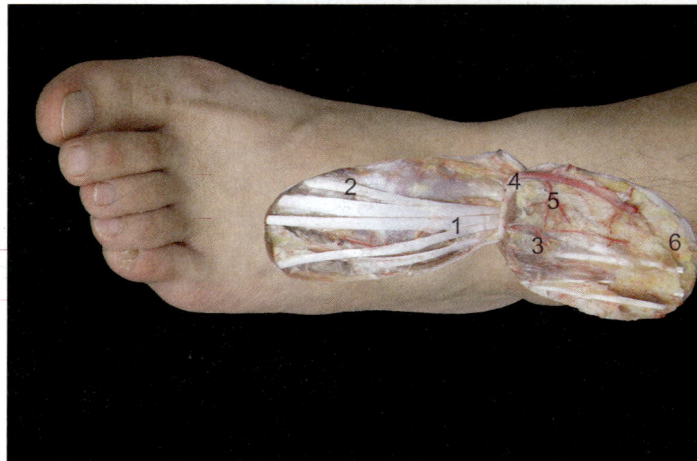

1. Extensor digitorum longus
2. Extensor hallucis longus muscle
3. Extensor digitorum brevis
4. Anterior tibial artery and vein
5. Muscular branch
6. Flap

Figure 2-85   Transposition of the flap

The incision should extend proximally. The crural transverse ligament and the cruciate ligament should be separated, and an extensor digitorum brevis musculocutaneous flap harvested with pedicles of the anterior tibial artery and vein. The flap might be transferred locally to repair a wound on the medial malleolus.

Key points in applied anatomy

Firstly, the extensor digitorum brevis is situated in the lateral deep surface of the extensor digitorum longus. The extensor hallucis longus could be easily identified and used as a mark to identify the extensor digitorum brevis. Secondly, the proximal branch of the lateral tarsal artery is the main blood supplier of the flap and should be kept intact. Thirdly, since the lateral tarsal artery tends to be small in diameter, it is preferable that the dorsal pedal artery serve as the vascular pedicle of the flap. Fourthly, the deep peroneal nerve gives the extensor digitorum brevis muscular branches at the intermalleolus line to extend anteriorly outwards, and enter the muscle with the proximal branch of the lateral tarsal artery. When a long nerve is needed for a free flap pedicled with nerves and vessles, the nerve should be separated retrogradely along the muscular branch until it is long enough. Fifthly, in most cases, the dorsal pedal artery extends constantly along the lateral side of the extensor hallucis longus, but in some cases, its course might have altered, since there is a perforating branch of the peroneal artery that takes its place.

Abductor Hallucis Musculocutaneous Flap

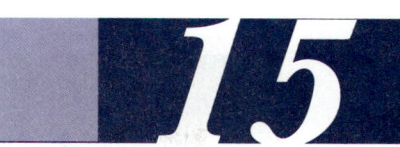

15

The abductor hallucis musculocutaneous flap depends on the medial plantar artery for blood supply. It is situated at the non weight-bearing region of the medial planta, but its anatomic structure is similar to that of the weight-bearing region. It has such advantages as a good blood circulation, a good sensory function but little affect on the function after the flap is dissected. An abductor hallucis musculocutaneous flap might be transferred to restore a soft tissue defect on the calcaneus, the malleolus or the lower leg. A free flap might be transferred to restore a muscular defect on the face that occurs subsequent to an injury or an operation. It might be transferred to restore the facial paralysis, too.

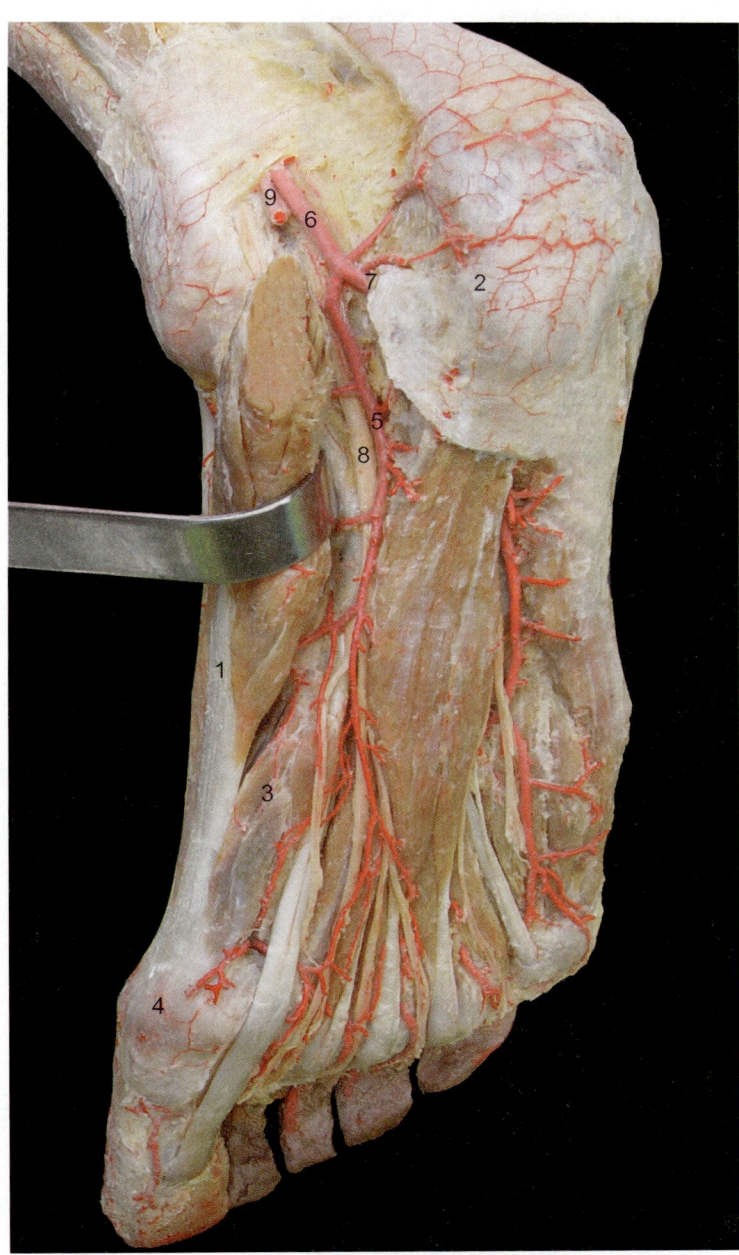

| Figure 2-86 | Applied anatomy |

The abductor hallucis muscle is situated at the medial planta. It starts from the medial process of the calcaneal tuberosity, the navicular tuberosity and the ligaments, converges into the medial head of the flexor hallucis brevis muscle, and terminate at the medial digital ligament and the base of proximal phalanx. It has the medial plantar artery as its nutrient vessel, which originates from the posterior tibial artery at the deep surface of the origin of the abductor hallucis muscle and extends forward through the deep surface of the muscle. Along the course, it gives muscular branches and cutaneous branches to nourish the abductor hallucis muscle and the overlying skin.

1. Abductor hallucis muscle
2. Calcaneal tuberosity
3. Flexor hallucis brevis muscle
4. Proximal phalanx
5. Medial plantar artery
6. Posterior tibial artery
7. Lateral plantar artery
8. Medial plantar nerve
9. Posterior tibial vein

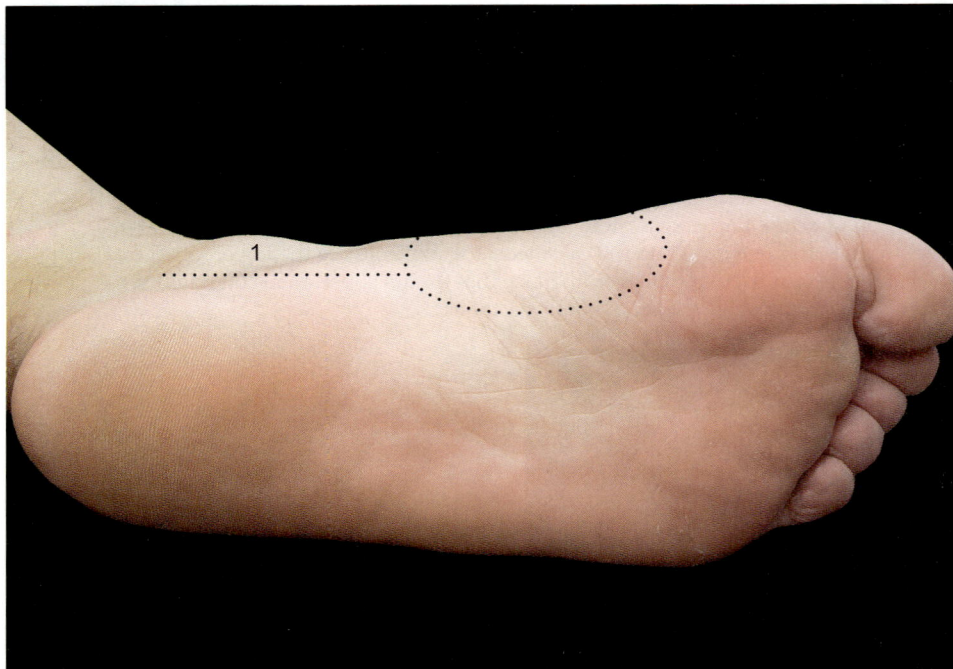

1. Medial malleolus

Figure 2-87   Design of the flap

The flap should be designed at the non-weight-bearing region of the medial planta, with its pivot point located at the cross point of the extension line anterior to the medial malleolus and the medial margin of the planta and with the abductor hallucis muscle as its axial line. The proximal incision line should be marked along the vessels.

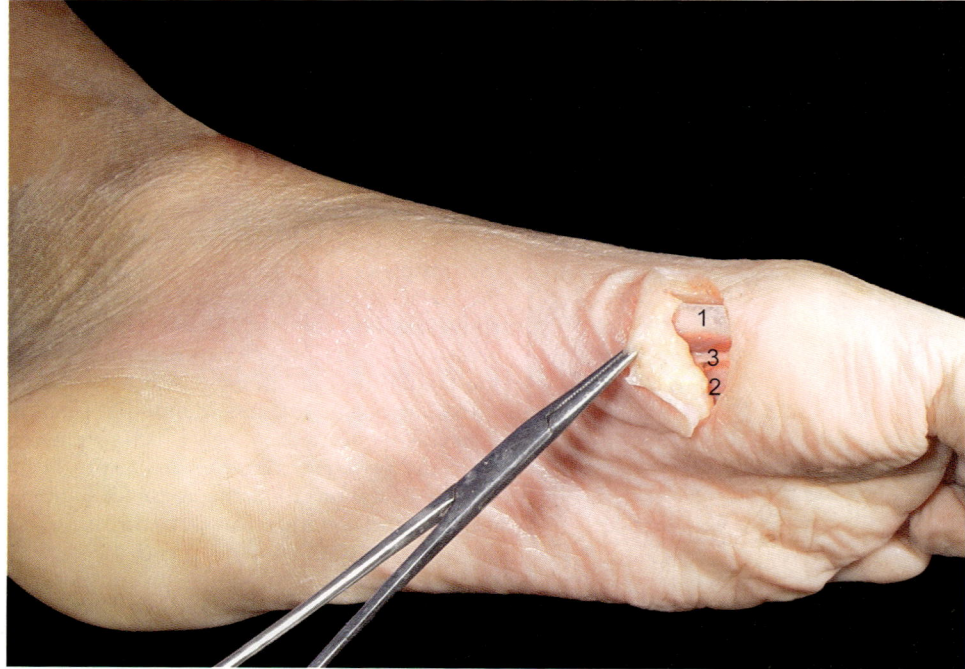

1. Abductor hallucis muscle
2. Flexor digitorum brevis
3. Medial plantar artery

Figure 2-88   Exposure of the vessels

The distal border of the flap should be incised first to expose the medial plantar artery in the septum between the abductor hallucis muscle and the flexor digitorum brevis.

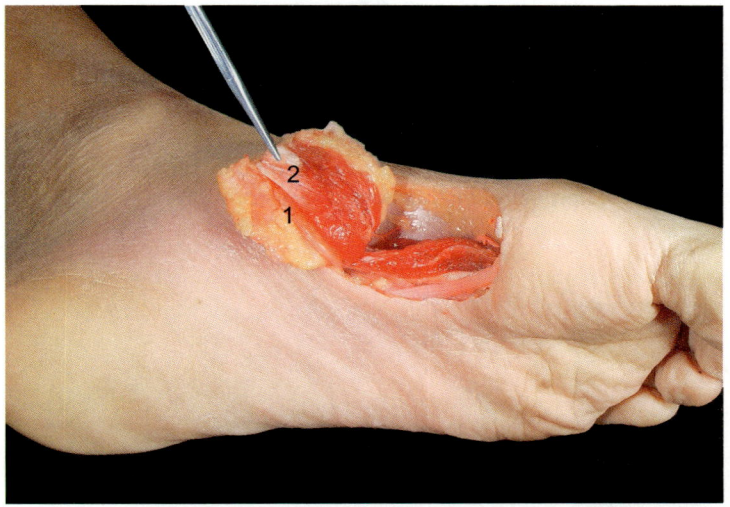

Figure 2-89   Dissection of the flap

The medial plantar artery should be cut off at the distal end of the flap. Along the artery, the dissection should extend proximally at the deep surface of the abductor hallucis muscle, and the muscle then elevated with the overlying skin.

1. Medial plantar artery
2. Abductor hallucis muscle

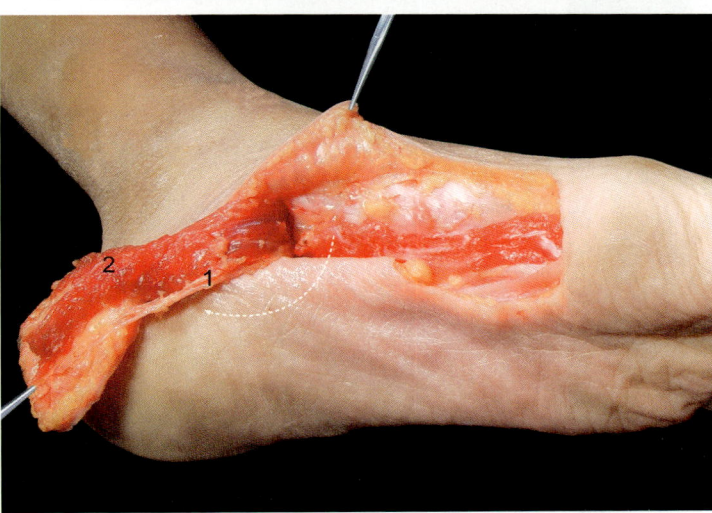

Figure 2-90   Dissection of the musculocutaneous flap

The proximal border of the musculocutaneous flap should be incised to separate the flap proximally. When an island flap is needed, the origin of the muscle should be divided. In any cases, the medial plantar artery situated beneath the deep surface of the muscle should be kept intact.

1. Medial plantar artery
2. Abductor hallucis muscle

Key points in applied anatomy

Firstly, the nerve that innervates the abductor hallucis muscle originates from the medial plantar nerve and accompanies closely either the trunk or the superficial branch of the medial plantar artery. The nerve should be carefully protected in the procedure. Secondly, when a long pedicle is needed, the nerve should be separated and traced to the place where the medial plantar artery originates. The nerval pedicle might be longer than 8.5 cm. When the nerve trunk is sharply split from the place where the medial plantar nerve bifurcates, an even longer pedicle could be harvested. Thirdly, only the non-weight-bearing skin should be included in the flap. The skin should be larger than the underlying muscle.

16

Flexor Digitorum Brevis Musculocutaneous Flap

The flexor digitorum brevis musculocutaneous flap based on the lateral plantar artery should be located at the non-weight-bearing region of the planta between the heads of the metatarsal bones and the calcaneus. A flap of this type tends to be large and might be transferred to restore a large soft tissue defect on the calcaneus.

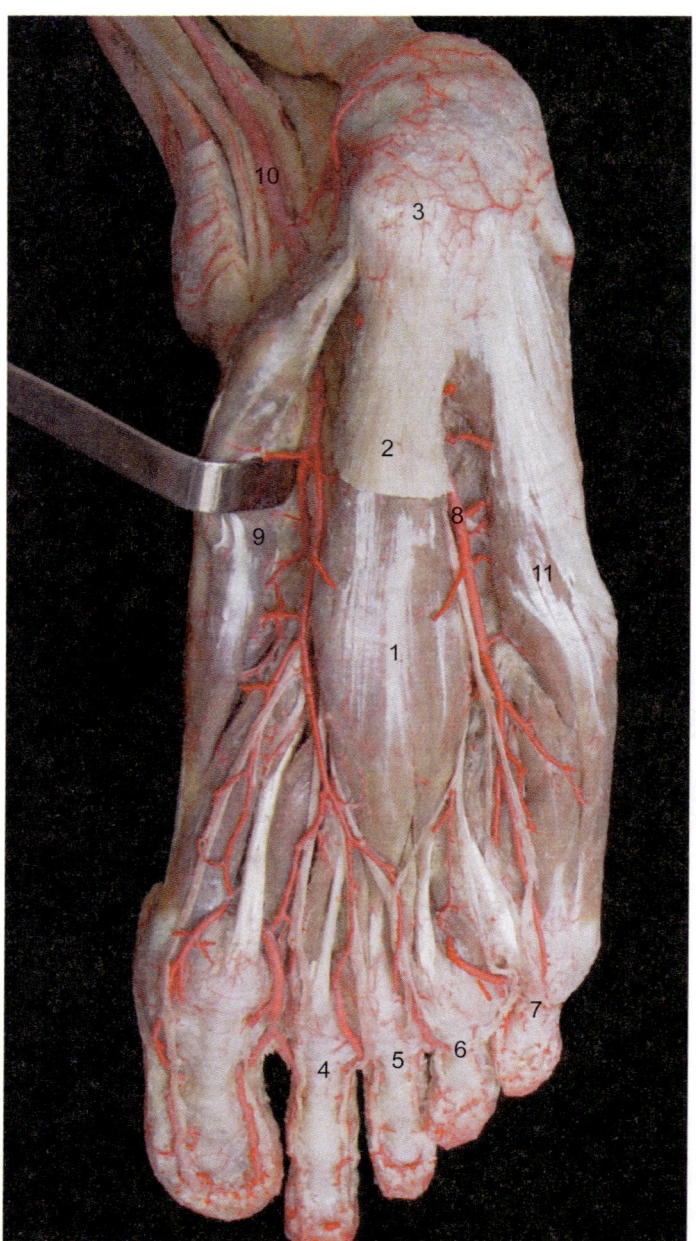

Figure 2-91   **Applied anatomy**

The flexor digitorum brevis is situated in the mid planta. It starts at the plantar aponeurosis and the medial process of calcaneal bone, and divides into 4 tendons that terminate at the 2nd, the 3rd, the 4th and the 5th middle phalanxes, respectively. Its nutrient vessels originate from the lateral plantar artery, which comes from the posterior tibial artery at the deep surface of the origin of the abductor hallucis muscle. Then the artery runs anteriorly outwards through the deep surface of the flexor digitorum brevis. In the septum between the flexor digitorum brevis and the abductor digiti minimi, the lateral plantar artery gives muscular branches to nourish the flexor digitorum brevis and the overlying skin.

1. Flexor digitorum brevis
2. Plantar aponeurosis
3. Calcaneal bone
4. 2nd middle phalanx
5. 3rd middle phalanx
6. 4th middle phalanx
7. 5th middle phalanx
8. Lateral plantar artery
9. Abductor hallucis muscle
10. Posterior tibial artery
11. Abductor digiti minimi

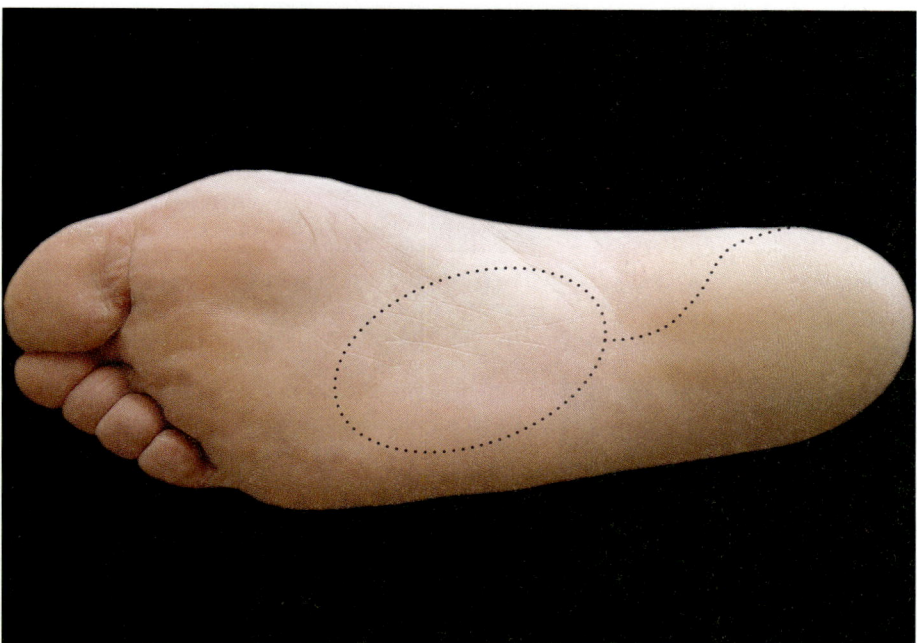

Figure 2-92   **Design of the flap**

The flap should be designed at the non-weight-bearing region of the mid planta, with its pivot point located at the cross point of the extension line anterior to the medial malleolus and the medial margin of planta, and with its axial line falling on the line from the cross point to the space between the 4th and the 5th metatarsal bones.

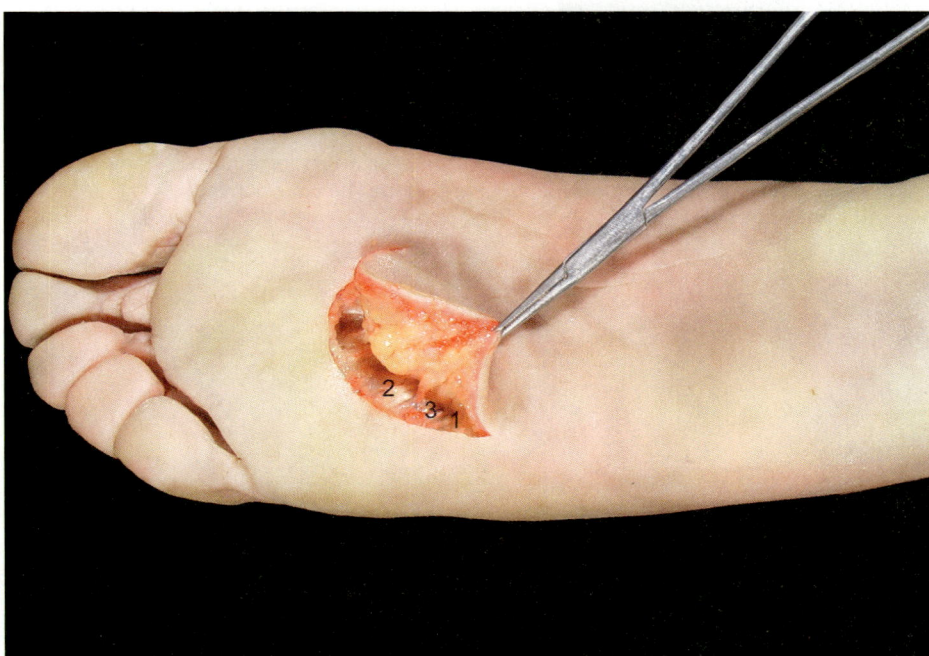

1. Abductor digiti minimi
2. Flexor digitorum brevis
3. 5th digital artery

Figure 2-93   **Exposure of the 5th digital artery**

As has been designed, the incision of the flap should begin with its distal border. Then the plantar aponeurosis should be separated to expose the 5th digital artery in the septum between the abductor digiti minimi and the flexor digitorum brevis.

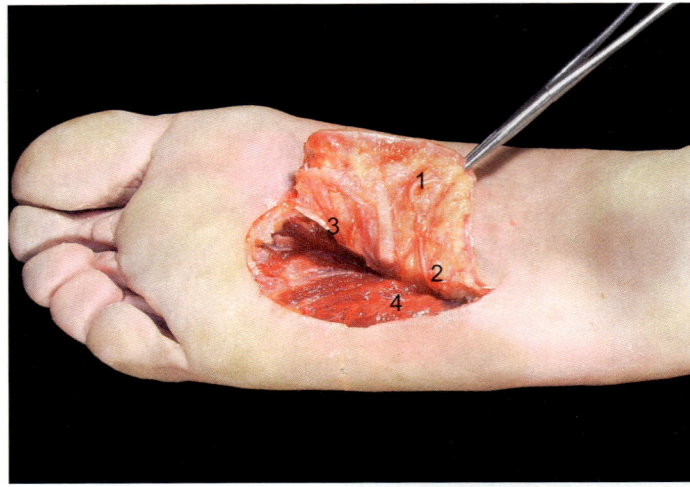

Figure 2-94 | **Dissection of the flap**

The 5th digital artery should be ligated and traced proximally to expose the lateral planter artery. The flap should be dissected retrogradely at the deep surface of the lateral plantar artery.

1. Digital artery
2. Lateral plantar artery
3. Flexor digitorum brevis
4. Abductor digiti minimi

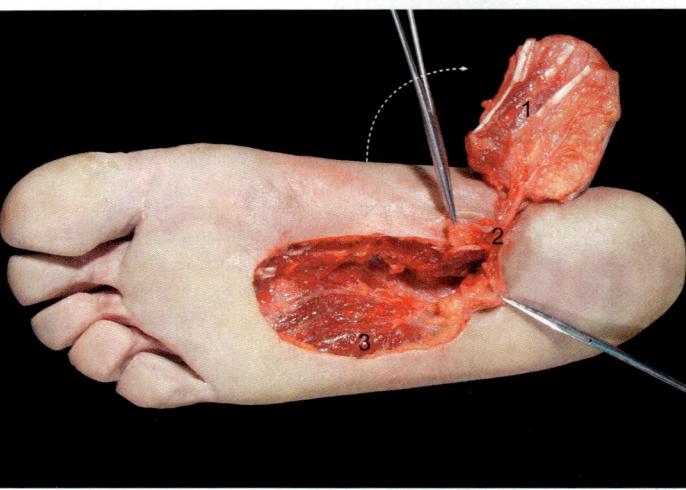

Figure 2-95 | **Elevation of the flap**

The separation of the flap should continue to the place where the lateral plantar artery originates from the posterior tibial artery. The skin between the donor and the recipient should be cut open and the flap transferred to cover a wound on the calcaneus.

1. Flexor digitorum brevis
2. Lateral plantar artery
3. Abductor digiti minimi

Key points in applied anatomy

Firstly, the nerval branches that are included in the flap should be kept intact to guarantee a good sensory function after the transplantation. Secondly, the lateral and the medial plantar arteries supply blood for the flexor digitorum brevis and the overlying skin, either will be a suitable pedicle. Which of them should be adopted depends on the conditions of the recipient site. Thirdly, the lateral plantar artery should be included in the flap during the operation. Fourthly, a free skin graft should be adopted if the donor wound is too large to be directly sutured.

Abductor Digiti Minimi Muscular Flap

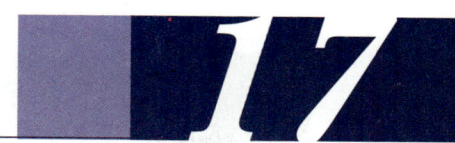

The abductor digiti minimi that gets its blood supply from the lateral plantar artery is situated in the lateral planta. Since the lateral planta plays a role in bearing weight, an abductor digiti minimi flap might be used only as a muscular one to restore a defect on the plantar region of the calcaneal bone or on the inferior part of the lateral malleolus. It might also be transferred to treat a calcaneal osteomyelitis.

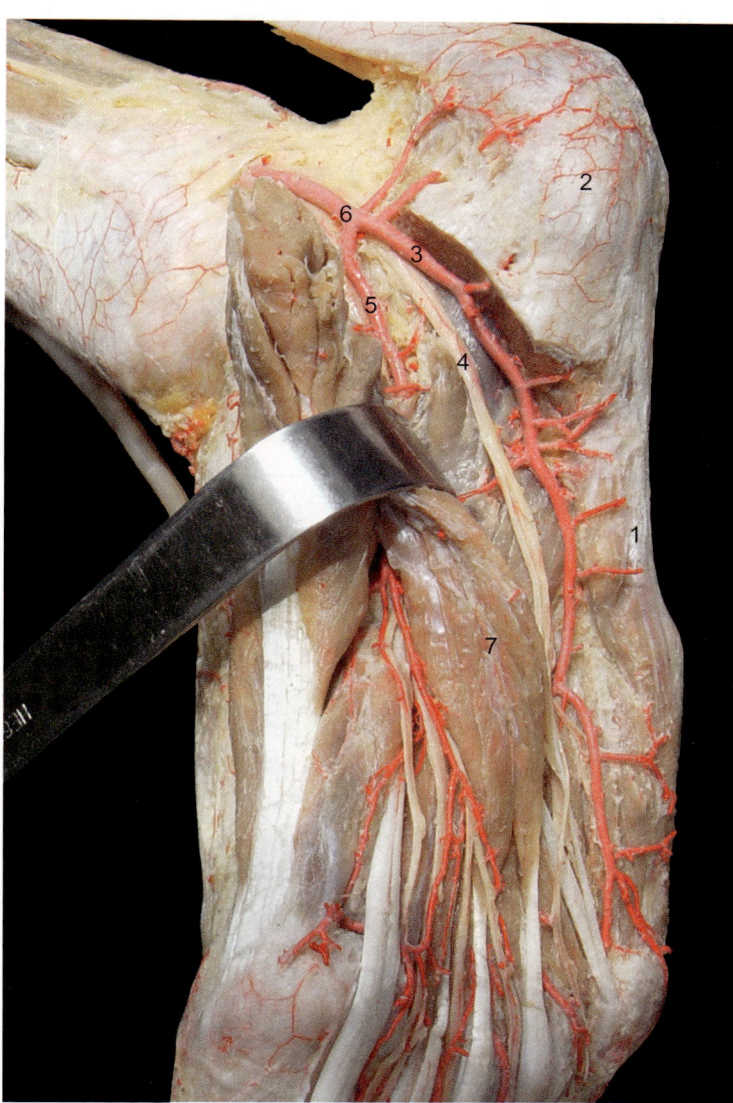

Figure 2-96	Applied Anatomy

The abductor digiti minimi is situated in the superficial layer of the lateral planta. It starts from the lateral processes of the calcaneal tuberosity, combines with the flexor digiti minimi brevis tendon and terminates at the lateral base of the 5th proximal phalanx. In most cases (91.37%) the artery of the flexor digiti minimi muscle originates from the branch of the lateral plantar artery. In a few cases, it originates from the dorsal pedal artery. In general, there are 2-6 arteries in the abductor digiti minimi that are 0.2-0.5 mm in diameter and anastomose with each other within the muscle. The veins in the muscle converge into the lateral plantar vein. There are 2-7 veins in the muscle that are 0.6 mm in diameter. The nerve in the muscle originates from the lateral plantar nerve at the medial surface of the calcaneus and runs laterally into the muscle at its proximal end, the nerve extends all the way through the muscle.

1. Abductor digiti minimi
3. Lateral plantar artery
5. Medial plantar artery
7. Flexor digitorum brevis

2. Calcaneal tuberosity
4. Lateral plantar nerve
6. Posterior tibial artery

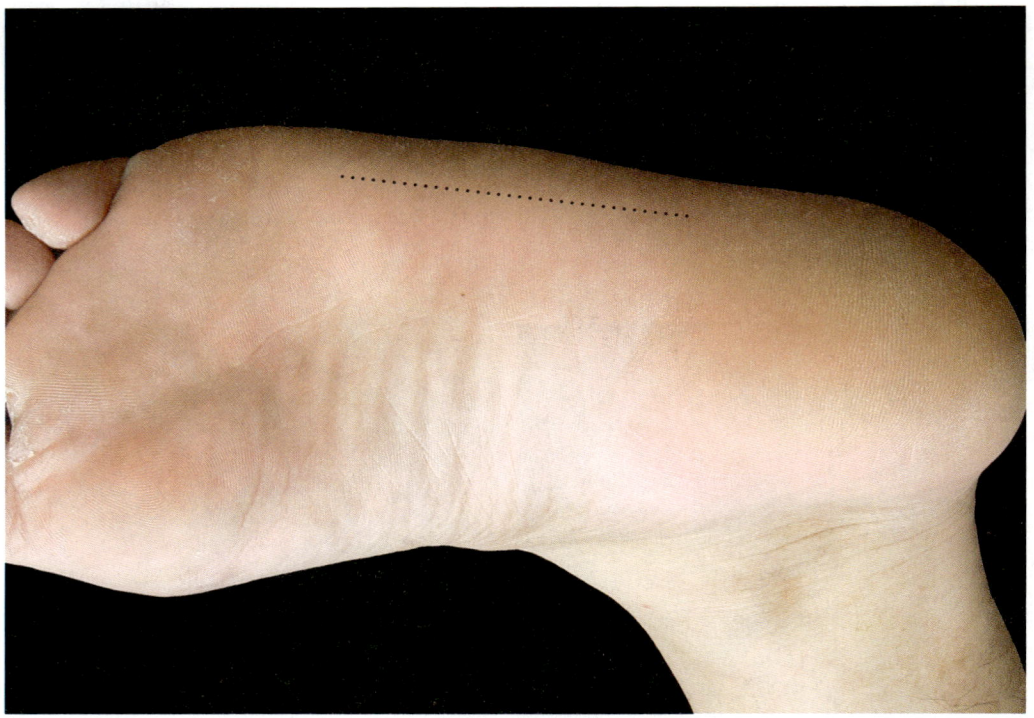

Figure 2-97	**Design of the incision**

A longitudinal incision should be made at the non-weight-bearing region of the lateral planta.

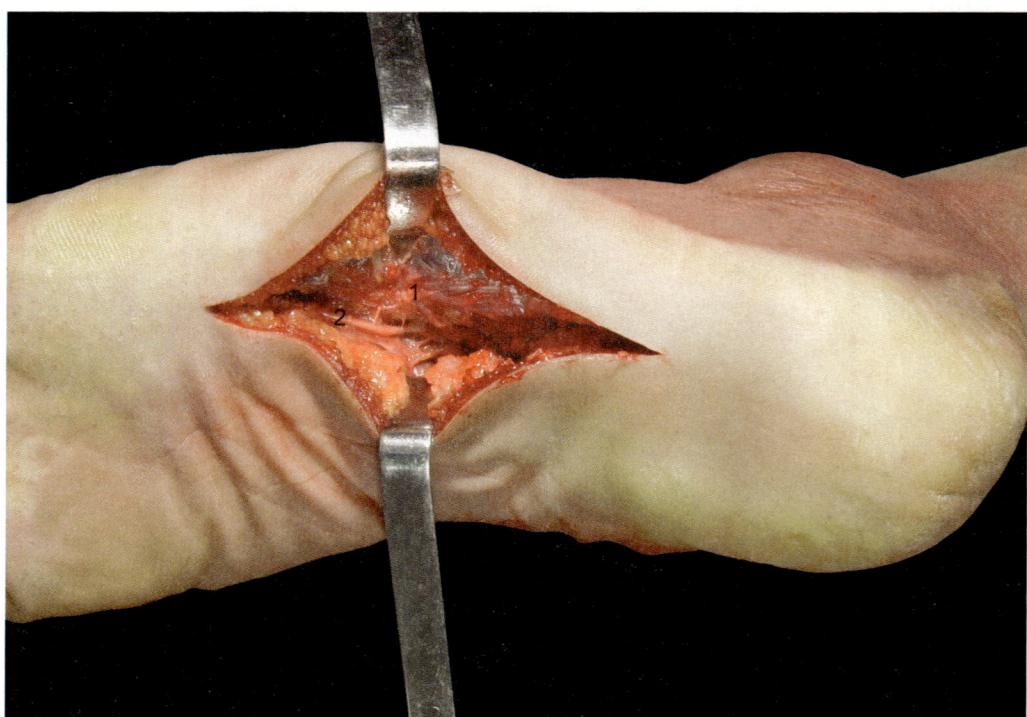

1. Abductor digiti minimi
2. Lateral plantar artery

Figure 2-98	**Exposure of the lateral plantar artery**

The skin should be incised to expose the abductor digiti minimi, and the lateral plantar artery that is situated medial to the abductor digiti minimi kept intact.

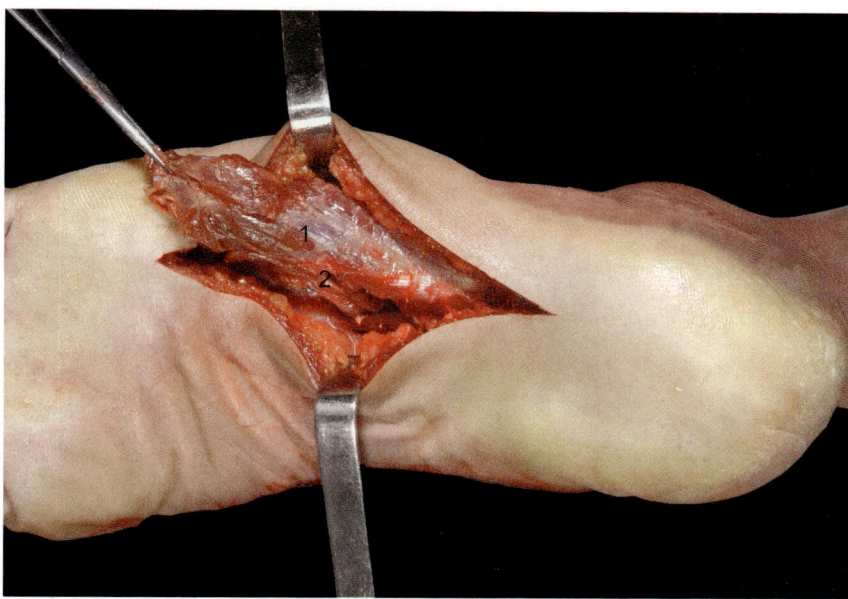

1. Abductor digiti minimi tendon
2. Lateral plantar artery

Figure 2-99   **Dissection of the muscular flap**

The abductor digiti minimi tendon should be cut at the base of the 5th proximal phalanx. The lateral plantar artery should be cut off and ligated after it sends the proximal branches into the muscle.

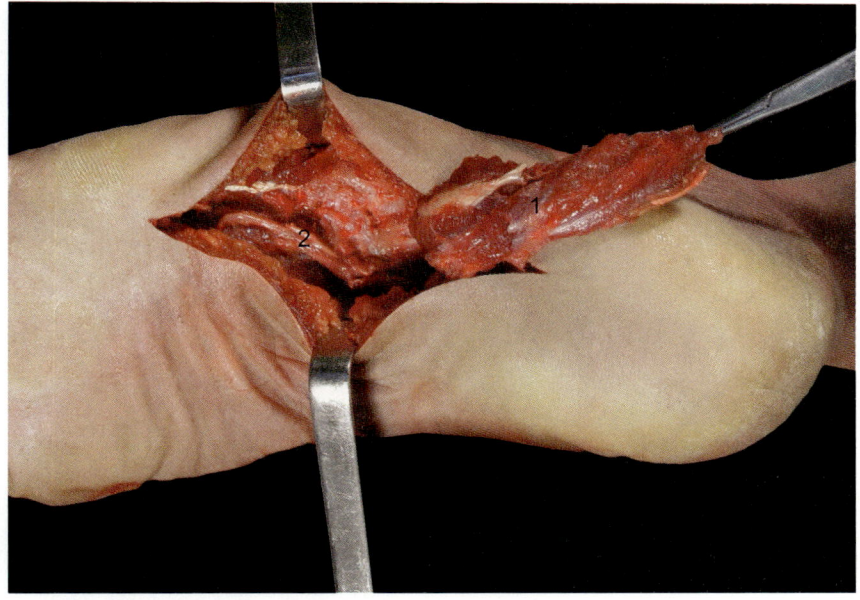

1. Abductor digiti minimi tendon
2. Lateral plantar artery

Figure 2-100   **Transposition of the muscular flap**

Once the muscular flap has been made, it might be transferred posteriorly.

Key points in applied anatomy

Firstly, in most cases (90%), the lateral plantar artery supplies blood for the abductor digiti minimi. The artery is closely accompanied by the lateral plantar nerve. It is suggested that the lateral plantar neurovascular branch be the priority of the pedicle of the abductor digiti minimi muscular flap. Secondly, the skin and the muscle should be kept stick to each other when the flap is being dissected.

Chapter **III**

Bone Flaps

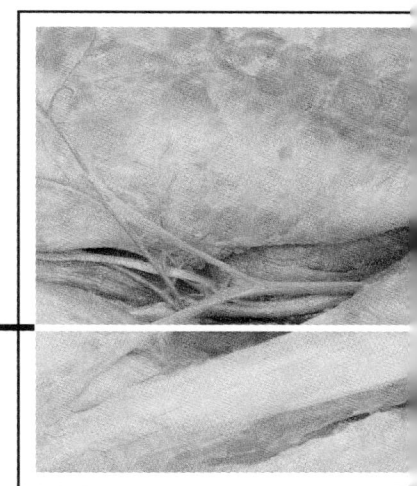

Blood Supply of Long Bone

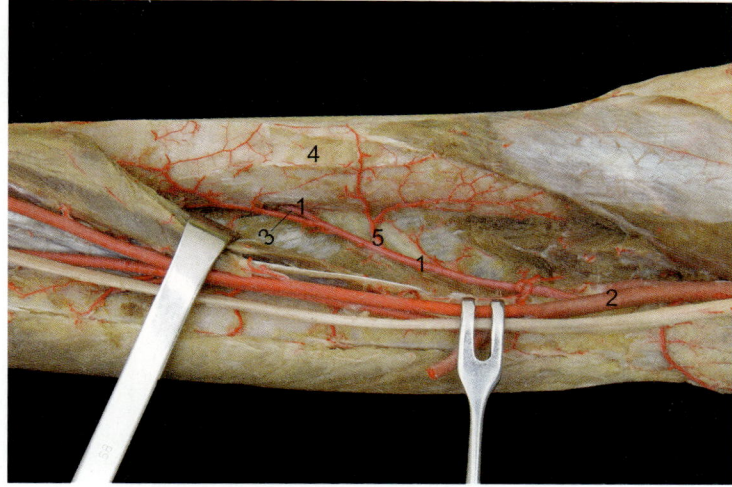

1. Nutrient artery
2. Posterior tibial artery
3. Nutrient foramen
4. Tibia
5. Periosteal branch of nutrient artery

Figure 3-1 Nutrient artery system

The nutrient artery (1-2 in general) of the long bone emerges from the adjacent arterial trunk and runs obliquely through the nutrient foramen into the bone. It enters the medullary cavity and bifurcates into ascending and descending branches. Both of the two extend respectively along the medullary membrane to the bilateral epiphyseal portions. Along the course, each sends branches into the medullary membrane to form a vascular network and cortical branches into the inner layer of the cortical bone. These branches might be categorized into either the 2nd or the 3rd generation group. The nutrient artery supplies blood for the long bone, which amounts to 50-70% of the total.

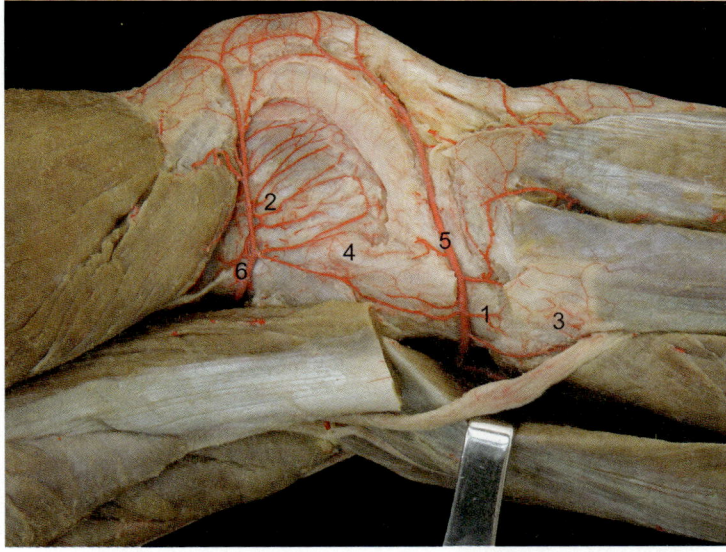

1. Epiphyseal artery
2. Metaphyseal artery
3. Fibular head
4. External epicondyle of femur
5. Lateral inferior genicular artery
6. Lateral superior genicular artery

Figure 3-2 Extremity artery system

The extremity artery system consists of the epiphyseal artery and the metaphyseal artery. They originate from the adjacent arterial trunks or the articular vascular net. Both arteries enter the bone and wind in the bone trabecula to reach the sub-layer of the articular cartilage, where they branch off and anastomose with each other to form arterial arches. They could not anastomose adequately before the epiphyseal cartilage plate is completely ossified. The blood from the extremity artery system amounts to 20-40% of the total.

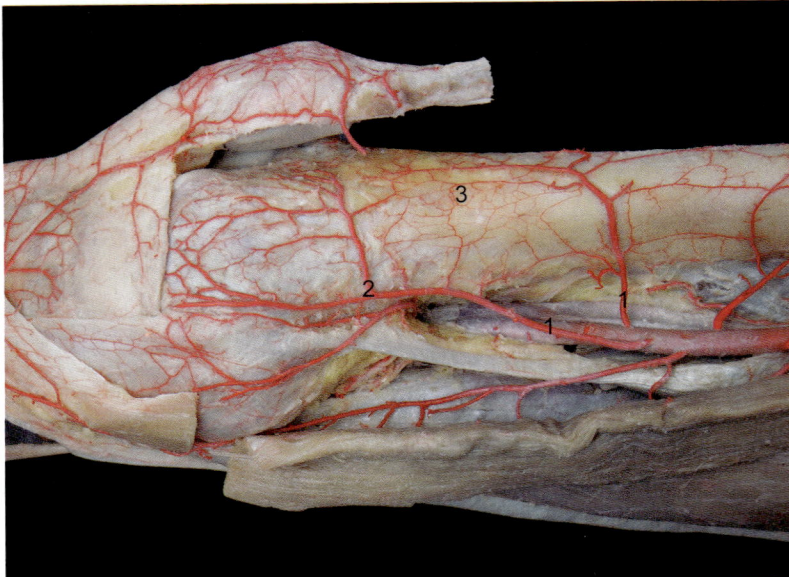

1. Periosteal branch
2. Metaphyseal artery
3. Arterial net

Figure 3-3   Periosteal artery system

The periosteum obtain their blood supply from the periosteal branches of the adjacent artery, the metaphyseal artery and some tiny arterial branches in the muscle, tendon, fascia and ligament attachment. The periosteal arteries branch off in the osseous membrane and anastomose with each other to form a vascular network. From the network they further send small branches into the cortical bone and fan out on its superficial layer. Some communicating branches perforate through the inner layer of the bone via Volkmann canal to communicate with the medullary arteries. The periosteal artery system supplies 10-20% of the blood for the long bone.

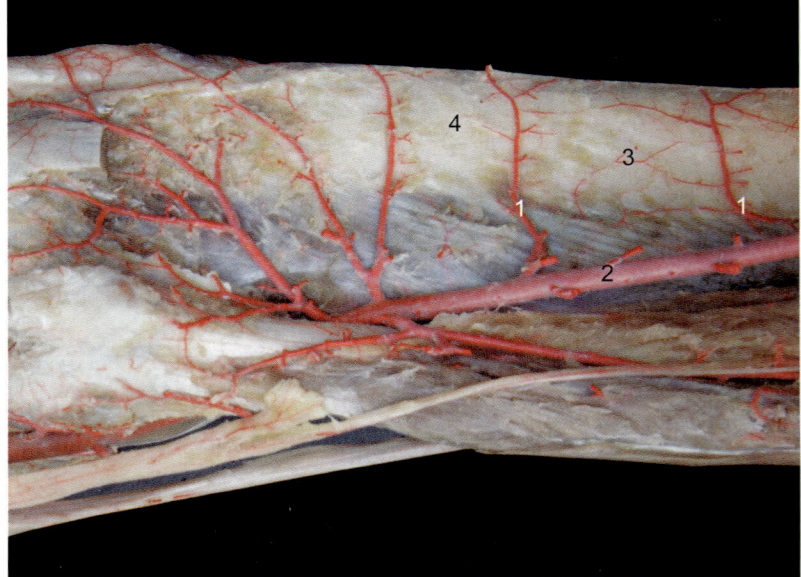

1. Musculoperiosteal artery
2. Anterior tibial artery
3. Arterial net
4. Tibia

Figure 3-4   Muscular, tendinous and fascial artery system

These arteries extend through the muscle, the tendon and the fascia, attaching closely to the osseous surface. They are called the musculoperiosteal artery, the tenoperiosteal artery and the fascioperiosteal artery respectively. All of them are small in diameter and anastomose extensively with the vessels in the periosteal vascular network. The artery system serves as the morphologic basis for designing the muscle-pedicled osseous flap, the fascia-pedicled osseous or periosteal flap.

Clavicular Periosteal (bone) Flap Pedicled with Thoracoacromial Vessels

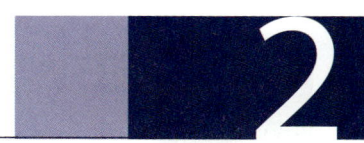

The clavicle lies horizontal under the skin of the basalis neck, and the whole length could be palpated beneath the body surface. It obtains its abundant blood supply from several vessels. There are also many groups of muscles attached to it. The clavicular periosteal (bone) flap based on the thoracoacromial vessels might be used for the treatment of comminuted proximal humeral fractures and ischemic necrosis of the humeral head .It has such advantages as donor and recipient sites located in same incision, easy operation, and direct donor site closure. Besides, local transposition could be performed free of vascular anastomosis.

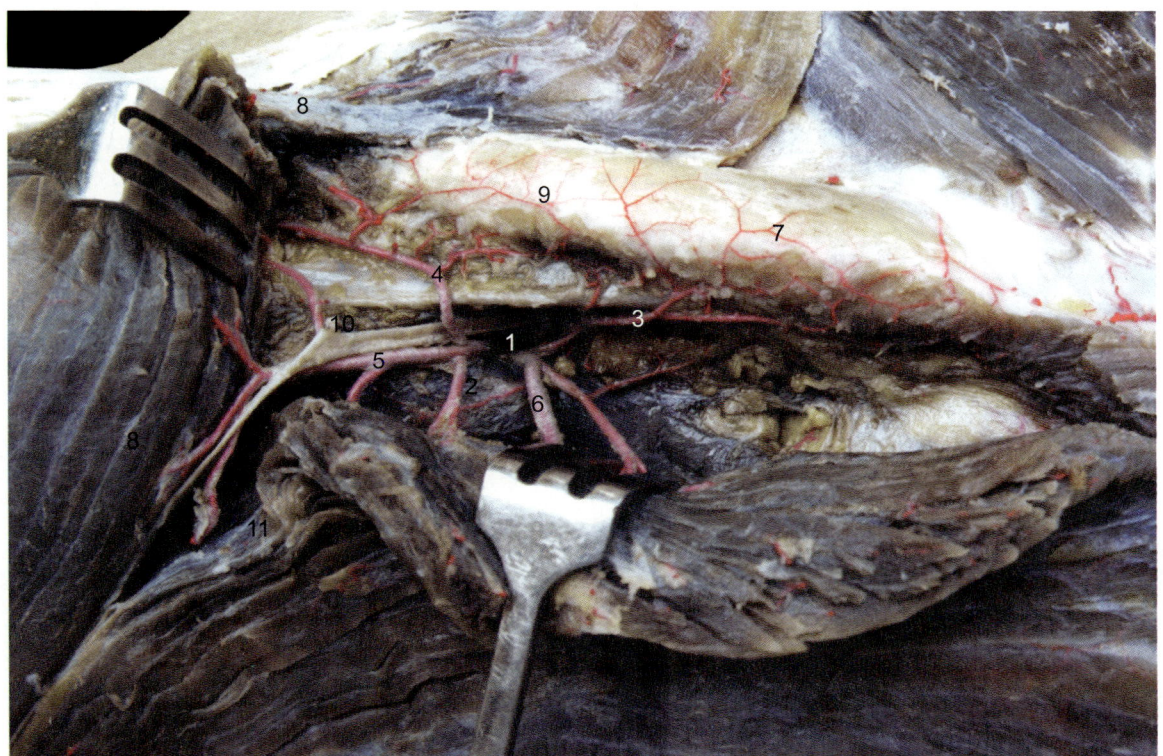

| Figure 3-5 | Applied anatomy |

The thoracoacromial artery perforates through the clavipectoral fascia at 2-3cm to the coracoid process on the superior pectoralis minor. It divides into a clavicular branch, an acromial branch, a deltoid branch and a pectoral branch. The clavicular branch ascends medially to distribute on the middle-medial segment periosteum of the clavicle and the subclavius muscle. The acromial branch runs outwards under the deep surface of the deltoid, and gives 3-5 periosteal branches (0.3-0.5mm in diameter) into the middle and lateral sections of the clavicle before it converges into the acromial vascular network. The deltoid branch is the terminal branch of the trunk. It extends along the cephalic vein in the groove between the deltoid and the pectoralis.

1. Thoracoacromial artery	**2.** Pectoralis minor	**3.** Clavicular branch	**4.** Acromial branch
5. Deltoid branch	**6.** Pectoral branch	**7.** Clavicle	**8.** Deltoid
9. Periosteal branch	**10.** Cephalic vein	**11.** Pectoralis major	

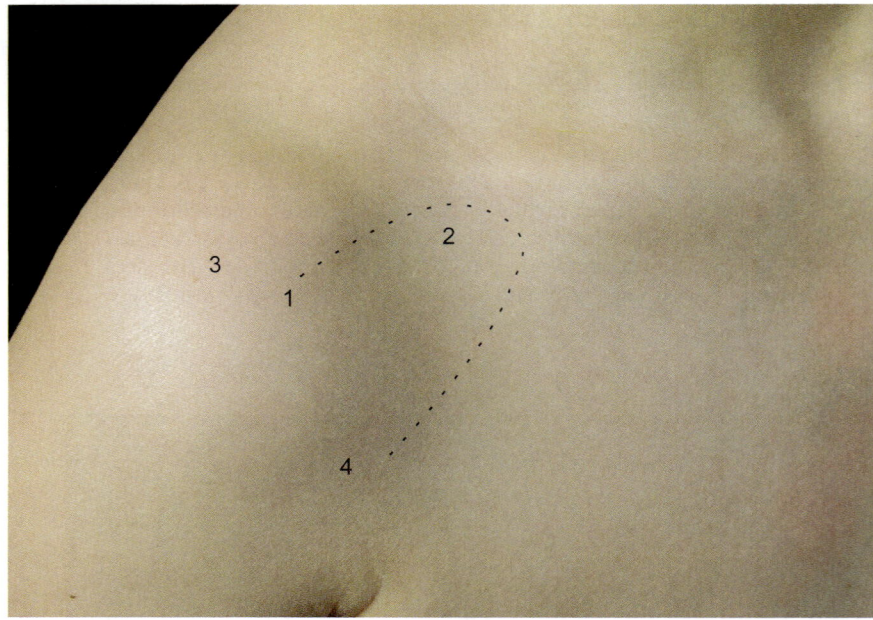

1. Acromioclavicular
   joint
2. Clavicle
3. Acromion
4. Intermuscular groove
   between deltoid and
   pectoralis major

Figure 3-6   Design of the incision

The patient is placed in a supine position, the scapular region of the operative side padded up for about 30 degree and the head turned contralaterally to extend the distance between the neck and the shoulder. The incision should begin with the anterior portion of the acromioclavicular joint and continue medially along the anterior lateral half of the clavicle. Then it should turn laterally downwards to the coracoid process and further extend along the intermuscular groove to the point above the insertion of the deltoid muscle.

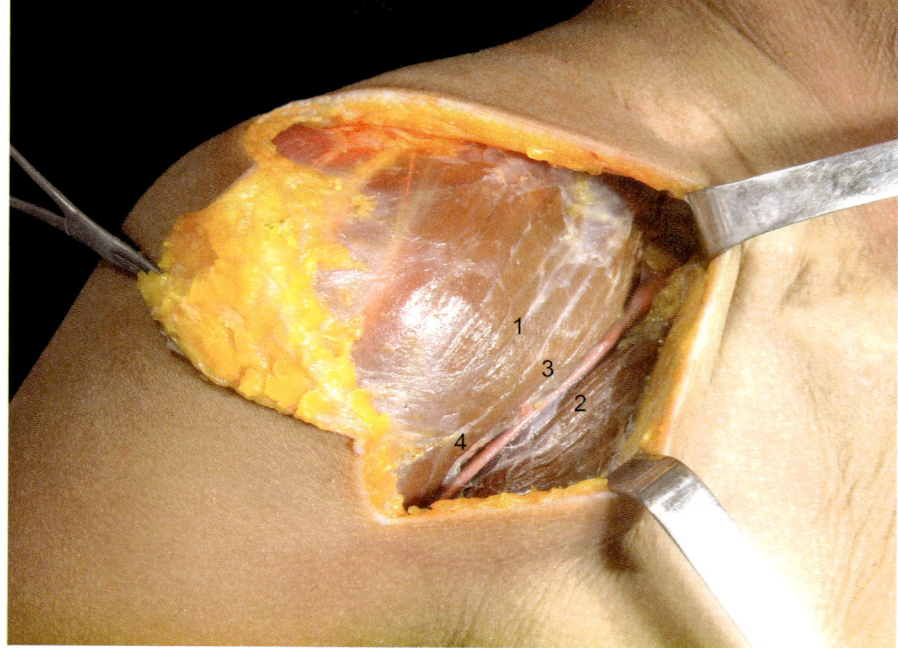

1. Deltoid
2. Pectoralis major
3. Cephalic vein
4. Deltoid branch of
   thoracoacromial
   artery

Figure 3-7   Exposure of the muscle

The skin and the subcutaneous tissue should be incised one by one to expose the cephalic vein and the deltoid branch of thoracoacromial artery in the intermuscular groove between the deltoid and the pectoralis major.

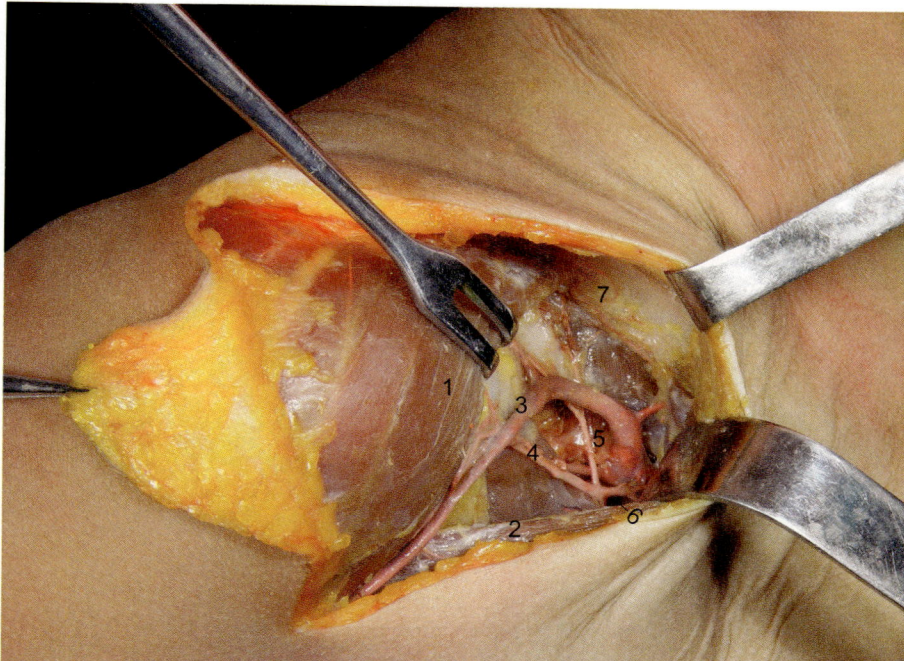

1. Deltoid
2. Pectoralis major
3. Cephalic vein
4. Deltoid branch
5. Acromial branch
6. Clavicular branch
7. Clavicle

Figure 3-8   Exposure of the vessels

The deltoid should be pulled laterally upwards and the pectoralis major medially downwards. The incision should trace along the deltoid branch to the origin of the clavicular branch of the thoracoacromial artery.

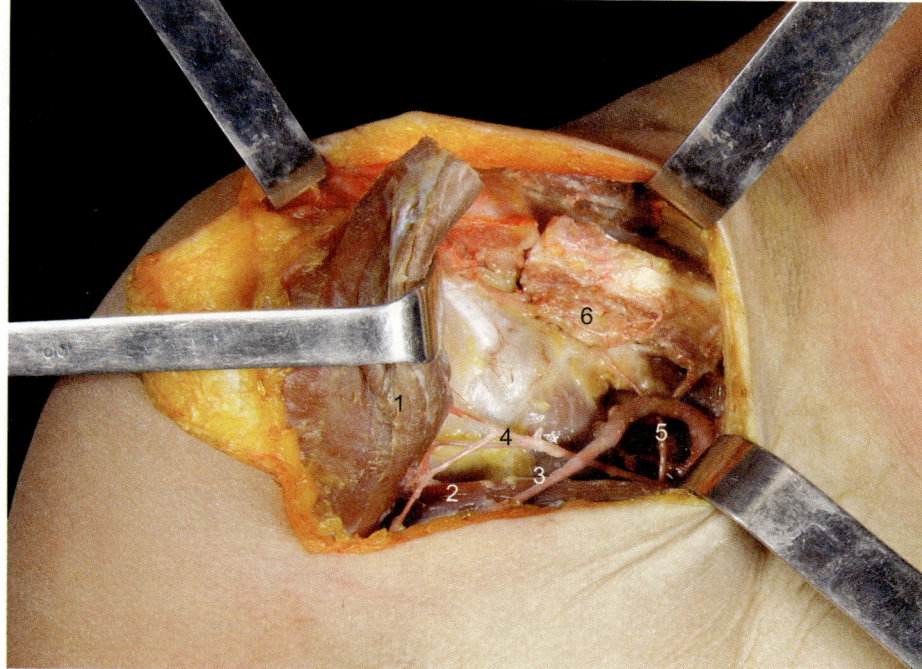

1. Deltoid
2. Pectoralis major
3. Cephalic vein
4. Deltoid branch
5. Acromial branch
6. Clavicular periosteal (bone) flap

Figure 3-9   Dissection of the bone flap

The clavicular branch should be further dissected to its terminal on the clavicle. Then the periosteal (bone) flap based on this branch could be harvested as was preoperatively designed.

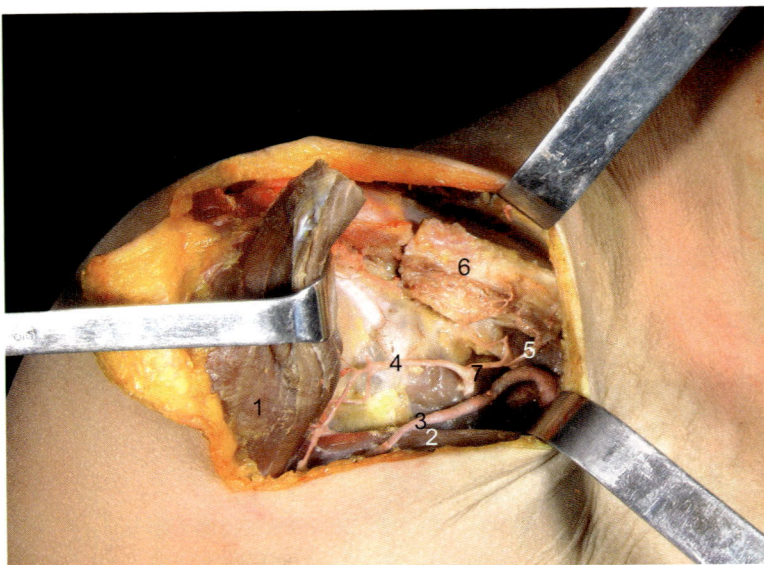

1. Deltoid
2. Pectoralis major
3. Cephalic vein
4. Deltoid branch
5. Acromial branch
6. Clavicular periosteal (bone) flap
7. Thoracoacromial artery

Figure 3-10	Separation of the vessels

The thoracoacromial artery trunk should be ligated before it gives the clavicular branch and the deltoid branch.

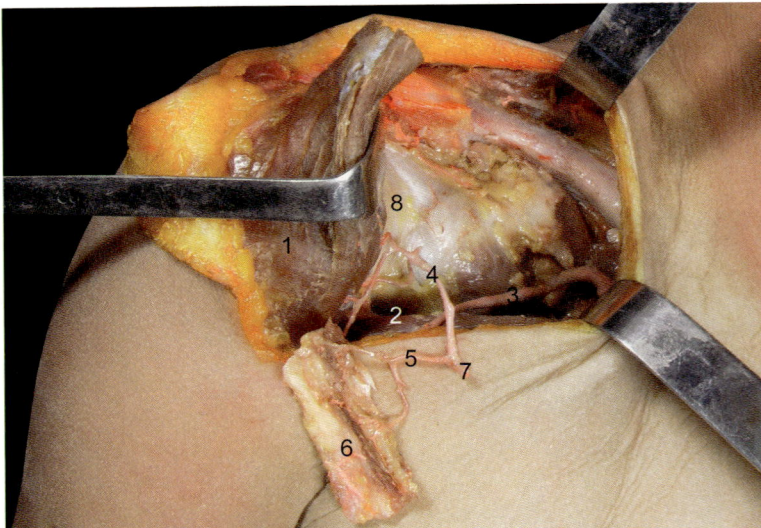

1. Deltoid
2. Pectoralis major
3. Cephalic vein
4. Deltoid branch
5. Acromial branch
6. Clavicular periosteal (bone) flap
7. Thoracoacromial artery
8. Humeral head

Figure 3-11	Transposition of the flap

After the fracture is restored and fixed, the periosteal (bone) flap with a vascular pedicle might be transferred to the recipient site on the humeral head or the proximal humerus.

Key points in applied anatomy

Firstly, when the periosteum is being stripped off, the subclavian vessels should be given great attention to avoid damages. Secondly, the deltoid branch should be separated towards the distal part (even into the deltoid muscle) so that the pedicle could be long enough for a smooth rotation without twist and compression. Thirdly, the trunk of the thoracoacromial artery should be ligated before it bifurcates into the clavicular branch and the deltoid branch. Fourthly, the vascular net in the periosteum of the clavicle, the cephalic vein and the anterior pectoral nerve should be protected during the operation. Fifthly, the cephalic vein in the muscular groove might serve as an important mark for recognizing the deltoid branch of the thoracoacromial artery.

Scapular Spinal Bone Flap Pedicled with Acromial Branch of Thoracoacromial Artery

The spine of the scapula bone flap based on the acromial branch of the thoracoacromial artery is located in a concealed, superficial donor region. It has advantages such as an easy operation, a direct suture of the donor incision and an alternative pedicle (the antegrade blood supply from the acromial branch and the retrograde blood supply from the deltoid branch—the acromial branch could be used). The flap could be transferred locally to repair non-union in the proximal humerus and the lateral segment of the clavicle. The flap based on the retrograde blood supply from the deltoid branch to the acromial branch might have a pedicle long enough to reach the superior-middle segment of the humerus for the restoration of non-union or defect.

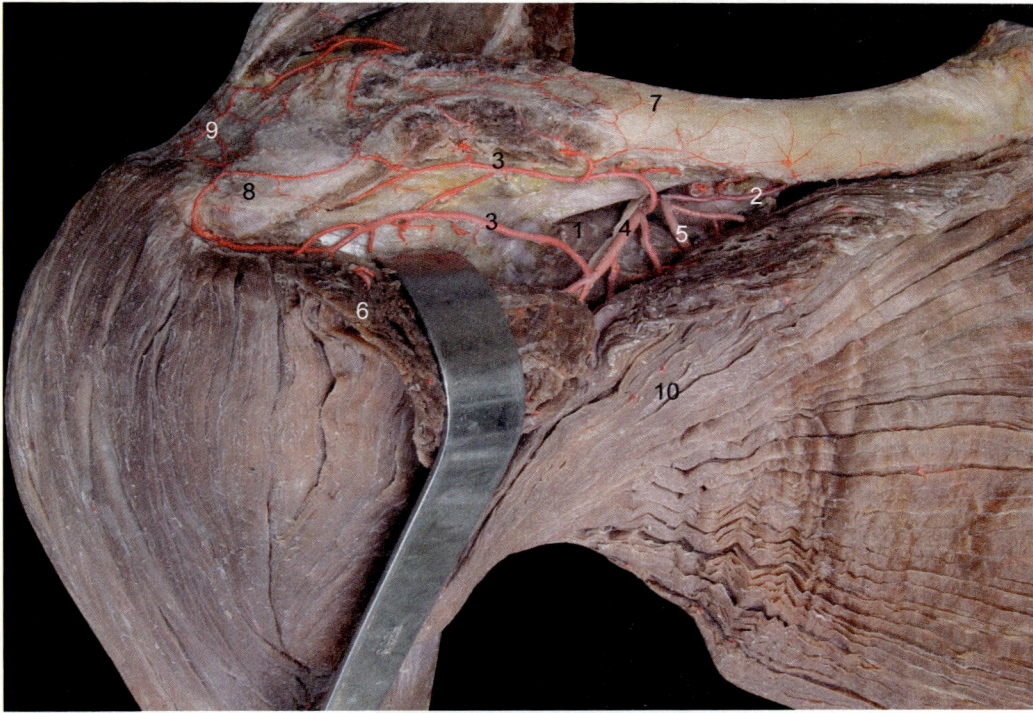

| Figure 3-12 | Applied anatomy |

The thoracoacromial artery might originate from different sources. It runs medially forwards across the superior pectoralis minor and perforates through the clavipectoral fascia at 2-3cm to the coracoid process. It divides into a clavicular branch, an acromial branch, a deltoid branch and a pectoral branch. There are generally 1-2 acromial branches that extend laterally upwards beneath the clavicular portion of the deltoid and close to the clavicle. The acromial branch runs for 1.5cm from its origin to the acromioclavicular joint. In most cases (86.7%), the acromial branch turns around the anterior or the lateral border of the acromion to join the acromial vascular net. In a few cases (13.3%), the branch crosses over the acromion at 4.6mm to the acromioclavicular joint and converges into the acromial vascular net. The trunk of the acromial branch is 1.5mm in diameter (on average).

1. Pectoralis minor	2. Clavicular branch	3. Acromial branch
4. Deltoid branch	5. Pectoral branch	6. Clavicular portion of deltoid
7. Clavicle	8. Acromion	9. Acromial vascular net
10. Pectoralis major		

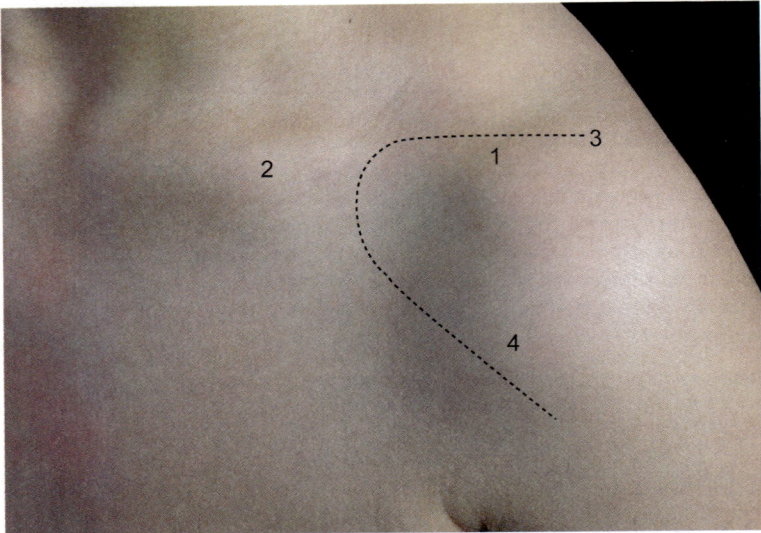

1. Acromioclavicular joint
2. Clavicle
3. Acromion
4. Deltoid

| Figure 3-13 | Design of the incision |

The patient is set in a lateral position, with the donor site above and the upper limb over the chest. The incision could be designed as follows: Firstly, as for the restoration of the proximal segment of the humerus, an inverted "U-shaped" incision should be made, which begins at 6-7cm below the anterior acromioclavicular joint and extends upwards across the anterior 1/3 portion of the deltoid and then to the top of acromioclavicular joint and continues along the posterior 1/3 portion of deltoid to 5-6cm below the acromioclavicular joint. If the reception site is on the humeral head, a "Y-shaped" incision should be designed. A curved incision should firstly be made with the acromioclavicular joint as its center. It should begin with the lateral segment of scapular spine, continue around the acromioclavicular joint and terminate at the coracoid process. Then a vertical incision could be further made distally about 6-8cm long from the center of the curve. Secondly, as for the restoration of the lateral segment of the clavicle, a curved incision should be made with the acromioclavicular joint as its center.

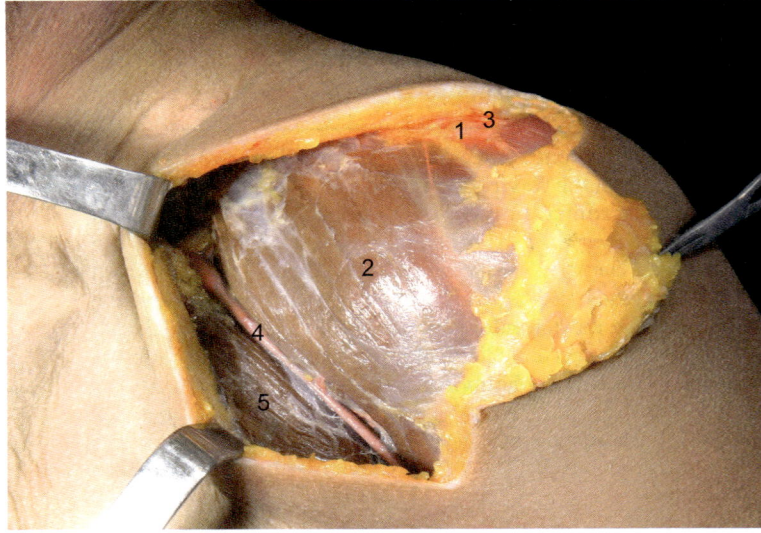

1. Acromion
2. Deltoid
3. Acromial vascular net
4. Cephalic vein
5. Pectoralis major

| Figure 3-14 | Exposure of the muscle |

The skin and the subcutaneous tissue should be incised open and the skin flap elevated bilaterally to expose the acromioclavicular joint, the acromion and the deltoid muscle that originates from the anterior, the lateral and the posterior portions of the acromion, on the top of which lie the acromial branches of thoracoacromial artery that converge into the acromial vascular net.

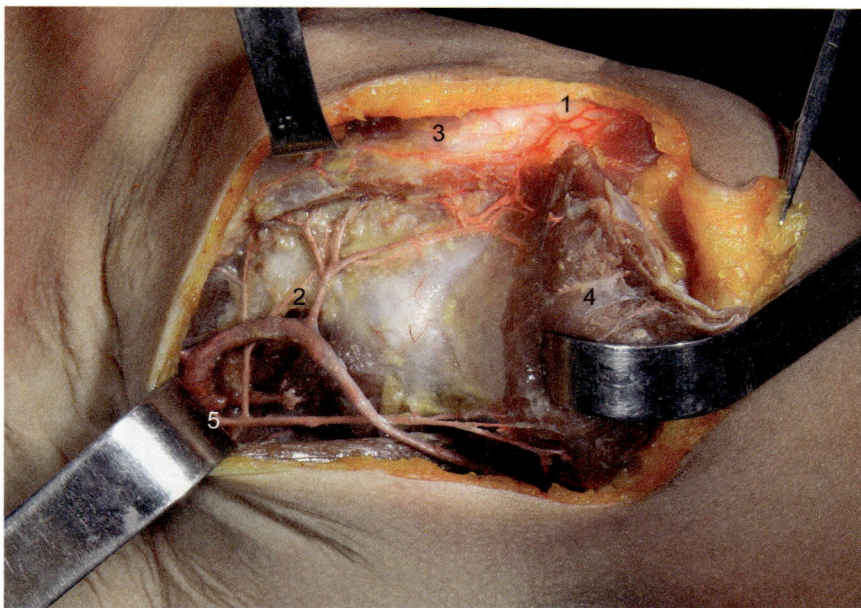

1. Acromion
2. Acromial branch
3. Clavicle
4. Deltoid
5. Thoracoacromial artery

| Figure 3-15 | Exposure of the vessels |

The dissection should trace retrogradely along the acromial branches to its origin near the lateral-middle 1/3 junction of the clavicle.

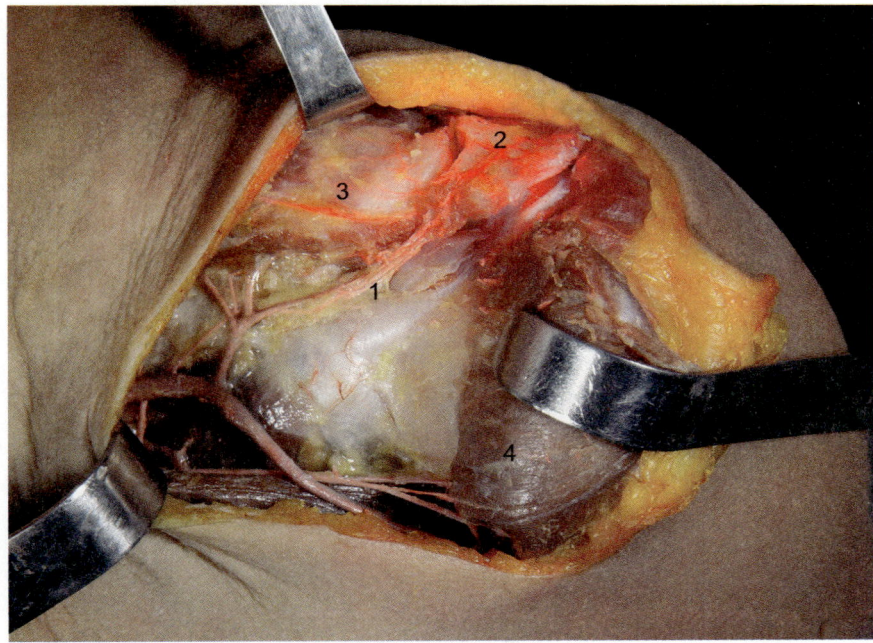

1. Acromial branches of thoracoacromial artery
2. Bone flap
3. Clavicle
4. Deltoid

| Figure 3-16 | Dissection of the bone flap |

As has been designed, the spine of the scapula bone flap should be dissected with the acromial branches of the thoracoacromial artery long enough for a transplantation.

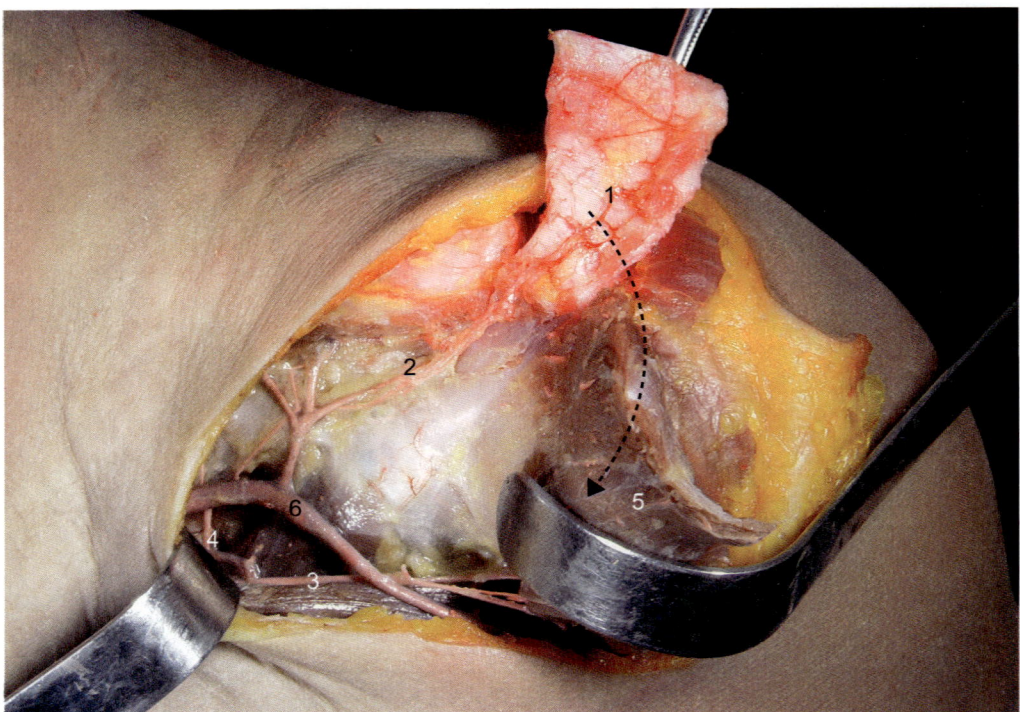

| Figure 3-17 | Transposition of the flap |

Then the humeral fracture should be repositioned and fixed properly before the flap with its pedicle could be transferred to the recipient site. If the arterial trunk were ligated before it gives off the acromial branches and the deltoid branches, the vascular pedicle could be long enough for the flap to be transferred to the region distal to the humeral head or even the lower segment of the humerus.

1. Bone flap
2. Acromial branch of thoracoacromial artery
3. Deltoid branch
4. Trunk of thoracoacromial artery
5. Deltoid
6. Cephalic vein

Key points in applied anatomy

Firstly, the dissection of the bone flap should be close to the middle segment of the scapular spine so as to guarantee the connection between the scapular notch and the acromion. Secondly, the dissected apocoptic trapezius muscle, supraspinous muscle and infraspinous muscle should be fixed on the stump of the bone to reduce the impact on the function. Thirdly, the fracture should be restored and fixed carefully and so should the bone flap be stripped to avoid damaging the subclavian vessels just beneath the bone structure. Fourthly, when the vascular pedicle is being dissected, the surrounding connective tissue sleeve should be retained to protect the acromial vascular net. Fifthly, alternative pedicle (either the acromial branch or the retrograded deltoid branch) could be adopted to augment the rotating arch of the vascular pedicle.

Spine of Scapula Bone Flap Pedicled with Acromial Branch of Suprascapular Artery

4

The spine of scapula bone flap based on the acromial branch of the suprascapular artery is located in a concealed, superficial donor region. It has such advantages as an easy operation and a direct suture of the donor incision. A flap pedicled with the antegrade blood supply from the acromial branch of the suprascapular artery might be transferred locally to repair non-union in the lateral segment of the clavicle.

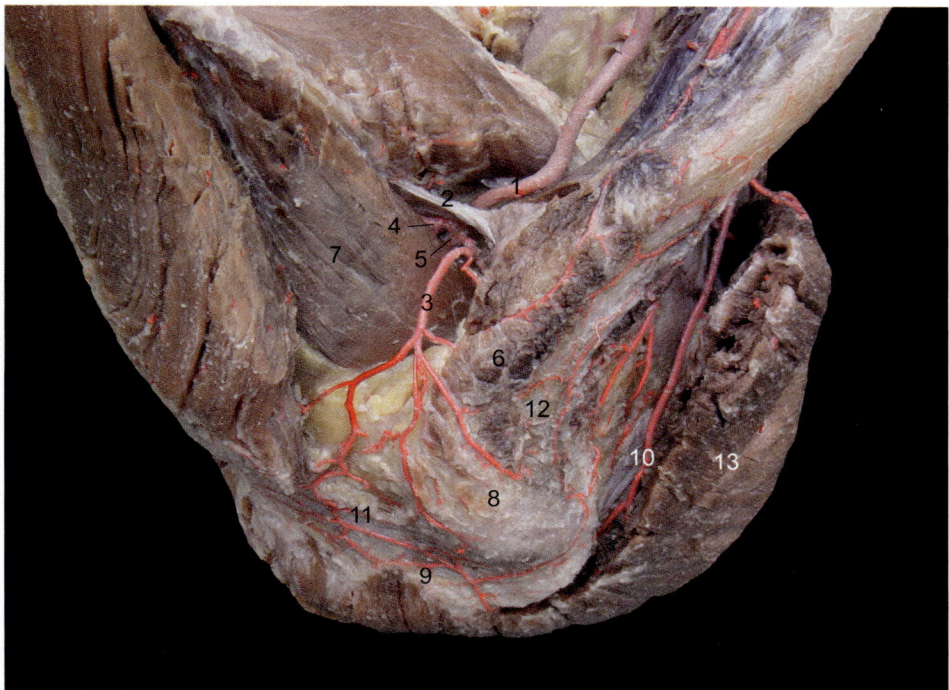

| Figure 3-18 | Applied anatomy |

The suprascapular artery emerges from different sources. It runs laterally downwards across the superficial layer of the anterior scalenus muscle and the phrenic nerve. It turns backwards at the middle 1/3 segment of the clavicle to the superior border of the scapula, where it divides into the acromial branch, the supraspinous branch and the infraspinous branch. The acromial branch extends outwards in the septum between the trapezius muscle and the supraspinous muscle and perforates through the acromial attachment of the trapezius muscle at 0.3-0.5cm to the posterior portion of the acromioclavicular joint. It reaches the acromion and anastomoses extensively with the acromial branch of the thoracoacromial artery to form an acromial vascular net. The branch is (4.6±1.1) cm in length (from its beginning to the acromion) and (1.7±0.4) mm in diameter.

1. Suprascapular artery
2. Superior transverse scapular ligament
3. Acromial branch
4. Supraspinous branch
5. Infraspinous branch
6. Trapezius muscle
7. Supraspinous muscle
8. Acromioclavicular joint
9. Acromion
10. Acromial branch of thoracoacromial artery
11. Acromial vascular net
12. Clavicle
13. Deltoid

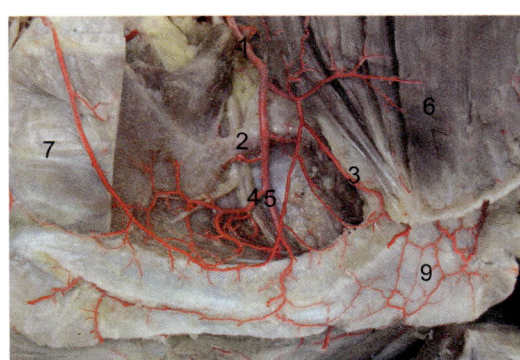

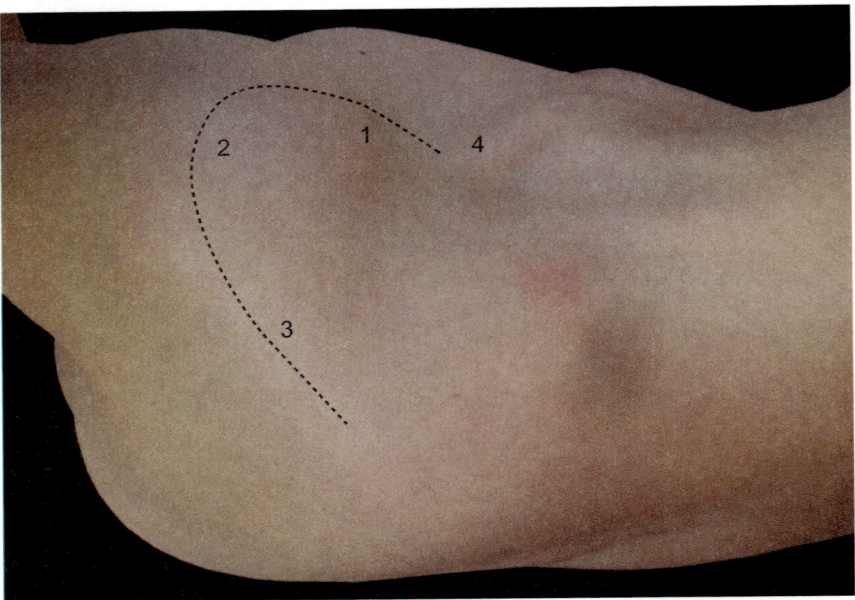

Figure 3-19 Design of the incision

The patient is placed in a supine position and the scapular region of the operative side padded up for about 30 degree. A curved incision should be designed from the posterior border of the acromion to the coracoid process via the anterior portion of the acromion.

1. Acromioclavicular joint   **2.** Acromion   **3.** Scapular spine   **4.** Clavicle

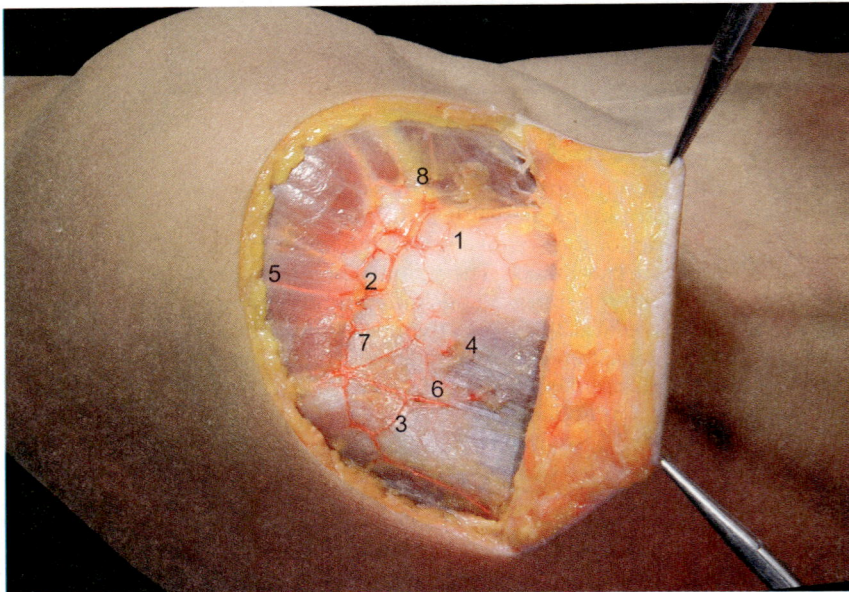

1. Acromioclavicular joint
2. Acromion
3. Scapular spine
4. Trapezius muscle
5. Deltoid
6. Acromial branch of
   suprascapular artery
7. Acromial vascular net
8. Acromial branch of
   thoracoacromial artery

Figure 3-20   Exposure of the acromion

The skin and the subcutaneous tissue should be incised open one by one, and the skin flap elevated bilaterally to expose the fractured clavicle, the acromioclavicular joint, the acromion and the muscular attachment of the trapezius and the deltoid from the scapular spine. At 0.3-0.5cm to the posterior portion of the acromioclavicular joint, the acromial branch of the suprascapular artery could be found extending superficially through the acromial attachment of the trapezius muscle to join the acromial vascular net.

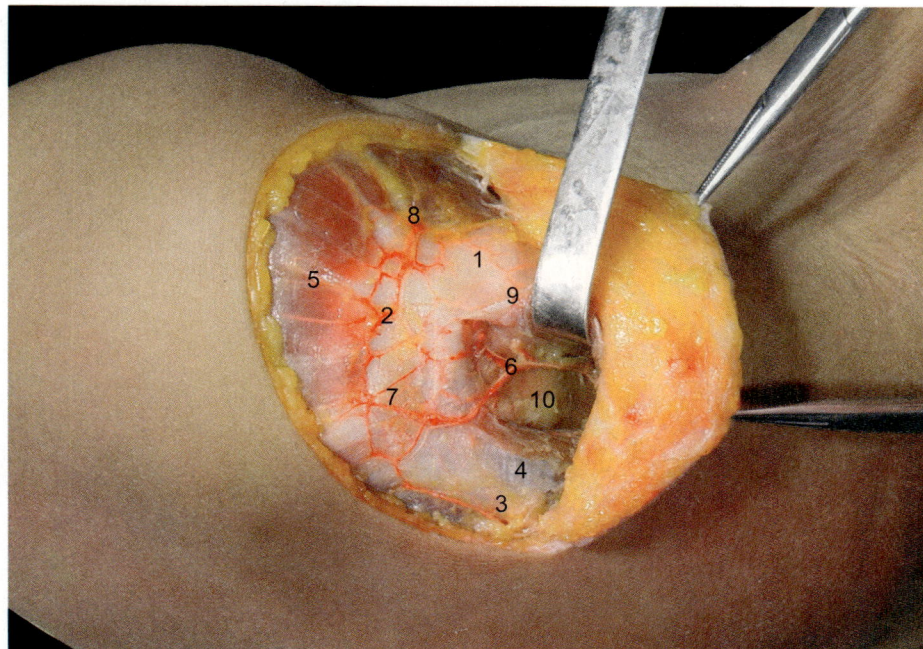

1. Acromioclavicular joint
2. Acromion
3. Scapular spine
4. Insertion of trapezius muscle
5. Deltoid
6. Acromial branch of suprascapular artery
7. Acromial vascular net
8. Acromial branch of thoracoacromial artery
9. Trapezius muscle (turned forward)
10. Supraspinous muscle

Figure 3-21   Exposure of the vessels

The dissection should trace along the vascular bundle of the acromial branches of the suprascapular artery to its origin near the lateral-middle 1/3 junction of the clavicle.

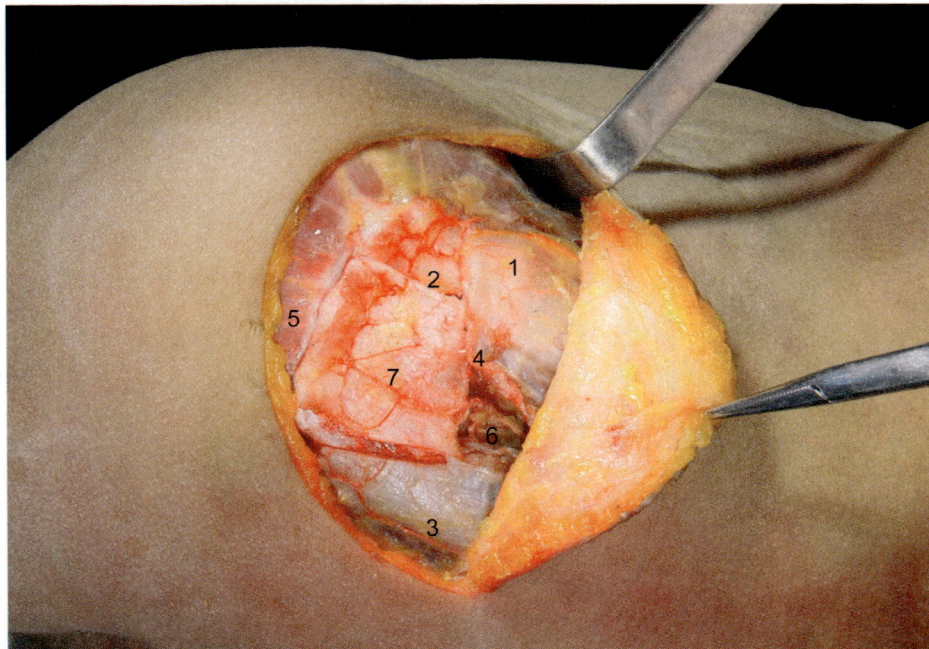

1. Acromioclavicular joint
2. Acromion
3. Scapular spine
4. Trapezius muscle
5. Deltoid
6. Acromial branch of suprascapular artery
7. Bone flap

Figure 3-22   Dissection of the bone flap

The attachment of the deltoid and the trapezius should be separated along the superior and the inferior borders of the acromion. The lateral spinal flap should be harvested as is required (the flap might be extended to the middle of the scapular spine) and protected with wet saline gauze for a transposition.

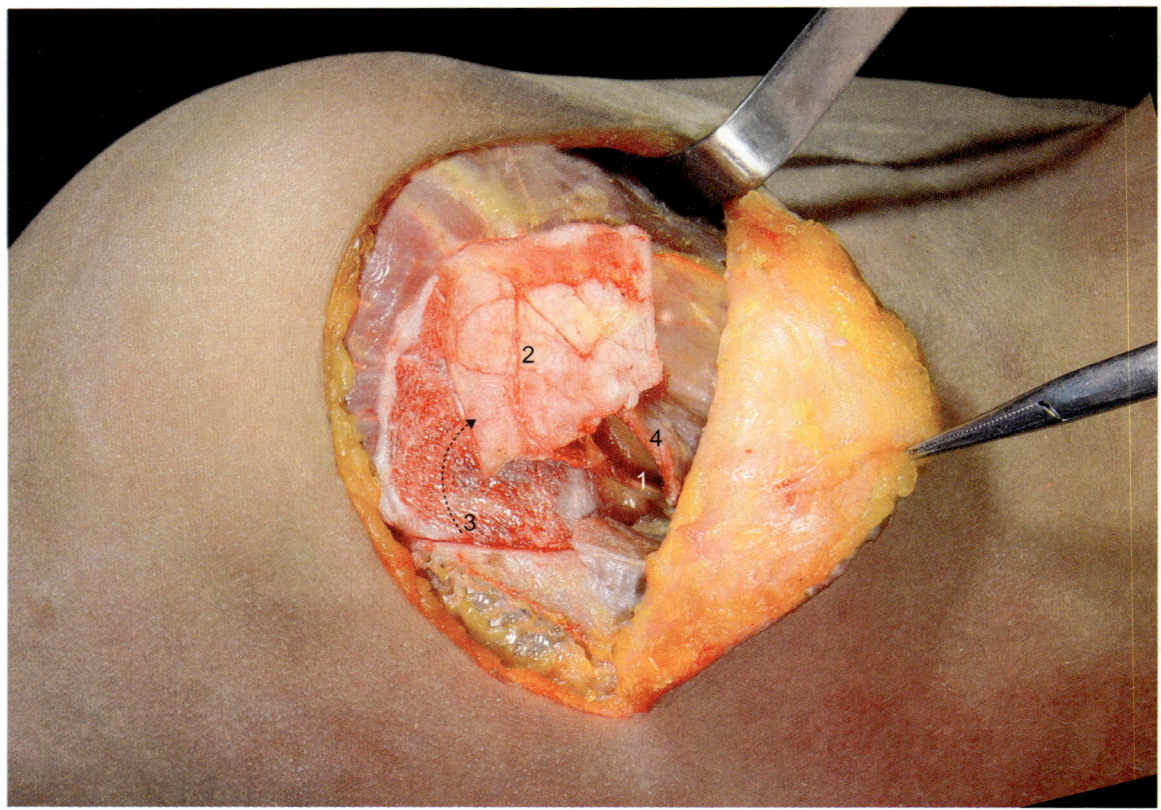

Figure 3-23   Transposition of the flap

The fracture should be repositioned and fixed properly before the bone flap could be transferred to the recipient site.

1. Acromial branch of suprascapular artery
2. Bone flap
3. Donor site
4. Trapezius muscle

Key points in applied anatomy

Firstly, the flap should be designed as close to the middle segment of the scapular spine as possible to guarantee the osseous connection between the scapular notch and the acromion. Secondly, the apocoptic trapezius muscle, the supraspinous muscle and the infraspinous muscle should be fixed on the stump of the bone to reduce the negative impact on the functions. Thirdly, when the fracture is being restored and fixed and the bone flap stripped off, the subclavian vessels should be given attention to avoid damages. Fourthly, when the vascular pedicle is being dissected the perivascular connective tissue sleeve should be retained for about 1.0cm thick.

Spine of Scapula Bone Flap Pedicled with the Acromial Branch of Transverse Cervical Vessels

5

The spine of scapula bone flap based on the acromial branch of the transverse cervical artery is located in a concealed, superficial donor region. It has such advantages as easy operation, and a long-constant vascular pedicle. The flap might be used for free bone grafting. It might also be transferred locally for the posterior cervical vertebral fusion.

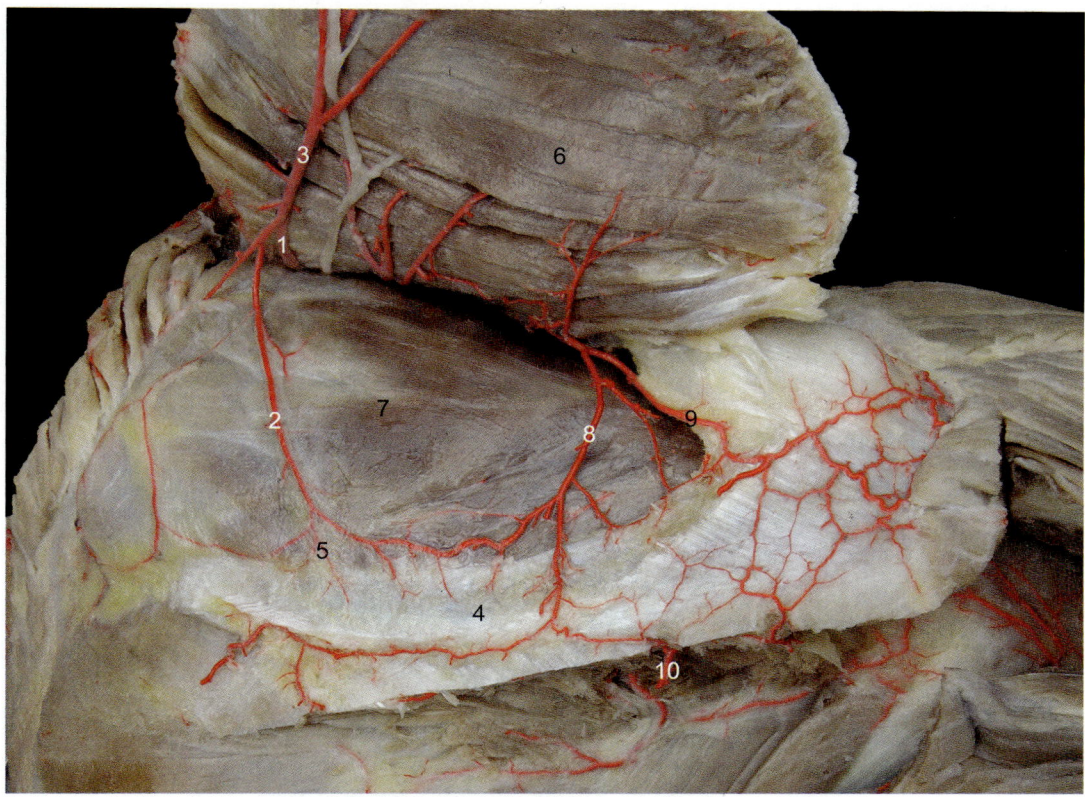

Figure 3-24	Applied anatomy

The transverse cervical artery runs outwards along the anterior trapezius muscle, the internal jugular vein and the posterior sternomastoid muscle to cross the cervical basal part along the superior border of the clavicle. It enters the trapezius muscle at 3.4cm above the intersection between the anterior trapezius muscle and the clavicle, and extends to the anterior levator scapular muscle to bifurcate into the superficial and the deep branches at 1.5cm above the superior angle of the scapula. The initiation of the superficial branch is 2.1mm in diameter and 1.7cm in length. The superficial branch further divides into the spinal branch and the trapezius muscular branch. The spinal branch runs laterally downward through the trapezius muscle to the superior scapular spine and comes out at 4.1cm to its medial border. It extends outwards along the spine and terminates at the middle spine process. Along its course, the artery sends 4-9 osseous branches (0.2-1.0mm in diameter) to distribute on the spine and anastomose with the supraspinous branch of the deep transverse cervical artery and the supra-/infra-spinous branches of the suprascapular artery.

1. Superficial branch of transverse cervical artery
2. Supraspinous branch (superficial branch of transverse cervical artery)
3. Trapezius muscular branch (superficial branch of transverse cervical artery)
4. Scapular spine   **5.** Osseous branch
6. Trapezius muscle   **7.** Supraspinous muscle
8. Supraspinous branch of suprascapular artery
9. Acromial branch of suprascapular artery
10. Infraspinous branch of suprascapular artery

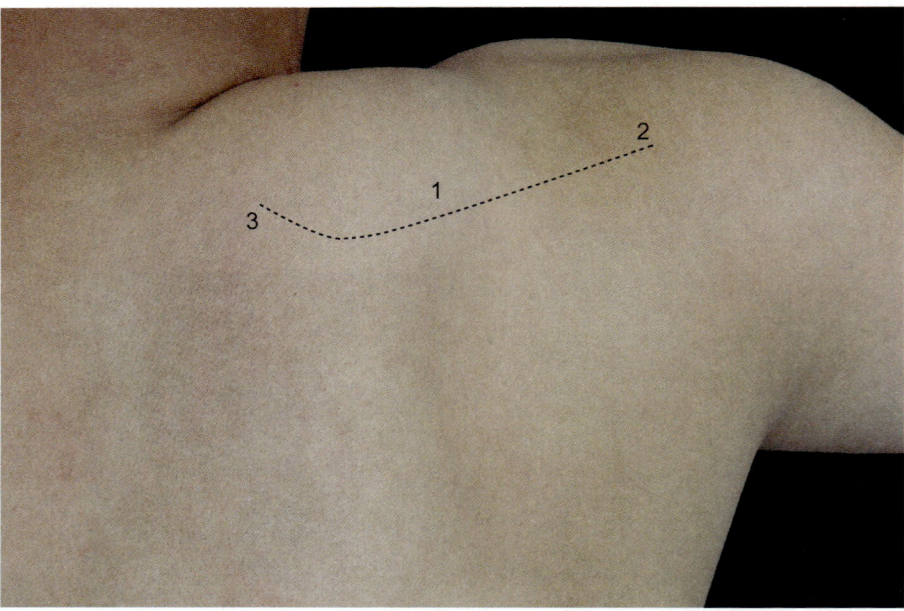

Figure 3-25	Design of the incision

The patient is in lateral position, with the donor region on the top and the upper limb on a bracket. A double-curved incision should be designed beginning with the laterosuperior portion of the acromion, extending along the scapular spine, and turning to the superior angle of the scapula at the mid-point.

1. Scapular spine
2. Acromion
3. Superior angle of scapula

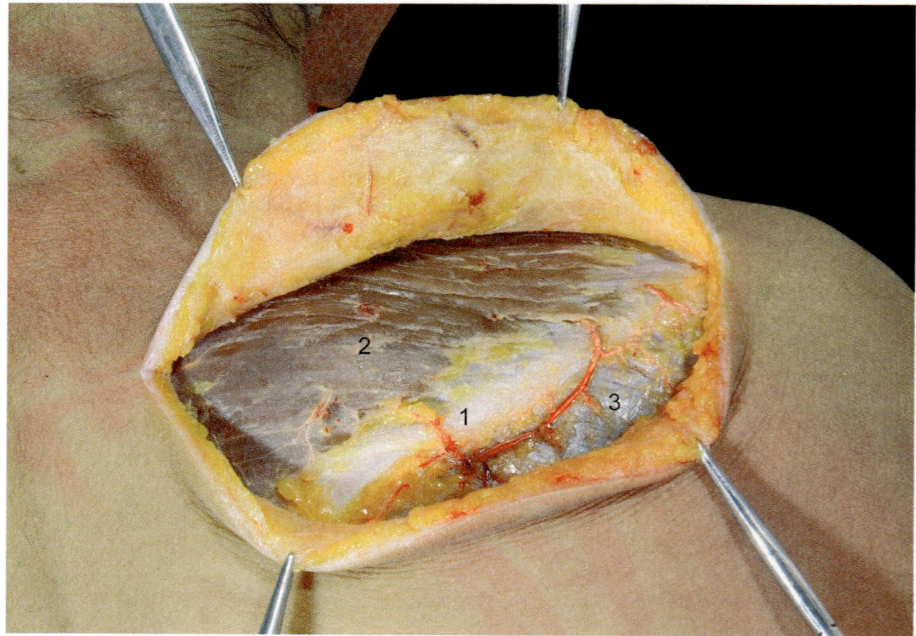

1. Scapular spine
2. Trapezius muscle
3. Deltoid

Figure 3-26	Exposure of the scapular spine

The skin and the subcutaneous tissues should be incised open to expose the scapular spine and the muscles attaching to it.

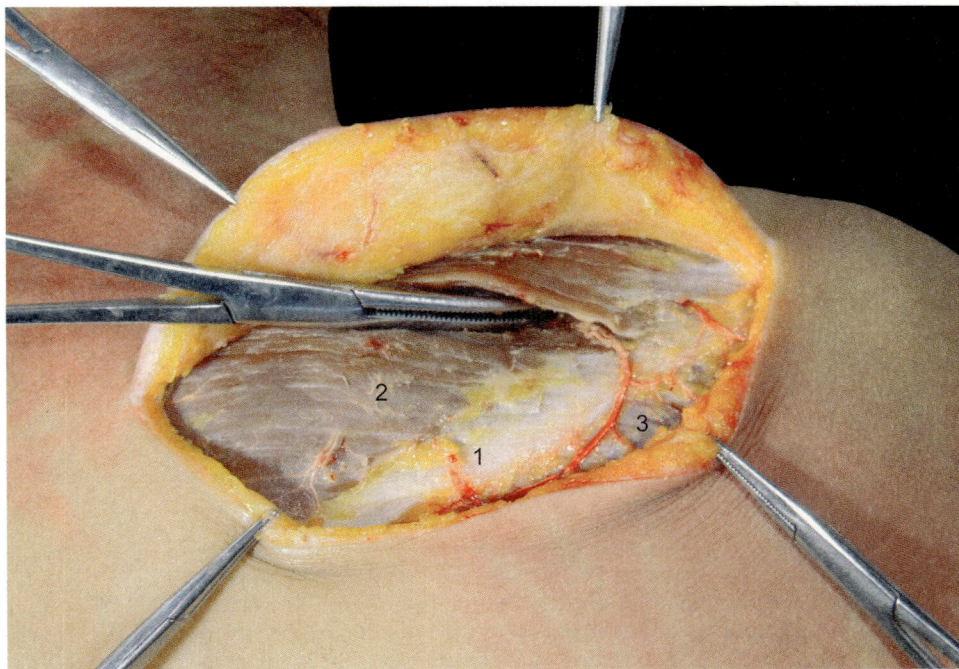

1. Scapular spine
2. Trapezius muscle
3. Deltoid

Figure 3-27 Separation of the trapezius muscle

The trapezius muscle should be separated at 3-4cm above the scapular spine and medial to the midpoint of the scapular spine.

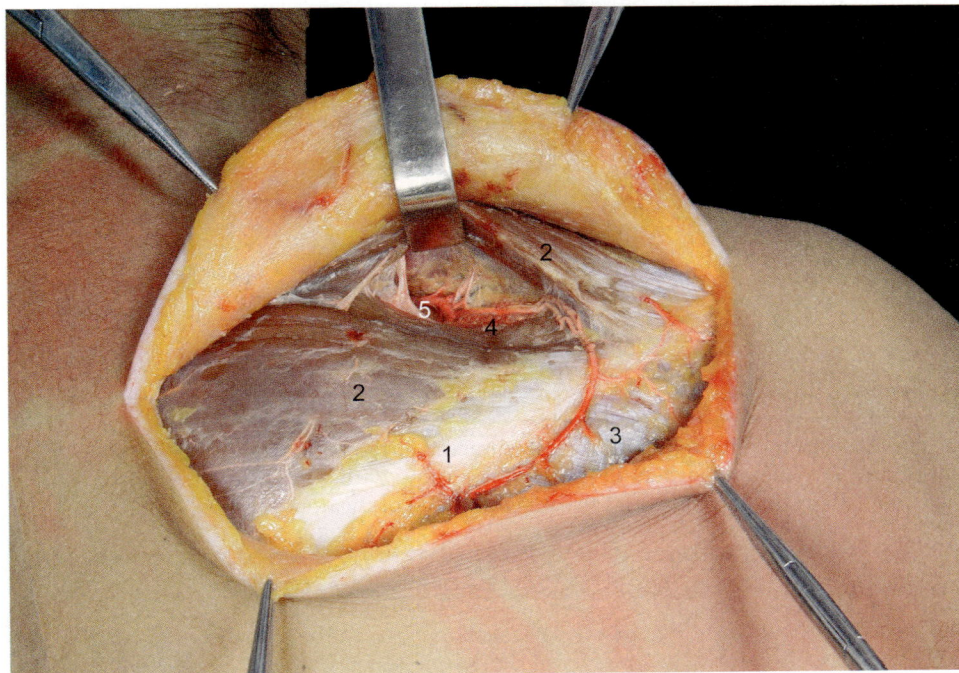

1. Scapular spine
2. Trapezius muscle
3. Deltoid
4. Spine of scapula branch
5. Superficial branch of transverse cervical artery

Figure 3-28 Exposure of the vessels

The dissection should continue to expose the spina scapulae branch and its further branches at the deep layer of the trapezius muscle and then trace medially upwards along the vascular bundle to the part where the superficial branch of the transverse cervical artery sends the spina scapulae branch.

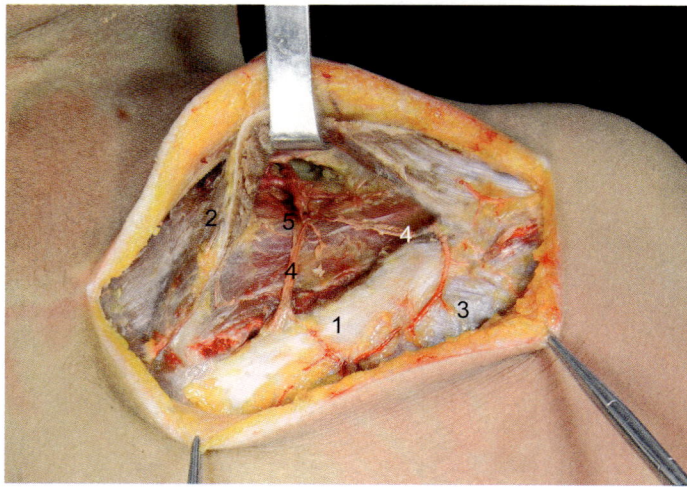

1. Scapular spine
2. Trapezius muscle
3. Deltoid
4. Spina scapulae branch
5. Superficial branch of transverse cervical artery

Figure 3-29   Separation of the vessels

The separation of the vascular plexus would be done bi-directionally, the distal direction to the osseous branches into the scapular spine and the proximal direction to the origin of the pedicle. If a long pedicle is expected, the separation should be done retrogradely towards the arterial trunk. If the flap is based on the spina scapulae vessel, the separation of it should trace along the spina scapulae branch to the shared trunk at the trapezius muscular branch.

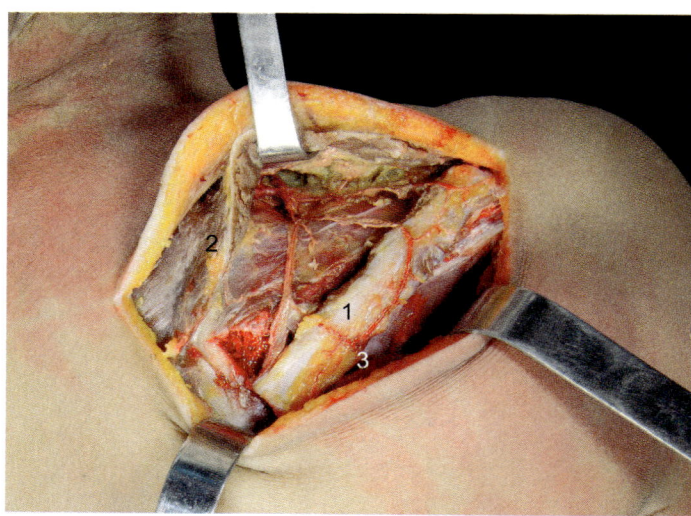

1. Spine of scapula bone flap
2. Trapezius muscle
3. Deltoid

Figure 3-30   Retrieval of the bone flap

The trapezius muscle, the supra-/infra-spinous muscles and the attachments of the deltoid muscle should be cut along the superior and the inferior borders of the scapular spine with the muscular sleeves (1cm thick) retained. The bone flap should be chiseled to satisfy the need of the donor region.

Key points in applied anatomy

Firstly, when the bone flap is being harvested, the osseous connection between the scapular notch and the acromion should be retained to guarantee the integrity of the acromioclavicular joint. Secondly, the apocoptic muscle should be fixed to the stump of the bone to reduce the impact on the muscular functions. Thirdly, when a reverse-flow flap based on the trapezius muscular branch or the scapular branch is being designed, the superficial branch or the transverse cervical artery should be ligated before it divides into the spina scapulae branch and the trapezius muscular branch. Fourthly, if the trapezius muscular branches are small in diameter, a bit of the perivascular muscular bundles should be retained to keep them intact. Fifthly, the bone flap should be transferred with its pedicle untwisted and un-stretched.

Spine of Scapula Bone Flap Pedicled with Infraspinous Branch of Suprascapular Vessels

6

The a infraspinous branch of the suprascapular artery is characterized with a superficial position, a constant course, a long pedicle and an easy dissection. It has been chosen as one of most popular pedicles of the spina scapulae bone flap. The kind of flap could be used for free grafting or transferred locally to repair the defect on the proximal humerus. It might also be designed as an osseous flap or osseomyocutaneous composite one to meet the requirement of the recipient.

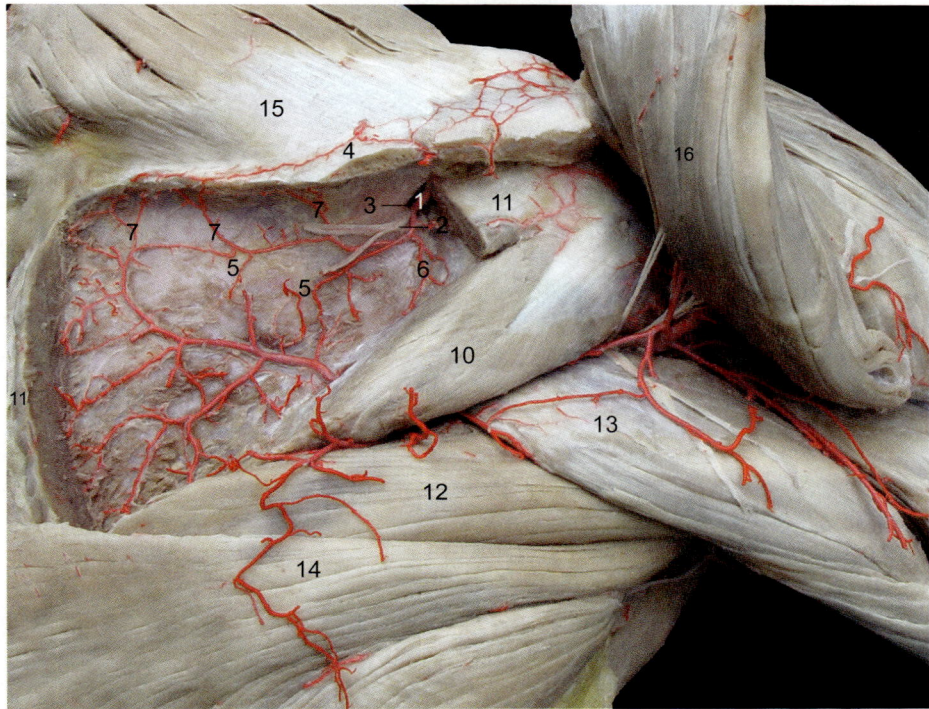

1. Suprascapular artery
2. Infraspinous branch
3. Scapular notch
4. Scapular spine
5. Muscular branch
6. Anastomotic branch
7. Spine of scapula branch
8. Deep branch of circumflex scapular artery
9. Large anastomotic branch
10. Teres minor muscle
11. Infraspinous muscle
12. Teres major muscle
13. Long head of triceps brachii muscle
14. Latissimus dorsi muscle
15. Trapezius muscle
16. Posterior portion of deltoid

Figure 3-31 Applied anatomy

The suprascapular artery emerges and runs laterally downwards into the supraspinous fossa through the superior transverse scapular ligament, where it sends the supraspinous branches. Its trunk winds around the scapular notch to the infraspinous fossa and extends as the infraspinous branch. The infraspinous branch perforates through the scapular notch at 2.5cm to the inferior scapular spine, and extends transversely inwards. Along its course it sends muscular branches, anastomotic branches and 4-6 spina scapulae branches (about 0.9mm in diameter) . These branches disperse over the superficial periosteum of the inferior or the basal scapular spine, each of which covers 1.5-2.0cm in general from the origin of the osseous branches to the base of the scapular spine. The anastomotic branches emerge constantly from the initiations of the infraspinous branches and run laterally downwards along the superficial periosteum to anastomose with the deep branches of the circumflex scapular artery or the posterior humeral circumflex artery. In a few cases (3.3%), the anastomotic branch is large in caliber and takes the place of the infraspinous branch, which is 1.8mm in diameter (on average) at its initiation and covers 3.5cm from the scapular notch to its first spina scapulae branch.

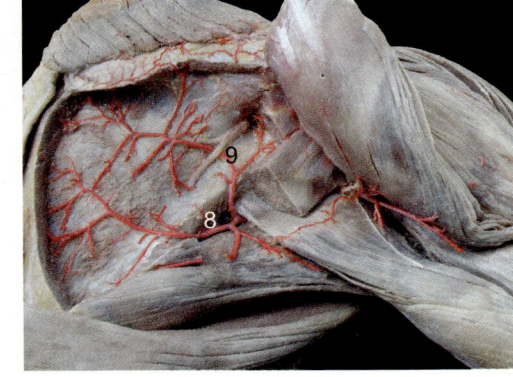

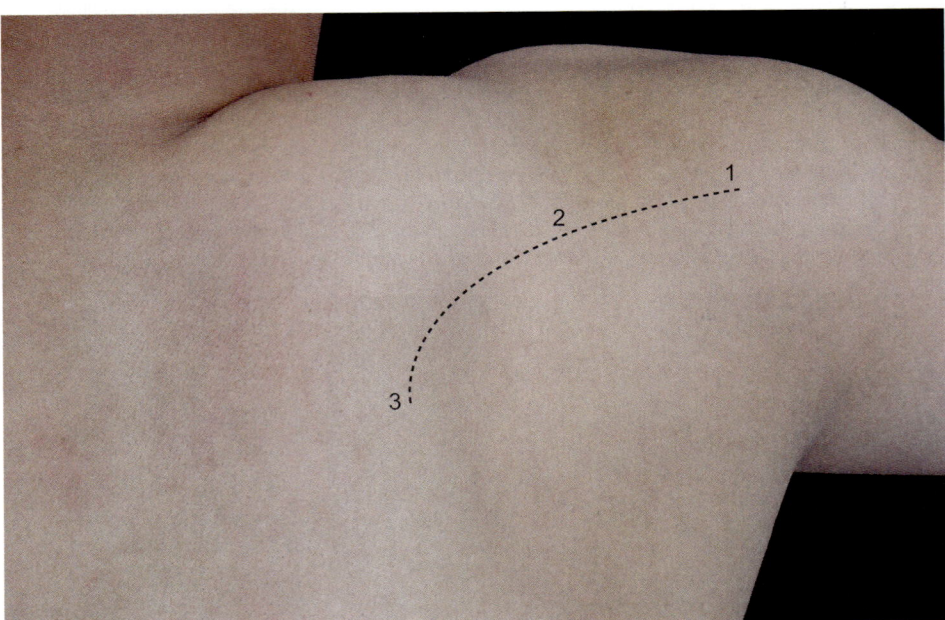

| Figure 3-32 | Design of the incision |

The patient is in a lateral position, the donor region on the top and the upper limb placed on a bracket. The incision should begin with the acromion, continue along the scapular spine to its medial border and turn downwards along the medial border of the scapula for about 5-6cm.
1. Acromion
2. Scapular spine
3. Medial border of scapula

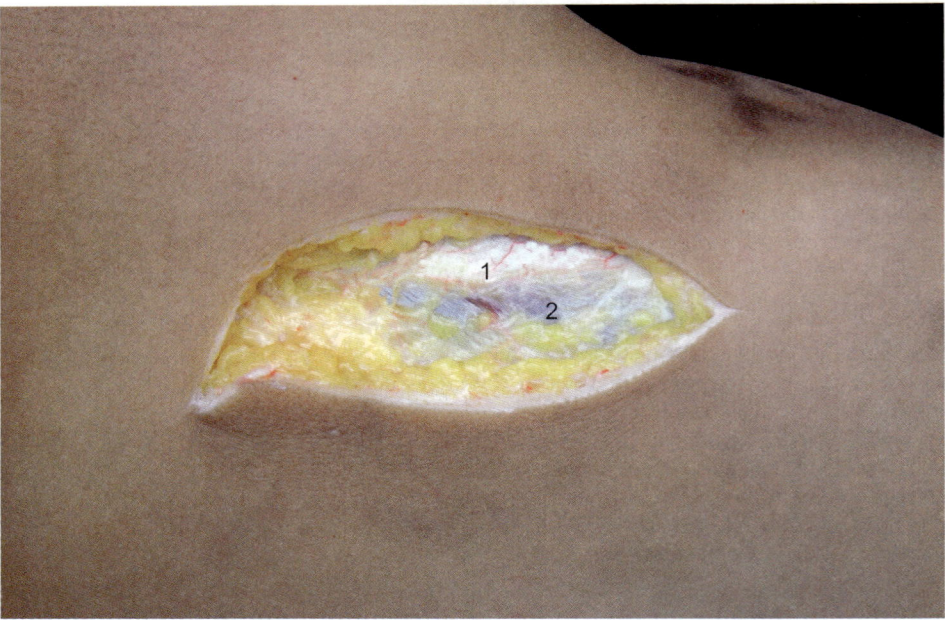

| Figure 3-33 | Exposure of the scapular spine |

The skin and the subcutaneous tissues should be incised open to expose the scapular spine and the muscles attaching to it.
1. Scapular spine
2. Deltoid

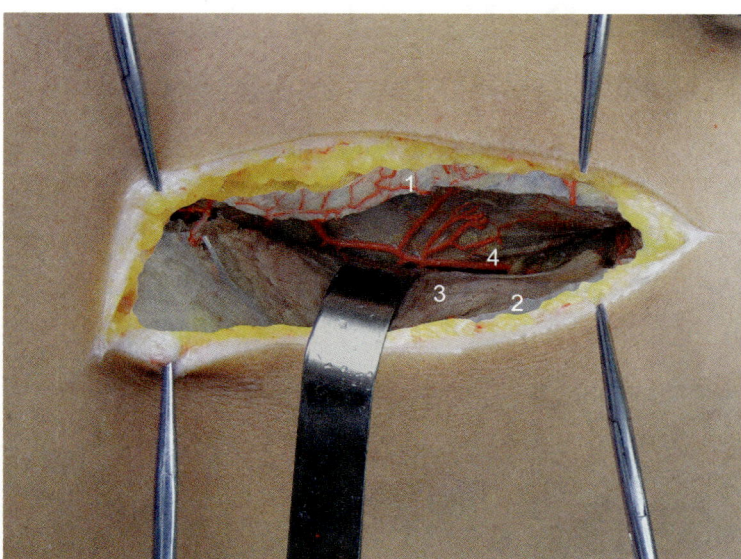

1. Scapular spine
2. Deltoid
3. Infraspinous muscle
4. Infraspinous branch

Figure 3-34   Exposure of the vessels

The deltoid muscle and the trapezius muscle should be separated along their attachment to the inferior border of the scapular spine. The infraspinous muscle should be cut along the inferior border of the scapular spine and the medial scapular border and pulled outwards to the scapular notch to expose the infraspinous branch.

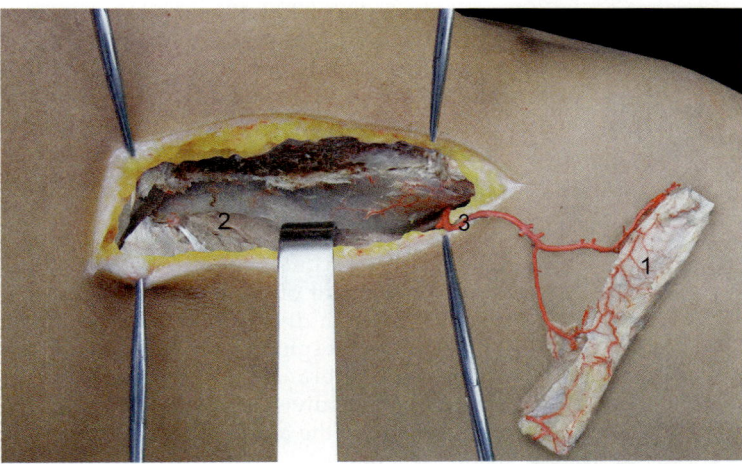

1. Spine of scapula bone flap
2. Infraspinous muscle
3. Infraspinous branch

Figure 3-35   Transposition of the bone flap

The superior attachment of the trapezius muscle on the scapular spine should be further divided and the supraspinous muscle stripped away to expose the supraspinous fossa. Then the bone flap should be chiseled to meet the requirements of the recipient site.

Key points in applied anatomy

Firstly, when the bone flap is being harvested, the osseous connection between the scapular notch and the acromion should be retained to guarantee the integrity of the acromioclavicular joint. Secondly, the divided apocoptic muscle should be fixed onto the stump of the bone to reduce the impact on the muscular functions. Thirdly, the flap should be transferred with the pedicle untwisted and unstretched. Fourthly, when the vascular pedicle is being dissected in the procedure, great attention should be given to the infraspinous branch of the suprascapular nerve, whose trunk should be pulled away from the superficial vascular surface. Only branches that wind through the deep surface of the vessels might be divided.

Bone Flap of Lateral Border of Scapula Pedicled with Circumflex Scapular Vessels

7

The circumflex scapular artery might serve as the pedicle of the bone flap of the lateral border of the scapula. The artery has such advantages as a large vascular caliber, a constant position, and a concealed donor region. An operation of this type could be easily done in the muscular septum and the incision of the donor skin directly sutured. If a composite flap is to be harvested, it is possible to choose an independent vascular pedicle for each of the bone flap and the osseous cutaneous flap. This type of flap could be used for free grafting or transferred to repair the non-union and defect on the proximal humerus or the shoulder arthrodesis.

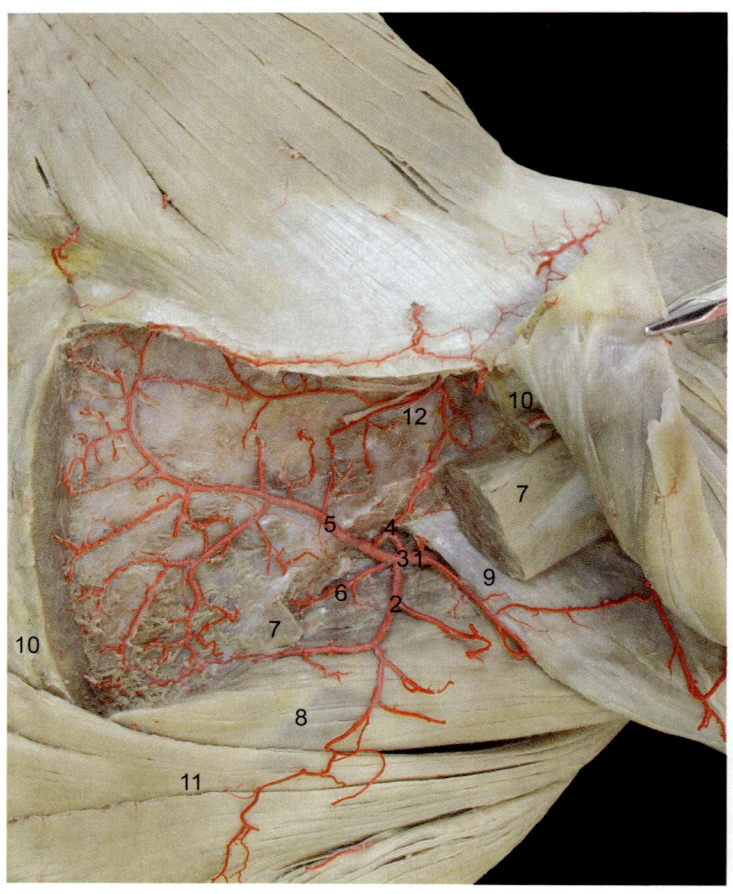

Figure 3-36   Applied anatomy

The infrascapular artery emerges from the axillary artery and immediately bifurcates into the thoracodorsal artery and the circumflex scapular artery. The thoracodorsal artery enters the latissimus dorsi muscle whereas the circumflex scapular artery perforates through the trilateral space and divides into the superficial and the deep ones. The superficial branch extends as the fasciocutaneous artery through the muscular septum and sends 1-3 branches into the infraspinous fossa and the adjacent fascia and skin. The deep branch is short in its trunk and runs closely to the superior segment of the lateral border of the scapula, where it divides into the anastomotic branch, the infraspinous fossa branch and the inferior angle branch. These branches give many small subdivisions to disperse over the dorsolateral or the anterolateral region of the lateral scapula.

1. Circumflex scapular artery
2. Superficial branch of circumflex scapular artery
3. Deep branch of circumflex scapular artery
4. Anastomotic branch
5. Infraspinous fossa branch
6. Inferior angle branch
7. Teres minor muscle
8. Teres major muscle
9. Long head of triceps brachii muscle
10. Infraspinous muscle
11. Latissimus dorsi muscle
12. Infraspinous branch of suprascapular artery

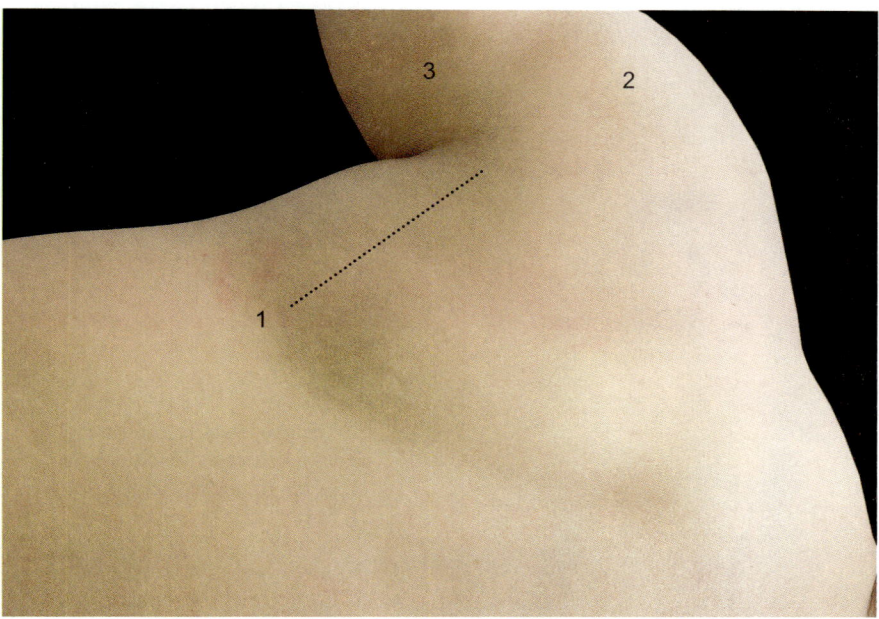

Figure 3-37   Design of the incision

The patient should be placed in a lateral position, and the incision made from the body surface projection of the trilateral space to the inferior angle of the scapula.
1. Inferior angle of scapula
2. Deltoid
3. Long head of triceps brachii muscle

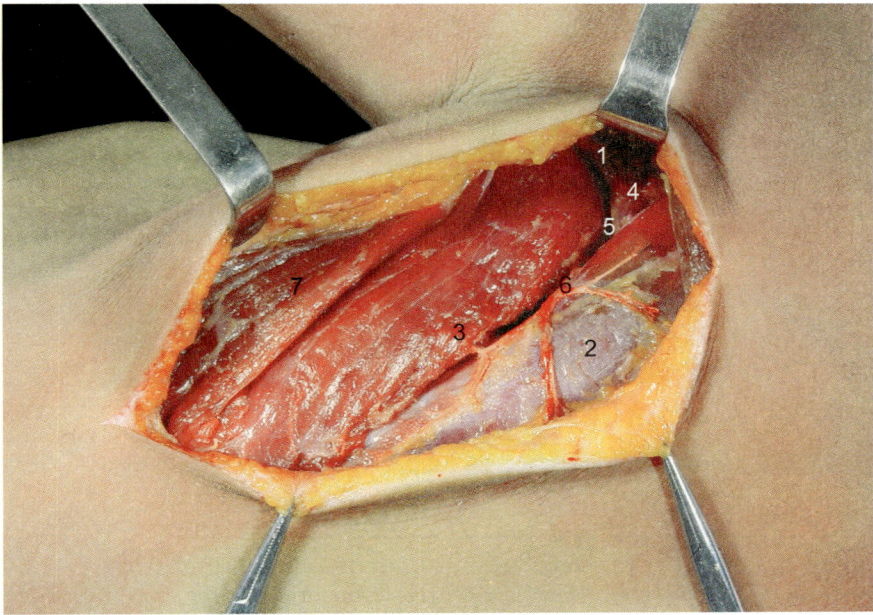

1. Deltoid
2. Teres minor muscle
3. Teres major muscle
4. Triceps brachii (long head)
5. Trilateral foramen
6. Cutaneous branch of circumflex scapular artery
7. Latissimus dorsi muscle

Figure 3-38   Exposure of the muscles

The skin and the subcutaneous tissues should be incised open, and the posterior margin of the deltoid muscle pulled forwards to expose the trilateral foramen, the cutaneous branch or the trunk of the circumflex scapular artery that perforates through the foramen.

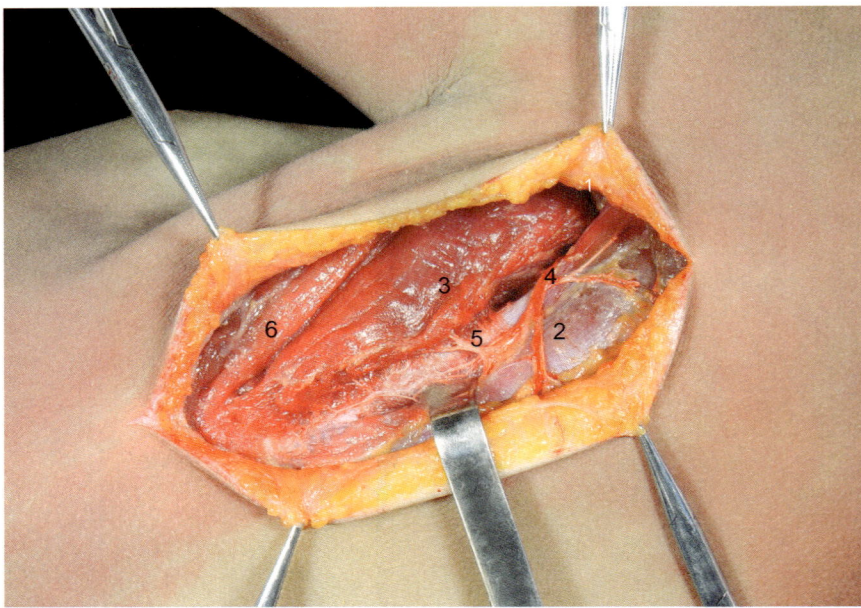

1. Triceps brachii (long head)
2. Teres minor muscle
3. Teres major muscle
4. Superficial branch of circumflex scapular artery
5. Scapula (lateral border)
6. Latissimus dorsi muscle

Figure 3-39   Exposure of the vessels

The circumflex scapular artery perforates through the trilateral foramen and its superficial or deep branches should be identified carefully. The arterial trunk, together with its concomitant vein, runs across the surface of the teres minor muscle, where it is 2.5mm in diameter. There are loose perivascular connective tissues that need to be carefully dissected.

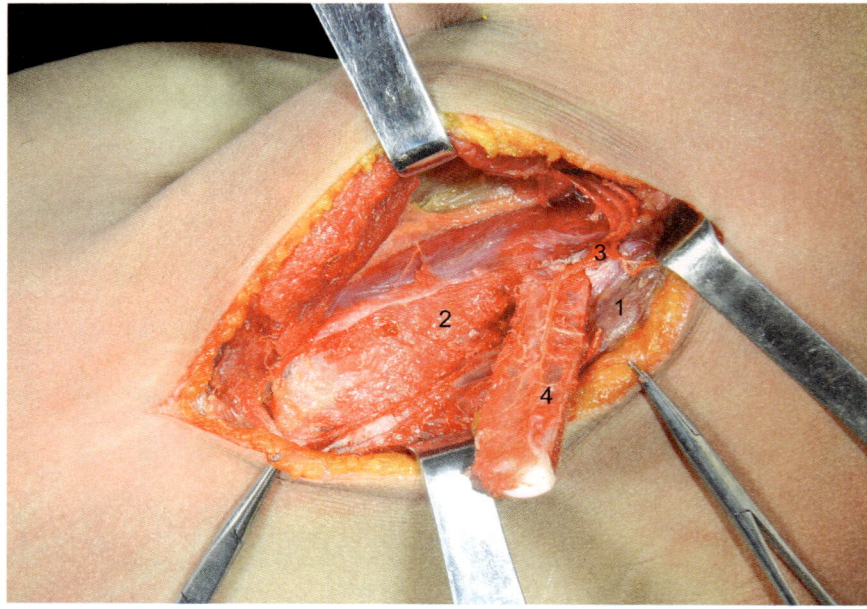

1. Teres minor muscle
2. Teres major muscle
3. Circumflex scapular artery
4. Bone flap

Figure 3-40   Dissection of the bone flap

The superficial branch from the circumflex scapular artery should be identified and cut off. The dissection of the flap then should trace along the proximal superficial branch to the origin of the circumflex scapular artery and enter the deep osseous branches. Then the bone flap should be chiseled in the lateral border of the scapula from 1cm below the glenoid cavity to the inferior scapular angle. The harvested bone flap might be transferred through the enlarged trilateral foramen to another incision in the axillary fossa, where the thoracodorsal artery should be ligated and cut off. The circumflex scapular artery should be traced to the origin of the infrascapular artery, based on which, the bone flap could be made with a vascular pedicle of 5.5-9.0cm long.

Bone Flap of Lateral Border of Scapula Pedicled with Thoracodorsal Vessels

8

The thoracodorsal artery might serve as a pedicle of the bone flap based on the lateral border of the scapula. It has such advantages as a large vascular caliber, a constant course and a long vascular pedicle. To meet the requirement of the recipient sites, the flap might be designed as a bone flap or a composite osteomyocutaneous flap consisting of parts of the scapula, the latissimus dorsi muscle and the adjacent skin. This type of flaps could be used for free grafting or transferred locally for the repair of the non-union, the defect on the proximal or middle segment of the humerus or the shoulder arthrodesis.

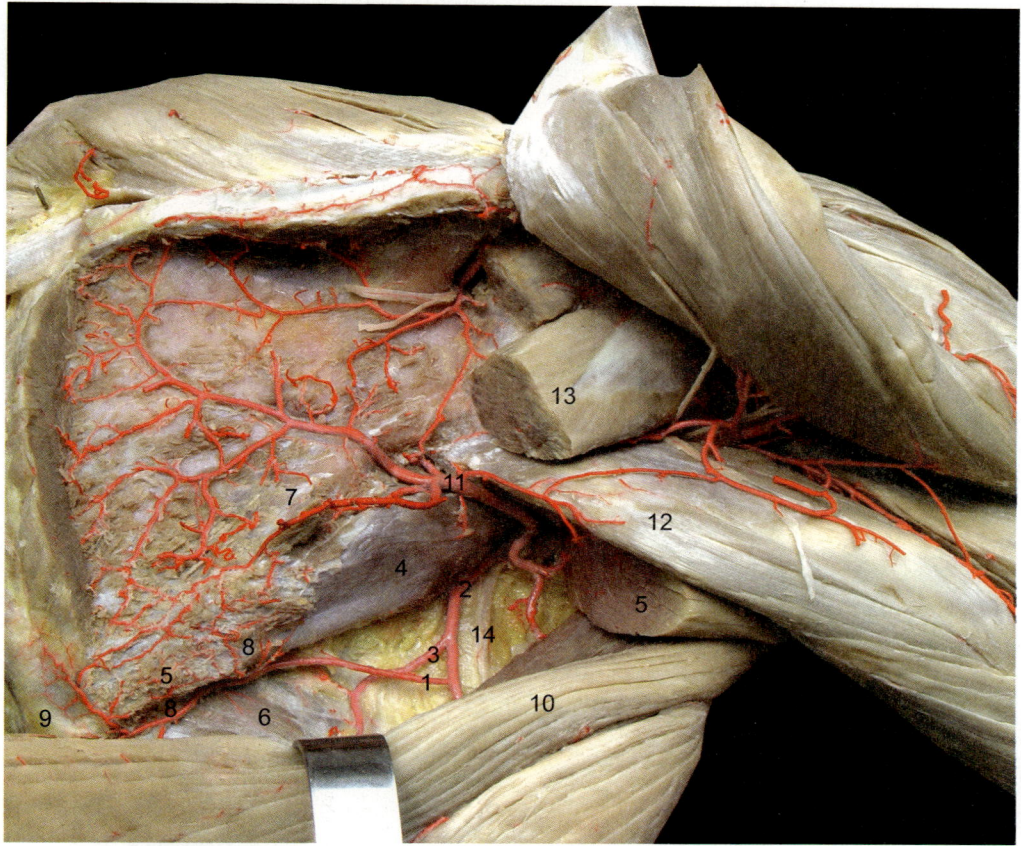

| Figure 3-41 | Applied anatomy |

The scapular branch originates from the thoracodorsal artery at 4.1cm from the initiation of the trunk. In most cases (80%), it might emerge from the common trunk of the scapular branch and the anterior serratus muscular branch. The common trunk is 1.9mm in length and 2.1mm in diameter. In a few cases (20%), it might emerge only from the thoracodorsal artery. In most cases (87.5%), there is only one scapular branch; but in a few cases (12.5%), there are 2. After its origin, the scapular branch runs in the septum between the lateral margin of the infrascapular muscle and the teres major muscle and the anterior serratus muscle. It extends closely to the middle-inferior segment of the lateral scapula and sends 4-9 musculoperiosteal branches (0.3-0.8mm in diameter) to disperse over the dorsolateral and the anterolateral regions of the middle-inferior segment of the scapula and over the inferior scapular angle.

1. Scapular branch of thoracodorsal artery
2. Thoracodorsal artery
3. Anterior serratus muscular branch
4. Subscapular muscle
5. Teres major muscle
6. Anterior serratus muscle
7. Lateral border of scapula
8. Musculoperiosteal branch
9. Inferior angle of scapula
10. Latissimus dorsi muscle
11. Circumflex scapular artery
12. Long head of triceps brachii
13. Teres minor muscle
14. Thoracodorsal nerve

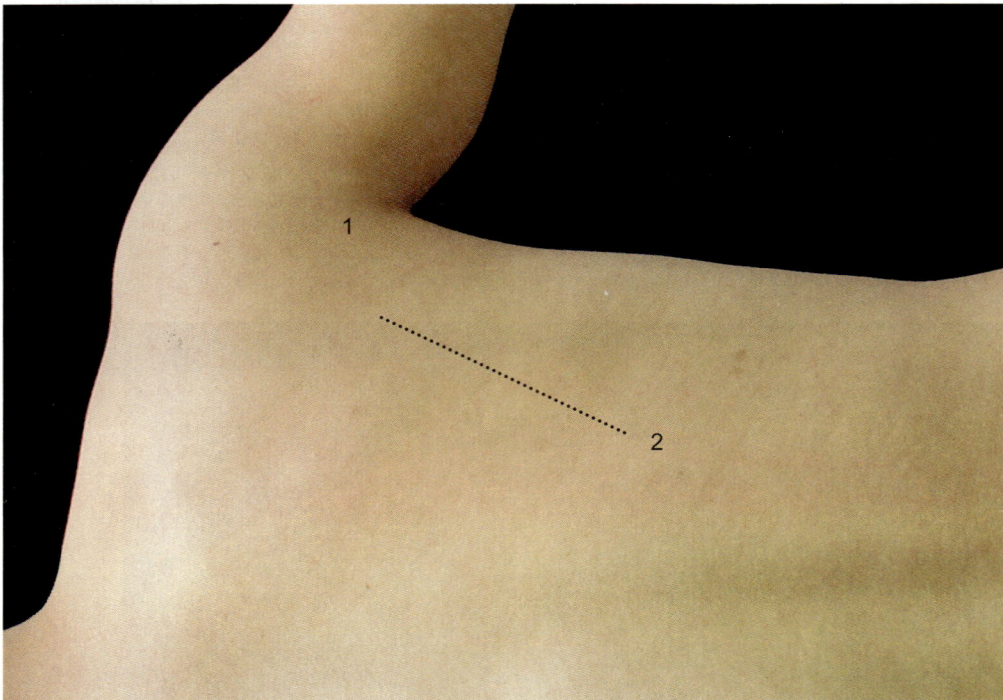

1. Posterior axillary fold
2. Inferior angle of scapula

| Figure 3-42 | Design of the incision |

Take the harvest of a pure bone flap for example. The patient should be placed in lateral position and a longitudinal incision done along the posterior axillary fold onto the inferior scapular angle.

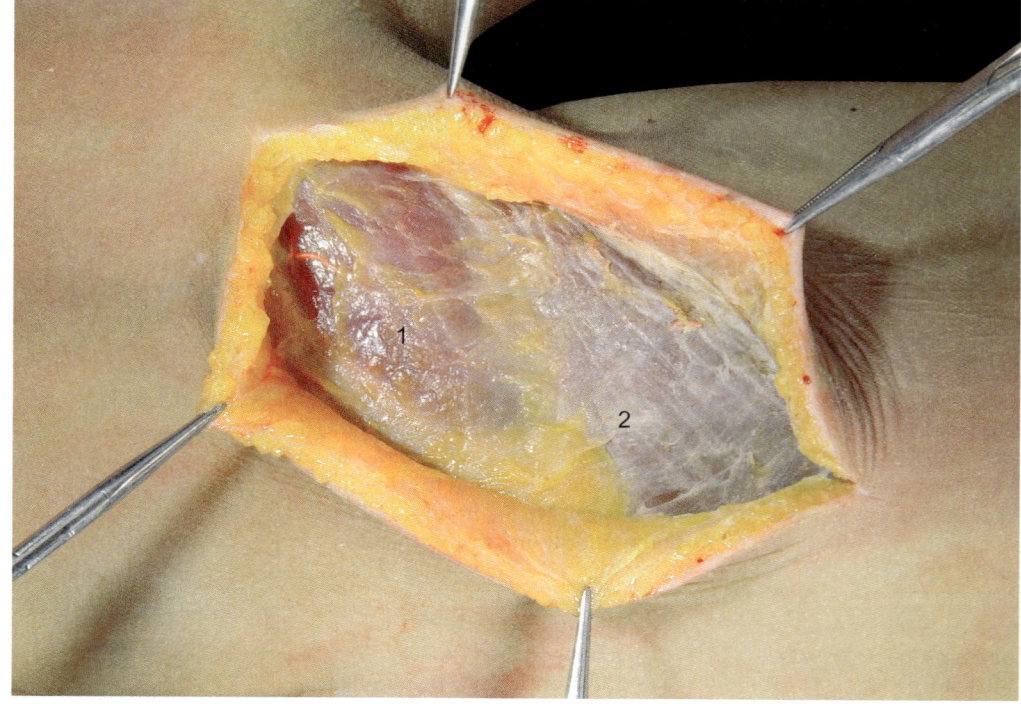

1. Teres major muscle
2. Latissimus dorsi muscle

| Figure 3-43 | Exposure of the muscles |

The skin should be incised open to expose the teres major and the latissimus dorsi muscles.

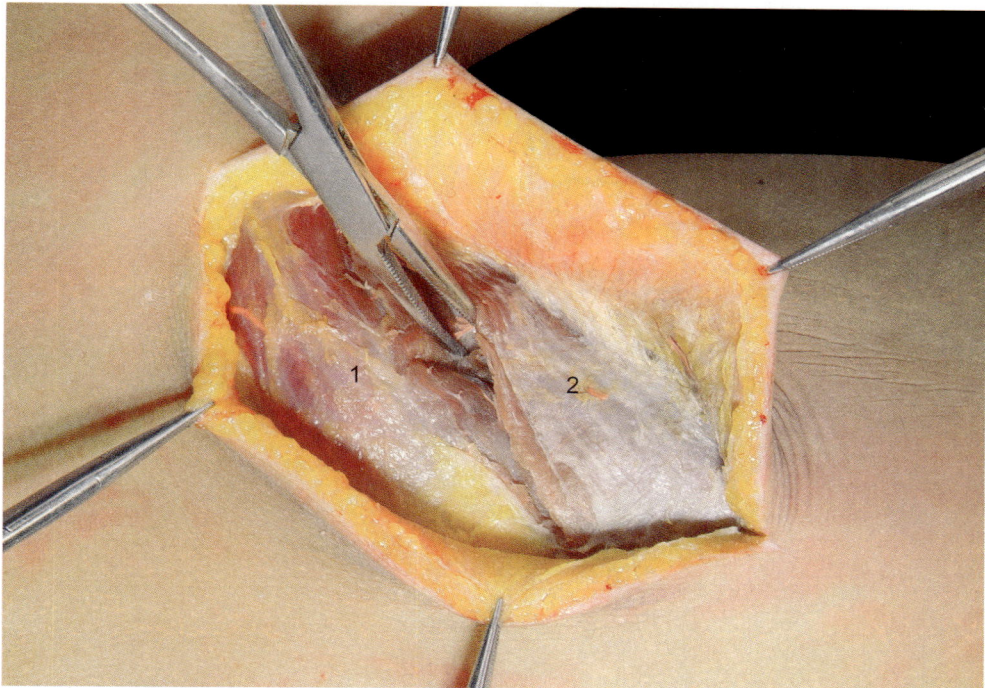

1. Teres major muscle
2. Latissimus dorsi muscle

Figure 3-44   Separation of the muscles

The septum between the teres major and the latissimus dorsi muscles should be bluntly separated.

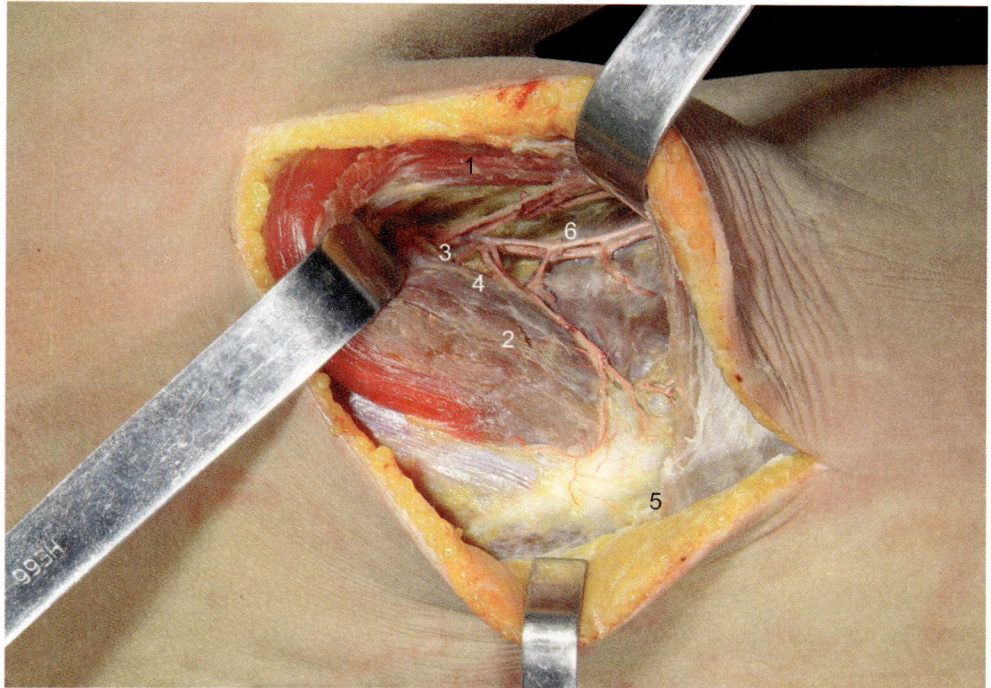

1. Latissimus dorsi muscle
2. Teres major muscle
3. Thoracodorsal artery
4. Scapular branch
5. Inferior angle of scapula
6. Anterior serratus muscle

Figure 3-45   Exposure of the vessels

The supra-posterior teres major should be pulled outwards and the latissimus dorsi muscles inwards to look for the thoracodorsal artery in the upper deep layer of the septum between the two muscles (just below the circumflex scapular artery). The dissection should trace medially backwards along the vascular trunk to look for the scapular branch, which might be situated about 4cm from the origin of the thoracodorsal artery.

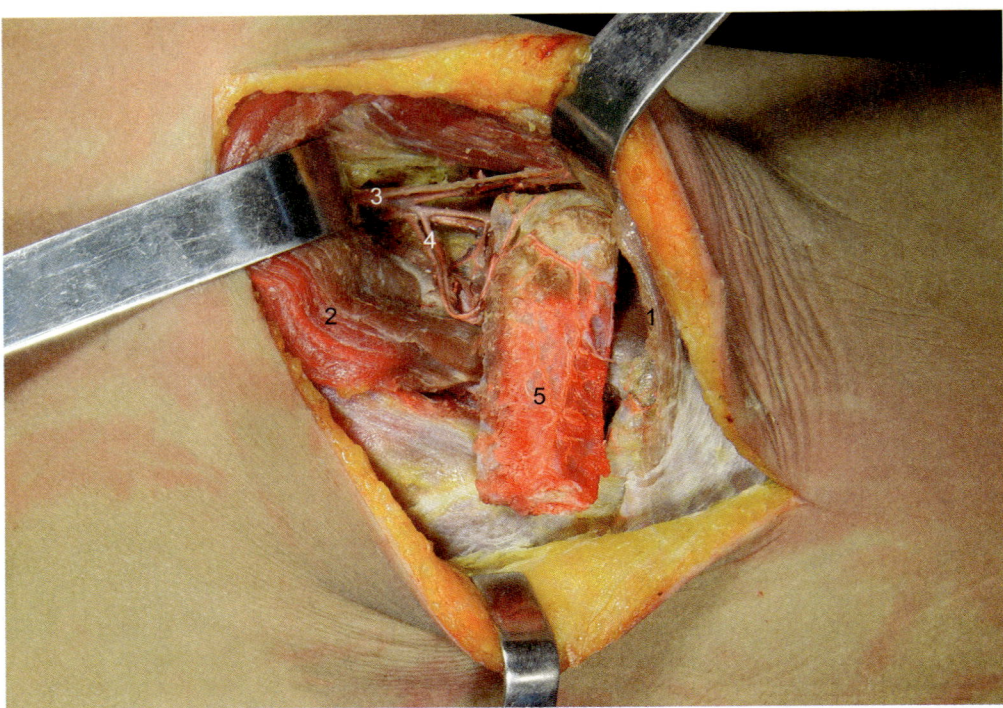

| Figure 3-46 | Dissection of the bone flap |

The teres major muscle should then be divided obliquely at the middle-inferior segment of the dorsal scapula and superiorly at the part where its divisions enter the muscle to keep intact the myo-osseous branches. The divisions of the scapular branch to the anterolateral region of the lateral scapula should also be carefully protected, with some of the infrascapular muscular bundles included in the flap. The anterior serratus muscle should be finally cut from its attachment on the inferior angle of the scapula. The middle-inferior segment of the lateral scapula then could be chiseled with a size of (6-8)×3cm.

1. Latissimus dorsi muscle
2. Teres major muscle
3. Thoracodorsal artery
4. Scapular branch
5. Bone flap

Key points in applied anatomy

Firstly, when the attachment of the teres major/minor muscle on the bone flap area was cut, the muscular sleeve (0.5cm thick) should be retained on the flap to protect the periosteal branches. Secondly, the superior border of the flap should be harvested below the infra-glenoid tubercle to prevent the humeral articular capsule from being damaged. Thirdly, the vascular pedicle should include some connective tissue in it and be separated from the accompanying thoracodorsal nerve. Fourthly, the apocoptic muscle should be sutured with the stump of the bone to reduce the impact to the muscular functions. Fifthly, the functional exercise of the shoulder over-head abduction should be carried out 10 days after the operation to prevent limitations on the motion.

Humeral Periosteal Flap Pedicled with Medial Descending Branch of Anterior Circumflex Humeral Vessels

9

The medial descending branch of the anterior circumflex humeral artery has advantages such as a constant course, an easy dissection, and an operation in a single incision. A flap based on this pedicle could be used to treat the ischemic necrosis of the humeral head and the bone non-union or a small defect in surgical neck of the humerus.

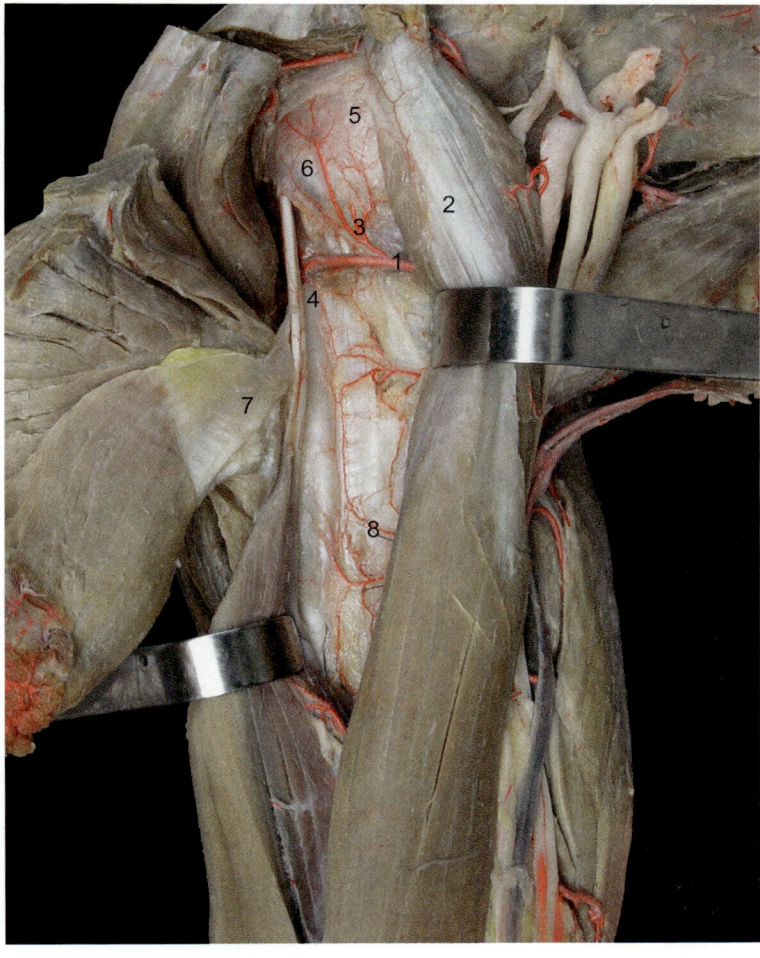

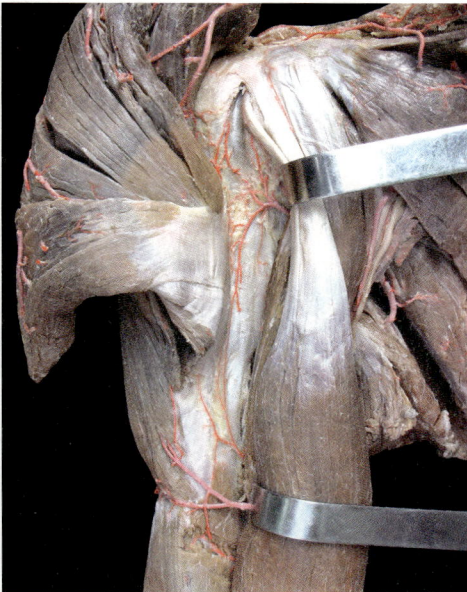

Figure 3-47	Applied anatomy

The anterior circumflex humeral artery runs in the deep layer of the coracobrachial muscle and the short head of the biceps brachii muscle, and enters the lateral margin of the intertubercular sulcus via the surgical neck of the humerus to bifurcate into the ascending and the descending branches. The ascending branch disperses over the humeral head and the lesser tubercle. The descending branch further divides into the medial and the lateral branches to run along the insertion of the pectoral major muscle, attaching bilaterally to the periosteum. The medial descending branch descends to anastomose with the direct periosteal branch of the lateral brachial artery. The trunk of the lateral brachial artery extends outwards to the medial insertion of the deltoid and sends upwards the direct periosteal branches (0.6mm in average diameter) into the periosteum of the bare area of the anteromedial segment of the humerus (equal to the region between medial insertion of deltoid and region above the origin of brachial muscle). Its terminals anastomose with the medial descending branches of the anterior circumflex humeral artery.

1. Anterior circumflex humeral artery
3. Ascending branch
5. Head of humerus
7. Insertion of pectoralis major
2. Short head of biceps brachii muscle
4. Medial descending branch
6. Lesser tubercle
8. Direct periosteal branch of lateral brachial artery

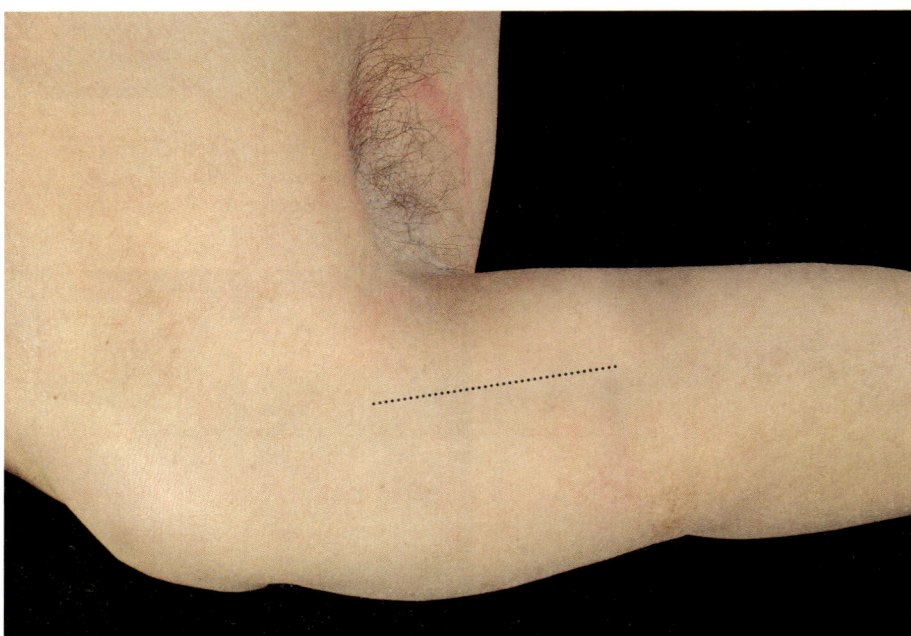

| **Figure 3-48** | Design of the incision |

The patient is in a supine position with a flat pillow padded under the posterior shoulder and the upper limb on the chest. The incision should extend downwards along the anterior deltoid and the lateral biceps brachii. Both the superior and the inferior ends of the incision might be adjusted properly to the lesion.

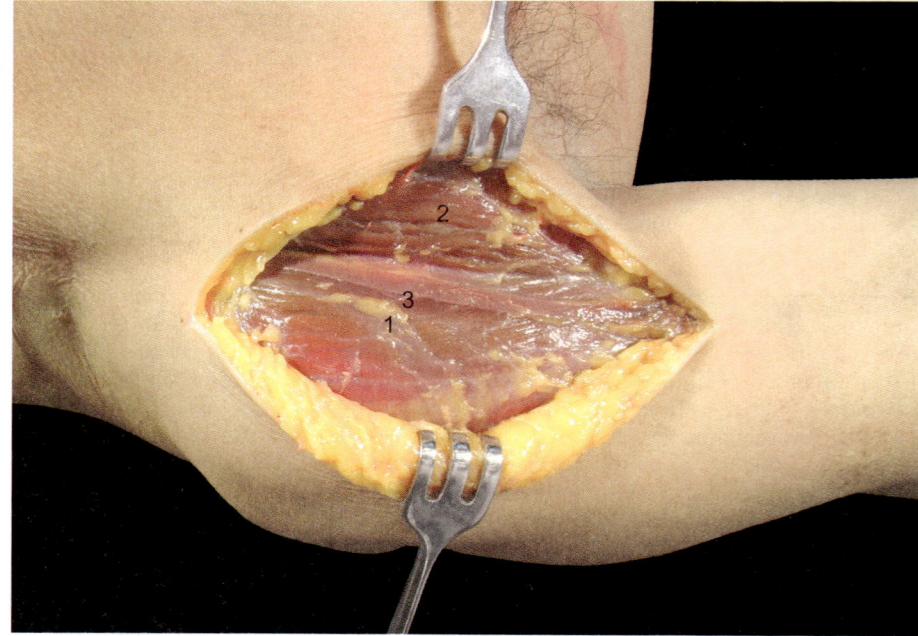

1. Deltoid muscle
2. Pectoralis major
3. Cephalic vein

| **Figure 3-49** | Exposure of the cephalic vein |

The skin and the subcutaneous tissues should be incised open to expose the cephalic vein in the intermuscular groove between the deltoid and the pectoralis major.

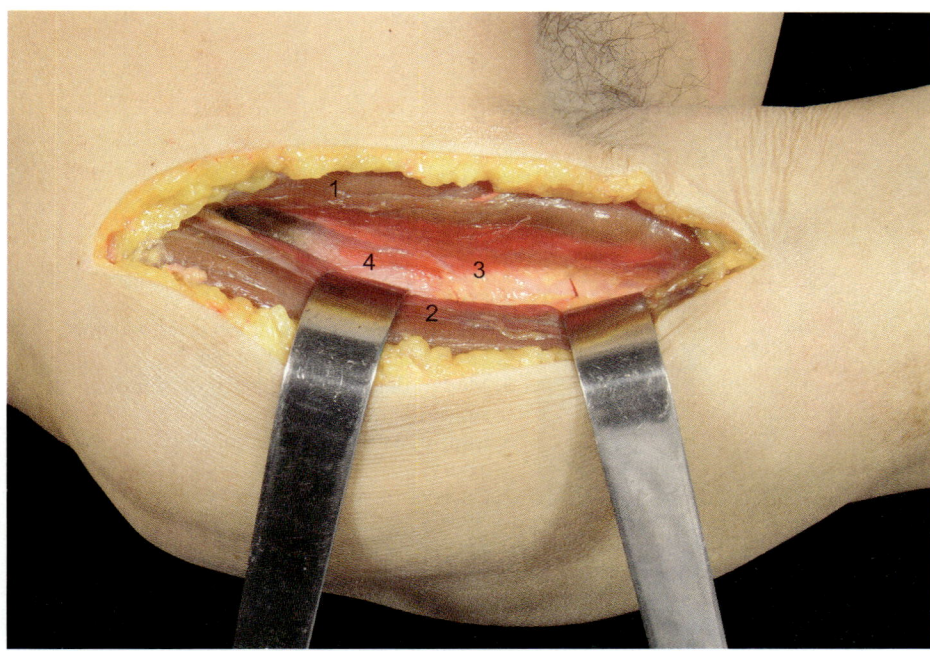

1. Pectoralis major
2. Deltoid muscle
3. Tendinous insertion of pectoralis major
4. Long head tendon of biceps brachii

Figure 3-50   Division of the tendon

The deltoid in the superior segment of the incision should be pulled outwards to expose the tendinous insertion of the pectoralis major, and the tendon then cut off.

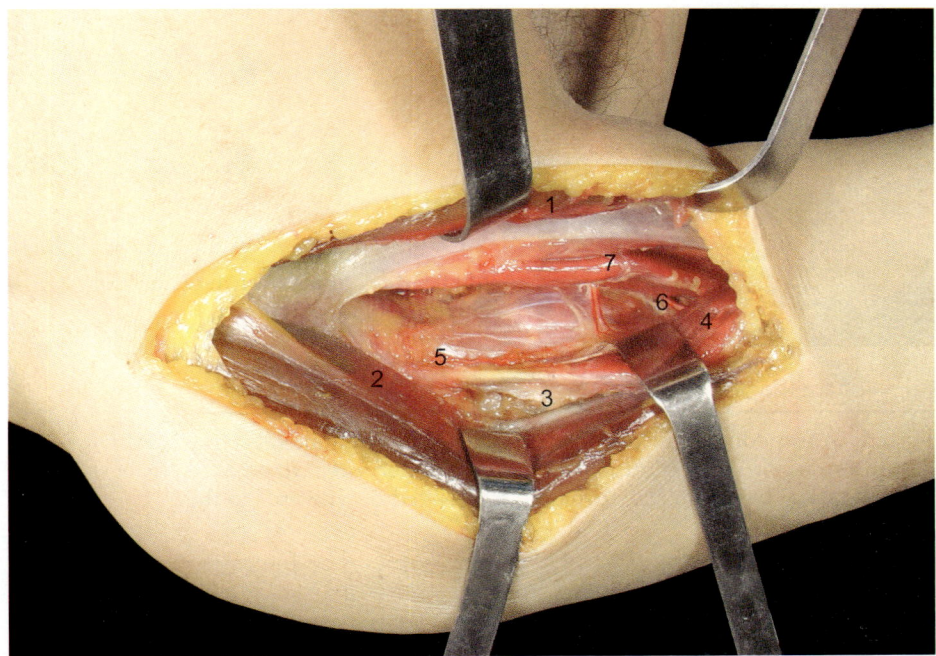

1. End of pectoralis major
2. Deltoid muscle
3. Tendinous insertion of pectoralis major
4. Long head of biceps brachii
5. Medial descending branch of anterior circumflex humeral artery
6. Intermuscular spatial branch of brachial artery
7. Coracobrachial muscle

Figure 3-51   Exposure of the vessels

In the inferior segment of the incision, the biceps brachii and the brachial muscle should be pulled bilaterally to expose the medial descending branch of the anterior circumflex humeral artery and the anastomotic branch of the direct periosteal branch of the lateral brachial artery (i.e. the ascending branch of the intermuscular spatial branch of brachial artery).

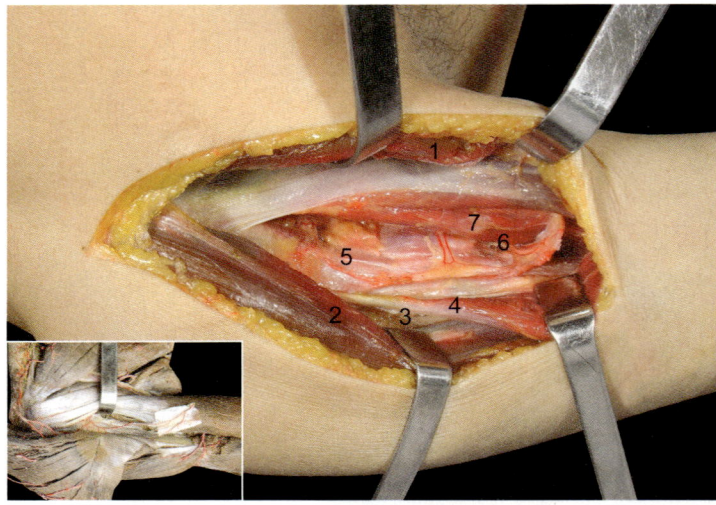

1. End of pectoralis major
2. Deltoid muscle
3. Tendinous insertion of pectoralis major
4. Long head of biceps brachii
5. Medial descending branch of anterior circumflex humeral artery
6. Intermuscular spatial branch of brachial artery
7. Coracobrachial muscle

Figure 3-52   Dissection of bone periosteal flap

Either the medial descending branch of the anterior circumflex humeral artery or the direct branch of the lateral brachial artery could be chosen as the pedicle of the bone flap, but it all depends on the site of the lesion. When the medial descending branch is to be used, the periosteum should be separated bilaterally and stripped medially to protect the vascular pedicle.

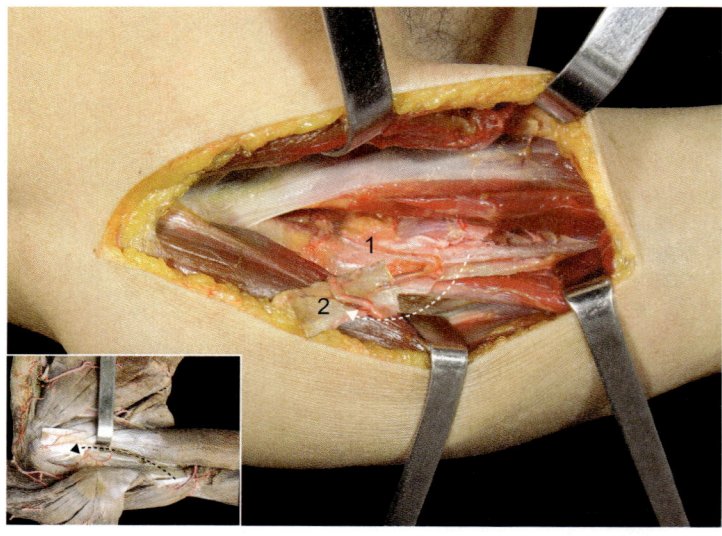

1. Medial descending branch of anterior circumflex humeral artery
2. Periosteal flap

Figure 3-53   Transposition of the flap

The periosteal flap based on the medial descending branch of the anterior circumflex humeral artery could be transferred upwards to the superior segment of the humerus. The periosteal flap based on the direct periosteal branch of the lateral brachial artery could be transferred downwards to the middle-inferior junction of the humerus.

Key points in applied anatomy

Firstly, besides the anteromedial bare segment of the humerus, the periosteum donor could include the periosteum covered with the brachial muscle and the deltoid. The flap might be 7×3cm in size. Secondly, the lateral descending one should be chosen as the pedicle if the medial descending branch is absent and replaced by the lateral descending branch, which anastomoses with the direct periosteal branch of the lateral brachial artery below the tendinous insertion of the pectoralis major. Thirdly, the direct periosteal branch of the lateral brachial artery often follows a different course, namely, in the muscular substance of the brachial muscle.

Humeral Periosteal Flap Pedicled with the Lateral Descending Branch of Anterior Circumflex Humeral Vessels

10

The lateral descending branch of the anterior circumflex humeral artery has such advantages as a constant course and an easy dissection. Besides, the flap based on it lies in the covered area of the deltoid on the lateral proximal segment of the humerus, where run neither important vessels nor nerves. The flap could be used safely for the treatment of the ischemic necrosis of the humeral head, the bone non-union or small defect in surgical neck of the humerus.

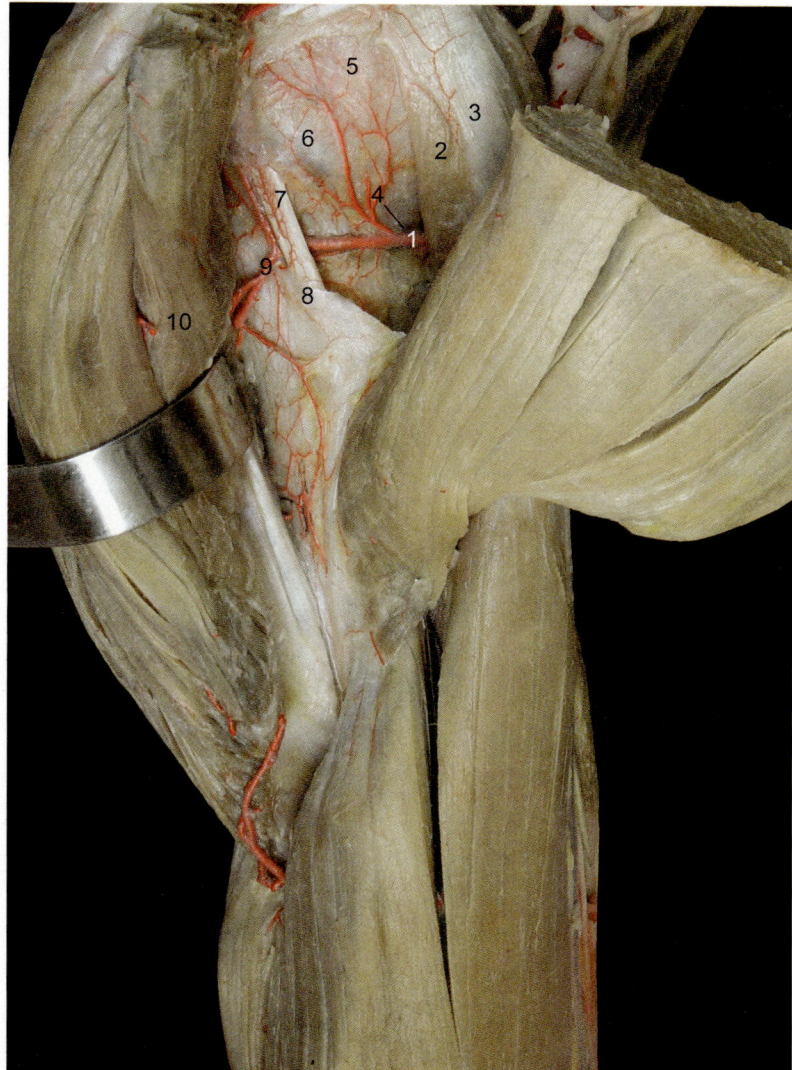

1. Anterior circumflex humeral artery
2. Coracobrachial muscle
3. Short head of biceps brachii muscle
4. Surgical neck of humerus
5. Head of humerus
6. Lesser tubercle
7. Long head of biceps brachii tendon
8. Pectoral major muscle
9. Lateral descending branch
10. Anterior portion of deltoid

| Figure 3-54 | Applied anatomy |

The anterior circumflex humeral artery emerges from the axillary artery and extends along the deep layers of the coracobrachial muscle and the short head of the biceps brachii muscle. It turns outwards around the surgical neck of the humerus and sends branches into the humeral head and the lesser tubercle. The trunk passes through the deep layer of the long head of the biceps brachii tendon and bifurcates into the ascending and the descending branches at the insertion of the pectoral major muscle. The descending branch further divides into the medial and the lateral ones to descend medially and laterally. The lateral one descends along the pectoral major muscle to disperse over the anterior deltoid covered area on the lateral proximal humerus. The distance between its origin and the vertex of the greater tuberosity of the humerus is 4.1cm, the diameter of the caliber at its origin 1.2mm and the length of pedicle 6.0cm.

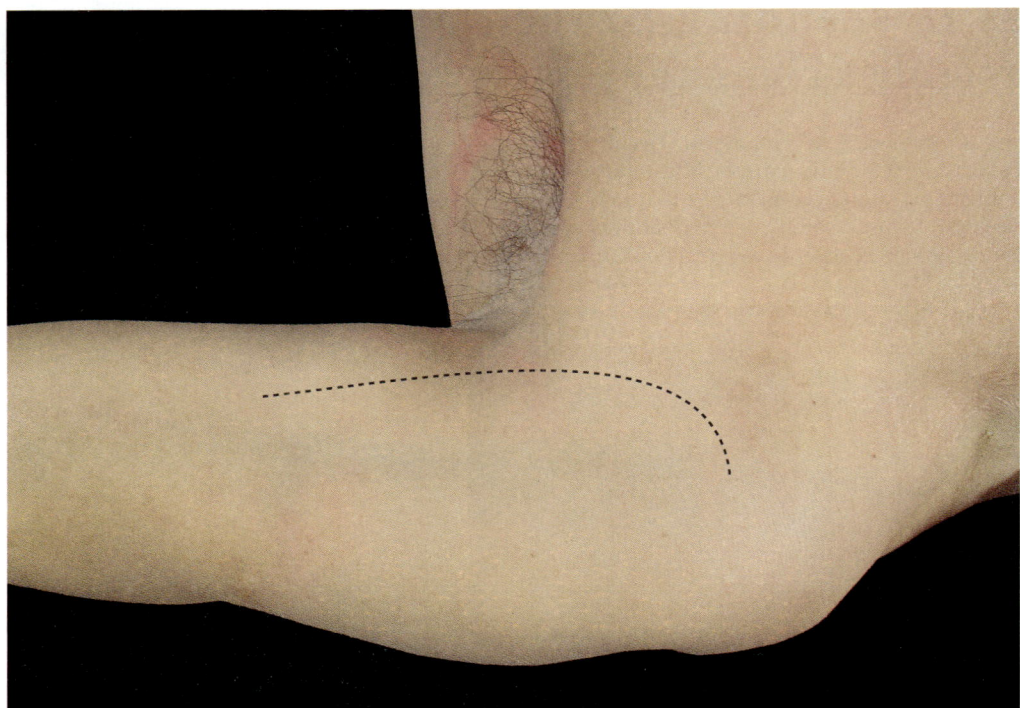

Figure 3-55   Design of the incision

The patient is placed in supine position with a flat pillow padded under the posterior shoulder and the upper limb on the chest. A "7" shape-like incision should be made at the anterior shoulder.

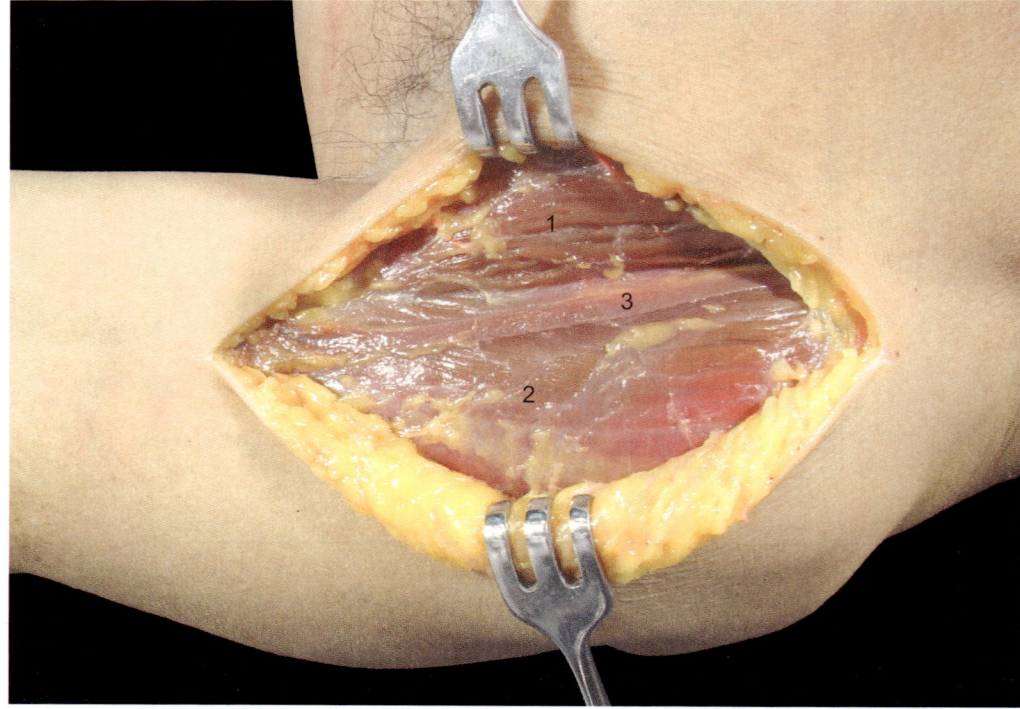

1. Pectoralis major
2. Deltoid muscle
3. Cephalic vein

Figure 3-56   Exposure of the cephalic vein

The skin and the subcutaneous tissues should be incised open to expose the cephalic vein in the intermuscular groove between the deltoid and the pectoralis major.

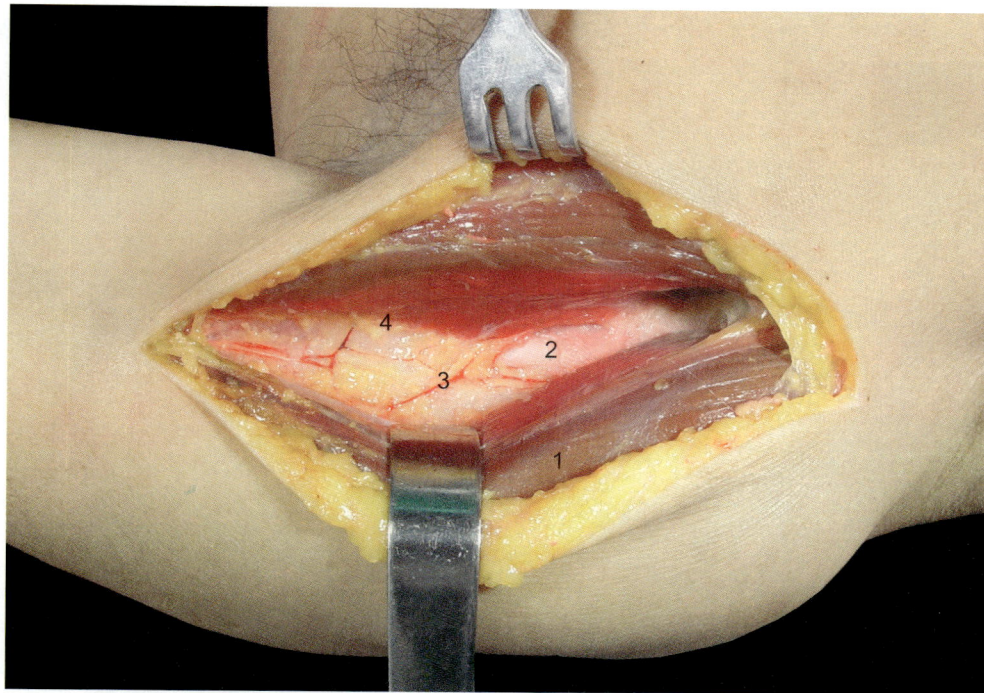

1. Anterior portion of deltoid
2. Long head of biceps brachii tendon
3. Lateral descending branch
4. Insertion of pectoralis major tendon

Figure 3-57   Exposure of the vessels

The anterior portion of the deltoid should be pulled outwards to search along the lateral of the tendon for the anterior circumflex humeral artery that perforates through the long head of the biceps brachii tendon and its lateral descending branch.

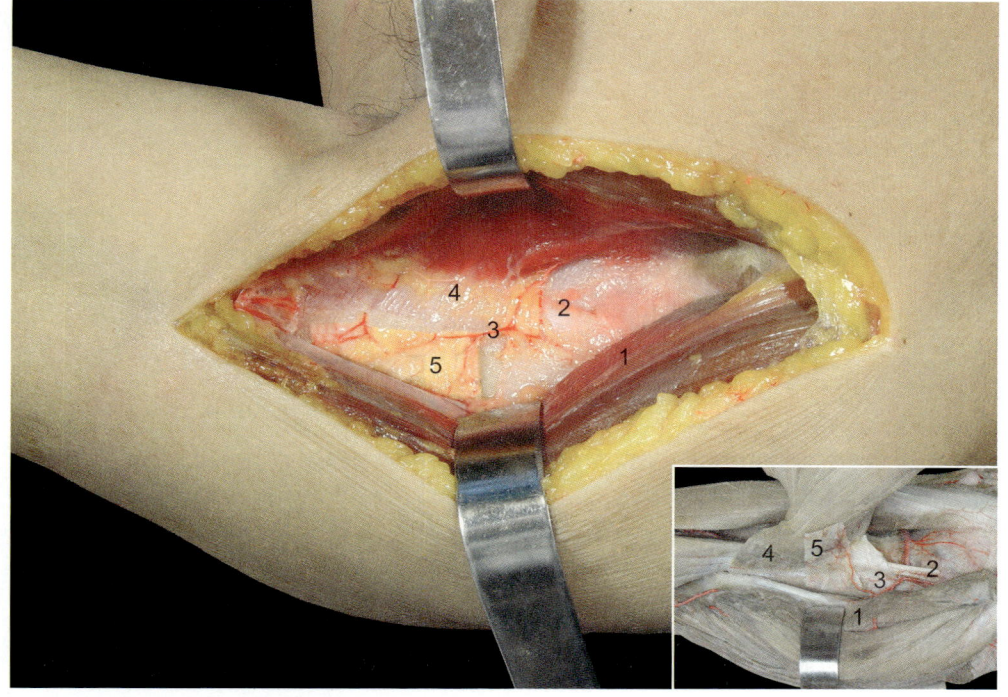

1. Anterior portion of deltoid
2. Long head of biceps brachii tendon
3. Lateral descending branch
4. Insertion of pectoralis major tendon
5. Periosteal flap

Figure 3-58   Dissection of periosteal (bone) flap

A stripe-like periosteal flap could be stripped along the vascular distribution as has been designed.

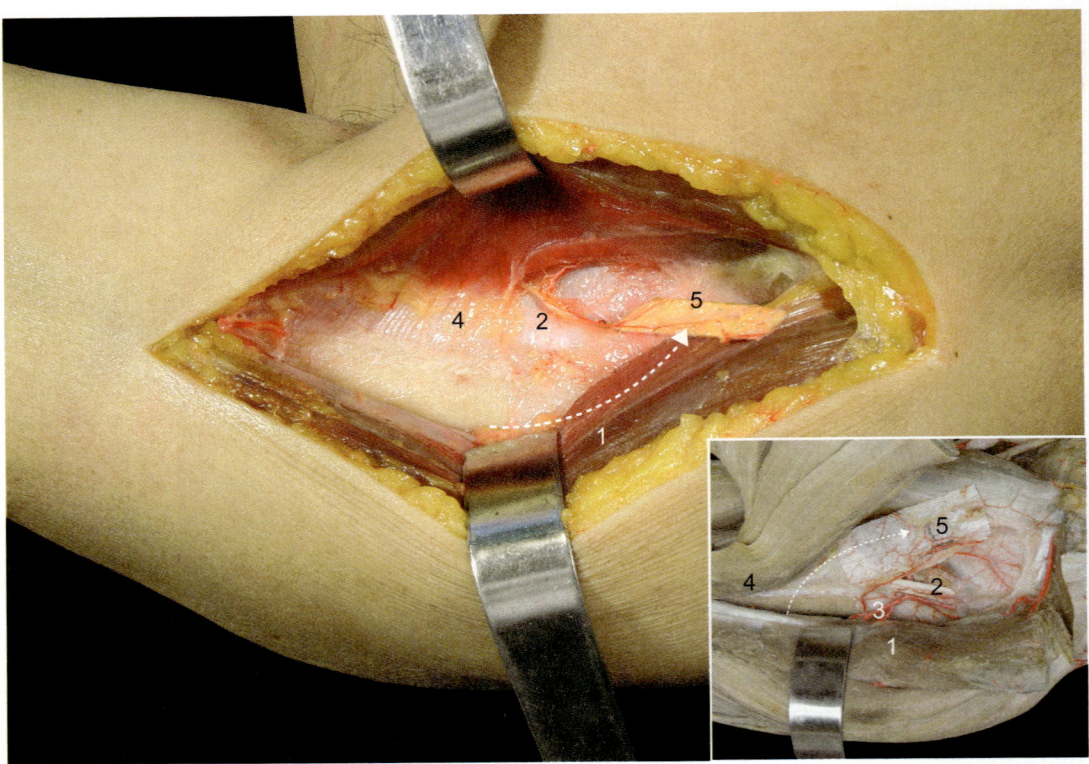

| Figure 3-59 | Transposition of the flap |

A periosteal flap based on the lateral descending branch of the anterior circumflex humeral artery might be transferred upwards for the treatment of the ischemic necrosis of the humeral head and the bone non-union in the proximal humerus.

1. Anterior portion of deltoid
2. Long head of biceps brachii tendon
3. Lateral descending branch
4. Insertion of pectoralis major tendon
5. Periosteal flap

Key points in applied anatomy

Firstly, if the defect on the proximal humerus is too large to be covered with a flap of this type, a double-lobe periosteal flap should be designed to solve the problem. Since the medial descending branch of the anterior circumflex humeral artery joins the vascular net on the anteromedial region of the middle segment of the humerus, the incision should be extended along the lateral margin of the biceps brachii muscle. Then the septum between the biceps brachii and the brachial muscle should be separated and the insertion of the pectoralis major tendon cut off to expose the medial descending branch. A double-lobe periosteal flap might be chiseled along the vascular distribution. Secondly, enough muscular sleeve should be kept on the surface of the periosteum to avoid getting the pedicle damaged when the flap is being stripped or the vessels separated.

Humeral Periosteal Flap Pedicled with Posterior Circumflex Humeral Vessels

11

The posterolateral region of the greater tuberosity of the humerus obtains its blood supply from the greater tuberal osseous branch of the posterior circumflex humeral artery. An osteal flap based on the artery has such advantages as a sufficient blood supply, an easy dissection and a constant vascular course. A flap based on it could be transferred to repair the ischemic necrosis of the humeral head.

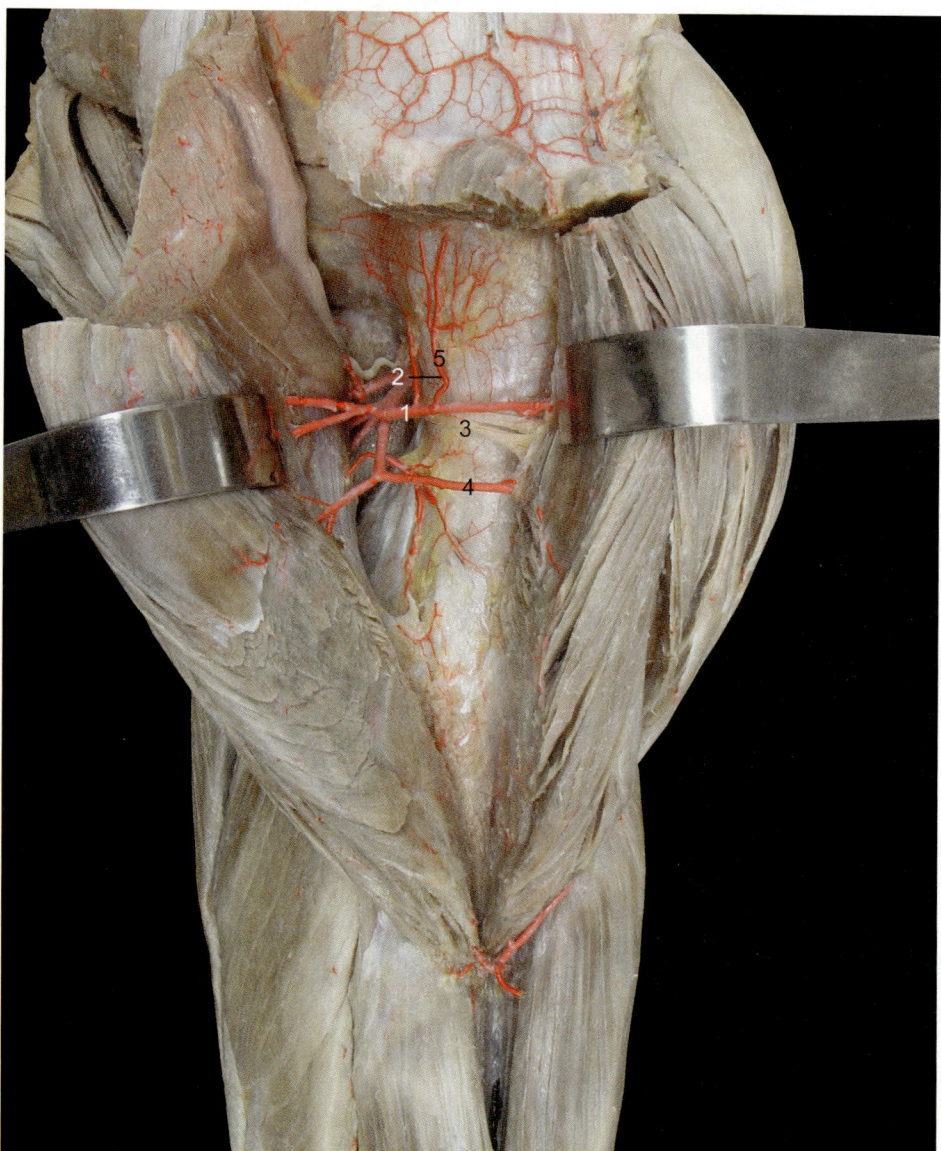

1. Posterior circumflex humeral artery
2. Surgical neck of humerus
3. Axillary nerve
4. Deltoid muscular branch
5. Greater tuberal osseous branch

| Figure 3-60 | Applied anatomy |

The posterior circumflex humeral artery emerges from the axillary artery, attaching tightly to the surgical neck of the humerus. The artery, with the axillary nerve, perforates through the quadralateral space to the deep layer of the deltoid at 5.6cm below the top of the greater tubercle, where it sends the deltoid muscular branch and the greater tuberal osseous branch. The trunk of the vessel continues anteriorly to anastomose with the anterior circumflex humeral artery. Along its course to the top of the greater tubercle, the greater tuberal osseous branch gives 2-5 periosteal branches to fan out over the posterolateral region of the greater tubercle. At its initiation, the artery is 1.2mm in diameter (on average) and the flap about 5.0×3.0cm in size. The trunk of the posterior circumflex humeral artery is 8.2cm in length and 2.4mm in diameter (on average).

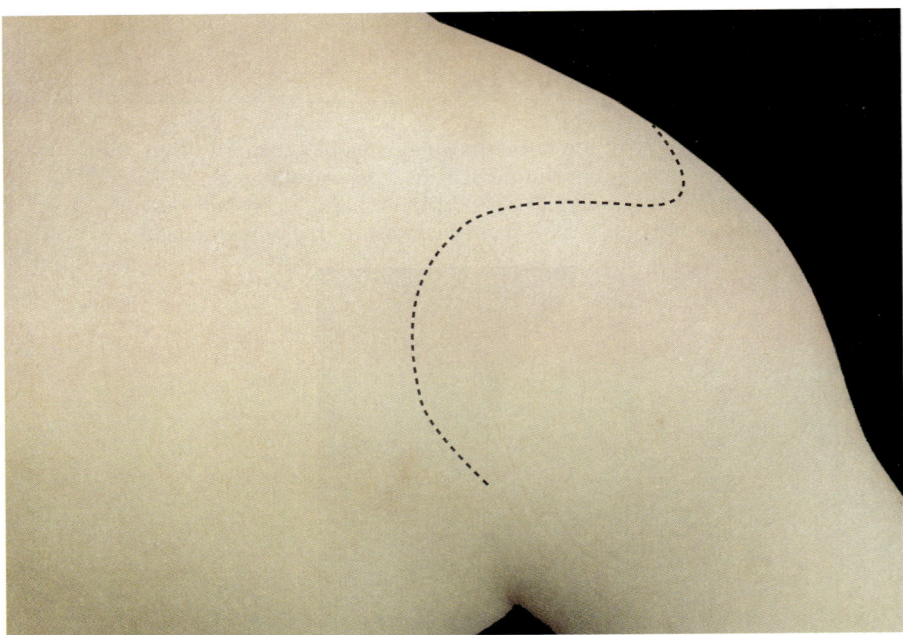

Figure 3-61   Design of the incision

A posterior shoulder incision is to be designed. The incision should begin with the acromioclavicular joint and trace across the acromion onto the scapular spine. It should then turn laterally downwards to 4.0cm above the posterior axillary fold.

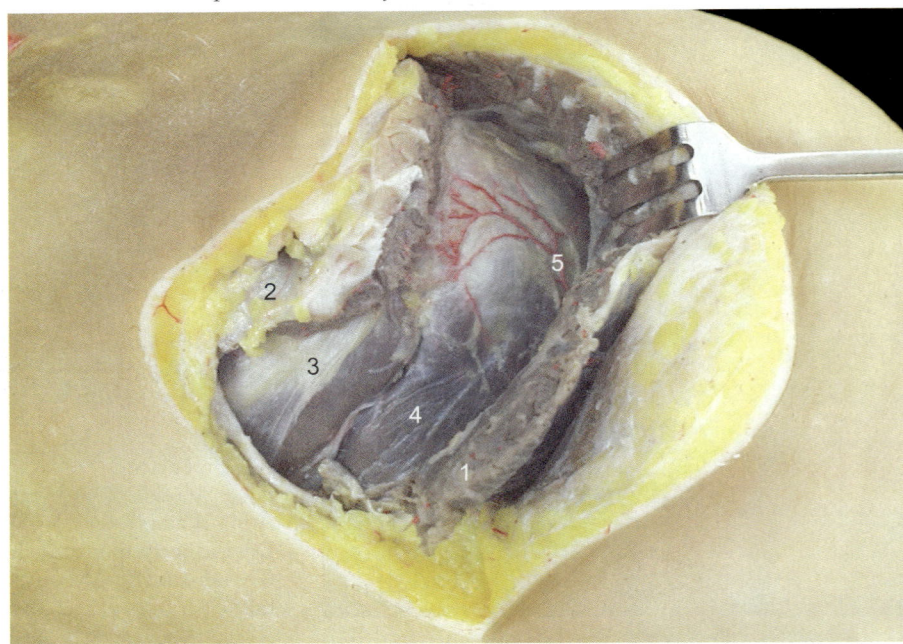

1. Posterior border of deltoid
2. Supraspinous muscle
3. Infraspinous muscle
4. Teres minor
5. Greater tuberal osseous
   branch

Figure 3-62   Exposure of the vessels

The skin, the subcutaneous tissues and the deep fascia should be incised open one by one to expose the posterior margin of the deltoid muscle, get it separated forwards and cut off at 1.0cm below its attachment. Then the deltoid should be pulled forwards to the acromioclavicular joint to expose the supraspinous muscle, the infraspinous muscle and the teres minor muscle. At the inferior border of the teres minor muscle (i.e. the exit of quadralateral space) are the posterior circumflex humeral artery and the plexus of axillary nerve. The axillary nerve should be separated from the vessels and the braches of the posterior circumflex humeral artery (muscular and greater tuberal osseous ones) carefully protected.

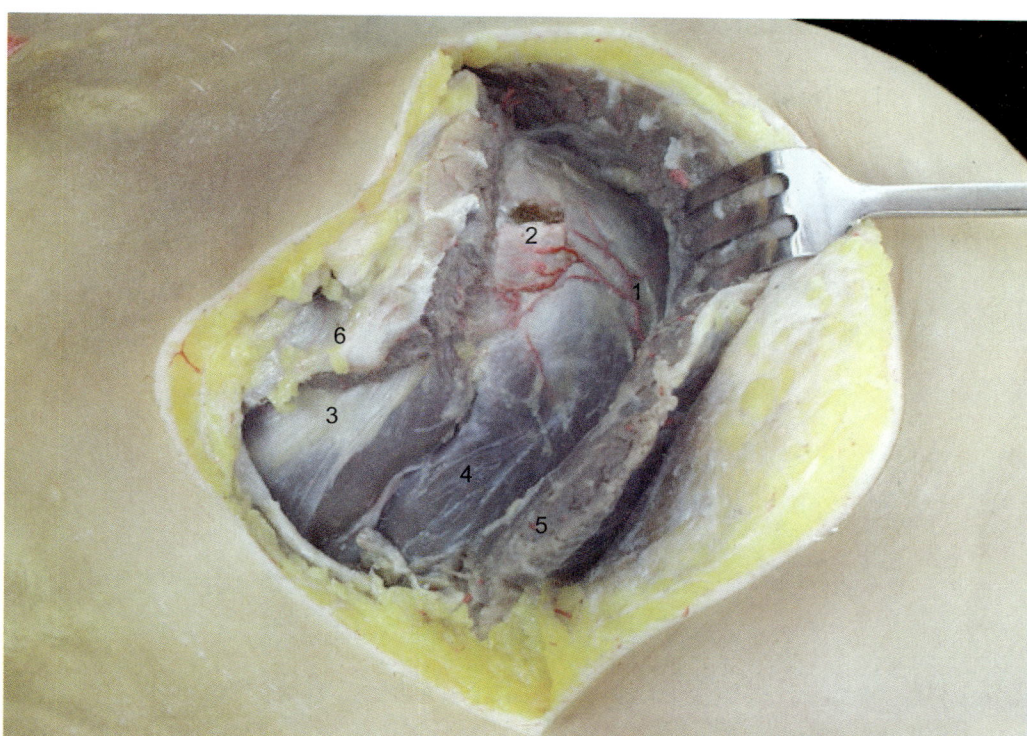

1. Greater tuberal osseous branch
2. Periosteal flap
3. Infraspinous muscle
4. Teres minor
5. Posterior border of deltoid
6. Acromion

Figure 3-63   Dissection of periosteal flap

On the posterolateral region of the greater tubercle, the periosteal flap should be harvested with the greater tuberal osseous branches as its axis. It might be about 5.0×3.0cm in size.

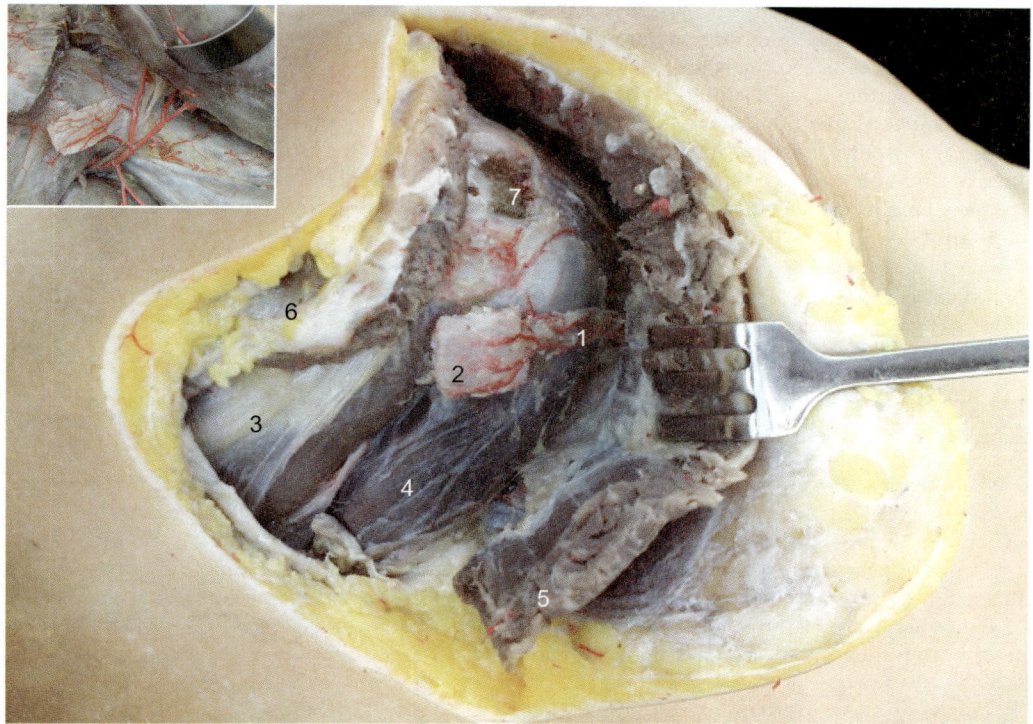

1. Greater tuberal osseous branch
2. Periosteal flap
3. Infraspinous muscle
4. Teres minor
5. Posterior border of deltoid
6. Acromion
7. Donor site

Figure 3-64   Transposition of the flap

The periosteal flap based on the posterior circumflex humeral artery might be transferred to repair a lesion in the humeral head.

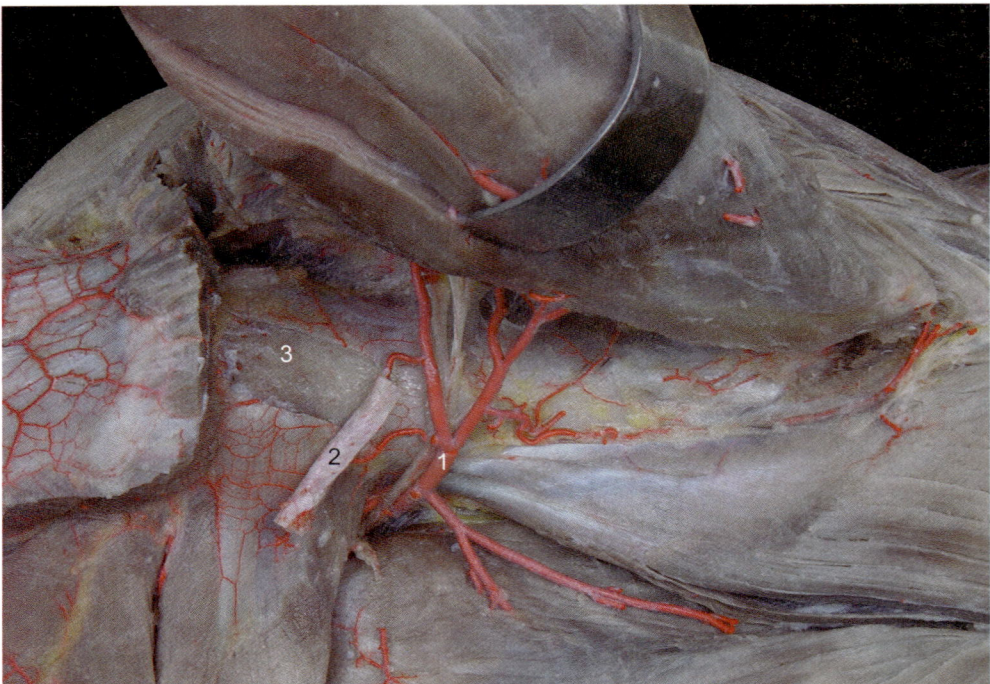

| Figure 3-65 | Implantation of the flap |

The deltoid muscular branches and the distal trunk of the posterior circumflex humeral artery should be carefully ligated. The germinative layer should be turned outwards, rolled up into a short cigarette-like "stick" and fixed with fine sutures. The infraspinous muscle and the teres minor muscle should be cut off closely to their insertion. The articular capsule should be separated longitudinally to expose the posterior region of the humeral head. An osseous cavity (1.5-2.0 cm deep) should be drilled from the middle line of the anatomical neck (equal to the posterosuperior region of the top of the greater tubercle) to the central zone of the humeral head. The granulation tissue and the dead bone in the humeral head should be debrided. If the humeral head is collapsed, it should be restored with a special metal stick to pole the articular surface in the drilled cavity. The cavity should be filled with some of cancellous bones harvested from the greater tubercle. The periosteal "stick" should be implanted into the cavity and its outside border sutured and fixed with the surrounding soft tissues. Finally the articular capsule, the cut infraspinous muscle and the teres minor muscle should be sutured.

1. Posterior circumflex humeral artery
2. Periosteal flap
3. Donor site of periosteal flap

Key points in applied anatomy

Firstly, the posterior circumflex humeral artery perforates through the quadralateral space at 6.2cm (on average) to the acromion to reach the posterolateral region of the humeral head, and so it should be separated bluntly along the posterior border of the deltoid for at most 5.0cm beneath the acromion to avoid damaging the neurovascular bundle. Secondly, the posterior circumflex humeral artery perforates through the quadralateral space closely to the inferior border of the teres minor muscle, and so the muscle should be cut off at its insertion to facilitate a smooth transfer of the vascular pedicle. The vessels should be protected carefully in the procedures. After the flap is transferred, the ends of the teres minor muscle should be sutured properly to avoid getting the pedicle twisted and pressed. Thirdly, if the pedicle is not long enough to be inserted into the humeral cavity, the trunk of the posterior circumflex humeral artery should be chosen as the pedicle. In this case, the distal continuation of the arterial trunk and its deltoid muscular branch should be separated and ligated. If the greater tuberal osseous branch emerges from the deltoid muscular branch, the muscular branch should be cut off and ligated after it gives the osseous branch to guarantee the blood supply in the flap.

Middle Humeral Periosteal Flap
Pedicled with Lateral Brachial Vessels

The middle humeral periosteal flap based on the lateral brachial artery is located in the middle portion of the anterolateral surface of the humerus. It has such advantages as an easy operation, a long vascular pedicle, a large vascular caliber and a constant vascular course. A periosteal flap might be transferred to repair non-union or defect in the inferior 1/3 segment of the humerus. A compound periosteal-cutaneous flap could be harvested to restore a compound tissue defect.

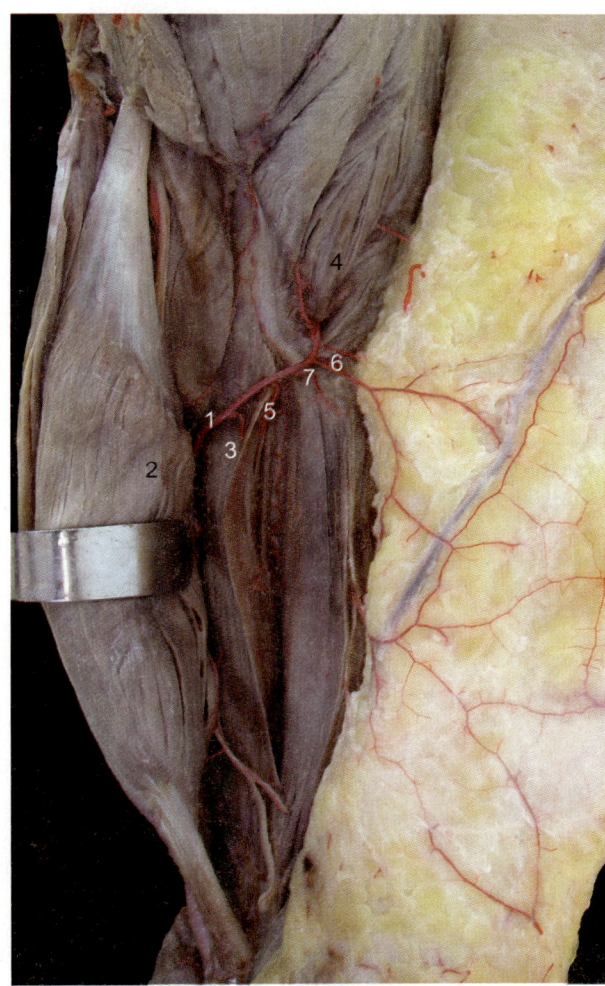

1. Lateral brachial artery
2. Biceps brachii muscle
3. Brachial muscle
4. Deltoid muscle
5. Descending branch
6. Cutaneous branch
7. Direct periosteal branch

| Figure 3-66 | Applied anatomy |

The lateral brachial artery emerges from the brachial artery at 13.6cm above the medial condyle of the humerus. In most cases (86.7%), it runs outwards closely to the bone surface between the biceps brachii muscle and the proximal end of the brachial muscle. In a few cases (13.3%), it runs through the origin of the brachial muscle and in other cases (6.7%) it runs through the insertion of the coracobrachial muscle to the insertion of the deltoid. The artery (1.6mm in diameter) runs for 3.8cm on average before it divides into the ascending branch, the descending branch, the cutaneous branch and the direct osseous branch. The direct osseous branch (0.6mm in diameter) ascends along the deep layer of the deltoid to nourish the adjacent periosteum and anastomose with the branches of the posterior circumflex humeral artery. The ascending branch runs through the insertion of the deltoid to enter the deep layer of the deltoid or into the muscle. Along the course it sends branches to disperse over the inferior portion of the deltoid and the periosteum beneath the muscle. The descending branch runs downwards through the proximal end of the brachial muscle to disperse over the proximal portion of the muscle and the periosteum beneath it.

233

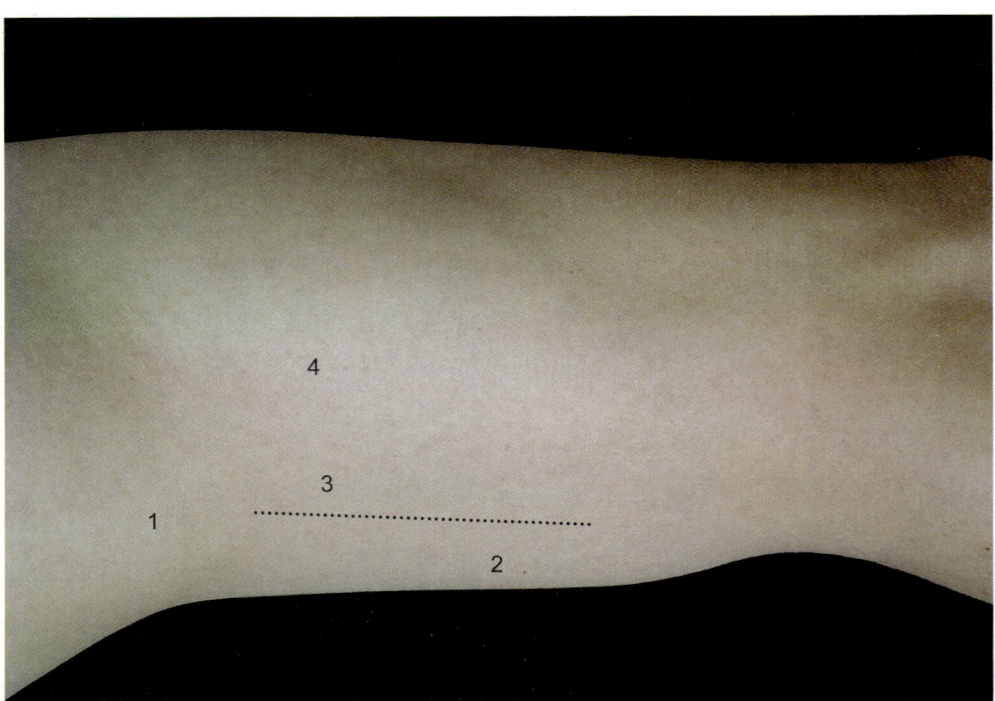

| **Figure 3-67** | Design of the incision |

A longitudinal incision should be made along the anterior border of the deltoid insertion on the superior-middle segment of the lateral arm. The length of the incision depends on the requirement of the recipient site.

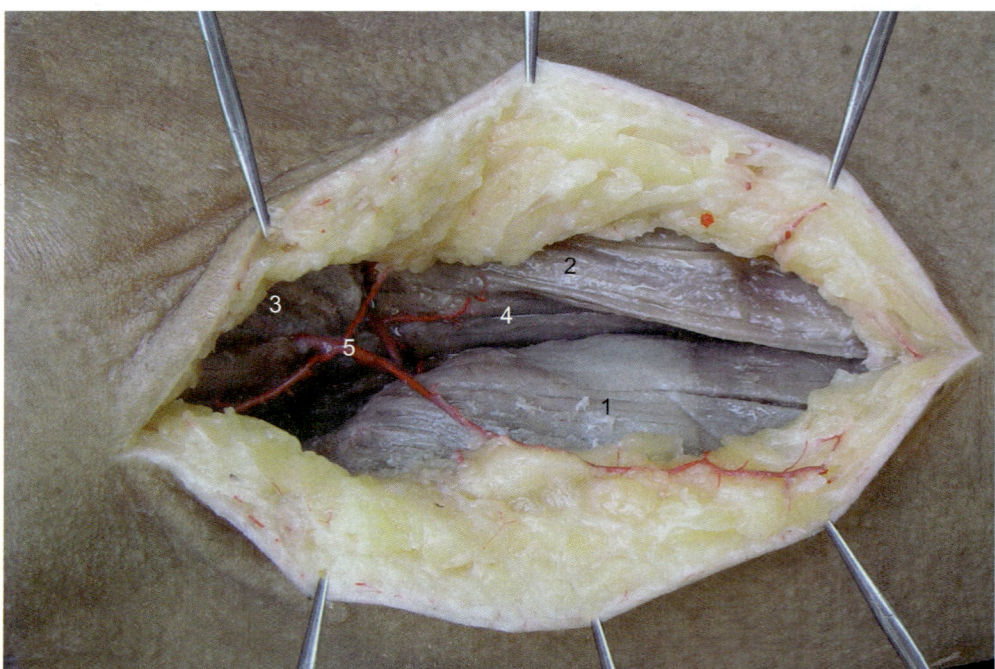

1. Biceps brachii
2. Triceps brachii
3. Deltoid
4. Brachial muscle
5. Lateral brachial artery

| **Figure 3-68** | Exposure of the vessels |

The skin, the subcutaneous tissues and the deep fascial should be incised open and the incision should extend to the lateral intermuscular septum between the biceps brachii and the triceps brachii. The septum should be dissected and the two muscles pulled bilaterally to expose the aimed pedicle located between the insertion of the deltoid and the origin of the brachial muscle.

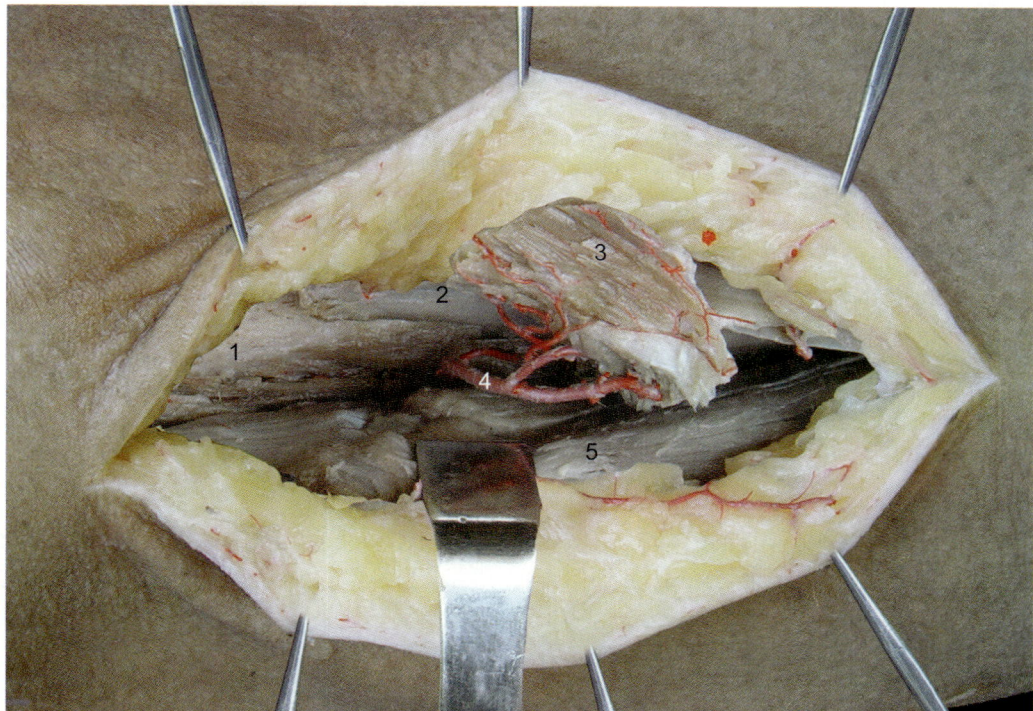

| Figure 3-69 | Dissection of the periosteal (bone) flap |

Part of the muscular attachment, together with the insertion of the deltoid and the origin of the brachial muscle, should be cut off to enlarge the size of the periosteal flap. A proper muscular cuff should be retained on the flap. Then the properly-sized flap could be harvested for free grafting or transposition.

1. Deltoid
2. Brachial muscle
3. Periosteal flap
4. Lateral brachial artery
5. Biceps brachii

Key points in applied anatomy

Firstly, in about 40% cases, the nutrient vessels of the flap run in the septum between the brachial muscle and the coracobrachial muscle, and so enough muscular sleeves should be retained on the surface of the periosteum to guarantee its blood supply when the flap is being harvested. Secondly, the lateral brachial artery extends outwards via the anterior middle segment of the humerus, and sends direct osseous branches or muscular-osseous branches to disperse over the anterolateral surface of the bone. Its terminal branches run superficially out of the lateral intermuscular septum to disperse over the skin on the lateral arm. Based on these nutrient vessels, a compound periosteal-cutaneous flap could be harvested to restore a trauma of the connective tissue. Thirdly, if the flap is to be transferred to the inferior segment of the humerus for the treatment of the bone non-union or the limited bone defect, the flap should be designed in the same direction as the vessel but more closely to the proximal end, because this artery runs from the medioinferior to the laterosuperior in many cases (60%). In this way, the pedicle could be extended long enough to guarantee a smooth transfer of the flap to the inferior segment of the humerus.

13 Inferolateral Humeral Periosteal Flap

The blood supply in the lateral periosteum of the inferior humerus comes from the branches of the radial collateral artery. The radial collateral artery anastomoses with the radial recurrent artery near the lateral epicondyle of the humerus. Based on either of the two arteries, an inferolateral humeral periosteal flap could be transferred to repair the bone non-union or defect on the humerus or on the proximal segment of the radius and the ulna.

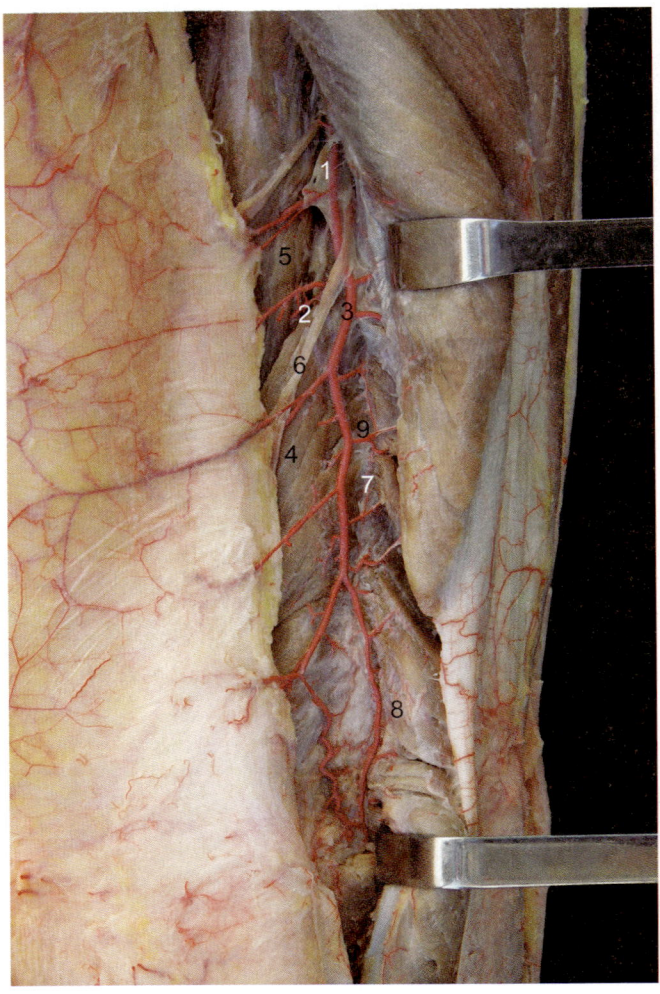

1. Radial collateral artery
2. Volar branch
3. Dorsal branch
4. Brachioradial muscle
5. Brachial muscle
6. Posterior antebrachial cutaneous nerve
7. Lateral epicondylic ridge
8. Lateral epicondyle
9. Musculoperiosteal branch

| Figure 3-70 | Applied anatomy |

The deep brachial artery bifurcates into the middle collateral artery and the radial collateral artery at the proximal end to the groove for the radial nerve and at 12.6cm above the lateral epicondyle of the humerus. The radial collateral artery descends laterally for 3.6 cm, accompanying the radial nerve, and further bifurcates into the volar branch and the dorsal branch above the origin of the brachioradial muscle. The volar branch is small in diameter and goes with the radial nerve through the lateral intermuscular septum into the septum between the brachioradial muscle and the brachial muscle. Along its course, it branches off to innervate the distal segment of the radial nerve and the adjacent muscles. The dorsal branch runs away from the groove for the radial nerve with the posterior antebrachial cutaneous nerve, and descends along the posterior surface of the lateral epicondylic ridge to the lateral intermuscular septum to anastomose with the distal branches of the radial recurrent artery. The dorsal branch covers 9.1cm on average and is 1.2mm in diameter at its origin. Along the course, the radial collateral artery and its dorsal branches send 6.5 (4-13) anteromedial branches and 7.1 (4-11) posteromedial musculoperiosteal branches to nourish the lateral periosteum of the distal humerus.

A. Inferolateral humeral periosteal flap pedicled with radial collateral vessels

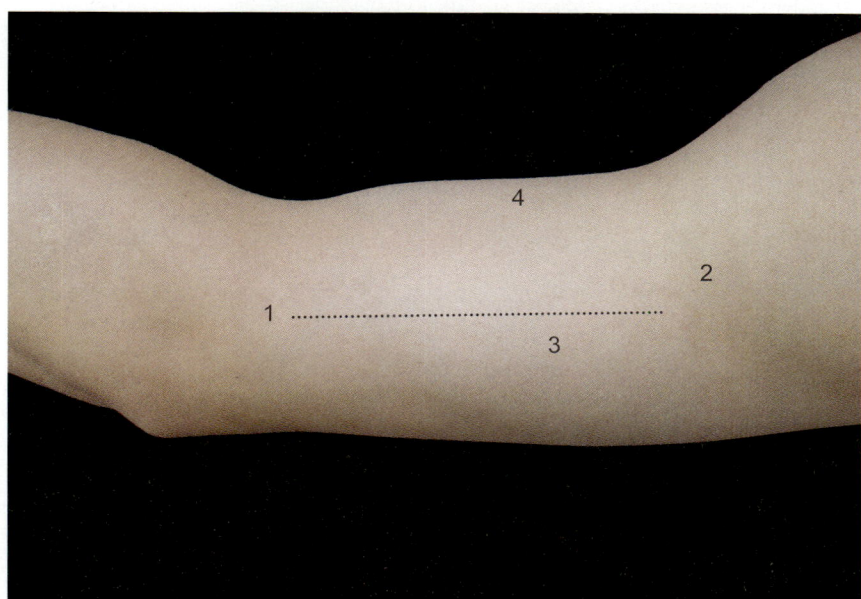

1. Lateral epicondyle
2. Deltoid
3. Triceps brachii
4. Biceps brachii

Figure 3-71   Design of the incision

The incision of the skin should begin with the posterior insertion of the deltoid and extend along the body surface projection line of the lateral intermuscular septum to the lateral epicondyle. The length of incision could be adjusted to the requirement of the recipient area.

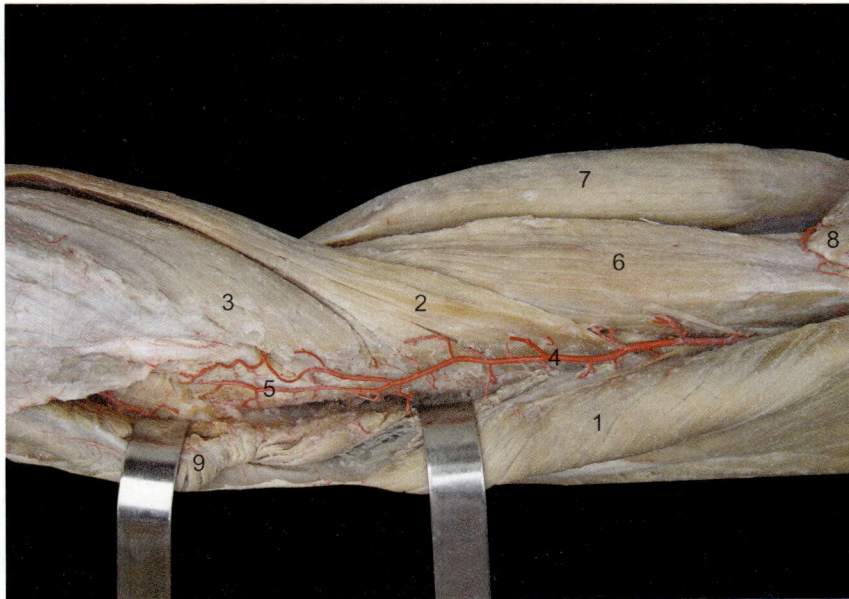

1. Triceps brachii
2. Brachioradial muscle
3. Extensor carpi radialis longus
4. Radial collateral artery
   (dorsal branch)
5. Periosteal branch
6. Brachial muscle
7. Biceps brachii
8. Deltoid
9. Anconeus

Figure 3-72   Exposure of the vessels

The skin, the subcutaneous tissues and the deep fascia should be incised open one by one to expose the lateral intermuscular septum. Along the posterior margin of the septum, the triceps brachii muscle should be separated bluntly and pulled backwards, and the proximal portion of the brachioradial muscle and the extensor carpi radialis muscle pulled forward to expose the radial collateral artery and its branches.

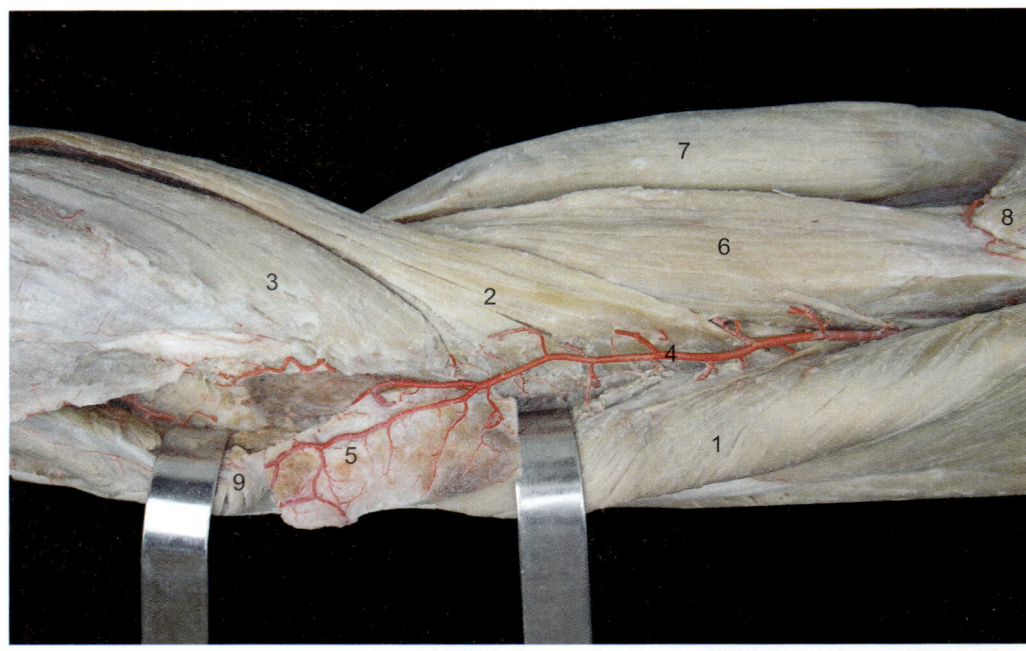

	1. Triceps brachii
	2. Brachioradial muscle
	3. Extensor carpi radialis longus
	4. Radial collateral artery (dorsal branch)
	5. Periosteal branch
	6. Brachial muscle
	7. Biceps brachii
	8. Deltoid
	9. Anconeus

Figure 3-73　　Dissection of the periosteal (bone) flap

A periosteal flap with a vascular pedicle could be harvested with a size about (7-8) ×(4-5) cm on the lateral distal 1/3 segment of the humerus. The flap might include part of the lateral epicondylic ridge if an osseous block is needed.

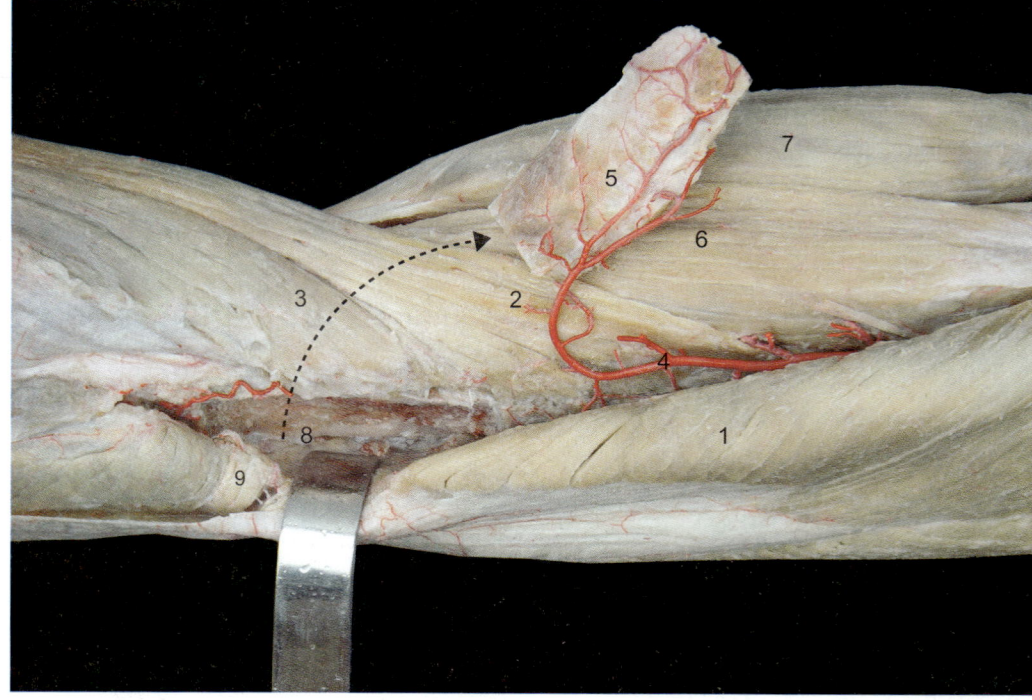

	1. Triceps brachii
	2. Brachioradial muscle
	3. Extensor carpi radialis longus
	4. Radial collateral artery (dorsal branch)
	5. Periosteal branch
	6. Brachial muscle
	7. Biceps brachii
	8. Donor site
	9. Anconeus

Figure 3-74　　Transposition of the flap

Then the bone flap should be transferred to the fracture or non-union region of the humerus. It should cover up the lesion area and be fixed with the surrounding soft tissues.

B. Inferolateral humeral periosteal flap pedicled with radial recurrent vessels

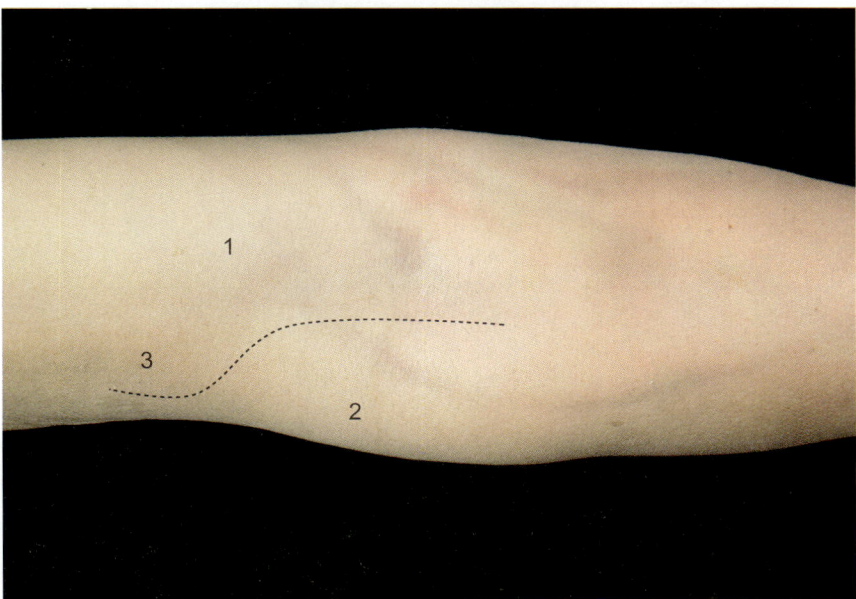

1. Biceps brachii
2. Brachioradial muscle
3. Brachial muscle

Figure 3-75   Design of the incision

An anterolateral approach of the elbow should be taken and the skin incised open from the middle-inferior junction of the lateral arm. The incision should extend downwards across the elbow onto the anterolateral region of the forearm. It might continue distally until it meets the requirement of the recipient site.

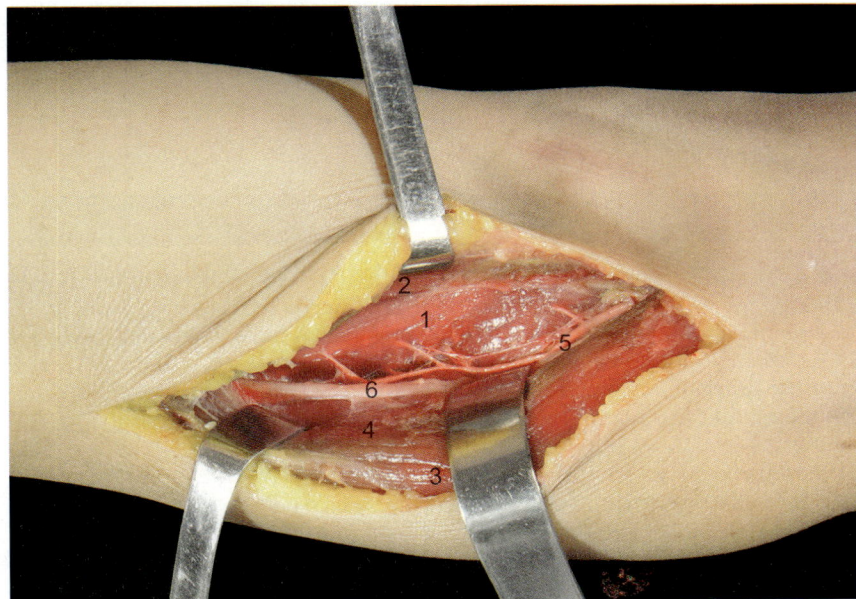

1. Brachial muscle
2. Biceps brachii
3. Brachioradial muscle
4. Extensor carpi radialis muscle
5. Radial recurrent vessels
6. Radial nerve

Figure 3-76   Exposure of the vessels

The skin, the subcutaneous tissues and the deep fascia should be incised open one by one. The brachial muscle, the biceps brachii muscle and the lateral antebrachial cutaneous nerve should be pulled medially and the brachioradial muscle and the extensor carpi radialis muscle pulled laterally to expose the radial recurrent vessels, the distal segment of radial nerve and its superficial or deep branch.

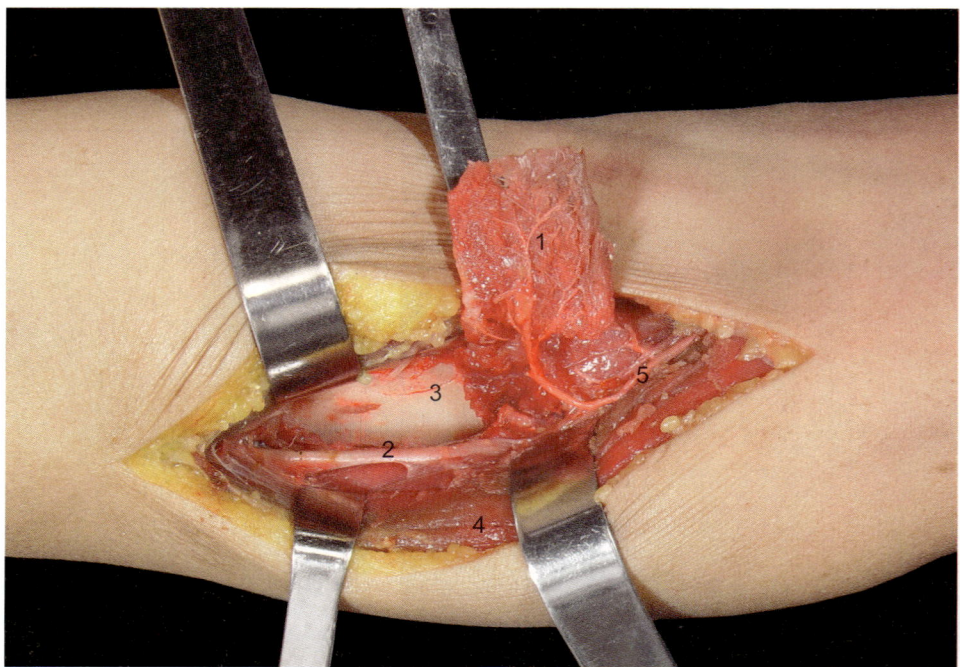

| Figure 3-77 | Dissection of the periosteal flap |

When the muscular attachment on the lateral border of the distal segment of the humerus is being cut off, a layer of muscular cuff should be retained on the surface of the periosteum. Then the periosteal flap should be harvested with a size about 7×4cm and transferred retrogradely to the middle-proximal segment of the radius or the ulna to restore the non-union of the bone.

1. Periosteal flap
2. Radial nerve
3. Humerus
4. Brachioradial muscle
5. Radial recurrent artery

Key points in applied anatomy

Firstly, the deep brachial artery and the radial collateral artery attach tightly to the radial nerve at the middle-distal segment of the humerus, and so the separation of the pedicle or the dissection of the flap should be done carefully to avoid damaging the nerve. Secondly, when the flap is being harvested, a slim layer of the muscle should be retained on the periosteum and part of the lateral intermuscular septum included for the safety of the nutrient vessels in the flap. Thirdly, when the flap is used to restore a non-union or defect on the middle segment of the humerus, it should be transferred to the lesion region beneath the radial nerve. In this way, it could facilitate the bone healing and offer a satisfactory soft tissue bed for the radial nerve as well. Fourthly, along the course from its origin to the distal anastomosis with the radial collateral artery, the radial recurrent artery neighbors on many important structures, especially on the distal segment of the radial nerve and its branches (i.e. the deep and the superficial branches, the brachioradial muscular branches and the extensor carpi radialis muscular branches), and so the vascular pedicle should be dissected very carefully to avoid damaging the radial nerve and its branches. Fifthly, the dorsal branch of the radial collateral artery descends along the lateral epicondylic ridge posterior to the lateral intermuscular septum, and sends periosteal or musculoperiosteal branches to perforate medially through the muscular attachment and disperse over the periosteum. When the muscular attachment is being cut to expose the periosteum, part of the lateral intermuscular septum and a slim layer of the muscle should be retained on the periosteum to protect the dorsal branch of the radial collateral artery and its periosteal branches.

Inferomedial Humeral Periosteal Flap

14

The blood supply in the medial periosteum of the inferior humerus comes from the branches of the inferior ulnar collateral artery, whose descending braches anastomose with the anterior branches of the ulnar recurrent artery around the medial epicondyle of the humerus. Both of the two arteries could serve as the pedicle of the inferomedial humeral periosteal flap that might be transferred locally to repair the bone non-union or defect on the humerus or on the proximal segment of the radius and the ulna.

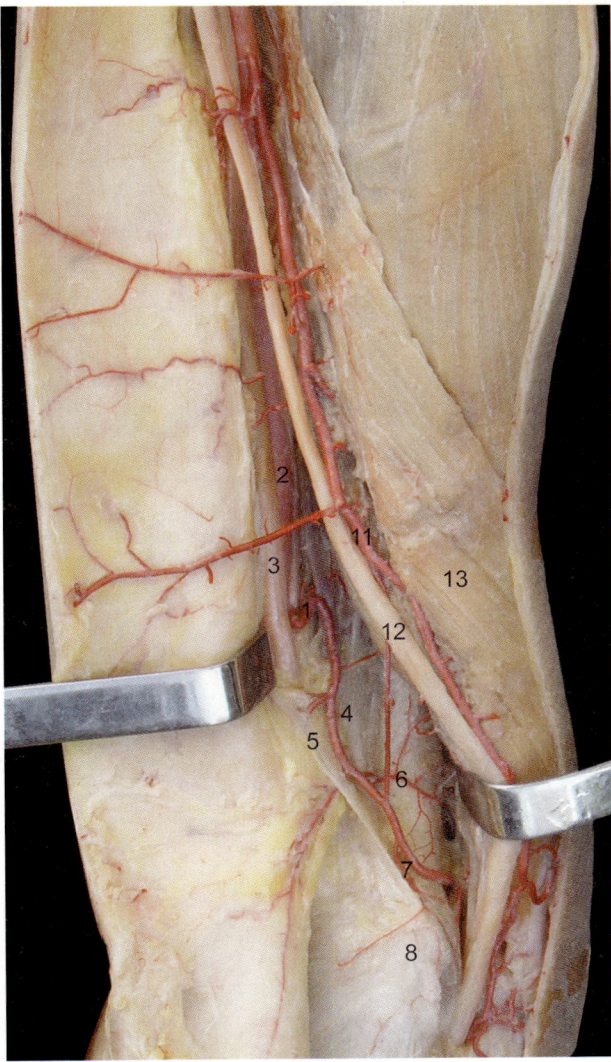

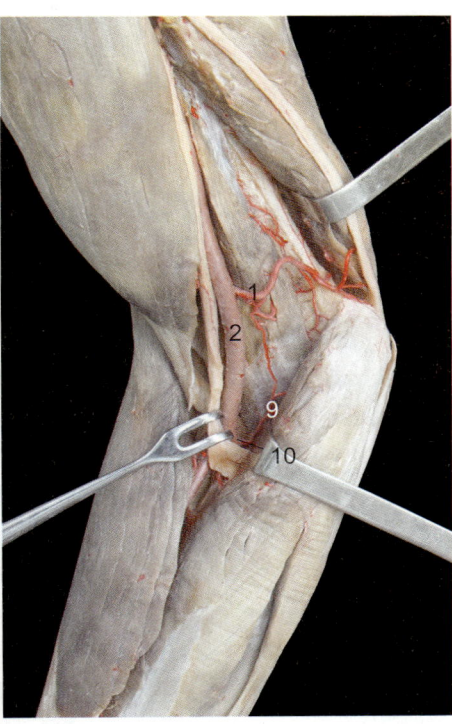

Figure 3-78	Applied anatomy

There are 1 to 2 inferior ulnar collateral arteries that emerge from the medial brachial artery at about 3.3cm above the connecting line between the medial and the lateral epicondyles of the humerus. The inferior ulnar collateral artery descends through the deep or the superficial surface of the median nerve and continues along the surface of the biceps brachii muscle to the anterior surface of the medial intermuscular septum. There it divides into the periosteal branch and the descending branch. The periosteal branch disperses over the anterior or the posterior periosteum of the medial distal humerus; the descending branch anastomoses with the anterior branch of the ulnar recurrent artery before the medial epicondyle. The ulnar recurrent artery emerges from the proximal ulnar artery at 5.5cm below the connecting line between the medial and the lateral epicondyles. Its anterior trunk ascends in the space between the humerus and the ulna via the pronator teres muscle to anastomose with the descending branch of the inferior ulnar collateral artery at the medial epicondyle of the humerus.

1. Inferior ulnar collateral artery
4. Biceps brachii
6. Periosteal branches
9. Ulnar recurrent artery
11. Superior ulnar collateral artery

2. Brachial artery
5. Medial intermuscular septum
7. Descending branches
10. Ulnar artery
12. Ulnar nerve

3. Median nerve
8. Medial epicondyle
13. Triceps brachii

A. Inferomedial humeral periosteal flap pedicled with inferior ulnar collateral artery

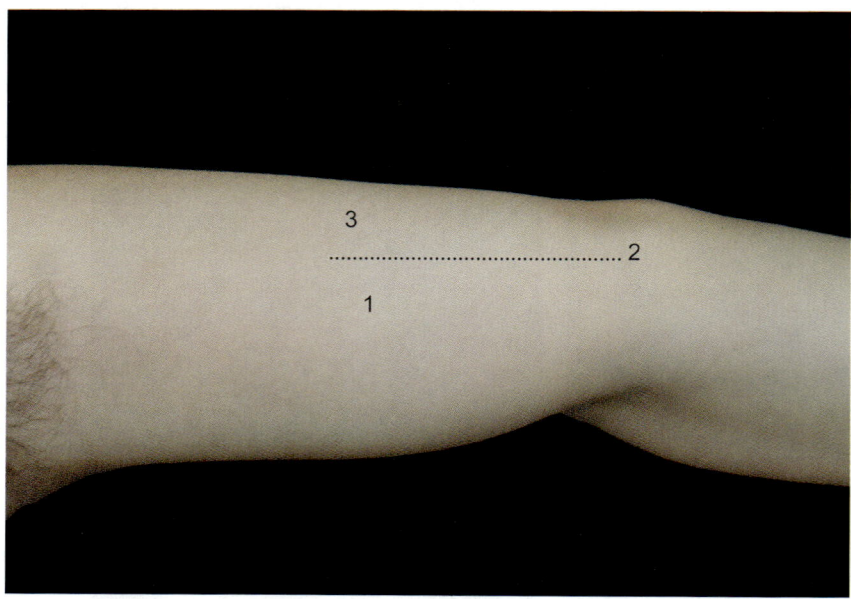

1. Biceps brachii
2. Medial epicondyle
3. Triceps brachii

Figure 3-79   Design of the incision

The patient should be placed in a supine position and a longitudinal incision made in the intermuscular groove posterior to the biceps brachii. Its inferior end might extend to the medial epicondyle and its superior end upwards for about 10cm.

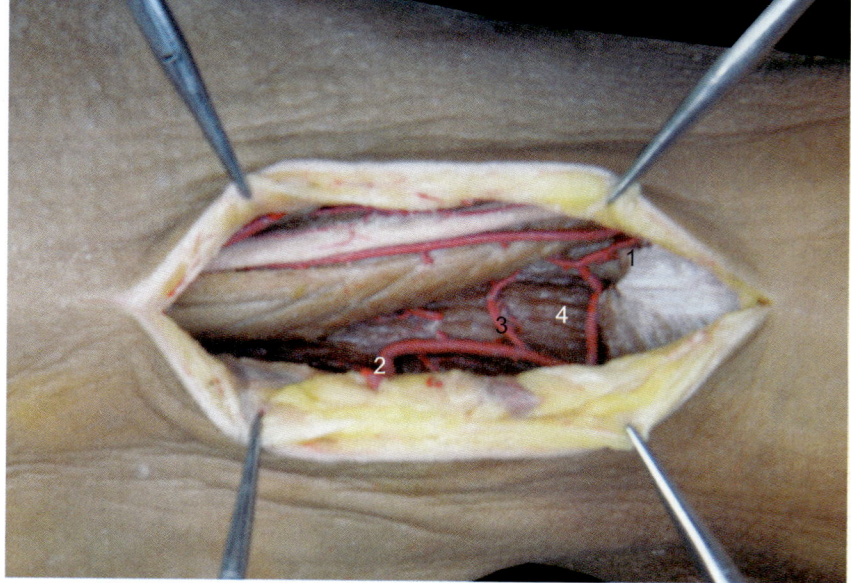

1. Medial epicondyle of humerus
2. Inferior ulnar collateral artery
3. Periosteal branches
4. Brachial muscle

Figure 3-80   Exposure of the vessels

The skin, the subcutaneous tissues and the deep fascia should be incised open and pulled bilaterally to expose the inferior ulnar collateral artery at 4cm above the medial epicondyle. The incision should trace along the periosteal branches into the bone.

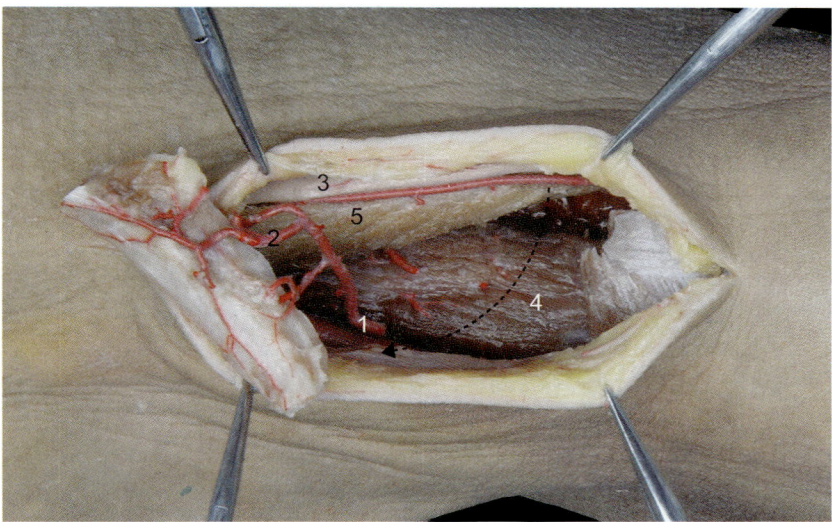

1. Inferior ulnar collateral artery
2. Periosteal branches
3. Ulnar nerve
4. Brachial muscle
5. Triceps brachii

| Figure 3-81 | Dissection of the periosteal flap |

The vascular pedicle should be exposed clearly and protected carefully. The biceps brachii and branchial muscle should be dissected bluntly along the anterior surface of medial intermuscular septum. The two muscles should be pulled outwards and the septum and the triceps brachii inwards to expose completely the inferior segment of humerus and its periosteum. The periosteal flap should be dissected from the medial border of the humerus, to which the septum attaches, to 1cm above the superomedial epichondyle of the humerus. The flap could cover an area of (5-6) ×1.0cm. The adjacent vessels should be cut and ligated before the bone flap is transferred into the recipient site.

B. Inferomedial humeral periosteal flap pedicled with ulnar recurrent artery

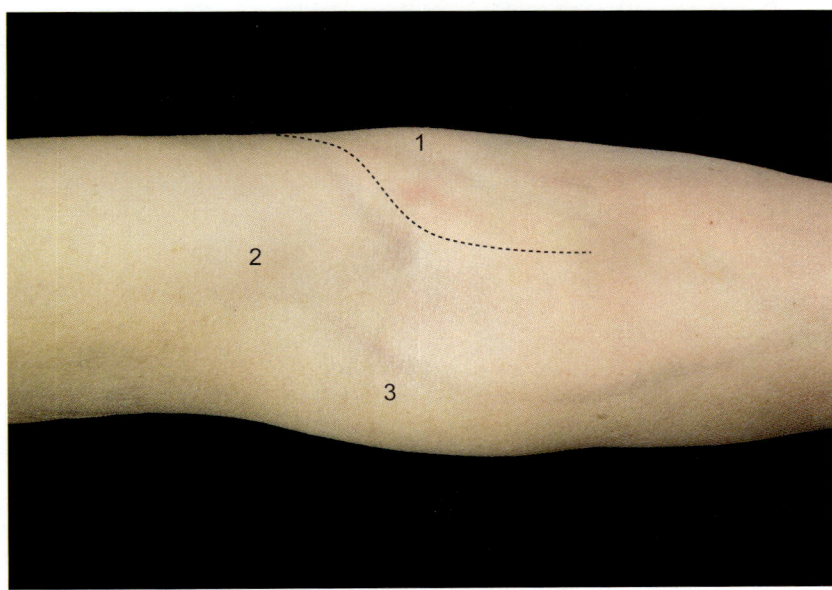

1. Medial epicondyle
2. Biceps brachii
3. Lateral epicondyle

| Figure 3-82 | Design of the incision |

The incision takes a medial approach of the elbow with the medial epicondyle as its anatomic mark. Its length should be adjusted to the location of the recipient site.

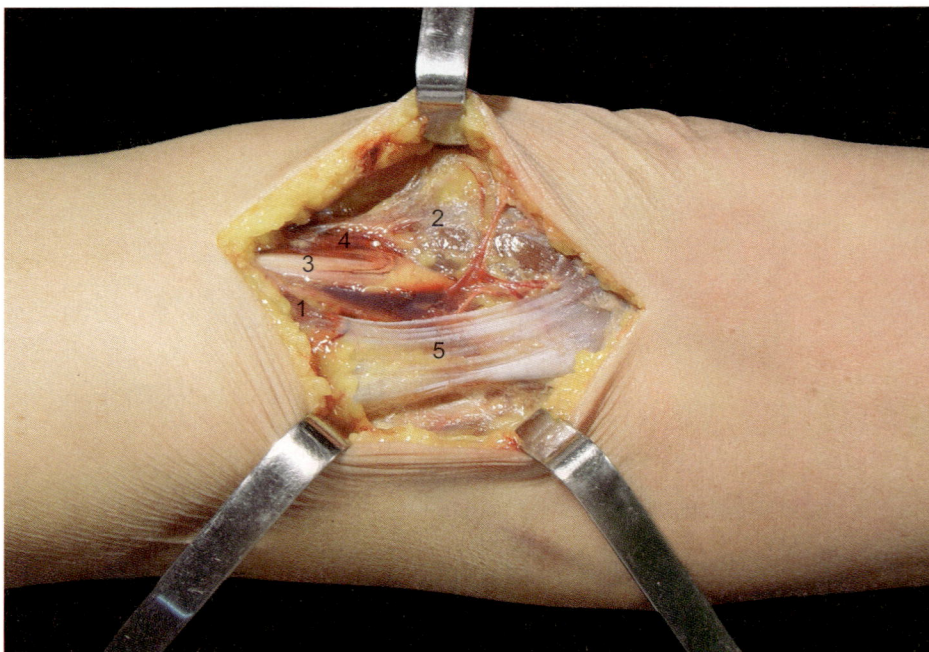

1. Biceps brachii
2. Pronator teres
3. Median nerve
4. Brachial artery
5. Aponeurosis of biceps
   brachii

| Figure 3-83 | Exposure of the incision |

The skin, the subcutaneous tissues and the deep fascia should be incised open to expose the biceps brachii, the pronator teres, the median nerve and the brachial vessels.

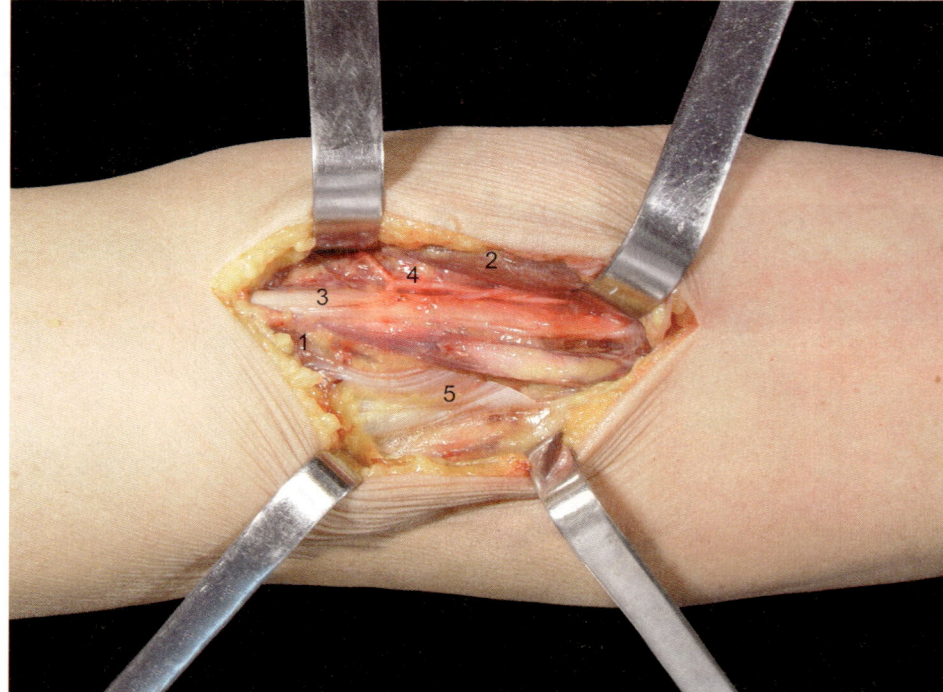

1. Biceps brachii
2. Pronator teres
3. Median nerve
4. Inferior ulnar collateral
   vessels
5. Aponeurosis of biceps
   brachii

| Figure 3-84 | Exposure of the vessels |

The biceps brachii and the brachial muscle should be dissected bluntly along the anterior surface of medial intermuscular septum. The two muscles should be pulled outwards, and the septum and the triceps brachii inwards to search for the inferior ulnar collateral artery at 4cm above the medial epicondyle. The artery might be situated medial to the median nerve and should be traced to its periosteal branches.

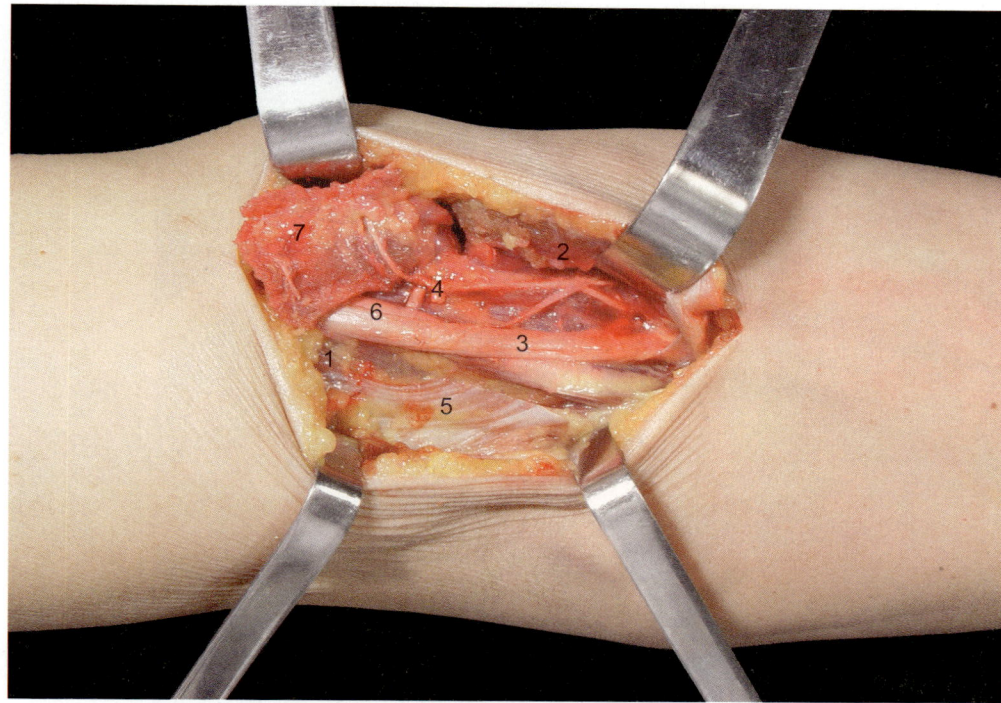

1. Biceps brachii
2. Pronator teres
3. Median nerve
4. Inferior ulnar collateral vessels
5. Aponeurosis of biceps brachii
6. Brachial artery
7. Periosteal flap (with relatively thick muscular sleeve)

| Figure 3-85 | Dissection of the periosteal flap |

The medial intermuscular septum should be cut longitudinally and medially to the vessels. A slim layer of the muscle should be retained on the bone surface. The flap should be dissected upwards from 1cm above the medial epicondyle until it is as large as is needed. The inferior ulnar collateral artery should be cut and ligated to form a retrograde blood flow from the ulnar recurrent artery.

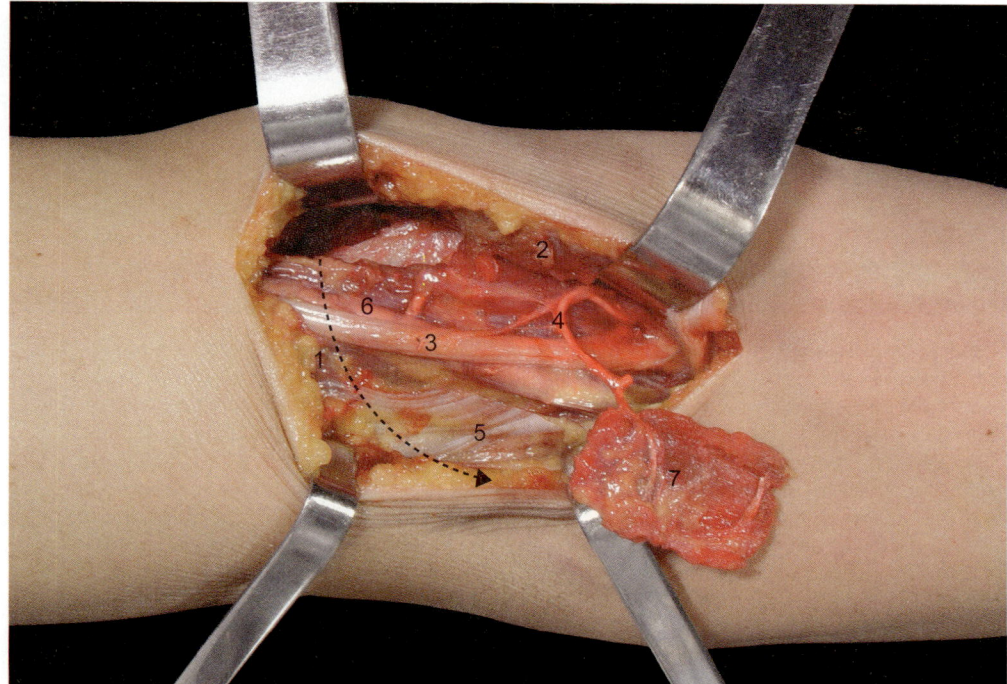

1. Biceps brachii
2. Pronator teres
3. Median nerve
4. Inferior ulnar collateral artery (vessels)
5. Aponeurosis of biceps brachii
6. Brachial artery
7. Periosteal flap

| Figure 3-86 | Transposition of the flap |

The flap should be elevated to separate the pedicle to its base. The dissected flap might be transferred downwards to the proximal-middle segment of the radius or the ulna.

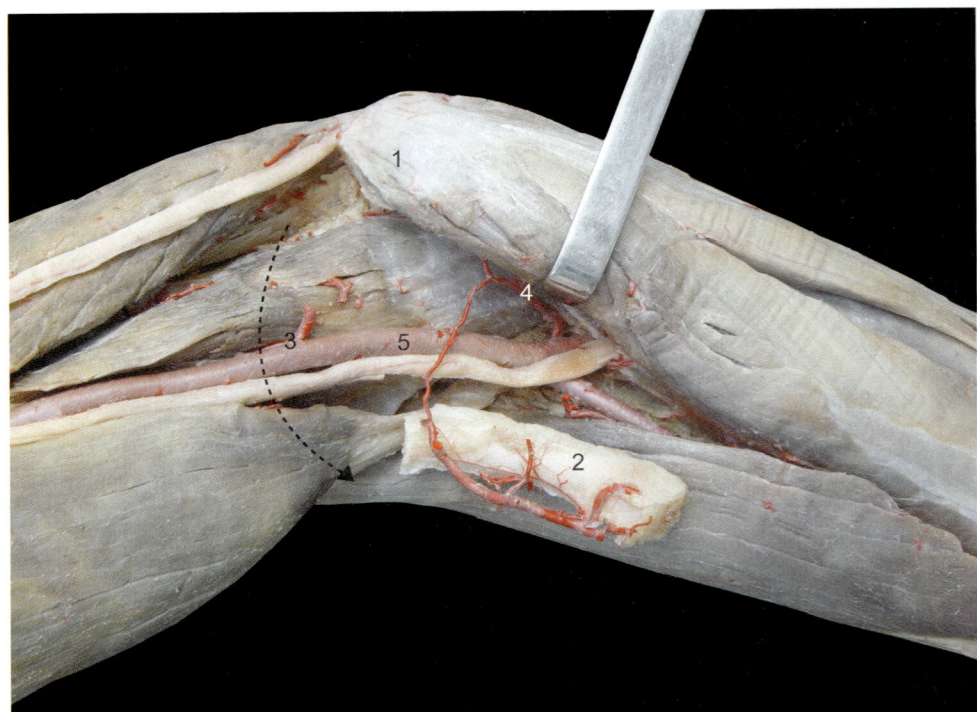

| Figure 3-87 | Dissection of the bone flap |

A bone flap should be designed upwards from 1cm above the medial epicondyle covering a size of 5cm×1cm. The trunk of the inferior ulnar collateral artery should be ligated and cut to make the bone flap pedicled with the ulnar recurrent artery. A flap of this type might be transferred downwards to repair a fracture or bone non-union of the radius or the ulna.

1. Medial epicondyle
2. Bone flap
3. Inferior ulnar collateral artery (vessels)
4. Ulnar recurrent artery (vessels)
5. Brachial artery

Key points in applied anatomy

Firstly, there are many important structures near the anterior and posterior surface of the middle-distal segment of the medial intermuscular septum. At the anterior surface, the inferior ulnar collateral artery runs medially to the median nerve; at the posterior surface, the superior ulnar collateral artery runs laterally to the ulnar nerve. Both of the two should be given great attention when the pedicle is being separated. Secondly, the periosteal branches of the inferior ulnar collateral artery extend through the attachment of the brachial muscle before it disperses over the anterior periosteum of the distal humerus. Likewise, the branches of the superior ulnar collateral artery extend through the attachment of the triceps brachii to the posterior distal humerus. When a flap is being harvested, a slim layer of the muscle should be retained on the periosteum, especially on the anterior humeral region, to protect the vessels in it. Thirdly, the ulnar recurrent artery is situated in the deep layer. Its anterior branch extends through the brachial head and the ulnar head of the pronator teres and along the cubital branches of the median nerve. So the separation of the vascular pedicle should not exceed downwards the cubital level to avoid damaging these nerval branches. Fourthly, the superior ulnar collateral artery runs along closely to the ulnar nerve. The length of the vascular pedicle should be adjusted to the required length. Over-lengthened pedicle would put the ulnar nerve at risk. Fifthly, the inferior border of the periosteal (bone) flap should be located at 1cm above the medial epicondyle without getting the periosteum in the groove of ulnar nerve involved.

Superior Ulnar Flap Pedicled with Posterior Interosseous Vessel

15

The superior ulnar flap pedicled with the recurrent branches of the posterior interosseous vessel has a size with its superior margin extending to the olecranon process of the ulna, its inferior margin to a certain position superior to the initiation of the recurrent branches of the posterior interosseous artery, its lateral margin to the ulnar interosseous crest and its inferior margin traversing the ulnar laterotergal margin to the half ulnar medial side near the laterotergal margin. The donor site has such advantages as a constant vascular anatomical location, a convenient operative exposure and safety. The ulnar flap might be transferred antegradely to repair the osseous nonunion on the middle-superior segment of the ulnar or retrogradely to repair the osseous nonunion on the inferior supracondylar part of the humerus.

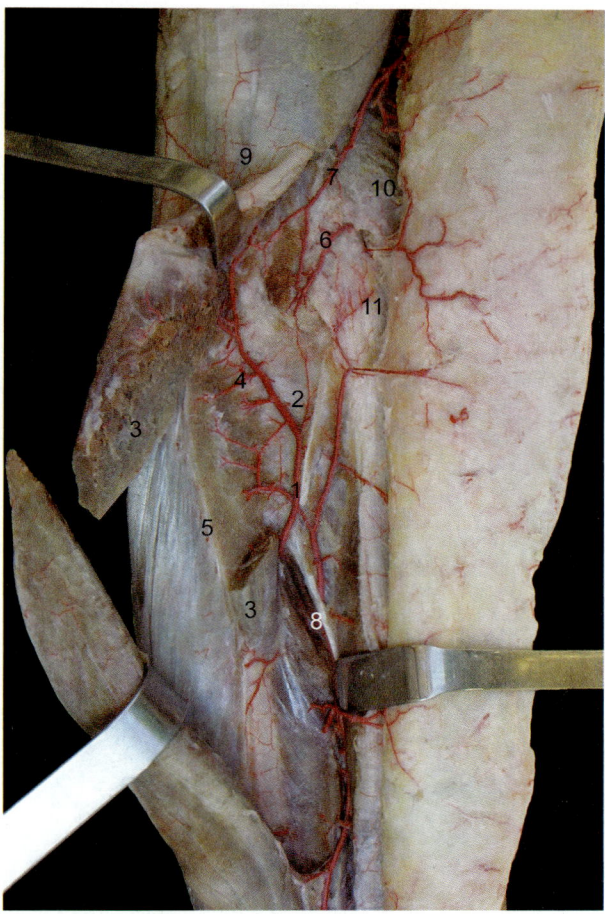 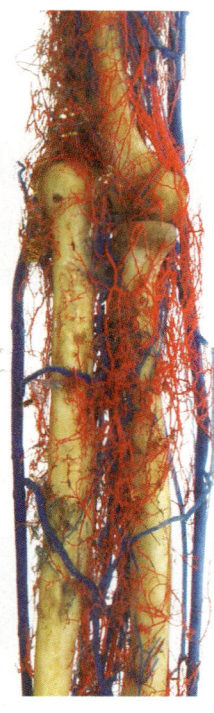

1. Interosseous recurrent artery
2. Supinator muscle
3. Anconeus muscle
4. Periosteal branches
5. Ulnar crest
6. Radial recurrent artery
7. Radial collateral artery
8. Posterior interosseous artery
9. Triceps brachii muscle
10. Extensor carpi radialis longus
11. Extensor carpi radialis brevis

Figure 3-88   Applied anatomy

The posterior interosseous artery enters the lateral forearm through the septum between the superior margin of the interosseous membrane and the oblique cord. It immediately gives the recurrent interosseous artery. It bifurcates at 6.9cm from the most prominent point of the ulnar olecranon process and 1.4cm from the ulnar crest. The recurrent interosseous artery runs upwards along the ulnar interosseous crest and the ulnar dorsolateral side through the septum between the supinator muscular surface and, the anconeus muscular deep surface. Along its course it sends 2-5 periosteal branches (0.5mm in diameter) to fan out over the laterotergal periosteum on the ulnar superior segment. The terminal branches of the recurrent interosseous artery anastomose constantly with the radial recurrent artery, the dorsal branch of radial collateral artery and the middle collateral artery on the posterolateral cubital articulation.

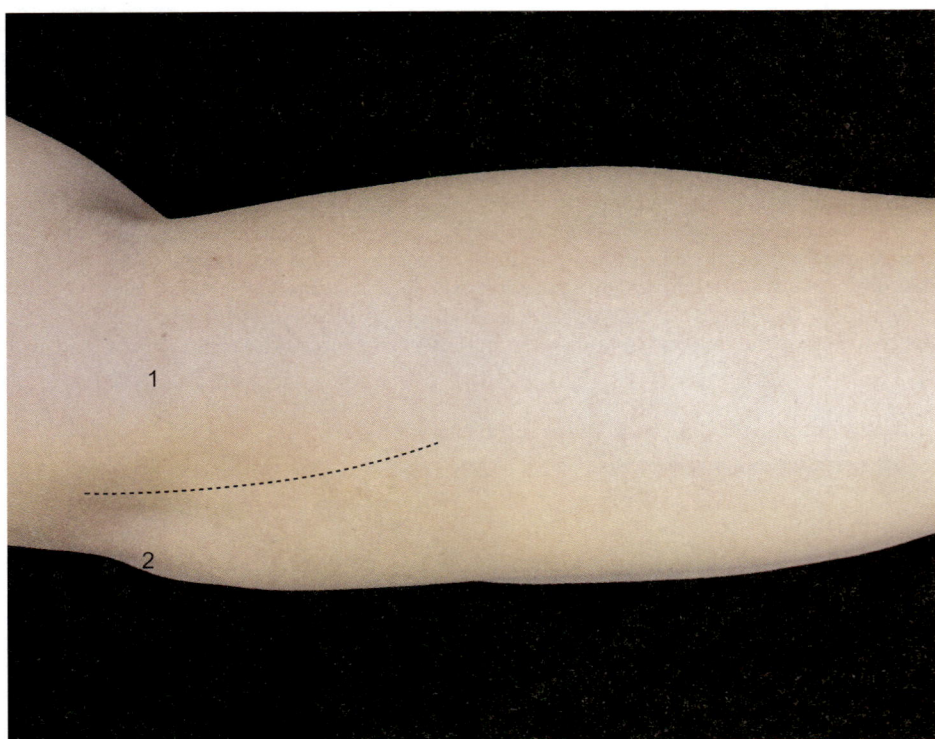

1. Lateral epicondyle
2. Olecranon

Figure 3-89   Design of the incision

The incision should be drawn upwards to the outer margin of the elbow along the ulnar laterotergal margin via the arch that is from the lateral epicondyle to the olecranon process, and drawn downwards to somewhere at 2-3cm from the distal starting point of posterior.

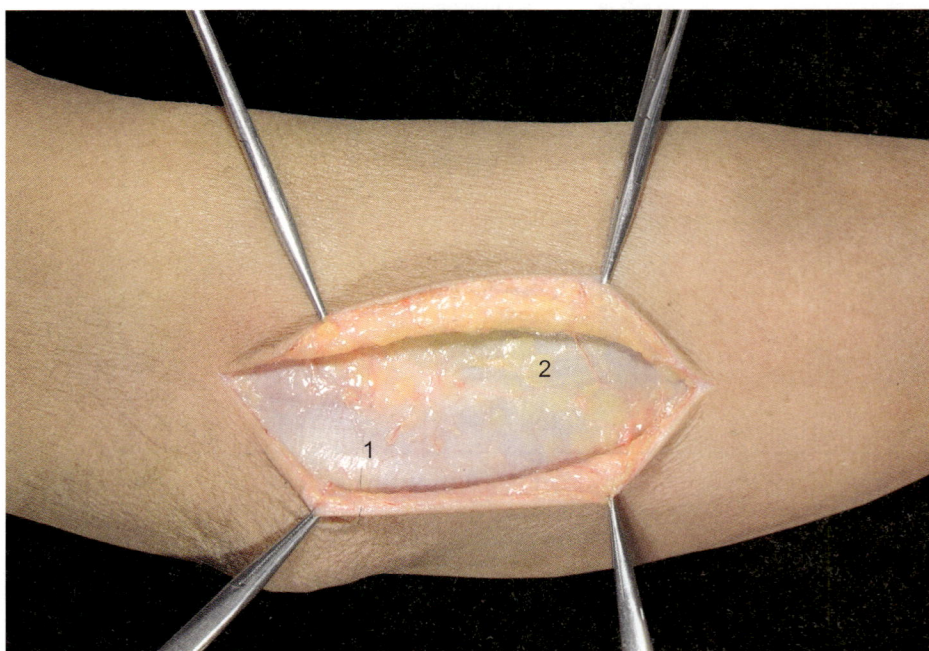

1. Anconeus muscle
2. Extensor digitorum muscle

Figure 3-90   Exposure for the incision

The skin and the subcutaneous tissue should be incised open to expose the anconeus muscle.

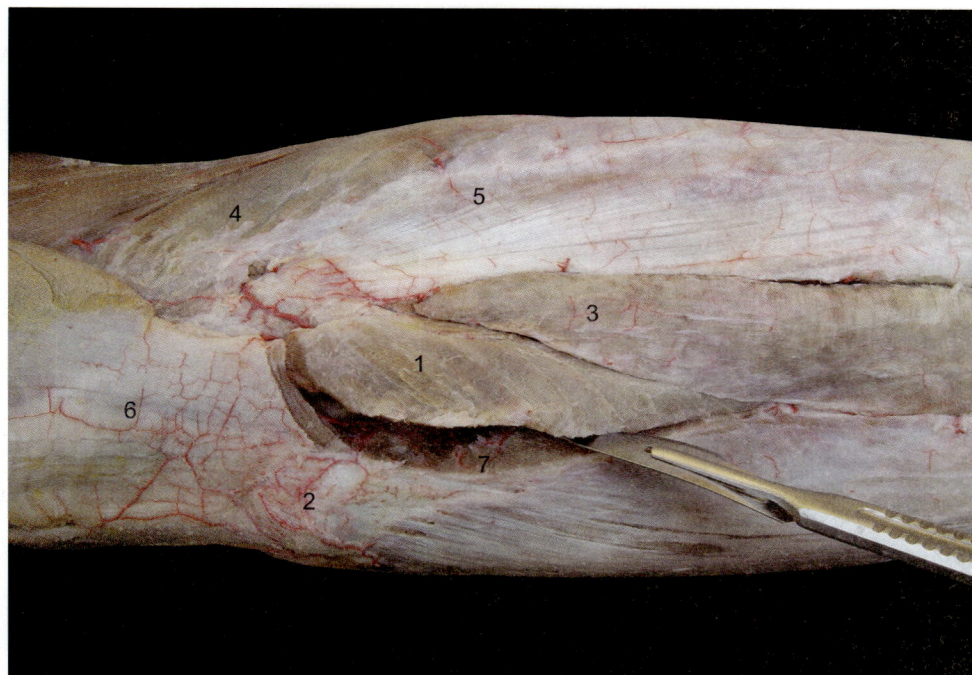

1. Anconeus muscle
2. Olecranon
3. Extensor digitorum muscle
4. Extensor carpi radialis longus
5. Extensor carpi radialis brevis
6. Triceps brachii muscle
7. Ulnar crest

Figure 3-91   Dissection of the anconeus muscle

The anconeus muscle should be dissected on the ulnar dorsum.

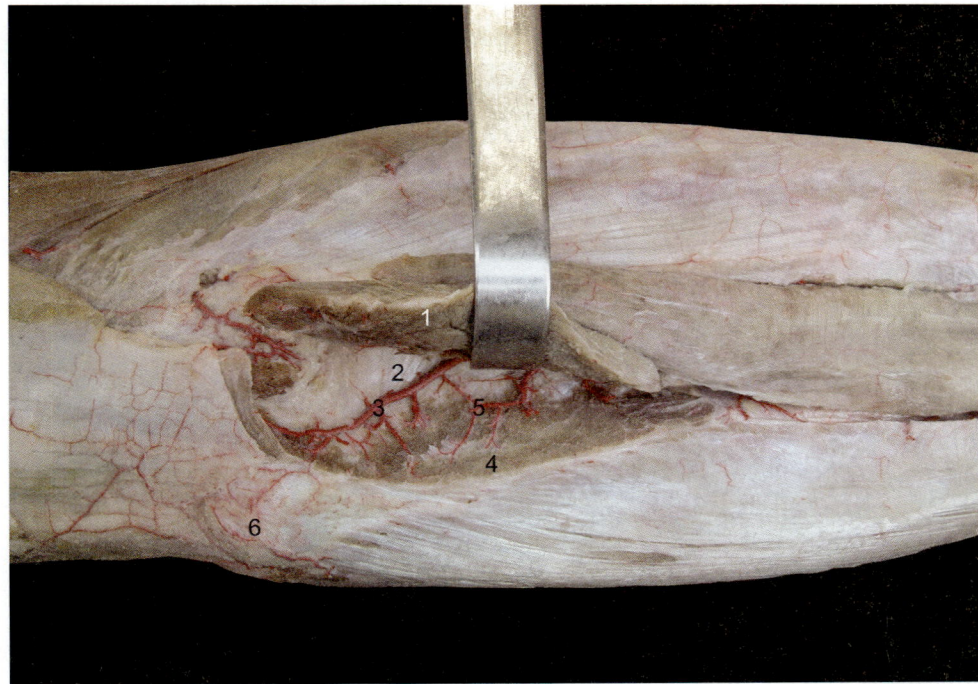

1. Anconeus muscle
2. Supinator muscle
3. Recurrent branch of posterior interosseus vessel
4. Ulnar crest
5. Periosteal branch
6. Olecranon

Figure 3-92   Exposure of the vessels

The anconeus muscle should be drawn radially to retain a lamellar muscular sleeve and to expose the supinator muscle, the posterior interosseus recurrent branch which ascends along the ulnar attaching part, the vascular pedicle and its periosteal branch. The initiation part of the periosteal branch should be dissected carefully to protect the periosteal branch. The supinator muscle might be incised near the ulnar crest.

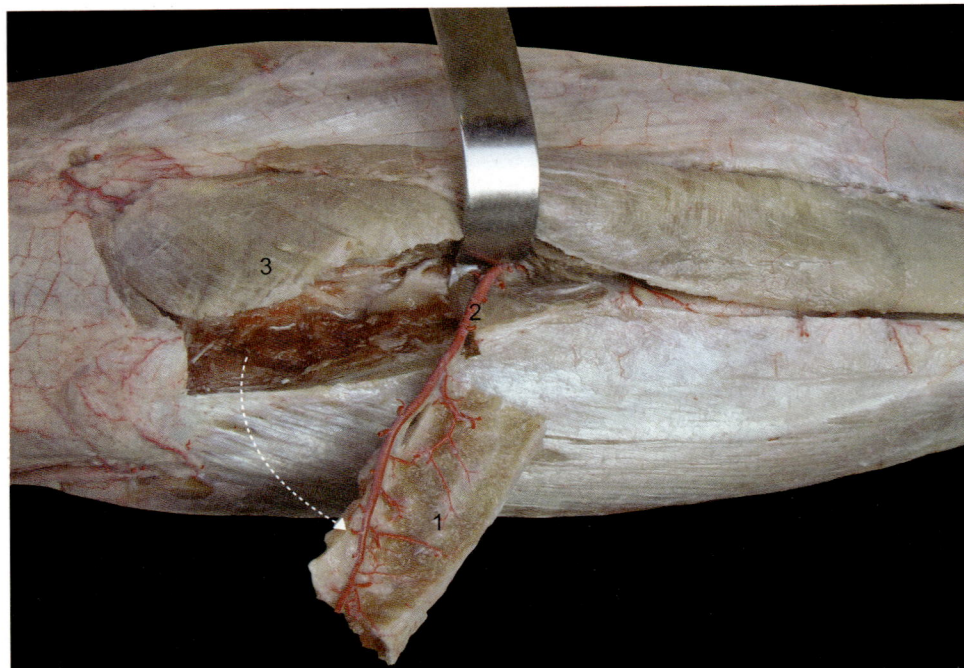

1. Bone flap
2. Recurrent branch of posterior interosseous vessel
3. Anconeus muscle

| Figure 3-93 | Anterograde transposition |

The bone flap should be harvested adjusted to the traumatic position after the osseous donor site is exposed. The terminal part of the interosseous recurrent vessel is ligated and then dissected at the proximal part of the bone flap. A properly long vascular pedicle should be dissected at the distal bone flap. The bone flap pedicled with the interosseous recurrent vessel might be transferred downwards to repair the trauma on the middle-superior segment of the radius and the ulna.

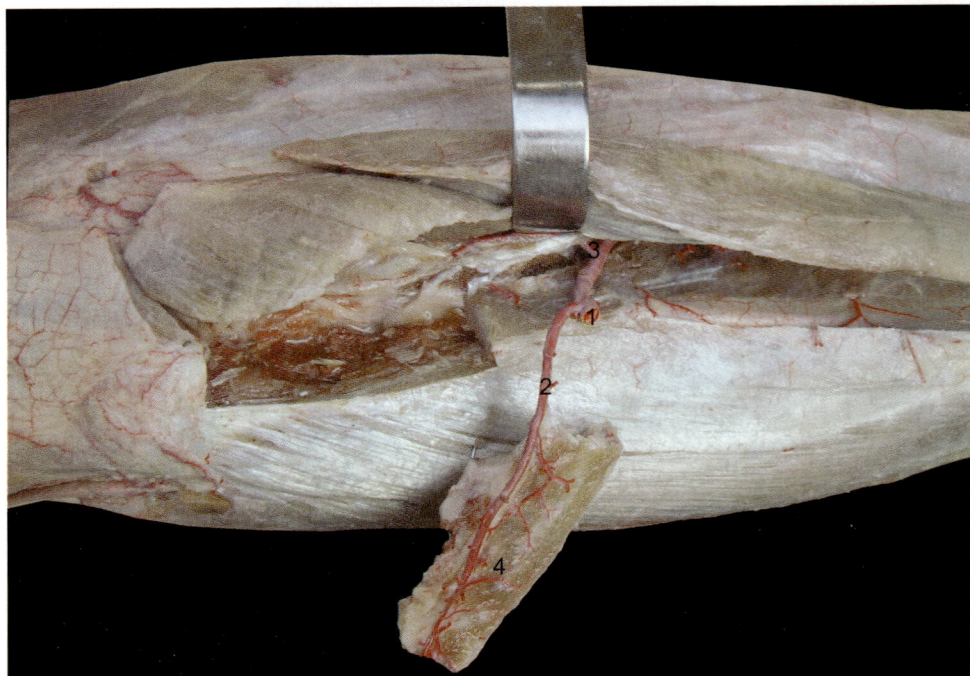

1. Main trunk of posterior interosseous vessel
2. Recurrent branch
3. Posterior interosseous vessel
4. Bone flap

| Figure 3-94 | Lengthen of the vascular pedicle |

The main trunk of the posterior interosseous recurrent vessel should be ligated before it sends the interosseous recurrent vessel. The bone flap pedicled with the posterior interosseous artery might be transferred to repair an osseous nonunion in the antebrachial inferior segment.

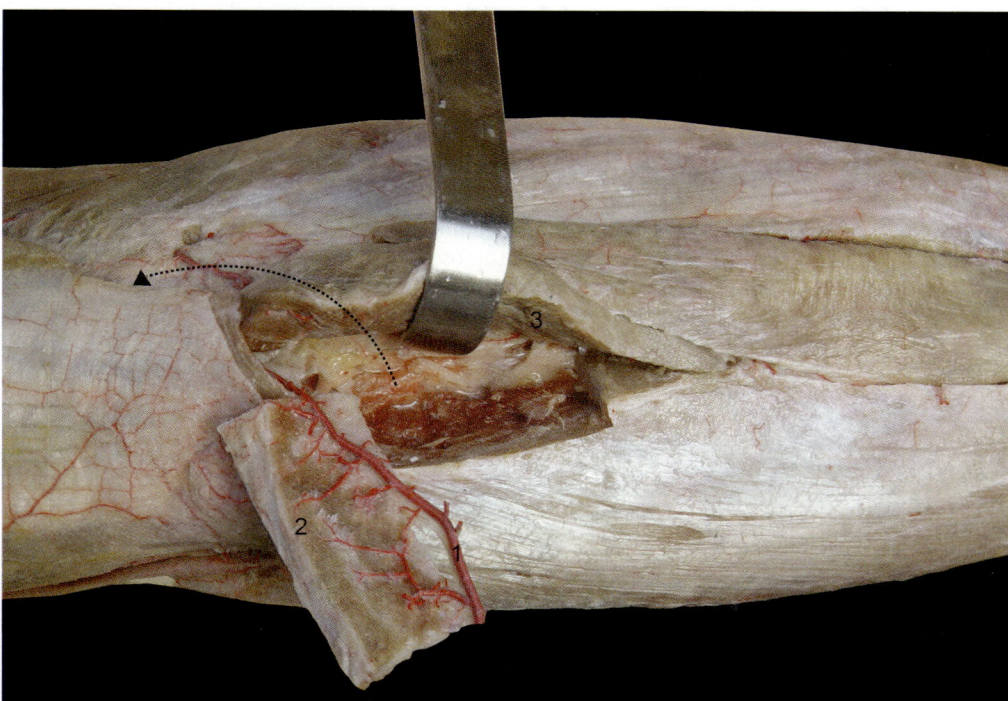

| Figure 3-95 | Retrograde transposition |

The initiation of the interosseous recurrent vessel should be ligated and dissected at the distal bone flap. A properly long vascular pedicle should be dissected at the distal bone flap. The bone (periosteal) flap pedicled with the interosseous recurrent vessel might be transferred retrogradely upwards to repair an osseous nonunion in the superior condyle of the humerus.

1. Recurrent branch of posterior interosseous vessel
2. Bone (periosteal) flap
3. Anconeus muscle

Key points in applied anatomy

Firstly, the supinator muscle should be incised between the two positions mentioned above to keep intact the vessels and the nerve when the recurrent interosseous artery or recurrent interosseous artery perforates through the interosseous membrane at 0.7cm from the position where the posterior interosseous nerve perforates through. Secondly, the superior margin of the bone (periosteal) flap should be incised at 1cm from the olecranon and the radial notch to prevent the adherent position of the cubital articular capsule from being incised. The cubital articular capsule should not be incised when the flap is being transferred retrogradely with the vascular pedicle located between the olecranon and the lateral condyle of the humerus on the surface of the cubital articular capsule. Thirdly, a muscular sleeve (2mm wide) should be retained on the surface of the periosteum when the anconeus muscle and the supinator muscle are being incised to avoid damaging the periosteal branch. Fourthly, the pedicled bone (periosteal) flap should carry with it partial fascia (1-2 cm wide) to protect the vascular pedicle when it is being retrogradely transferred.

16

Distal Ulnar (periosteal) Flap Pedicled with Posterior Interosseous Vessel

The pedicle of the posterior interosseous vessel has such advantages as a long pedicle, a large diameter and a constant course. Its distal part anastomoses with other vascular branches at the wrist. An antegrade or a retrograde bone (periosteal) flap might be designed according to the traumatic position. The distal ulnar (periosteal) flap pedicled with the proximal posterior interosseous vessel might be transferred retrogradely and proximally to repair the osseous nonunion on the middle-superior segment of the radius and the ulnar, or antegradely and distally to repair the osseous nonunion or defect of the carpal and the metacarpal bones.

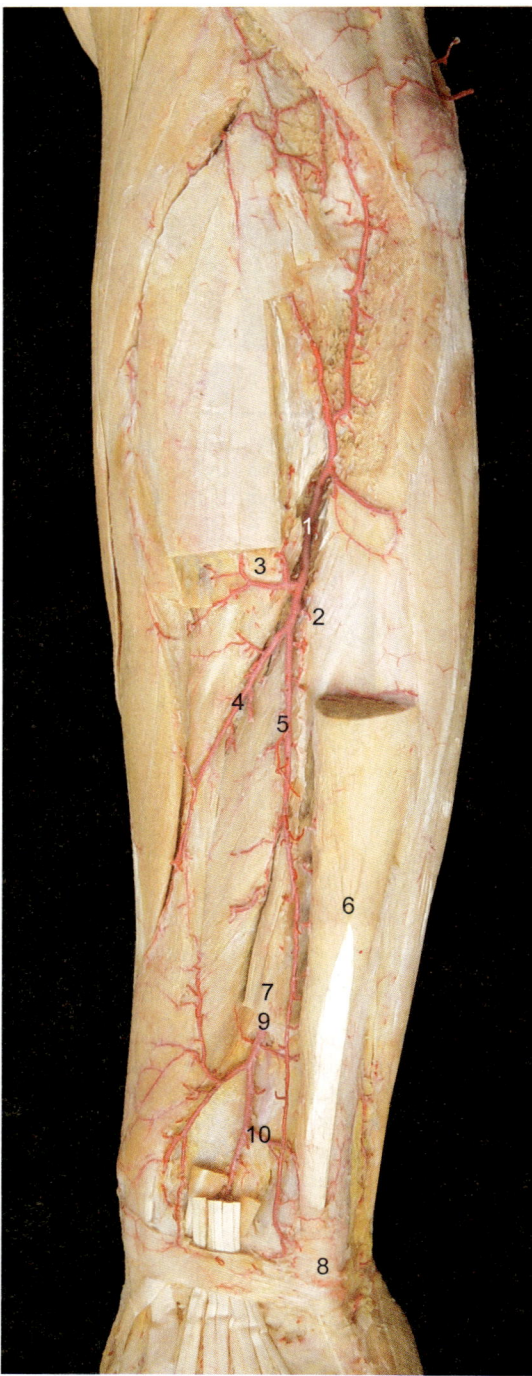

| Figure 3-96 | Applied anatomy |

The posterior interosseous artery emerges from the common interosseous artery, and perforates through the interosseous membrane via the septum between the abductor pollicis longus and the ulnar adherent part of the supinator muscle. Its main trunk runs downwards for about 1cm through the septum between the deep and the superficial layers of the antebrachial extensor muscles, and then gives laterally downwards the ulnar musculocutaneous branch to fan out over the muscles and the skin in the antebrachial posterior radial half. The main trunk of the posterior interosseous artery gives the radial musculocutaneous branch, namely, the ulnar musculocutaneous branch, then extends superficially to the deep fascia between the extensor carpi ulnaris and the extensor digiti minimi and keeps running downwards. Its distal part anastomoses with the dorsal carpal branch of the anterior interosseous artery that traverses inwards at 2.5cm (on average) superior to the ulnar styloid via the deep side of the extensor digiti minimi. Its anastomotic branch has a diameter of 0.8mm (on average) and an anastomosing frequency of 92%. The initiation part of the posterior interosseous artery has a diameter of 1.8mm on average. Its body surface projection falls on the middle-inferior segment of the connecting line between the lateral epicondyle of the humerus and the radial margin of the ulnar head. Its total length is 13.6cm on average.

1. Posterior interosseous artery
2. Abductor pollicis longus
3. Supinator muscle
4. Radial myocutaneous branch
5. Ulnar myocutaneous branch
6. Extensor carpi ulnaris muscle
7. Extensor digiti minimi muscle
8. Ulnar malleolus
9. Dorsal carpal branch of anterior interosseous artery
10. Anastomotic branch

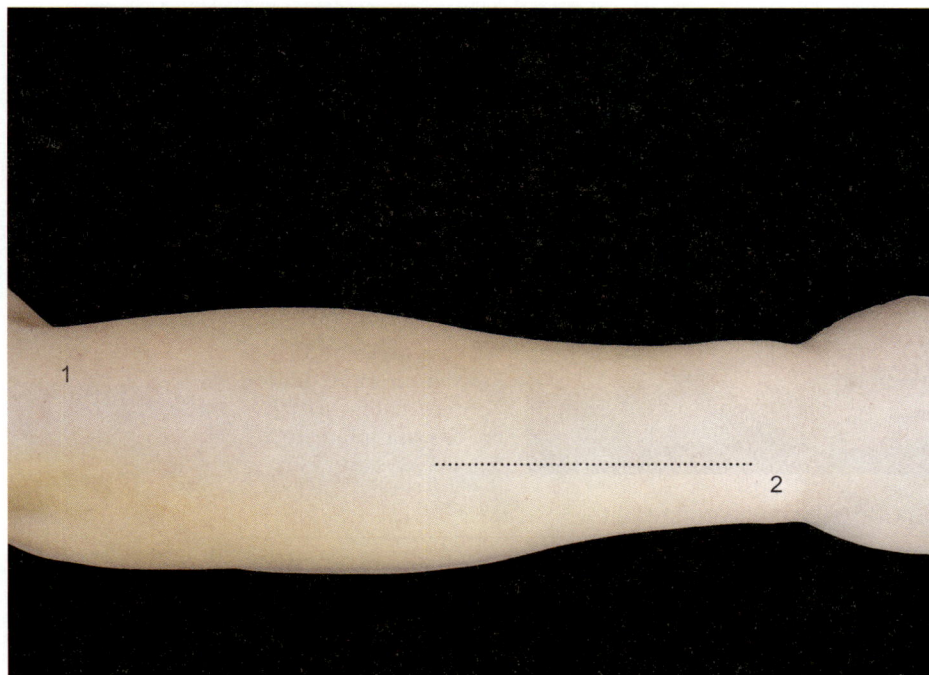

1. Lateral epicondyle of
   humerus
2. Ulnar head

| Figure 3-97 | Design of the incision |

The incision falls on the connecting line between the lateral epicondyle of the humerus and the radial margin of the ulnar head. It might be extended upwards from the radial side of the ulnar head and should be adjusted to the traumatic position.

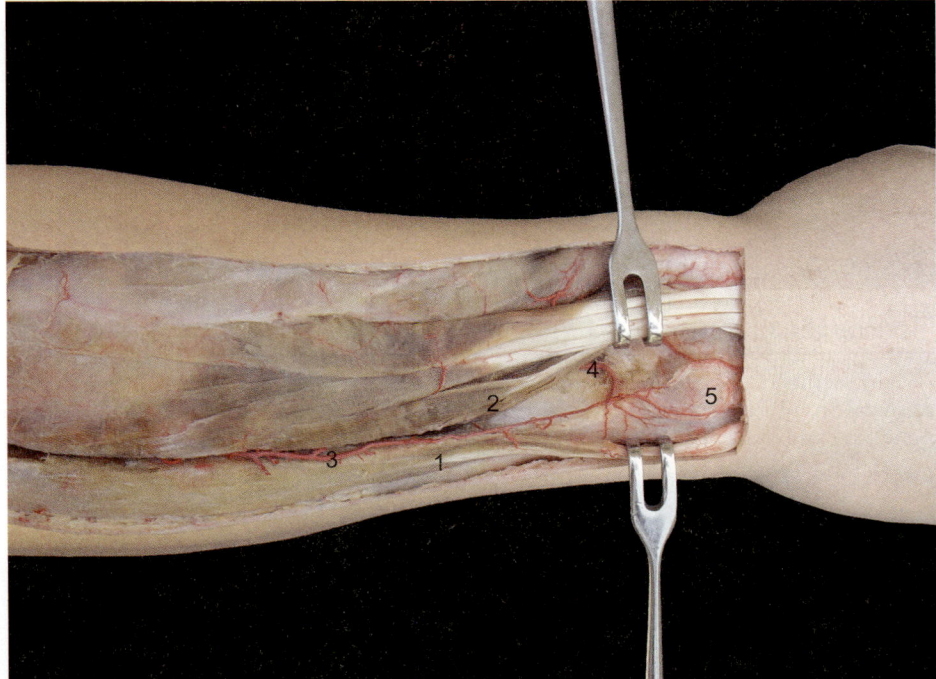

1. Extensor carpi ulnaris
   muscle
2. Extensor digiti minimi
3. Posterior interosseous
   vessel
4. Anastomotic branch
5. Radial capitulum

| Figure 3-98 | Exposure of the incision |

The skin and the subcutaneous tissue should be incised to expose the extensor carpi ulnaris muscle and the extensor digiti minimi. Respectively, the two muscles should be pulled laterally and medially to expose the posterior interosseous vascular pedicle inside the deep fascia between the two muscles.

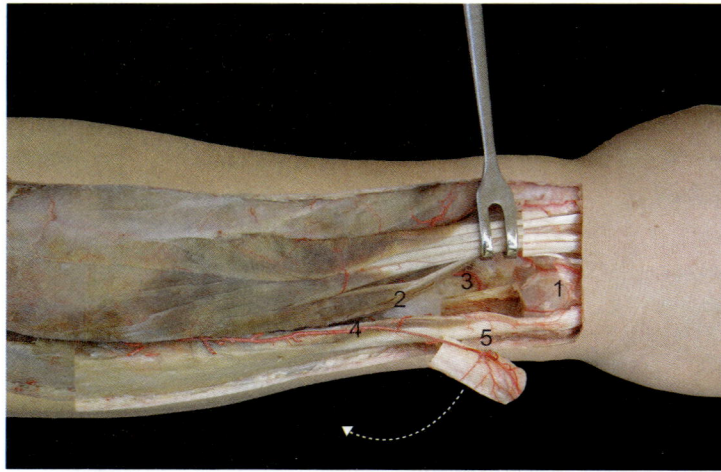

1. Ulnar capitulum
2. Extensor digiti minimi
3. Anastomotic branch
4. Posterior interosseous vessel
5. Extensor carpi ulnaris muscle

| Figure 3-99 | Dissection of the bone (periosteal) flap |

The anastomosis between the dorsal carpal branch of the anterior interosseous artery and the posterior interosseous artery should be ligated at 2.5cm above the ulnar styloid and on the deep surface of the extensor digiti minimi muscle tendon and distal from the ulnar. The bone (periosteal) flap of 1cm in width and 3.5cm in length should be chiseled from the radial half of the ulnar bone and might be transferred to the recipient site.

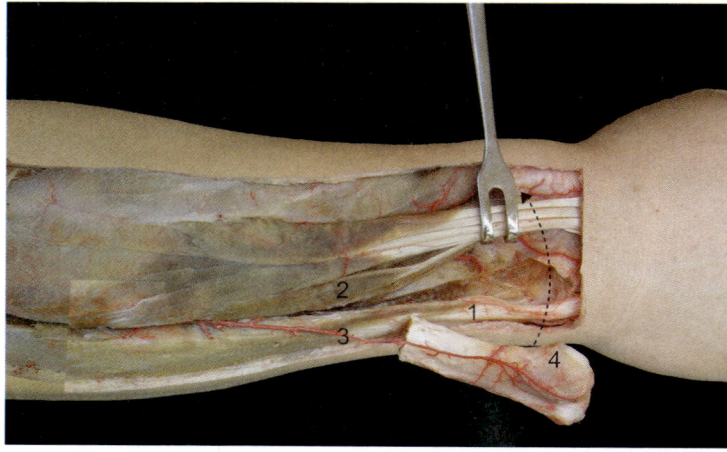

1. Extensor carpi ulnaris muscle
2. Extensor digiti minimi
3. Posterior interosseous vessel
4. Head of ulna

| Figure 3-100 | Transposition of the bone flap |

If both the radius and the ulna have osseous nonunion and the ulnar fracture is 5cm within the ulnar head, the whole ulnar segment distal from the fractured ulnar position might be inserted into the radial position of the osseous nonunion and defect.

Key points in applied anatomy

Firstly, the vascular pedicle should be dissected together with a deep fascia (1 cm wide) between the extensor carpi ulnaris muscle and the extensor digiti minimi to involve the vascular pedicle inside the deep fascia and in turn to protect the pedicle from being damaged. Secondly, the posterior interosseous nerve constantly accompanies the lateral posterior interosseous vessel at the middle-inferior 1/3 segment of the posterior forearm and keeps about 1cm away from the latter. The adjacent anatomical relationship of the vascular pedicle should be identified to prevent the nerve from being damaged. Thirdly, the anastomotic branches between the posterior interosseous artery and the dorsal carpal branch of the anterior interosseous artery are located at 2.5cm superior to the ulnar styloid, and so they should be ligated and incised on the side of the anterior interosseous vascular dorsal carpal branch to keep them far away from the ulnar bone, and in turn to protect the periosteal branch that emerges from the anastomotic branch.

Radial and Ulnar (periosteal) Flap Pedicled with Anterior Interosseous Vessel

17

The anterior interosseous vessel is the minor vessel for the forearm and the hand, and so the vascular pedicle might be harvested without sacrificing the main vascular trunk. It is suitable for repairing the damaged radial or ulnar vessels. It is so long and large that it might be included as a vascular pedicle in a suitable donor site for a bone (periosteal) flap according to the traumatic position. The antegrade bone (periosteal) flap pedicled with the anterior interosseous vessel is mainly used to repair the osseous nonunion and defect in the middle-superior segment of the radius and the ulna or the lesion in the inferior humeral segment. The retrograde bone (periosteal) flap pedicled with the anterior interosseous vessel is mainly used to repair the osseous nonunion and defect in the radial and ulnar distal part, and the osseous nonunion caused by the wrist fracture or the osseous ischemic necrosis.

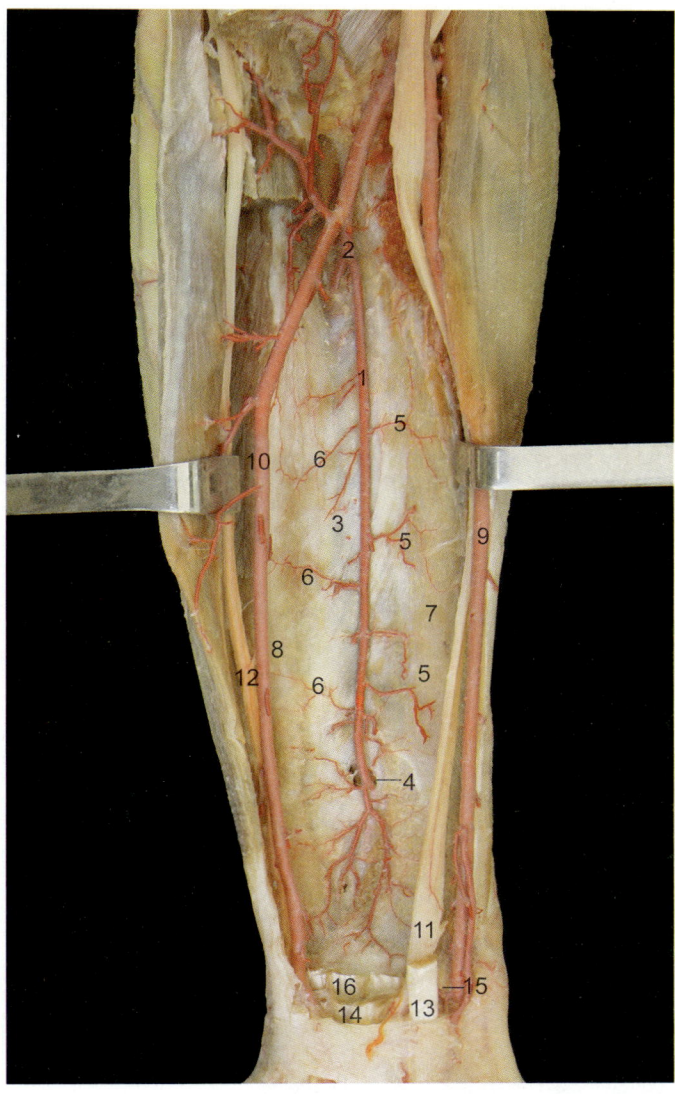

Figure 3-101 Applied anatomy

The anterior interosseous artery emerges from the common interosseous artery at 6.2cm to the connecting line between the medial and the lateral epicondyles of the humerus. Its initiation is 2.3mm in diameter. It perforates downwards through the deep surface of the long flexor muscle of the thumb and the deep flexor muscle of the fingers, and descends along the anterior aspect of the interosseous membrane. The anterior interosseous artery gives the dorsal carpal branch near the superior margin of the quadrate pronator muscle to perforate through the interosseous membrane to the posterior forearm. Its main trunk enters the deep surface of the quadrate pronator muscle. The anterior interosseous artery sends 5-8 radial periosteal branches laterally downwards into the radial palmar surface along its course from the initiation to the anterior wrist. It sends 5-11 ulnar periosteal branches medially downwards into the ulnar palmar surface via the septum between the interosseous membrane and the deep flexor muscle of fingers.

1. Anterior interosseous artery
2. Common interosseous artery
3. Interosseous membrane
4. Dorsal carpal branch
5. Radial periosteal branch
6. Ulnar periosteal branch
7. Radius
8. Ulna
9. Radial artery
10. Ulnar artery
11. Median nerve
12. Ulnar nerve
13. Flexor carpi radialis muscle
14. Flexor digitorum superficialis muscle
15. Flexor pollicis longus muscle
16. Flexor digitorum profundus muscle

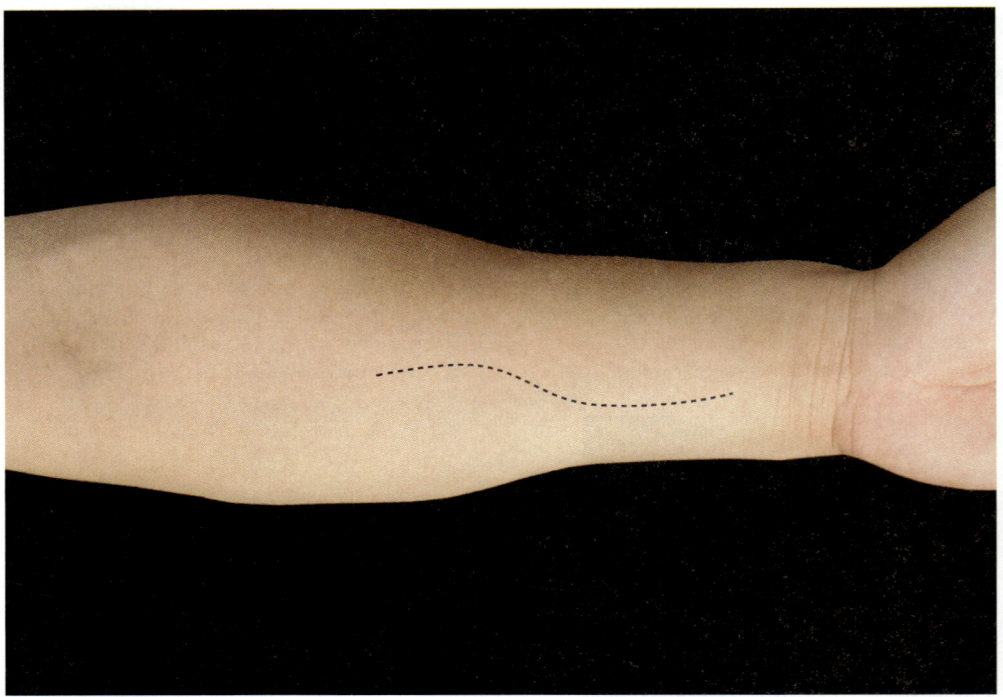

Design of the incision

The patient should be placed in supine position and a lazy S-shaped incision drawn on the middle-inferior part of the anterior forearm.

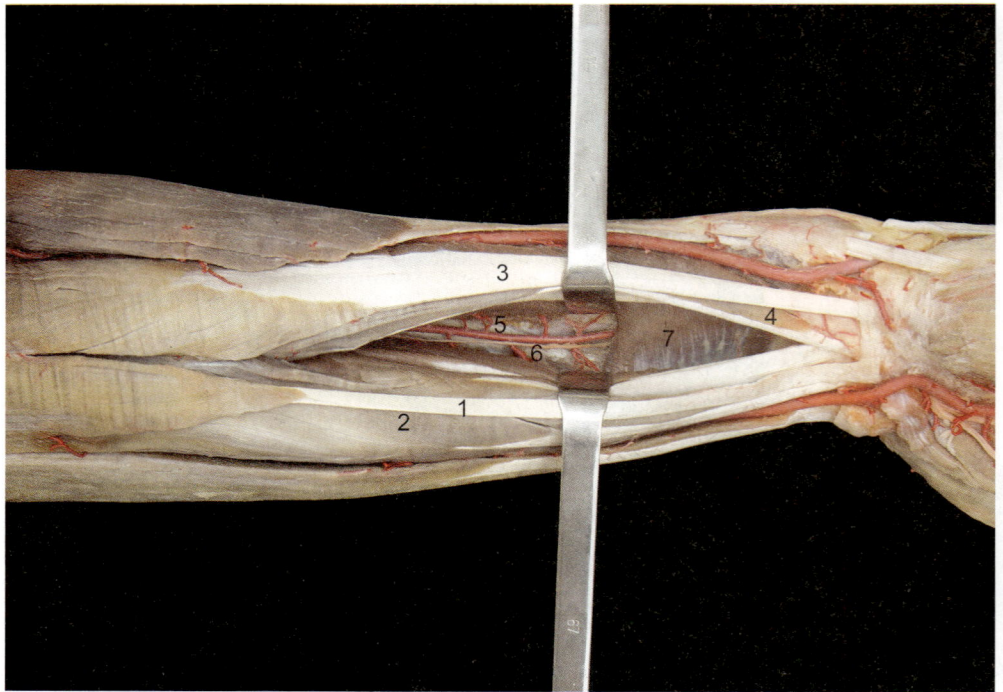

1. Long palmar muscle
2. Flexor digitorum superficialis muscle
3. Flexor carpi radialis
4. Flexor pollicis longus muscle
5. Anterior interosseous vessel
6. Anterior interosseous nerve
7. Quadrate pronator muscle

Figure 3-103   Exposure for vessels

The skin, the superficial and the deep fascia should be incised. The palmaris longus, the median nerve and the flexor digitorum superficialis muscle should be pulled to the ulnar side and the flexor carpi radialis muscle, the flexor pollicis longus muscle and the flexor digitorum profundus muscle pulled to the radial side to expose the anterior interosseous neurovascular bundle.

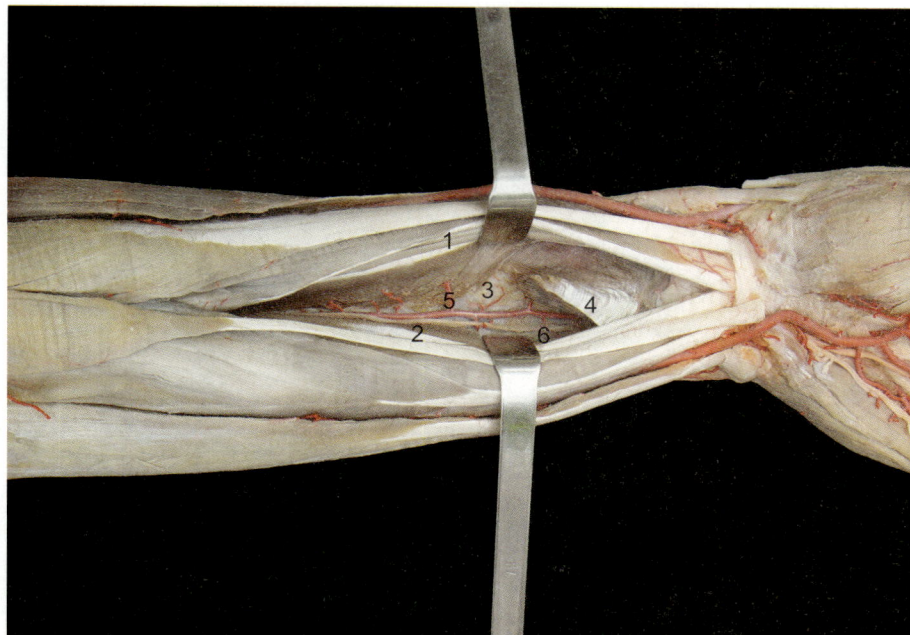

1. Flexor digitorum
   profundus muscle
2. Flexor pollicis longus
   muscle
3. Radius
4. Pronator quadratus
   muscle
5. Anterior interosseous
   vessel
6. Anterior interosseous
   nerve

Figure 3-104   Exposure of the periosteum

The flexor digitorum profundus muscle and the flexor pollicis longus muscle should be further dissected and pulled bilaterally to expose the required radial or ulnar segment. If the distal ulnar bone (periosteal) flap is necessary, a muscular sleeve (2-3 mm wide) of quadrate pronator muscular origin should be retained on the ulnar surface and the quadrate pronator muscle incised and turned to the radial side.

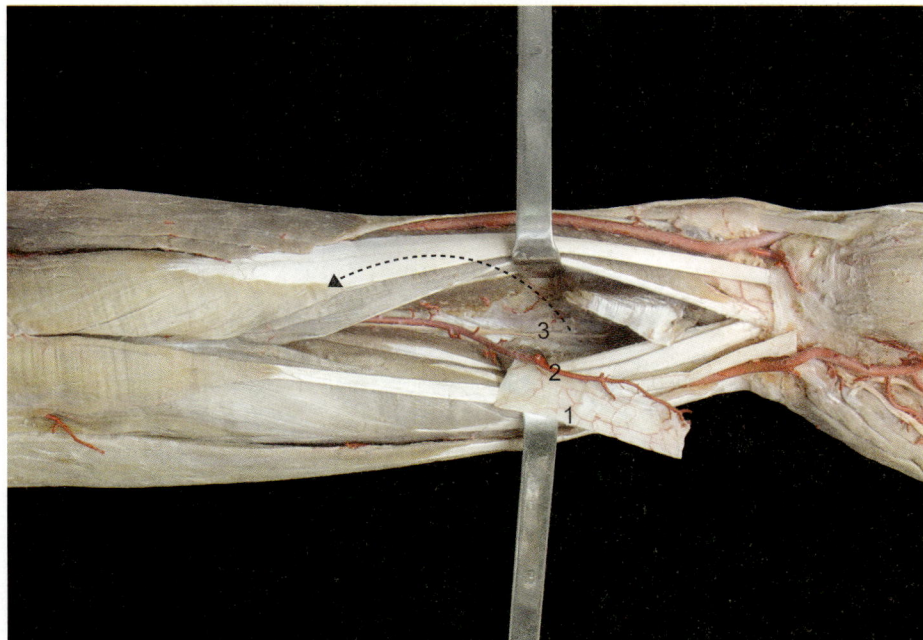

1. Bone (periosteal) flap
2. Anterior interosseous vessel
3. Anterior interosseous nerve

Figure 3-105   Anterograde transposition of the bone (periosteal) flap

A certain-sized bone (periosteal) flap and a piece of the interosseous membrane between the bone flap and the vascular pedicle should be incised, the vascular bundle ligated at the distal bone flap, and properly long vascular pedicle dissected at the proximal bone (periosteal) flap. With the lengthened incision and the expended tunnel, the pedicled bone (periosteal) flap might be transferred to the recipient site.

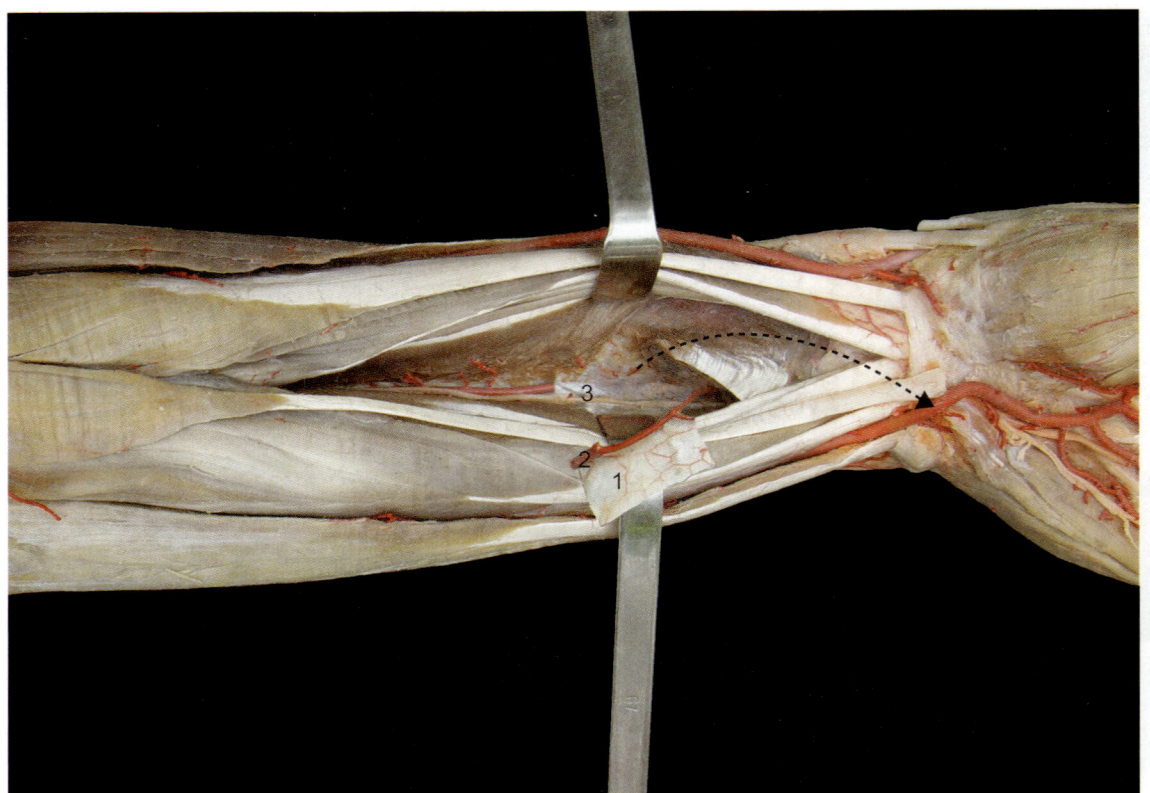

| Figure 3-106 | Retrograde transposition of the bone (periosteal) flap |

The vascular bundle should be ligated at the proximal bone (periosteal) flap and a properly long vascular pedicle dissected at the distal bone (periosteal) flap. The pedicled bone (periosteal) flap might be transferred downwards to repair the osseous nonunion or defect in the distal radial-ulnar segment, or be transferred to the prepared osseous slot of the scaphoid or the lunate bone.

1. Bone (periosteal) flap
2. Anterior interosseous vessel
3. Anterior interosseous nerve

Key points in applied anatomy

Firstly, the long and large interosseous vessel anastomoses with other vessels in the wrist. The bone (periosteal) flap based on the vessel might be transferred adjusted to the various traumatic positions. It might be transferred retrogradely to repair the distal antebrachial, carpal, and metacarpal bone. Secondly, an osseous segment of the bone (periosteal) flap and an interosseous membrane between the bone (periosteal) flap and the vascular pedicle should be incised during the operation to prevent the vascular and the periosteal branches from being damaged. Thirdly, when the periosteum carrying a muscular attachment is being dissected, a muscular sleeve (2-3mm wide) should be retained on its surface to prevent the vessel from being damaged. Fourthly, there are three types of bone (periosteal) flaps with the distal ulnar bone. They are classified as follows: the A-type bone flap might be shaped with the lateral half of the ulna splitted longitudinally; the B-type ulnar (periosteal) flap might be shaped with the periosteum splitted longitudinally along the anterior ulna and turned outwards to the interosseous crest and then back-inwards; the C-type bone flap might be shaped with the whole ulnar bone in the fractured distal segment harvested if there is a dislocation of the distal radioulnar joint, which will lead to the ulnar head resection.

Radial and Ulnar (periosteal) Flap Pedicled with Dorsal Carpal Branch of Anterior Interosseous Vessel

18

The main trunk of the dorsal carpal branch of the anterior interosseous vessel gives constantly ulnar and radial osseous cutaneous branches into the distal ulnar and the distal radial bones. Its distal part enters the carpal vascular net. The two bone might be harvested to obtain various bone or musculosseous flaps pedicled with the carpal vascular net. A flap of this type might be transferred distally to repair the scaphoid bone, the lunate aseptic necrosis and the metacarpal defection. The partial ulnar and radial bone might be incised together with the adjacent skin to obtain an osseous cutaneous flap for the reconstruction of thumb in the 1-stage. Because the vascular pedicle is located at the dorsum, this flap might be harvested easily for wrist surgery via a dorsal approach. In this case, it is unnecessary that the main trunk of the forearm be sacrificed.

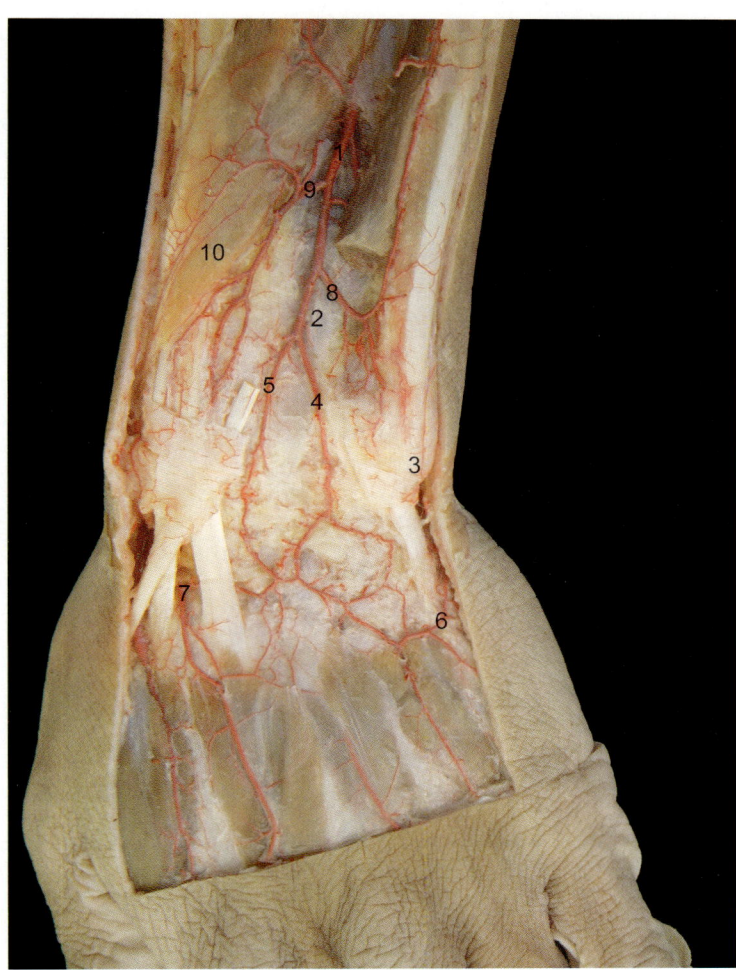

Figure 3-107	Applied anatomy

The dorsal carpal branch of the anterior interosseous artery descends under the deep surface of the extensor tendon, sticking to the interosseous membrane. It extends to (1.6± 0.8) cm above the ulnar malleolus and then bifurcates into the medial terminal and the lateral terminal branches, which anastomose with the dorsal carpal branches of the ulnar and the radial arteries, respectively. The proximal dorsal carpal branch gives constant ulnar and radial osseous cutaneous branches. The radial osseous cutaneous branch runs obliquely and distally along the ulnar margin of the extensor pollicis brevis. It perforates through the septum between the pollicis brevis and the long extensor muscles to fan out over the distal radial dorsum and anastomose with the radial styloid branch that emerges from the dorsal carpal branch of the radial artery. The radial osseous cutaneous branch is (2.5±7.3) cm in length and (1.0±0.2) mm in diameter. It is able to support a periosteal bone flap about 3.2×3.1×0.5cm in size. The ulnar osseous cutaneous branch runs along the ulnar capitulum via the extensor septum to fan out over the dorsal ulnar segment. It is (1.4±0.7) cm in length and (0.9±0.2) mm in diameter. It is able to support a periosteal bone flap about 3.2×3.1×0.3cm in size.

1. Dorsal carpal branch of anterior interosseous artery
2. Interosseous membrane
3. Ulnar malleolus
4. Medial terminal branch
5. Lateral terminal branch
6. Dorsal carpal branch of ulnar artery
7. Dorsal carpal branch of radial artery
8. Ulnar osseous cutaneous branch
9. Radial osseous cutaneous branch
10. Extensor pollicis brevis

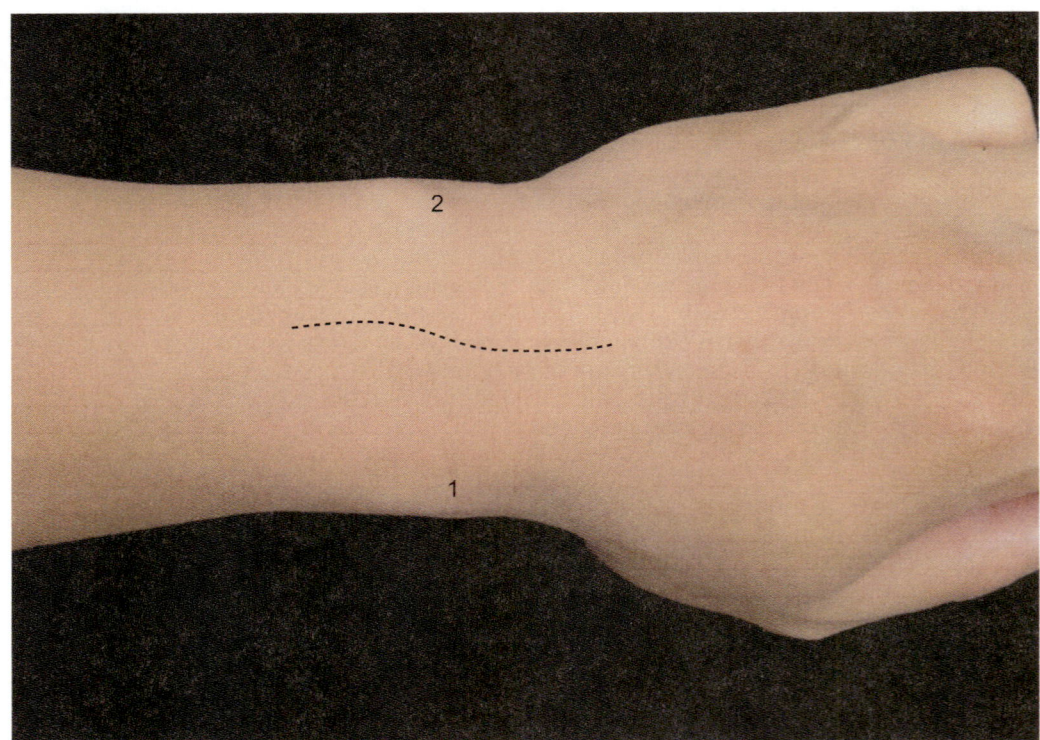

1. Radius
2. Ulnar capitulum

| Figure 3-108 | Design of the incision |

Take a scaphoid nonunion for example. An S-shaped incision should be drawn and extended upwards or downwards according to the traumatic situation on the dorsal wrist.

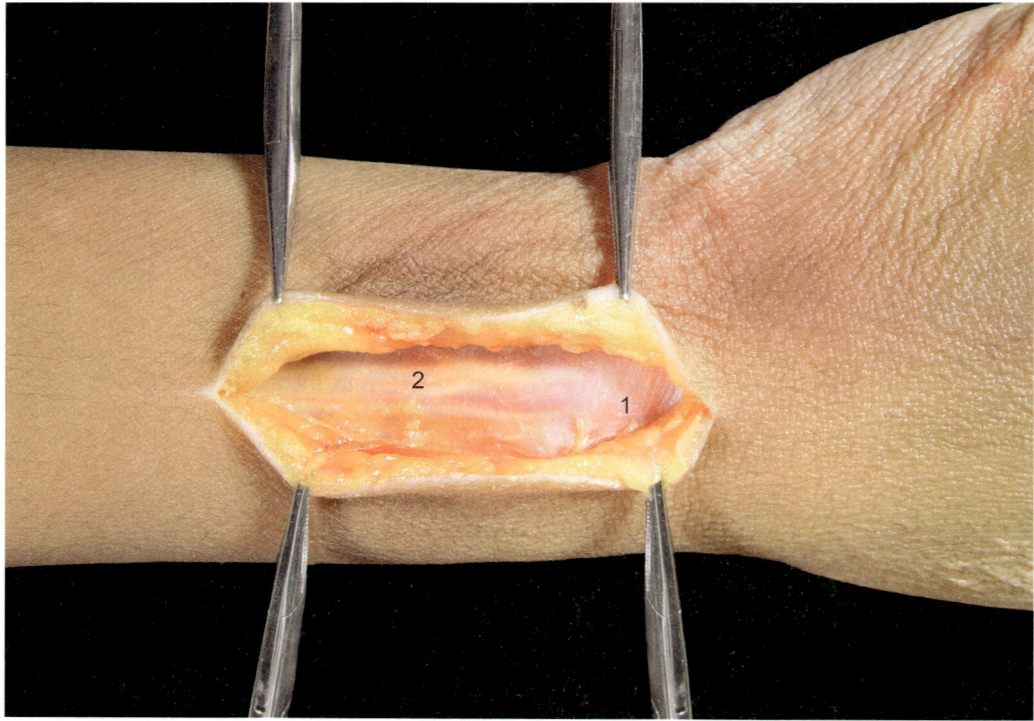

1. Dorsal carpal ligament
2. Tendon of extensor digitorum communis muscle

| Figure 3-109 | Exposure of the incision |

The skin and the subcutaneous tissue should be incised to expose the carpal dorsal ligament.

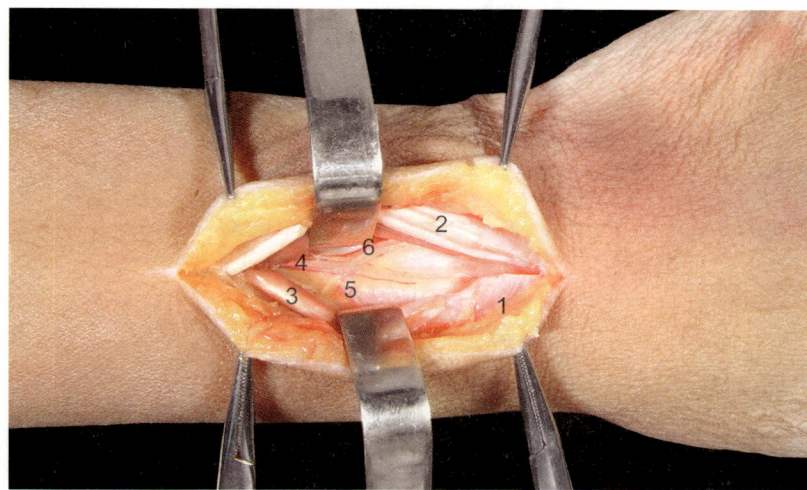

1. Dorsal carpal ligament
2. Extensor digitorium communis tendon
3. Extensor hallucis longus tendon
4. Dorsal carpal branch of anterior interosseous artery
5. Radial osseous cutaneous branch
6. Ulnar osseous cutaneous branch

Figure 3-110   Exposure of the vessels

The dorsal carpal ligament should be incised and the extensor hallucis longus tendon and the extensor digitorium communis tendons pulled bilaterally to expose the longitudinal dorsal carpal branch of the anterior interosseous artery. The incision should trace along the vessel to expose the radial or the ulnar osseous cutaneous branch as well as the medial and the lateral branches.

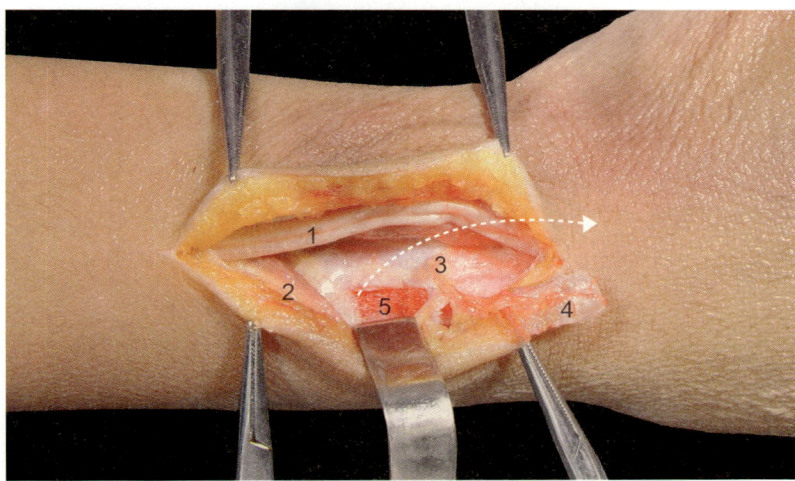

1. Extensor digitorium communis tendon
2. Extensor hallucis longus tendon
3. Dorsal carpal branch of anterior interosseous artery
4. Bone (periosteal) flap
5. Donor site

Figure 3-111   Incision of the bone (periosteal) flap

The preoperatively designed dorsal radial or ulnar bone (periosteal) flap should be harvested and protected with wet saline gauze. After the scaphoid osseous fracture is chipped and fixed properly, the dorsal carpal branch should be ligated before the origin of the radial or the ulnar osseous cutaneous branch. The bone (periosteal) flap might be transferred retrogradely and inserted in the scaphoid osseous slot.

Key points in applied anatomy

Firstly, a small osseous slot should be chiseled along the diseased bone so that the pedicled bone flap could be inserted after the bone fracture is chipped and fixed properly. The germinal layer of the bone (periosteal) flap should be scrolled outwards into a rounded barrel-shape and its margin fixed with several sutures before it is transferred and implanted into the osseous slot. Secondly, the connection of the vascular pedicle- periosteum-bone block should be kept intact during the operation. The superficial fascia of the bone flap and the periosteum should be a little larger than the bone block. Thirdly, the bone facture should be fixed with a kirschner wire or screw. If necessary, the surrounding fascia should be sutured to make the bone flap fixed.

19 Radial Styloid Bone Flap Pedicled with Recurrent Branch of Radial Artery

The radial styloidectomy is a traditional method to treat the osseous nonunion of the carpal scaphoid bone. Since the radial artery gives a recurrent branch to nourish the radial styloid, the nutrient vessel might be retained during the radial styloidectomy, and the pedicled styloid bone flap might be transferred to increase the blood supply of the recipient site, to repair the bone tissue, and to treat the osseous nonunion and ischemic necrosis caused by the fracture on the scaphoid bone.

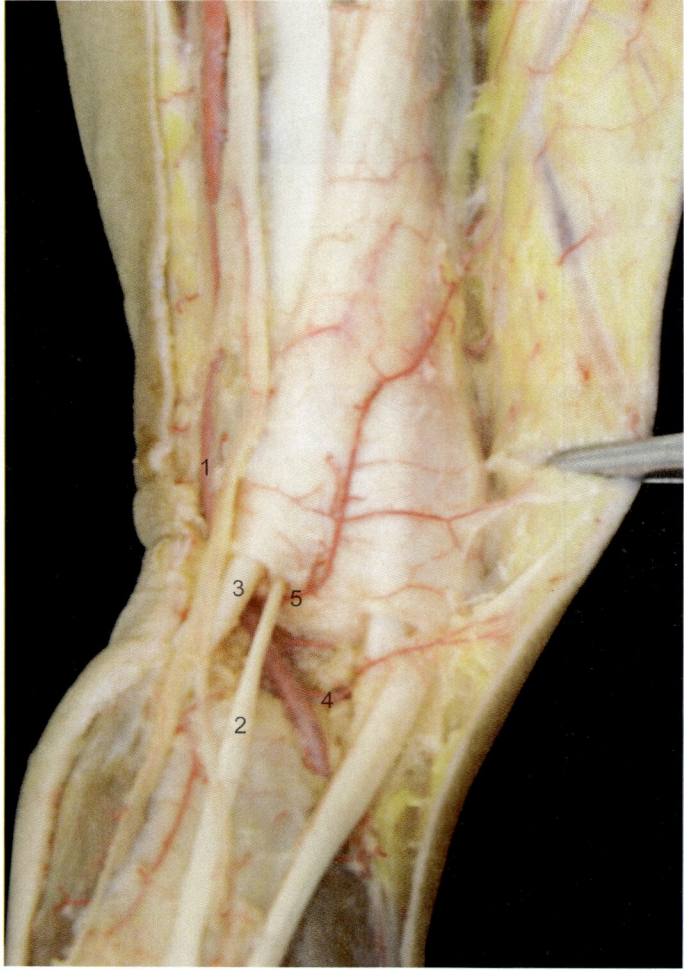

| Figure 3-112 | Applied anatomy |

The radial artery winds round the inferior styloid process via the anterior radial bone, and runs obliquely through the deep surface of the Abductor pollicis longus and the extensor pollicis brevis to the anatomical snuff-box in the wrist dorsum. There it gives ulnarly a relatively large dorsal carpal branch at 1.2cm beneath the styloid process. It gives superiorly 1-2 styloid recurrent branches to enter the radial styloid at the proximal dorsal carpal branch. The styloid branches are 1.2cm in length on average and 0.4mm in diameter at its origin. It has two accompanying veins. One is as large in diameter as the homonymous artery, and the other a little thinner.

1. Radial artery
2. Extensor pollicis brevis
3. Abductor pollicis longus
4. Dorsal carpal branch of radial artery
5. Recurrent branch of styloid process

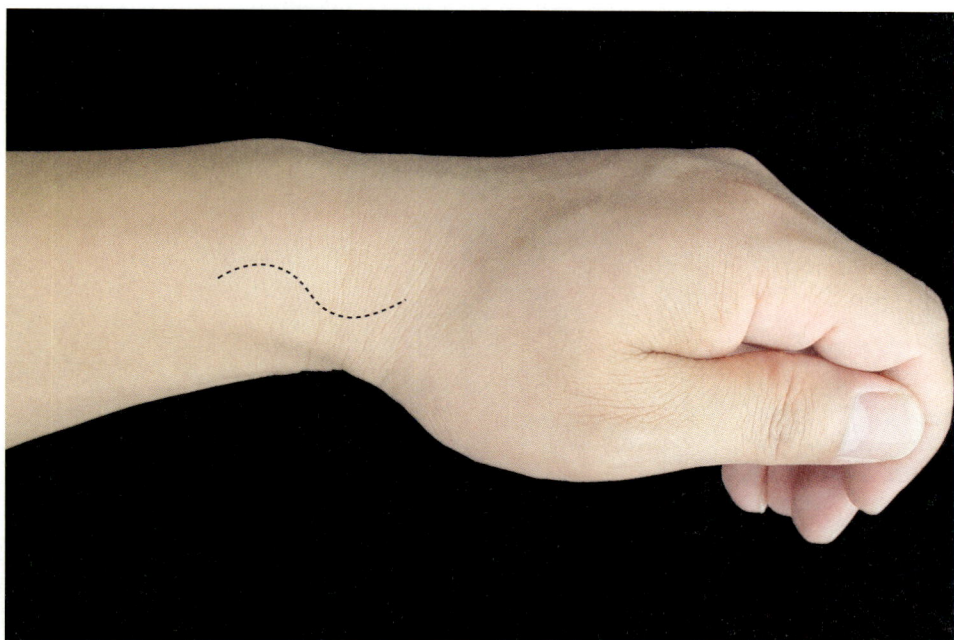

Figure 3-113   Design of the incision

A longitudinal or an S-shaped incision should be made (falling on the axial line of the anatomical snuff-box) on the lateral carpal articulations and might be extended slightly upwards and downwards if necessary.

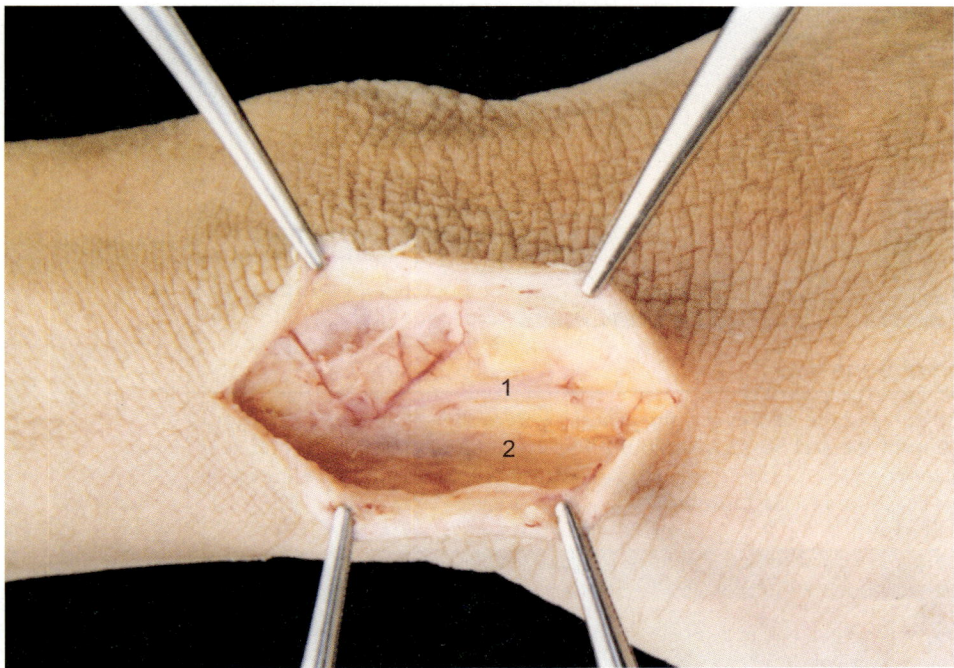

Figure 3-114   Exposure of the incision

The skin and the subcutaneous tissue should be dissected to expose the cephalic vein and the superficial branch of radial nerve.

1. Cephalic vein
2. Superficial branch of radial nerve

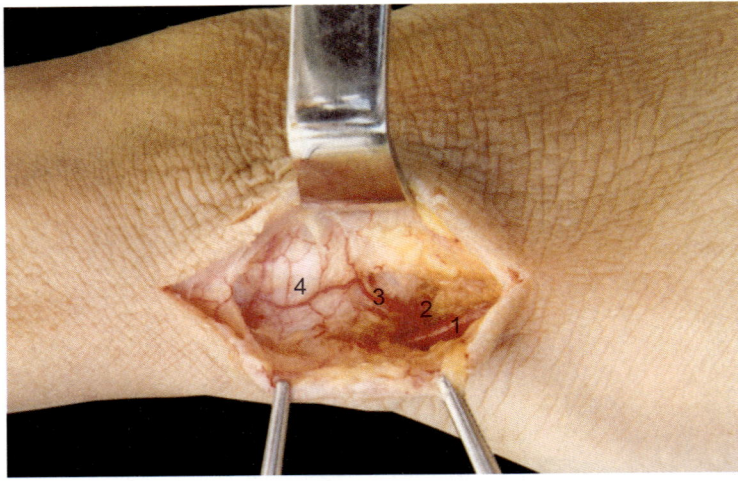

1. Radial artery
2. Dorsal carpal branch
3. Recurrent branch of styloid process
4. Styloid process of radius

| Figure 3-115 | Exposure of the vessel |

The superficial branch of the radial nerve and the cephalic vein should be pulled aside to expose the radial artery between the extensor hallucis longus and the extensor pollicis brevis tendon. The incision should be traced upwards to expose the dorsal carpal branch that emerges from the radial artery and the recurrent branch of the styloid process that emerges above the dorsal carpal branch.

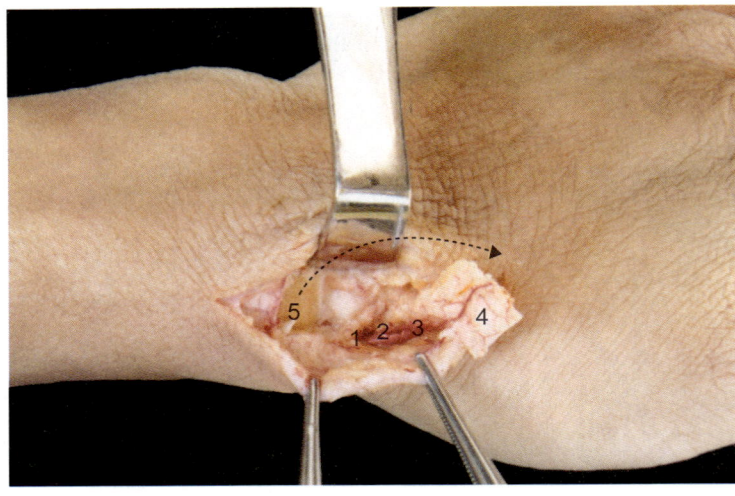

1. Radial artery
2. Dorsal carpal branch
3. Recurrent branch of styloid process
4. Bone flap of radial styloid process
5. Donor site

| Figure 3-116 | Incision of bone flap |

The position where the recurrent branch of the styloid process enters the styloid process should be identified so that a bone flap of the styloid process could be incised and clipped as a long strip-shaped one including most part of the periosteum. An osseous slot should be chiseled on the scaphoid so that the bone flap could be inserted into it.

Key points in applied anatomy

Firstly, the initiations of the superficial branch of the radial nerve and the cephalic vein are both located at the subcutaneous tissue under the course of incision, and so the skin incision should not be made too deeply. The superficial branch of the radial nerve and the cephalic vein should be pulled aside or the cephalic vein ligated before the dissection goes deeply downwards. Secondly, part of the dorsal nutrient foramen of the styloid process (about 0.5-1.5 cm from the point of styloid process) should be retained and the vascular net on the surface of the periosteum protected carefully so that the small vessels that enter the nutrient foramen could not get demage. Thirdly, the styloid bone flap should be incised with its incised osseous surface intersects and the axial line of the radial shaft at an angle of 80-90 degree. Its available range might exceed the fracture line of the scaphoid waist.

Metacarpal Bone Flap Pedicled with 2nd Dorsal Metacarpal Vessel

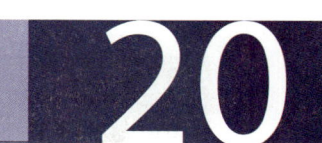

20

The 2nd dorsal metacarpal artery gives branches to nourish the metacarpal bone near the metacarpophalangeal articulations. The artery has such advantages as a constant course, a superficial location and a large diameter. It has two accompanying veins whose diameters are as large as or smaller than those of the homonymous arteries. Its affiliated bone flap has an abundant blood supply. The metacarpal bone flap pedicled with the 2nd dorsal metacarpal vessel might be transferred proximally to treat the scaphoid fracture and the lunate aseptic necrosis, or transferred retrogradely to repair the osseous nonunion and the phalanges defection .

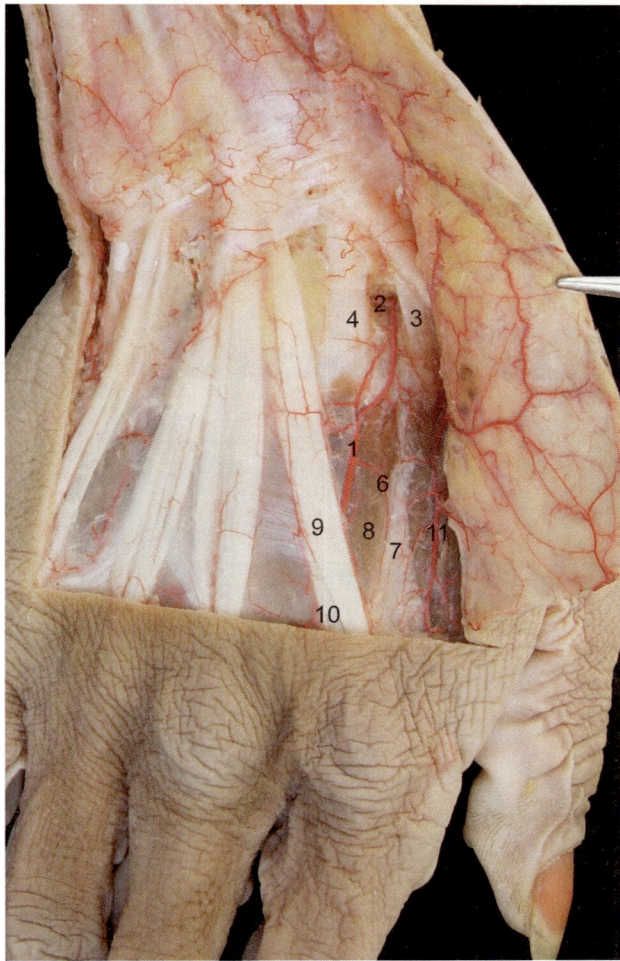

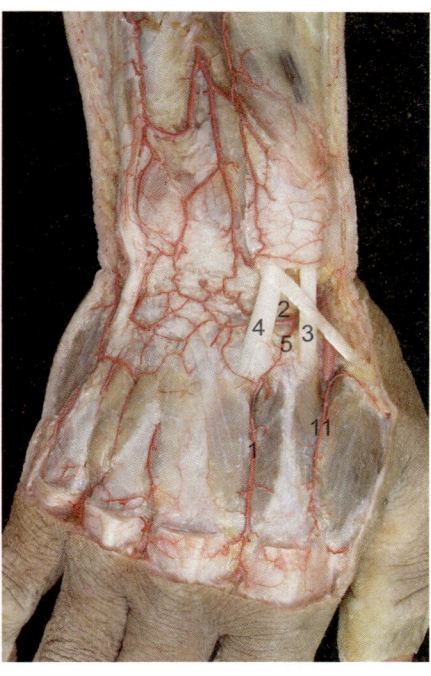

| Figure 3-117 | Applied anatomy |

The 2nd dorsal metacarpal artery is a main arterial trunk that extends on the 2nd dorsal intermetacarpal space. Its initiation is 1.2mm in diameter on average. Its terminal is 0.8mm in diameter on average. The artery anastomoses with the proper palmar digital artery or the common palmar digital artery. The 2nd dorsal metacarpal arteries might be classified into three categories. The first category refers to the dorsal carpal branch that emerges from the dorsal carpal branch of the radial artery and runs towards the 2nd intermetacarpal space through the septum between the long and the short tendons of the extensor carpi radialis brevis. The dorsal carpal branch converges into the 1st branch of the deep palmar arch at the proximal septum. It presents in most cases (69%) . The second category refers to the perforating branch. The 2nd dorsal metacarpal artery emerges from the 1st perforator of the deep palmar arch and anastomoses with the relatively small dorsal carpal artery. It presents in some cases (29%). The third category refers to the cases (2%) where no dorsal metacarpal arteries exist on the 2nd dorsal intermetacarpal space. The dorsal interosseous tissue gets its blood supply from the volar arterial branch.

1. 2nd dorsal metacarpal artery
2. Dorsal carpal branch of radial artery
3. Tendon of extensor carpi radialis longus
4. Tendon of extensor carpi radialis brevis
5. Anastomotic branch
6. Musculoperiosteal branch
7. 2nd metacarpal bone
8. Dorsal interossei muscle
9. Extensor tendon
10. Extensor indicis tendon
11. 1st dorsal metacarpal artery

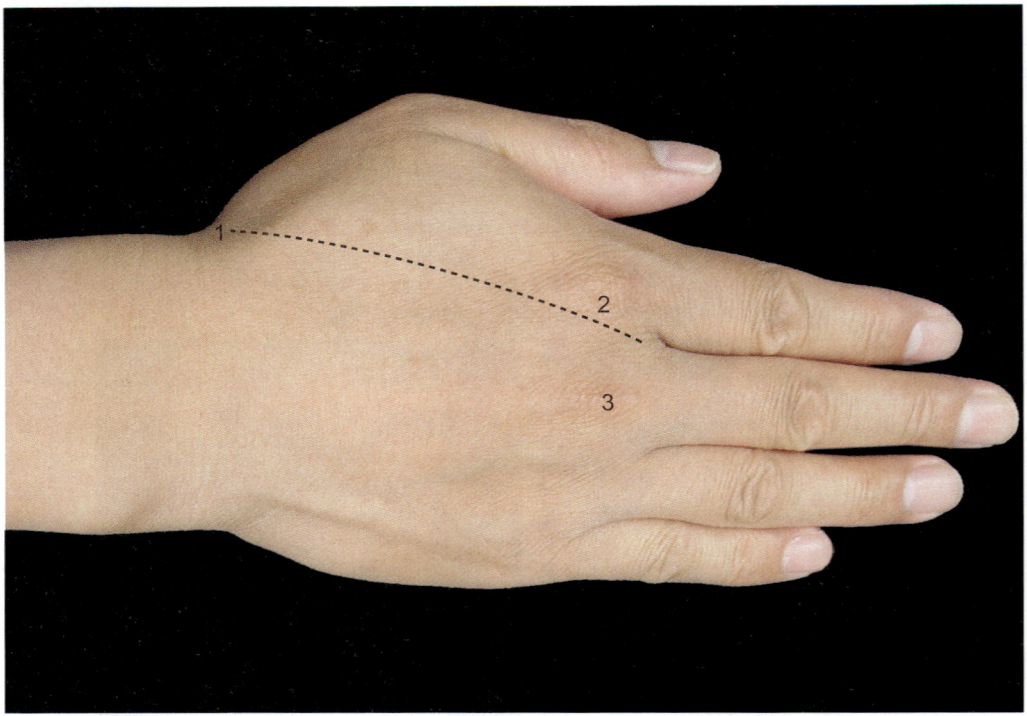

| **Figure 3-118** | Design of the incision |

A curved incision might be drawn from the anatomical snuff-box to the plane of the 2nd and the 3rd metacarpophalangeal joints.

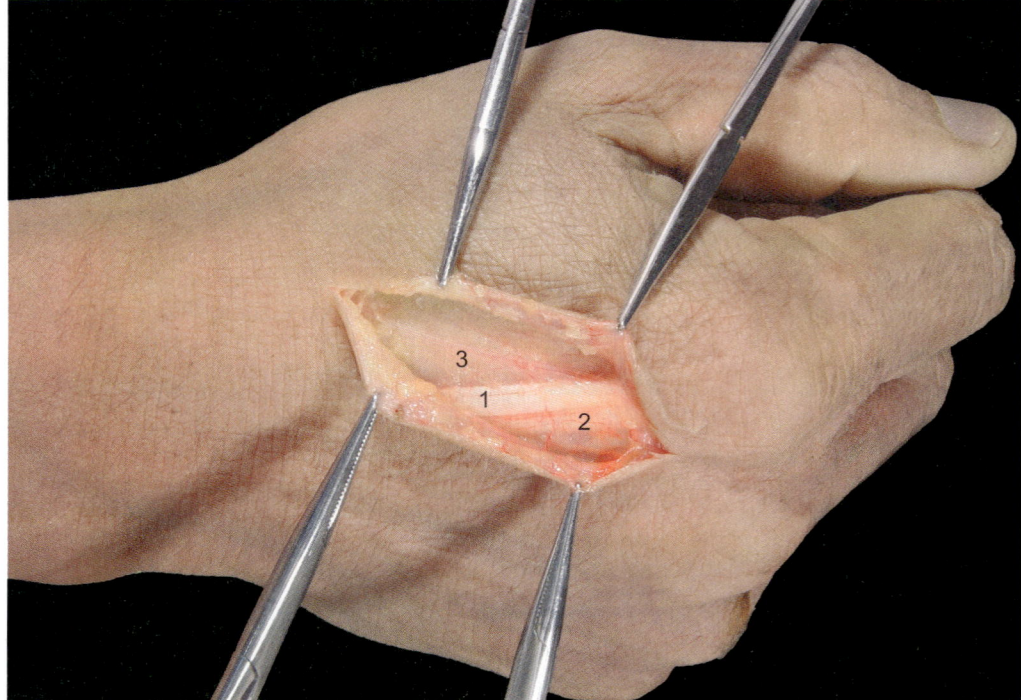

1. Extensor tendon
2. Extensor indicis tendon
3. Dorsal interossei muscle

| **Figure 3-119** | Exposure of the incision |

The distal incision should be made firstly to expose the extensor tendon and the extensor indicis tendon.

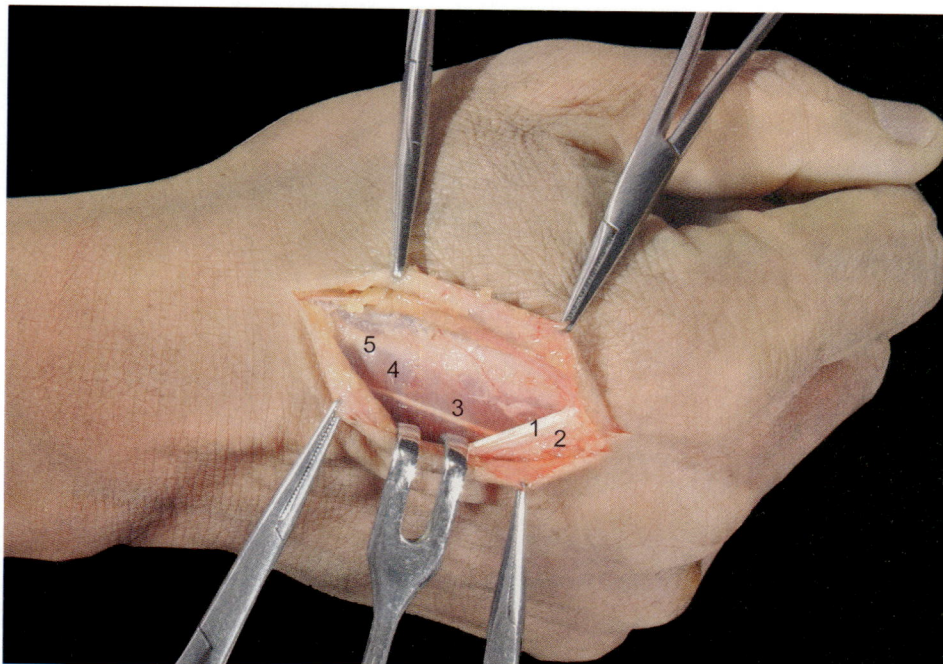

1. Extensor tendon
2. Extensor indicis tendon
3. 2nd dorsal metacarpal artery
4. Dorsal interossei muscle
5. Metacarpal bone

Figure 3-120   Exposure of the vessel

The extensor tendon and the extensor indicis tendon should be pulled ulnarly to trace the 2nd dorsal metacarpal artery in the septum between the long and the short tendons of the extensor carpi radialis brevis. The 2nd metacarpal artery that emerges from the dorsal carpal arterial arch should be dissected distally until it reaches the head of the metacarpal bone.

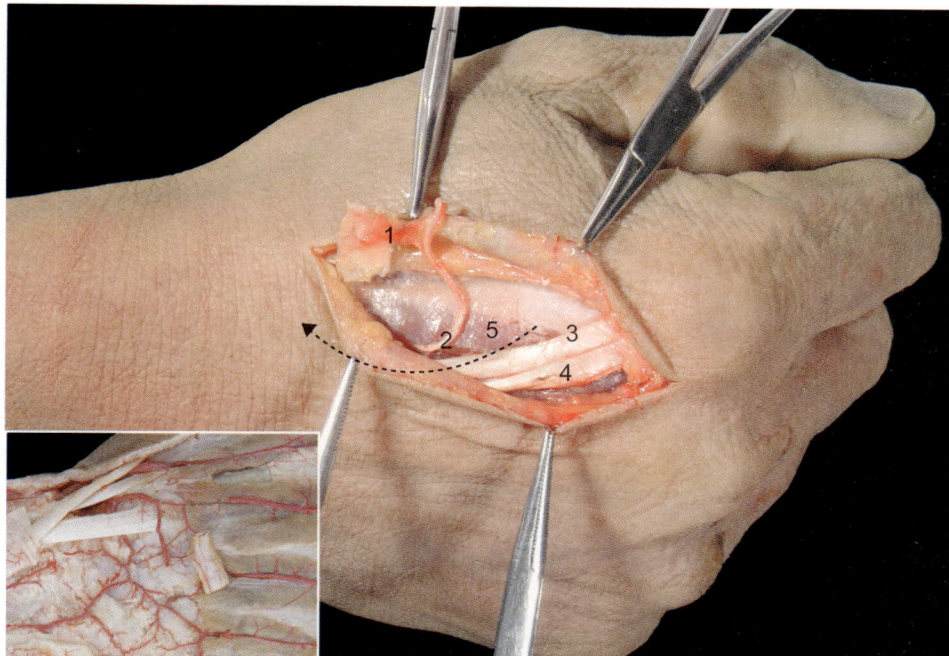

1. Metacarpal bone flap
2. 2nd dorsal metacarpal artery
3. Extensor tendon
4. Extensor indicis tendon
5. Dorsal interossei muscle

Figure 3-121   Transposition of the bone flap

A small bone block should be chiseled from the 2nd ulnar metacarpal bone and the vascular bundle ligated and incised at the distal end. An osseous slot should be chiseled when the scaphoid bone is satisfactorily reshaped. Then the metacarpal bone flap should be transferred and inserted into the prepared slot.

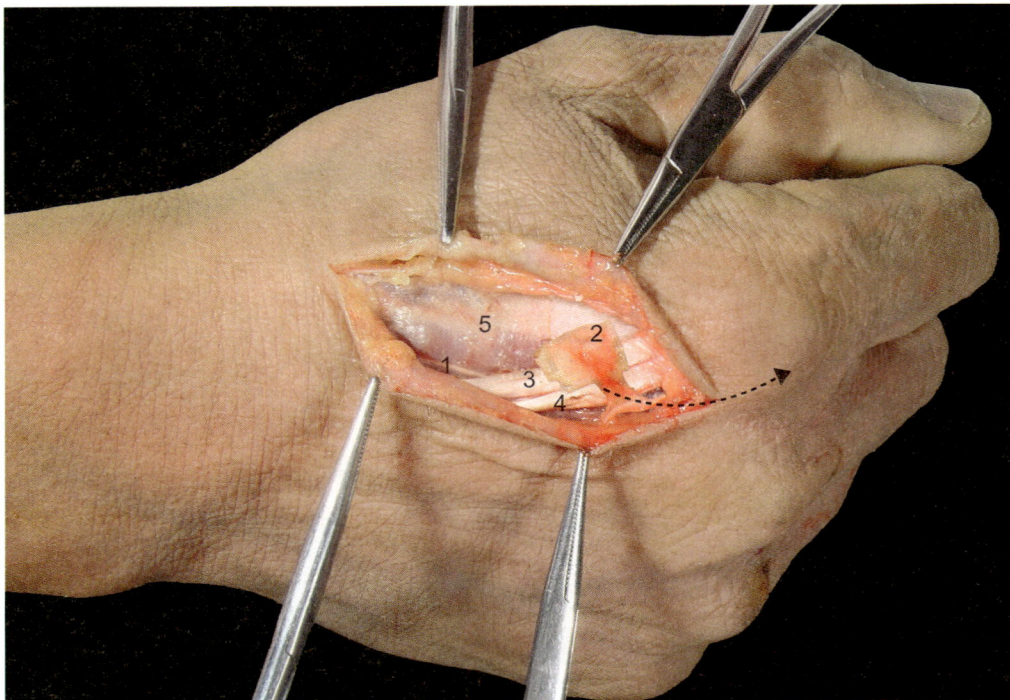

| **Figure 3-122** | Retrograde transposition of the flap |

The proximal vascular pedicle should be ligated and incised, and a small bone block chiseled from the 2nd ulnar metacarpal bone and transferred to repair the phalangeal defect.

1. 2nd dorsal metacarpal artery
2. Metacarpal flap
3. Extensor tendon
4. Extensor indicis tendon
5. Dorsal interossei muscle

Key points in applied anatomy

Firstly, the connection between the vascular bundle and the bone block should be carefully retained when the bone block is being chiseled. Secondly, the 1st or the 3rd dorsal metacarpal artery might be the option of a vascular pedicle when there is no 2nd dorsal metacarpal artery in some cases. Thirdly, the perforating branch of the deep palmar arterial arch should be ligated when the distal vascular pedicle is being transferred retrogradely. Fourthly, the bone flap should be incised with part of the interosseous muscle to protect the branch of the dorsal metacarpal artery that enters the bone flap and its accompanying vein. If necessary, a surgical flap should be harvested compounded with part of bone, muscle, tendon and dorsal metacarpal skin to repair the complicated defect on the fingers. A flap that is less than 2×2cm in size might be sutured directly, but the donor site a relatively large flap should be recovered with a free skin graft.

21

Iliac Bone Flap Pedicled with Deep Iliac Circumflex Vessel

The deep iliac circumflex vessel has such advantages as a large diameter, a long main trunk, a constant course and an abundant blood supply. The iliac bone flap pedicled with the deep iliac circumflex vessel has a tenacious lateral bone plate and a porous cancellous bone. It is 10×3.5cm in size, on average. It is slightly warped so that it might be conveniently molded. The iliac bone flap might be transferred proximally to repair the defect of the superior femur, the femoral neck fracture and the aseptic necrosis of the femoral head or transplanted to reconstruct a relatively large bone defect of the jaw and the pelvis.

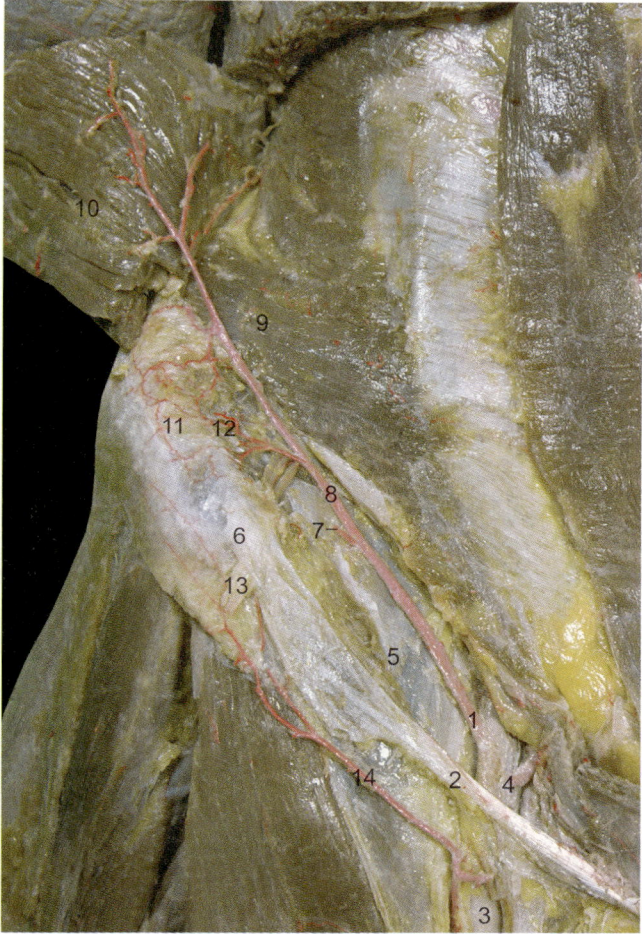

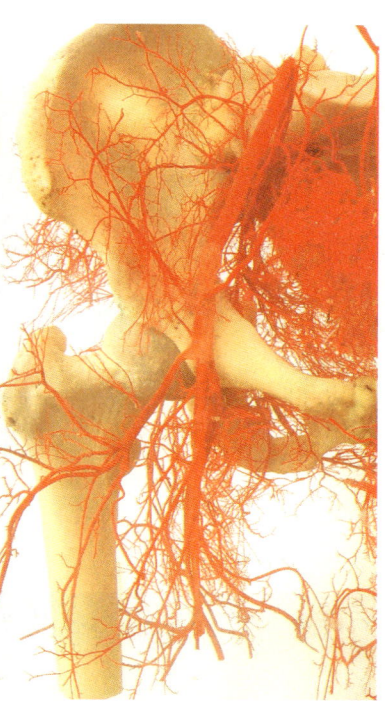

Figure 3-123 | Applied anatomy

The deep iliac circumflex artery emerges from the femoral artery or the external iliac artery above or beneath the inguinal ligament. It runs laterally upwards along the lateral half of the inguinal ligament in the septum between the deep surface of the abdominal muscle and the superficial layer of the transversalis fascia and bifurcates into the ascending branch (abdominal muscular branch) and the terminal branch at 3 cm or so to the medial superior iliac spine. The ascending branch runs upwards between the transverse abdominal muscle and the obliquus internus abdominis muscle to nourish the abdominal wall. The bracket-shaped terminal branch runs backwards between the iliac fascia and the iliac muscle at 2cm inferior to the anterior internal lip of iliac crest. Along the course, it gives several branches to nourish the anterior iliac crest and the surrounding skin. The lateral femoral cutaneous nerve perforates through the deep surface of the vessel to enter the lateral thigh at 2 cm intero-superior to the anterior superior iliac spine. The ilioinguinal nerve runs coincidently with the deep iliac circumflex artery or closely to it sometimes.

1. Deep iliac circumflex artery
2. Inguinal ligament
3. Femoral artery
4. External iliac artery
5. Superficial layer of transversalis fascia
6. Anterosuperior iliac spine
7. Ascending branch
8. Terminal branch
9. Transversus abdominis muscle
10. Obliquus internus abdominis muscle
11. Iliac crest
12. Iliac branch
13. Lateral femoral cutaneous nerve
14. Superficial iliac circumflex artery

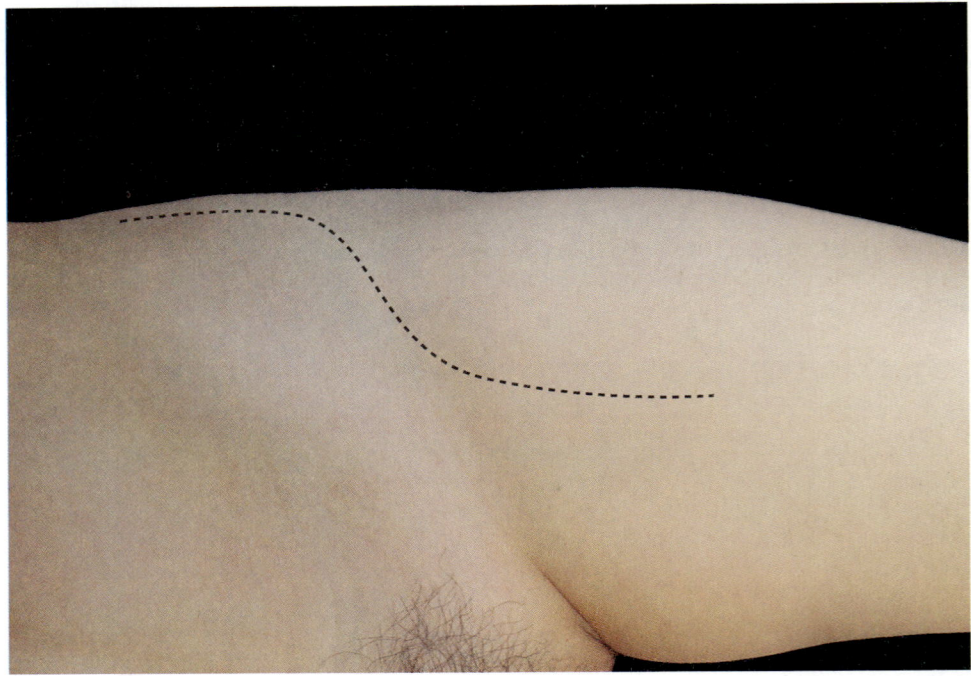

| Figure 3-124 | Design of the incision |

The incision should be drawn from the medial midpoint of the iliac crest to the midpoint of the inguinal ligament via the iliac crest and then bent towards the anterolateral thigh.

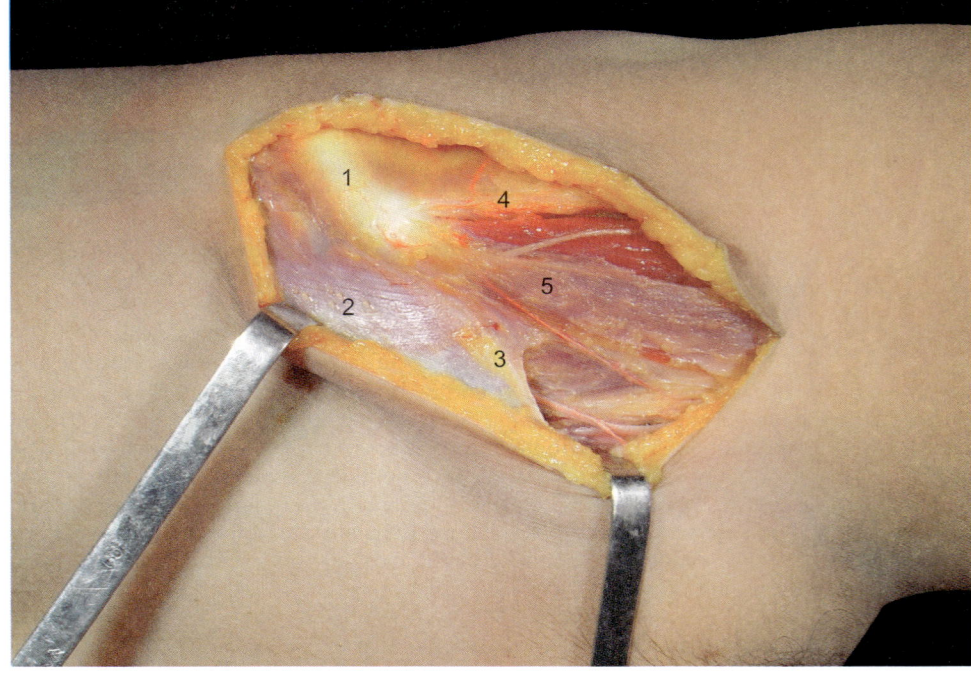

1. Iliac crest
2. Oblique externus abdominis muscle
3. Inguinal ligament
4. Tensor muscle of fascia lata
5. Sartorius muscle

| Figure 3-125 | Exposure of the muscle |

A curved incision from the iliac crest to the midpoint of the inguinal ligament should be made to expose the iliac crest, the oblique externus abdominis muscle and the inguinal ligament.

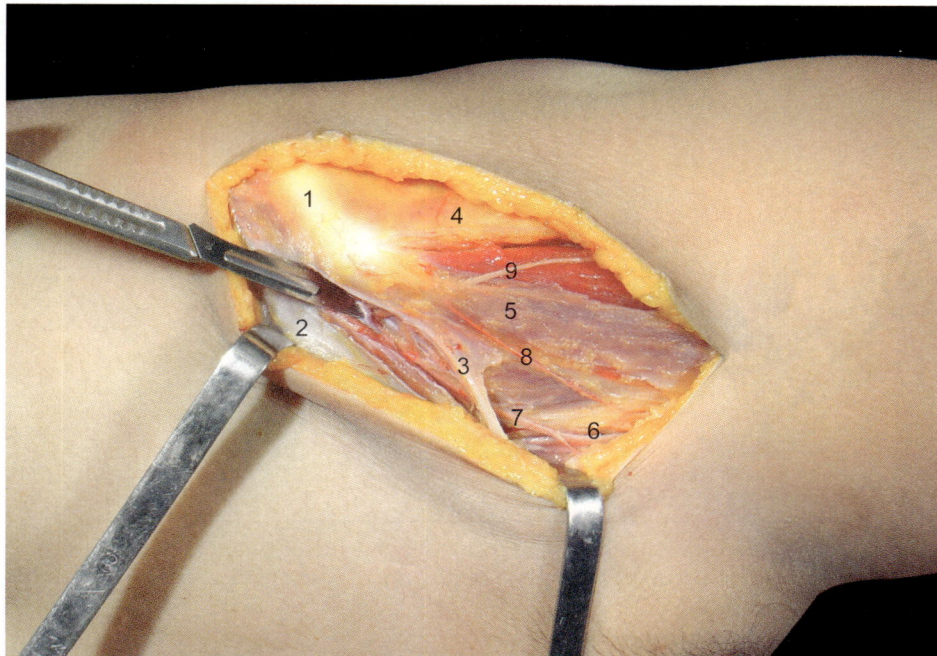

1. Iliac crest
2. Oblique externus abdominis muscle
3. Inguinal ligament
4. Tensor muscle of fascia lata
5. Sartorius muscle
6. Femoral artery
7. Deep iliac circumflex artery
8. Superficial iliac circumflex artery
9. Lateral femoral cutaneous nerve

Figure 3-126   Exposure of the vessel

The pulsating position of the femoral artery should be confirmed before the abdominal muscle is separated from the inguinal ligament. The inguinal ligament should be incised temporarily to expose the femoral artery and vein as well as the deep iliac circumflex veins so that the operation could be conducted smoothly, but it should be repaired at the end of the operation.

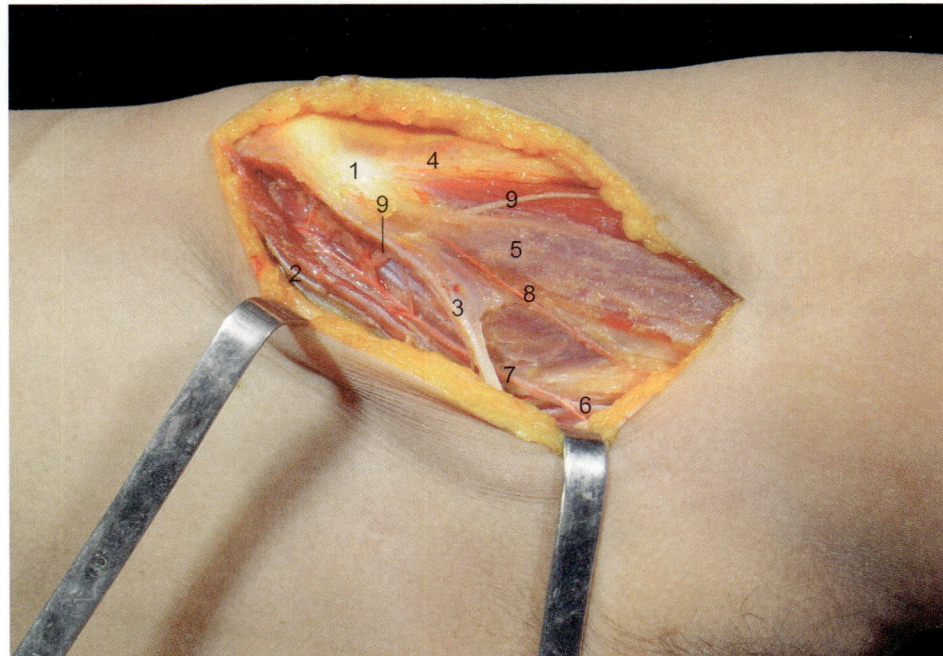

1. Iliac crest
2. Oblique externus abdominis muscle
3. Inguinal ligament
4. Tensor muscle of fascia lata
5. Sartorius muscle
6. Femoral artery
7. Deep iliac circumflex artery
8. Superficial iliac circumflex artery
9. Lateral femoral cutaneous nerve

Figure 3-127   Separation of the vessel

The vessel should be dissected distally along the deep iliac circumflex vessel to confirm whether the terminal branch enters the iliac bone. Then the deep branch that enters the abdominal muscle could be ligated and incised. The three layers of the abdominal muscles should be incised along the terminal branch. The lateral femoral cutaneous nerve is located at 2cm medial to the anterior superior iliac spine and runs beneath the vessel. The nerve should not be damaged.

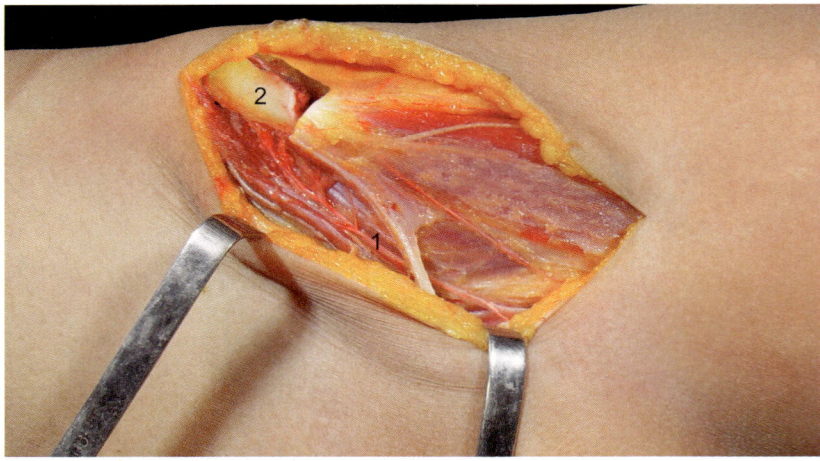

1. Deep iliac circumflex artery
2. Bone flap

| Figure 3-128 | Incision of the bone flap |

The incised abdominal muscle should be pulled inwards to expose and split downwards the medial periosteum of the iliac bone beneath the deep iliac circumflex vessels. The iliac bone block should be chiseled outwards as is required for the recipient site.

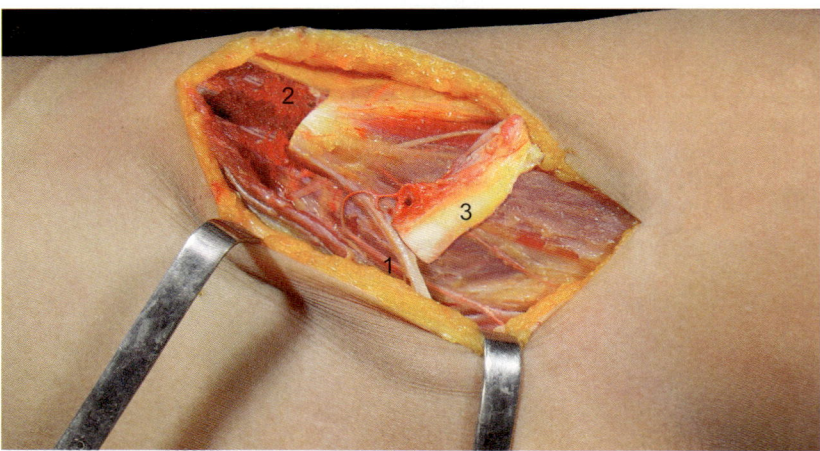

1. Deep iliac circumflex artery
2. Donor site
3. Bone flap

| Figure 3-129 | Transposition of the bone flap |

An anterolateral incision (Smith-Peterson) of the hip should be made downwards and the femoral neck fracture properly repositioned and fixed before the bone flap could be transferred to the recipient site and inserted into the osseous slot.

Key points in applied anatomy

Firstly, the iliac branch of the deep iliac circumflex artery is located at the muscular layer superior to and runs along the iliac crest. The muscular attachment to the superior iliac crest should be incised at 1.0-1.5cm superior to the iliac crest to prevent the vessel from being damaged. Secondly, the iliac flap should be designed at the distal vascular bundle, as distally as possible, so that the flap could be transferred easily to the recipient site. Thirdly, the periosteum should be larger than the bone flap so that it could be spread to cover the femoral neck fractured line and in turn to help the fracture heal up as soon as possible. Fourthly, the rotating arch should be large enough to protect the vascular pedicle from being twisted, stretched or pressed. Fifthly, the iliopsoas muscular surface at medialis anterior superior iliac spine should be dissected with great care to protect the lateral femoral cutaneous nerve from damages. Sixthly, when the transverse abdominal muscle and the obliquus internus abdominis muscle are being dissected, the ilioinguinal nerve and the iliohypogastric nerve should be carefully protected. Seventhly, the femoral triangle should be operated very carefully to protect the femoral artery and nerve from damages.

Iliac Bone Flap Pedicled with Superficial Iliac Circumflex Vessel

22

The small superficial circumflex iliac artery mainly nourishes its surrounding skin and muscle, and a relatively small proportion of the bone. The iliac flap has such advantages as a tenacious lateral bone plate, a porous cancellous bone, a slight warp and a convenient molding. It might be transferred adjacently to repair the defect of the superior femoral bone, the femoral neck fracture, the aseptic necrosis of femoral head or the big cutaneous deficiency.

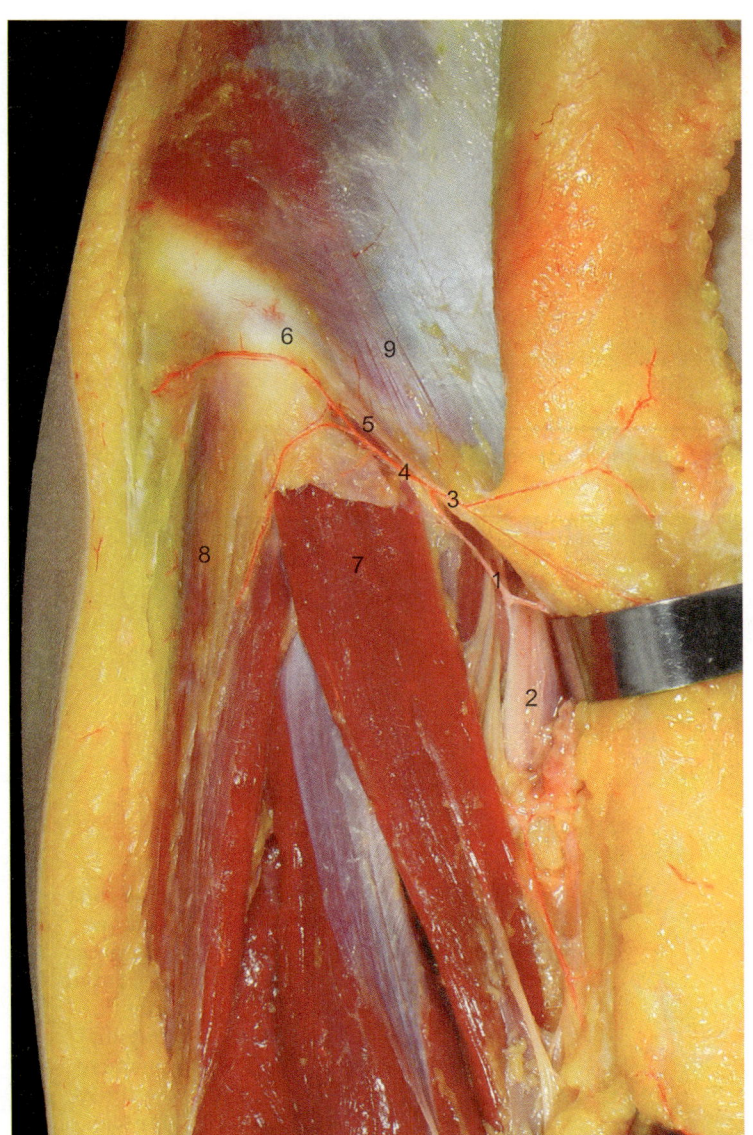

Figure 3-130   Applied anatomy

The initiation of the superficial circumflex iliac artery varies from case to case. Those which emerge from the femoral artery account for 75.1% of the total cases, those from the deep iliac circumflex artery 12.9%, those from the lateral femoral circumflex artery 8%, those from the deep femoral artery 3.5%, and those from the medial femoral circumflex artery 0.5%. Those that emerge from one single branch account for 75.1%, those from the double branch 3%, and those from the shared branch 18%. The superficial circumflex iliac artery is 1.3mm in diameter at its origin. Its main trunk bifurcates into the superficial branch and the deep branch immediately after it emerges. The superficial branch perforates through the femoral fascia and runs inferiorly upwards to the inguinal ligament, and then obliquely laterally downwards. It crosses the plane of the anterosuperior iliac spine and turns upwards to fan out over the lateral half of the inguinal groove and the adjacent skin of the anterior iliac crest. The deep branch runs downwards along the inguinal ligament at the deep fascial sub-surface and perforates through the deep fascia to become a terminal branch. The deep branch gives its affiliated branches before it perforates through the deep fascia to fan out over the adjacent muscle, the periosteum and the cortical bone of the anterior iliac crest.

1. Superficial iliac circumflex artery
2. Femoral artery
3. Superficial branch
4. Deep branch
5. Inguinal ligament
6. Anterosuperior iliac spine
7. Sartorius muscle
8. Tensor muscle of fascia lata
9. Aponeurosis of oblique externus abdominis muscle

273

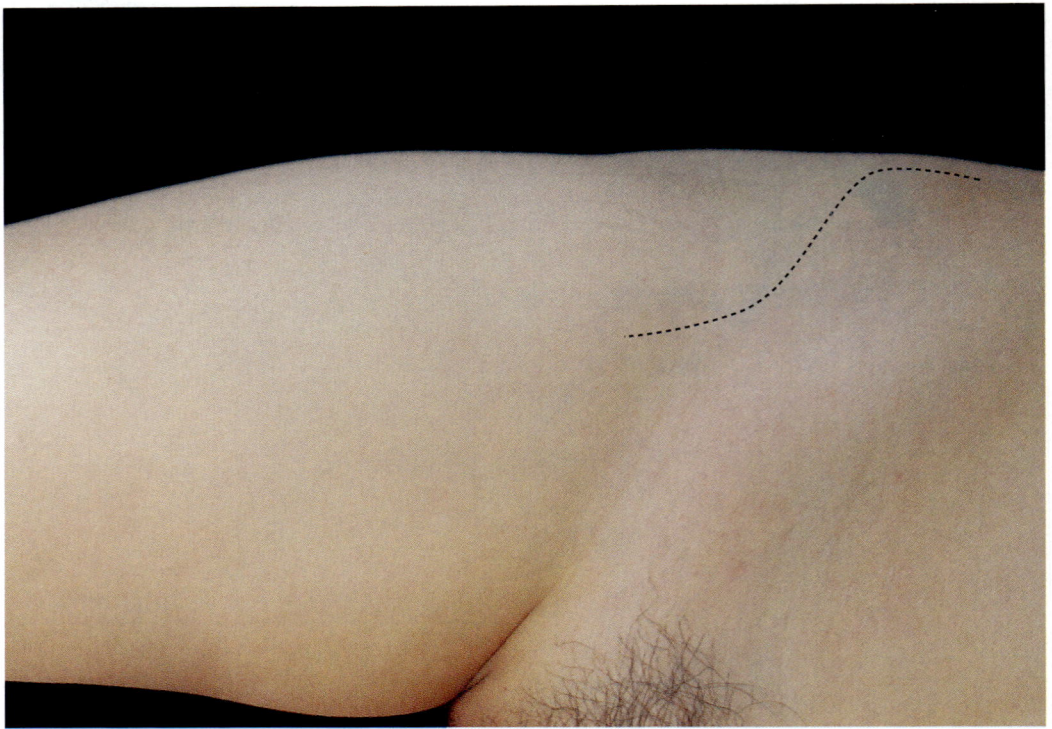

Figure 3-131   Design of the incision

The incision might be drawn along the iliac crest from the midpoint of the medial iliac crest to midpoint of the inguinal ligament and bent towards the anterolateral thigh.

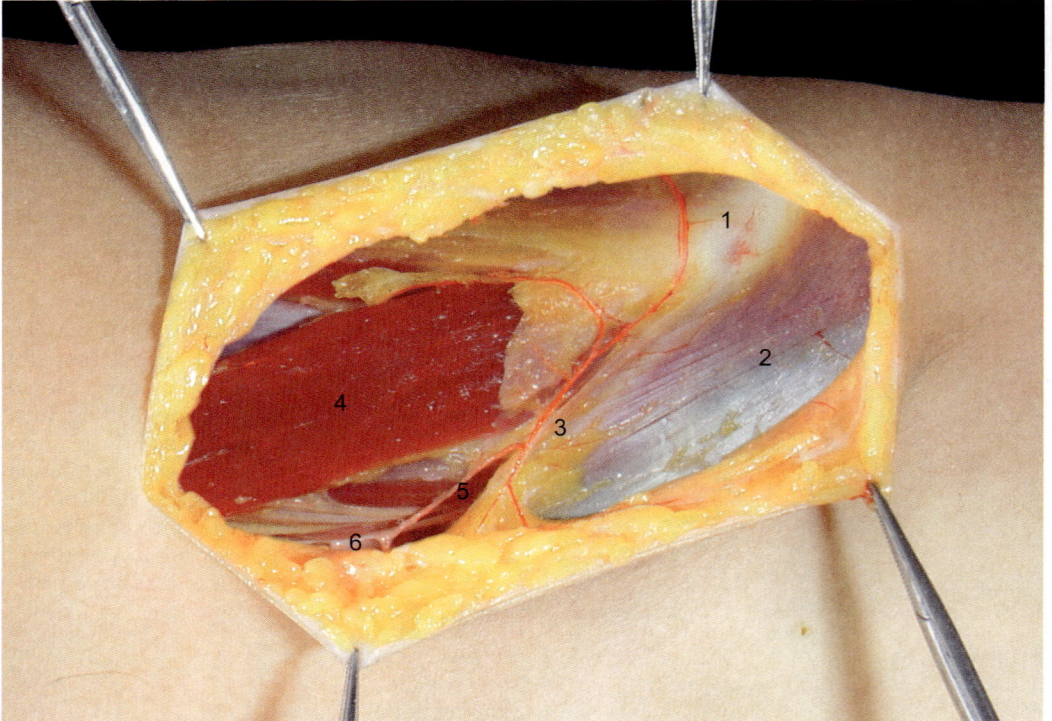

1. Iliac crest
2. Oblique externus abdominis muscle
3. Inguinal ligament
4. Sartorius muscle
5. Superficial iliac circumflex artery
6. Femoral artery

Figure 3-132   Exposure of the muscle

A curved incision should be made from the iliac crest to the midpoint of the inguinal ligament to expose the iliac crest, the oblique externus abdominis muscle and the inguinal ligament.

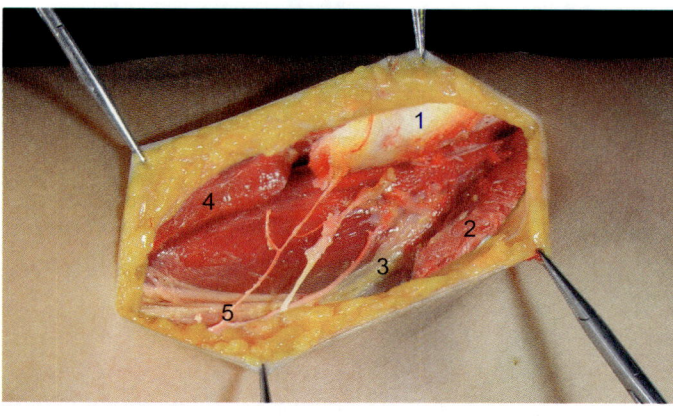

1. Iliac crest
2. Oblique externus abdominis muscle
3. Inguinal ligament
4. Sartorius muscle
5. Superficial iliac circumflex artery

Figure 3-133   Incision of the bone flap

The incised abdominal muscle should be pulled inwards and the deep iliac circumflex vessel ligated. The medial periosteum of the iliac bone should be incised downwards and decohered under the subperiosteum so that an iliac bone block could be chiseled outwards and obtained.

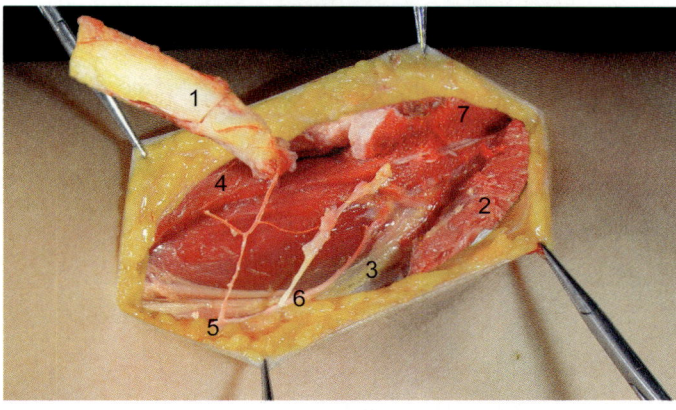

1. Iliac flap
2. Oblique externus abdominis muscle
3. Inguinal ligament
4. Sartorius muscle
5. Superficial iliac circumflex artery
6. Deep branch of superficial iliac circumflex artery
7. Donor site

Figure 3-134   Transposition of the periosteal flap

An anterolateral incision of the hip should be incised downwards to unfold the septum between the tensor muscle of the fascia lata and the sartorius muscle. The rectus femoris muscle should be incised and turned distally to the adjacent anterior inferior iliac spine. The hip articular capsule should be incised to expose the bone fracture and chisel an osseous slot on the femoral neck. The bone flap might be transferred to the recipient site and inserted into the slot via the deep surface of the sartorius muscle. The bone fracture should be fixed with a lag screw.

Key points in applied anatomy

Firstly, the superficial circumflex iliac artery is a cutaneous artery in most cases. It nourishes mainly a small area of the bone and the periosteum. It is suitable to be used as a surgical flap including skin, muscle and bone but a single bone flap for transplantation. Secondly, the deep branch of the superficial circumflex iliac artery extends towards the anterior superior iliac spine around the sartorius muscular membrane, and so the sartorius muscular membrane might be a significant marker for tracing the superficial circumflex iliac artery. Thirdly, when the iliac bone is being chiseled, the tensor muscle of the fascia lata on the outer plate and the part of the mesogluteal initiation should be retained to avoid damaging the superficial circumflex iliac artery which perforates through those tissues and to guarantee a reliable blood supply for the transplantation of the flap. Fourthly, the nutrient vessels should not be dissected when the osseous cutaneous flap is being harvested. Fifthly, the adjacent lateral femoral cutaneous nerve should be protected carefully when the anterior superior iliac spine is being dissected. Sixthly, the superficial circumflex iliac artery and vein extend in the same direction. The superficial circumflex iliac vein should be firstly located and then the deep branch of the superficial circumflex iliac artery traced in most cases.

23

Iliac Bone Flap Pedicled with Ascending Branch of Lateral Femoral Circumflex Vessel

The ascending branch of the lateral femoral circumflex artery runs towards the anterolateral iliac bone to supply the blood for the vicinity of the anterior superior iliac spine. It has a long vascular pedicle and a constant anatomical position so that the operation could be performed very conveniently under the same incision. It might be used mainly to treat the osseous nonunion of the femoral neck and the avascular necrosis of the femoral head.

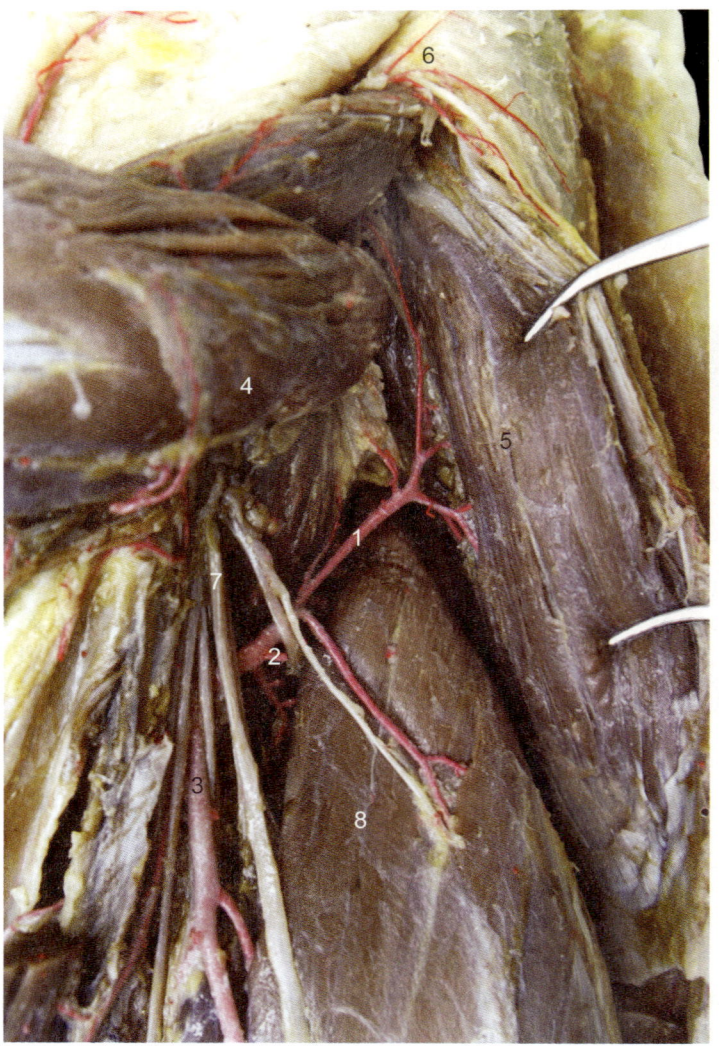

| Figure 3-135 | Applied anatomy |

The lateral femoral circumflex artery emerges from the deep femoral artery and divides into an ascending branch, a transverse branch and a descending branch. The ascending branch enters the tensor muscle of the fascia lata via the lateroposterior rectus femoris muscle to nourish the muscle and the surrounding skin. Its terminal branch anastomoses with the superficial iliac circumflex artery and the gluteal artery near the anterior superior iliac spine to support the iliac bone. The ascending branch is 3.1mm in diameter. It has its accompanying veins. In most cases (64.5%), it has two, which are 3.7mm and 2.6mm in diameter, respectively. In other cases (35.5%), it has only one, which is 5.2mm in diameter.

1. Ascending branch of lateral femoral circumflex artery
2. Transverse branch
3. Descending branch
4. Rectus femoris muscle
5. Tensor muscle of fascia lata
6. Anterior superior iliac spine
7. Femoral nerve
8. Intermediate great muscle

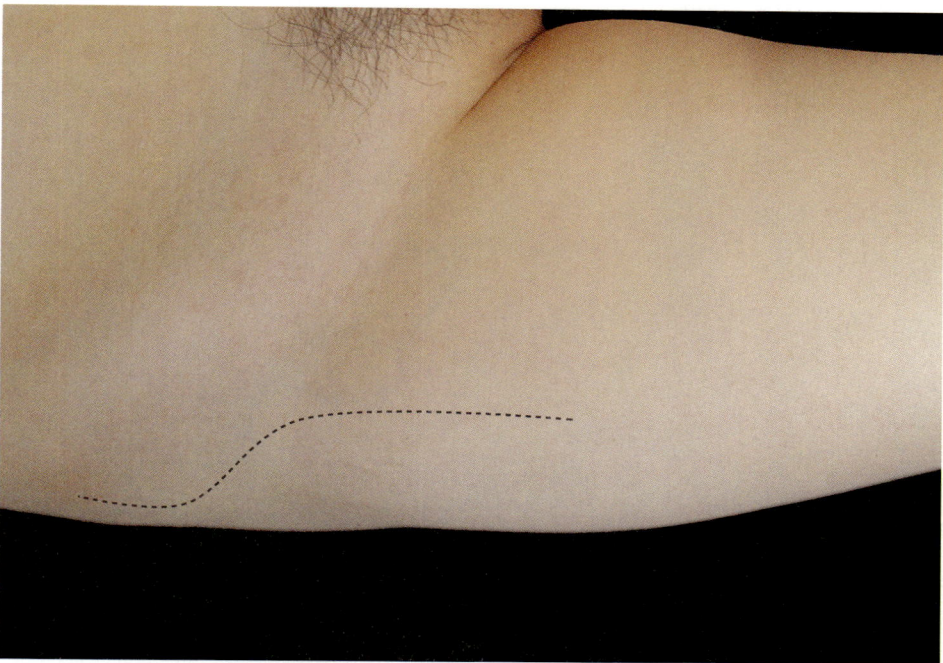

Figure 3-136   Design of the incision

The patient should be placed in supine position, with a flat pillow padded under the buttock. A Smith-Peterson incision should be drawn from the anterior iliac crest to the anterior superior iliac spine via the iliac crest. It then extends slightly outuards for 10-12cm towards the distal part. Its superior and inferior lengths and courses should be adjusted to the demanded sizes of the bone and the periosteal flap, the length of the vascular pedicle and the diseased part of the hip.

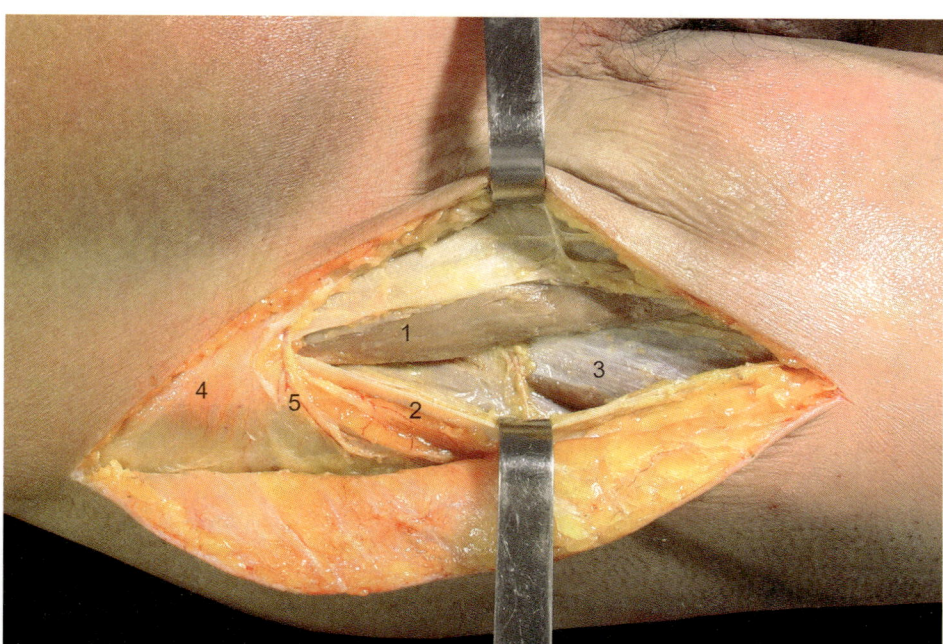

1. Sartorius muscle
2. Tensor muscle of fascia lata
3. Rectus femoris muscle
4. Anterior superior iliac spine
5. Cutaneous branches of superficial iliac circumflex artery (vessel)

Figure 3-137   Exposure of the muscle

The skin and the superficial and deep fascia should be incised, and the lateral femoral cutaneous nerve separated and pulled inwards to expose the sartorius muscle, the tensor muscle of fascia lata and the rectus femoris muscle.

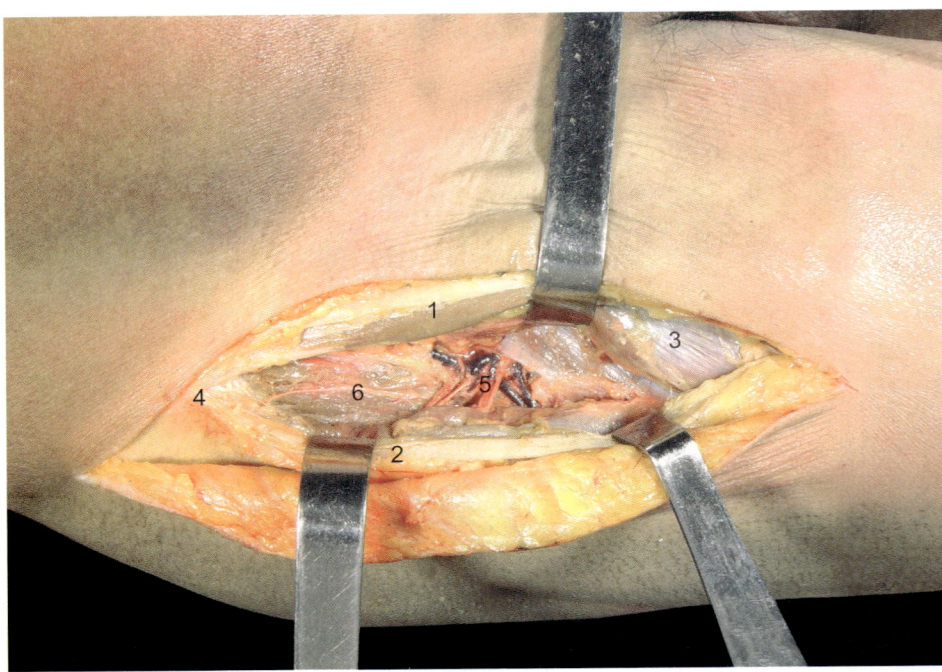

1. Sartorius muscle
2. Tensor muscle of fascia lata
3. Rectus femoris muscle
4. Anterior superior iliac spine
5. Ascending branch of lateral femoral circumflex artery
6. Iliac cristal branch

Figure 3-138   Exposure of the vessel

The deep fascia should be incised via the septum between the sartorius muscle and the tensor muscle of the fascia lata (the rectus femoris muscle might be incised and turned downwards) to expose the vascular bundle of the lateral femoral circumflex vessels. The incision should continue along the ascending branch to expose the vascular branch that enters the muscle and the terminal branch of the iliac crest.

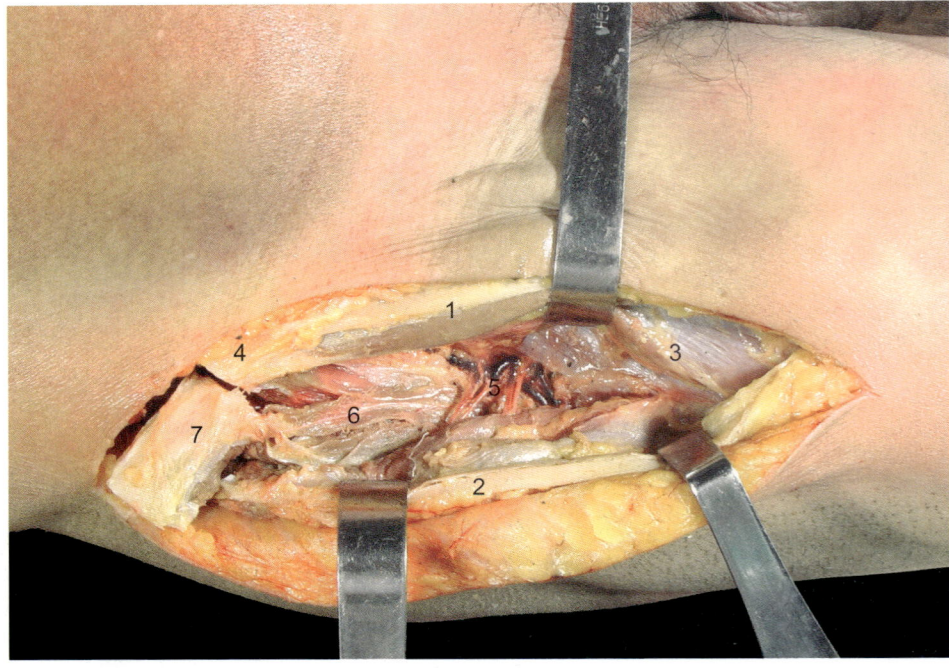

1. Sartorius muscle
2. Tensor muscle of fascia lata
3. Rectus femoris muscle
4. Anterior superior iliac spine
5. Ascending branch of lateral femoral circumflex artery
6. Iliac cristal branch
7. Bone flap

Figure 3-139   Incision of the bone flap

The internal surface of the anterior iliac bone should be stripped, but the lateral muscular attachment of the anterior superior iliac spine and the muscle (3cm) adjacent to the iliac crest should be retained. A proper size of the iliac bone flap should be dissected outwards from the iliac internal plate.

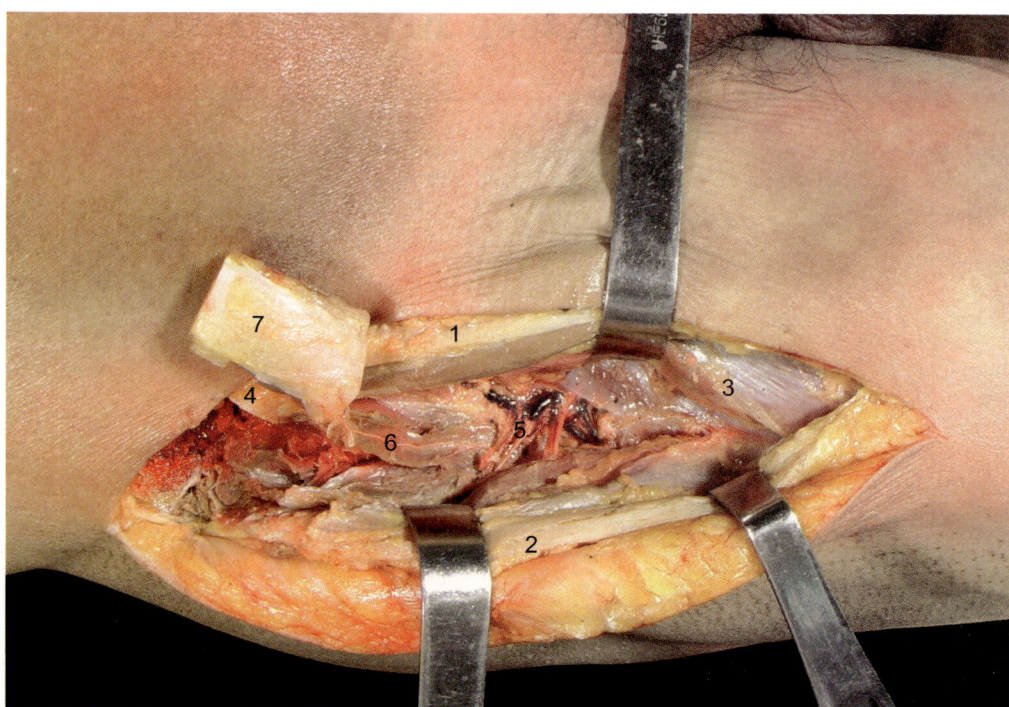

Figure 3-140   Transposition of the periosteal flap

The hip articular capsule should be incised to expose the fractured part of the femoral neck, and an osseous slot chiseled and embed with a pedicled bone block.

1. Sartorius muscle
2. Tensor muscle of fasciae lata
3. Rectus femoris muscle
4. Anterior superior iliac spine
5. Ascending branch of lateral femoral circumflex artery
6. Iliac cristal branch
7. bone flap

Key points in applied anatomy

Firstly, the ascending branch of the lateral femoral circumflex artery transverses over the deep layer of the rectus femoris muscle and extends upwards. When a relatively long vascular pedicle is required, the initiation of the rectus femoris muscle should be cut off and turned downwards so that the main trunk of the ascending branch could be dissected at its initiation. The dissection should be performed closely to the tendinous tissue to avoid damaging the iliac cristal branch. Secondly, there is a complicated relationship between the vastus lateralis muscular branches of the femoral nerve and the initial part of the ascending branch of the lateral femoral circumflex artery. The artery transverses over the femoral nerve at an angle of 70 degree. Both of them attach closely to each other by the connective tissue and should be dissected carefully to avoid getting them damaged. Thirdly, the iliac cristal branch varies in some cases. If the variation is too small, the bone flap should include the gluteus medius muscular branch to guarantee a blood supply through the two vessels.

Iliac Periosteal (bone) Flap Pedicled with Superior Deep Branch of Superior Gluteal Vessel

The superior deep branch of the superior gluteal vessel is the main source to nourish the lateral iliac surface. Based on it, an iliac flap might be made and transferred locally to repair the bone defect of the hip and the sacralis.

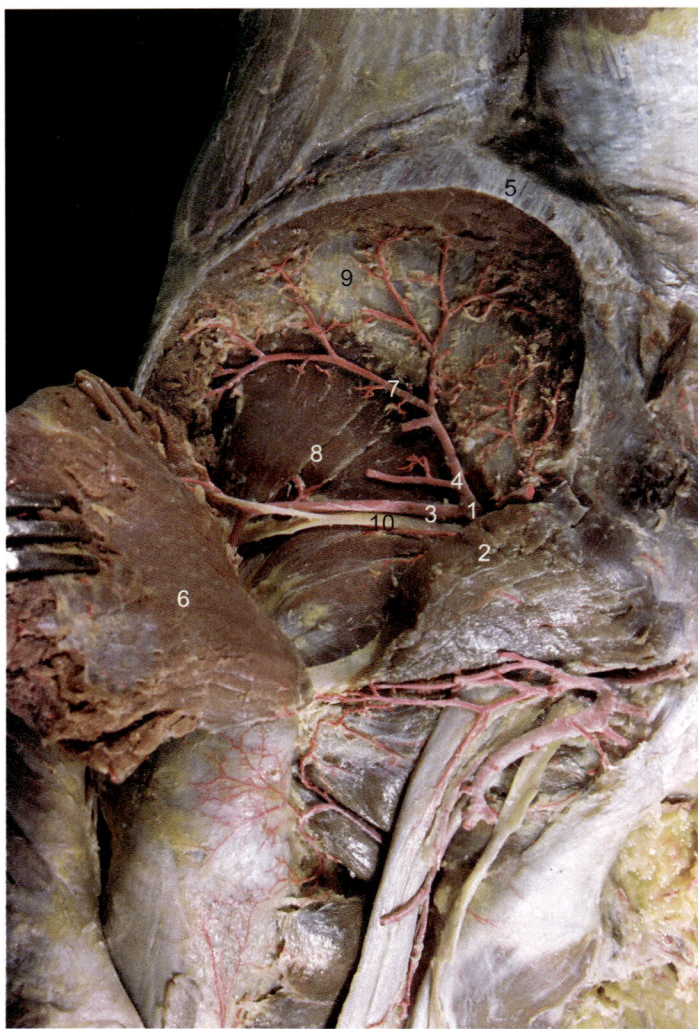

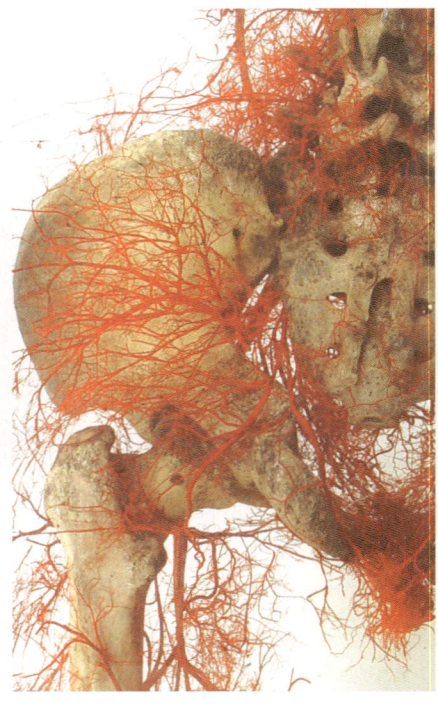

| Figure 3-141 | Applied anatomy |

The superior gluteal artery perforates through the superior margin of the pisiformis muscle and bifurcates immediately into a superficial branch and a deep branch. The superficial branch runs under the deep layer of the gluteus maximus muscle to nourish the gluteus maximus muscle and the gluteus medius muscle. The deep branch bifurcates into a superior branch and an inferior branch under the gluteus medius muscle. The superior deep branch runs along the superior margin of the gluteus minimus muscle, sticking tightly to the external lamina of ilium. It presents itself in an arc shape in the anterosuperior direction. It is 2-4cm from the external lip of the iliac crest and terminates at the lateral margin of the inferior anterior iliac spine.

1. Superior gluteal artery
2. Piriform muscle
3. Superficial branch
4. Deep branch
5. Gluteus maximus muscle
6. Gluteus medius muscle
7. Superior deep branch of superior gluteal artery
8. Gluteus minimus muscle
9. External lamina of ilium
10. Superior gluteal nerve

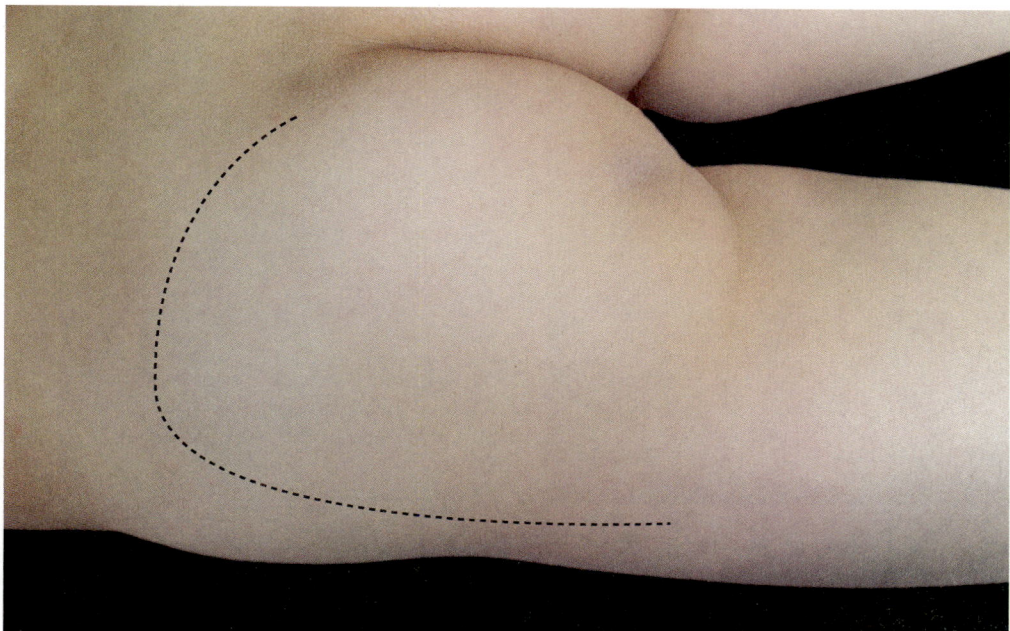

Figure 3-142   Design of the incision

The patient should be placed in the lateral position on its uninjured side. The incision should be drawn forwards from the posterior superior iliac spine to the anterior superior iliac spine along the iliac crest and then turned to the greater trochanter.

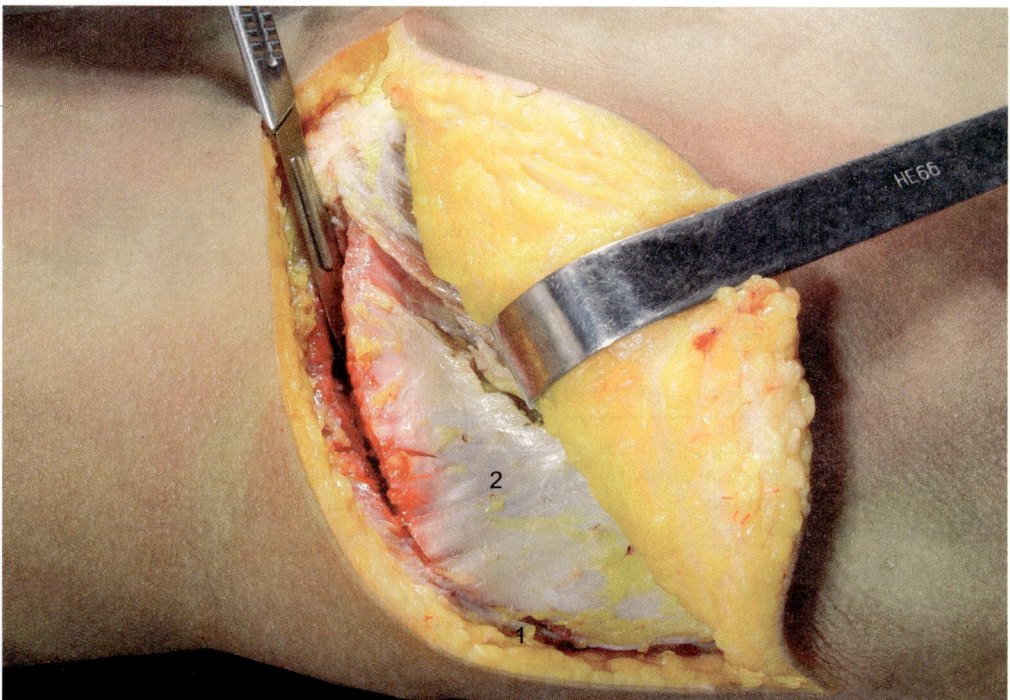

Figure 3-143   Exposure of the muscle

The skin should be incised to expose the gluteus medius muscle and the tensor muscle of the fascia lata. The initiations of both muscles should be cut off and a muscular pedicle retained for 2 cm long.

1. Gluteus medius muscle
2. Gluteus maximus muscle

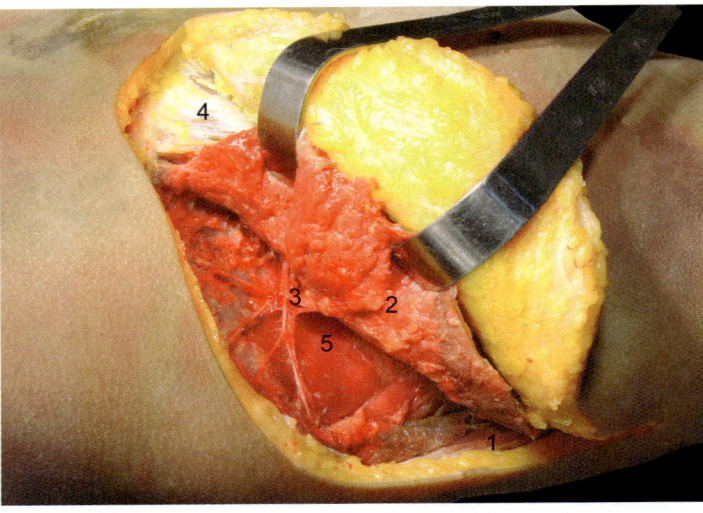

1. Tensor muscle of fascia lata
2. Gluteus medius muscle
3. Superior deep branch of superior gluteal vessel
4. Gluteus maximus muscle
5. Gluteus minimus muscle

Figure 3-144   Incision of the periosteal(bone) flap

The tensor muscle of the fascia lata should be drawn forwards and the gluteus medius muscle turned downwards to expose clearly the superior deep branch of the superior gluteal vessel.

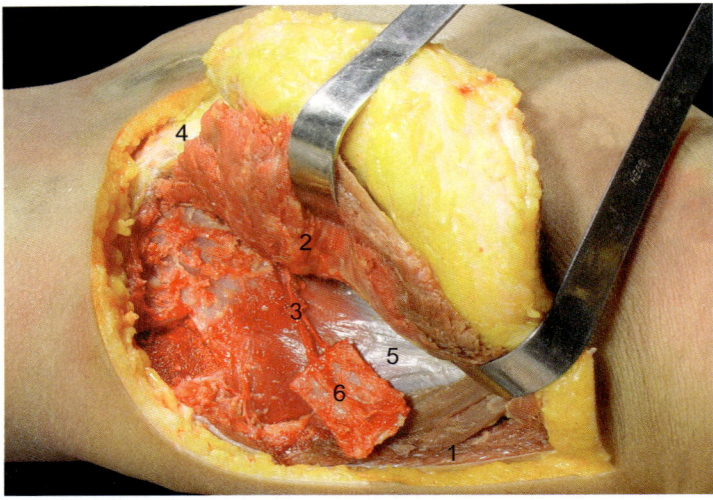

1. Tensor muscle of fascia lata
2. Gluteus medius muscle
3. Superior deep branch of superior gluteal vessel
4. Gluteus maximus muscle
5. Gluteus minimus muscle
6. Iliac flap

Figure 3-145   Chiselation and transposition of the bone flap

Then the inner lamina of the ilium should be stripped under the osseous membrane, and the iliac flap dissected at the gluteal surface in the vascular direction. The iliac flap based on the superior deep branch of the superior gluteal artery might be transferred downwards and fixed on the superior margin of the coxal cavity in the cotyloid shelf operation.

Key points in applied anatomy

Firstly, in the operation the anatomical layers should be identified carefully to avoid a deep incision and a subsequent damage of the superior deep branch of the superior gluteal vessel. The deep branch sticks tightly to the deep layer of the gluteus medius muscle. Secondly, the dissection should be performed along the vessels towards their initiations so that a properly long vascular pedicle could be obtained. Thirdly, the branch of the superior deep branch of the superior gluteal artery enters the iliac nutrient foramen at 1.5cm or so beneath the iliac crest, and so the soft tissue on the iliac gluteal surface, the periosteum and the vascular branches that enter the nutrient foramen should be protected carefully while the vessels are being dissected.

Trochiterian Bone Flap Pedicled with Deep Branch of Medial Femoral Circumflex Vessel or Anastomotic Branch of Inferior Gluteal Vessel

25

The area of the femoral greater trochanter has such advantages as a cancellous bone, an abundant blood supply, a multi-vascular distribution and a multi-muscular attachment. The trochiterian bone flap based on the deep branch of the medial femoral circumflex artery or the anastomotic branch of inferior gluteal artery might be transferred locally to treat the femoral neck fracture and the avascular necrosis of the femoral head.

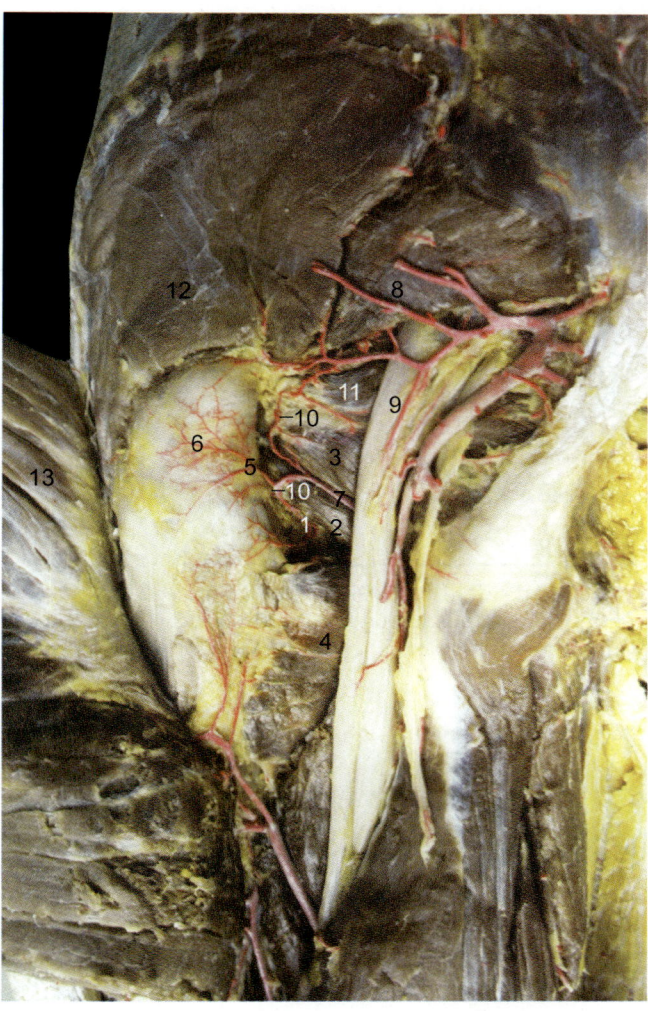

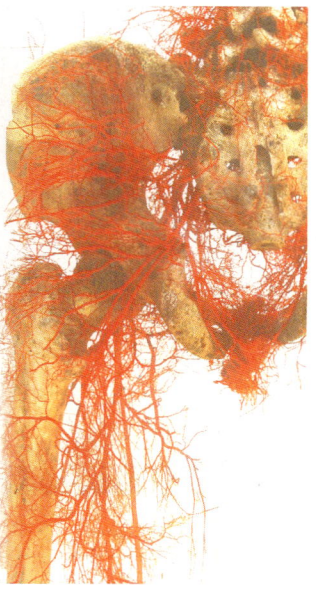

Figure 3-146	Applied anatomy

The deep branch of the medial femoral circumflex artery extends to the posterior hip joint via the septum between the short adductor muscle and the external obturator muscle. It runs laterally-upwards along the posterior basilar part of the femoral neck via the septum between the quadratus femoris muscle and the external obturator muscle. Its terminal part enters the inferior gemellus muscle and the deep layer of the internal obturator muscular tendon. It gives a great trochiterian branch at 6.2mm (on average) beneath the superior margin of the quadratus femoris muscle and 7.9mm from the intertrochanteric crest. It runs outwards and comes superficially via the septum between the quadratus femoris muscle and the inferior gemellus muscle, and transverses over the intertrochanteric crest to fan out over the posterolateral part of the greater trochanter in a claw-like shape. The anastomotic branch of the inferior gluteal artery emerges from the inferior margin of the piriform muscle and descends outwards along the superficial or the deep surface of the sciatic nerve to enter the connective tissue between the inferior gemellus muscle and the quadratus femoris muscle onto the basilar part of the femoral neck. In most cases (78%), its main trunk anastomoses directly with the deep branch of the medial femoral circumflex artery; in other cases (22%), its terminal part divides into several branches to anastomose or to anastomoses dictyoidly with the deep branch. The every branch emerges from the main trunk and distributes directly over the posterosuperior greater trochanter to form an anastomosis net.

1. Deep branch of medial femoral circumflex artery
2. Inferior gemellus muscle
3. Internal obturator muscular tendon
4. Quadratus femoris muscle
5. Trochiterian branch
6. Greater trochanter
7. Anastomotic branch of inferior gluteal artery
8. Piriformis muscle
9. Sciatic nerve
10. Direct anastomosis
11. Gemellus superior muscle
12. Gluteus medius muscle
13. Gluteus maximus muscle

A. Trochiterian bone flap pedicled with deep branch of medial femoral circumflex vessel

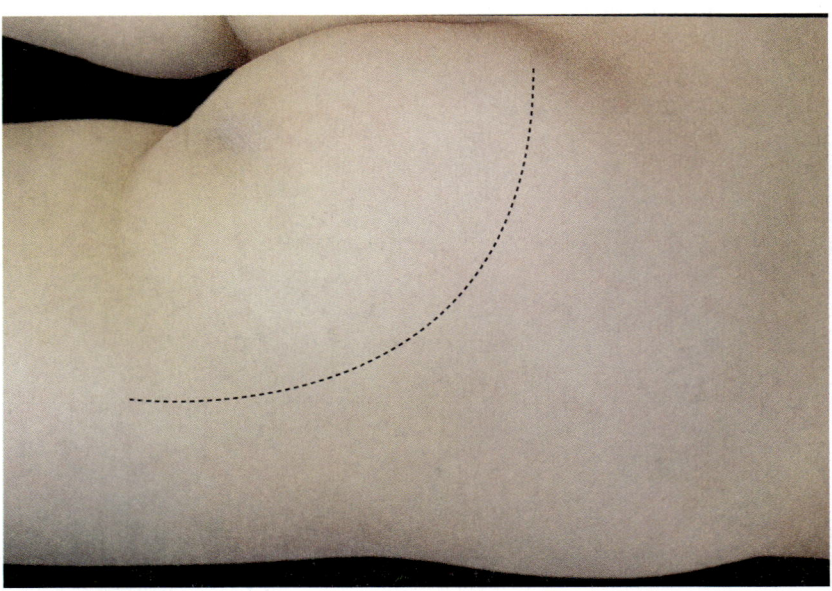

Figure 3-147	Design of the incision

The patient should be placed in the lateral position on the uninjured side. The incision should begin from 3cm beneath the lateroinferior superior iliac spine, continue along the gluteus maximus muscle to the posterosuperior greater trochanter and turn downwards about 5 cm long.

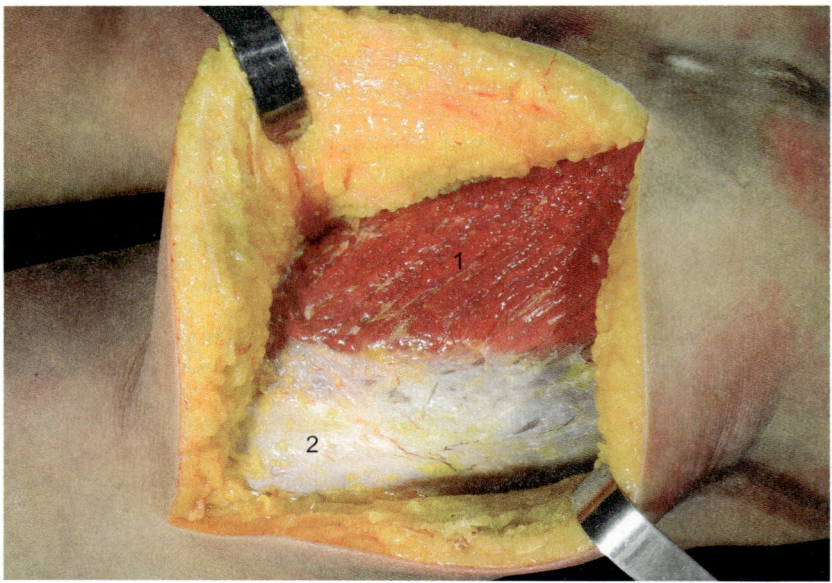

Figure 3-148	Exposure of the muscle

The skin and the subcutaneous tissue should be incised to expose the gluteus maximus muscle.
1. Gluteus maximus muscle
2. Iliotibial tract

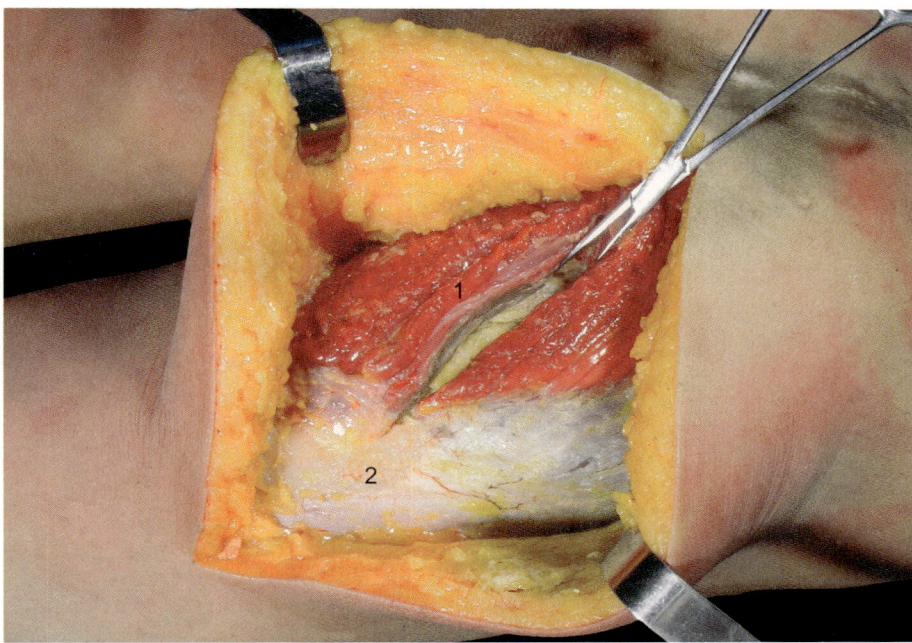

1. Gluteus maximus muscle
2. Iliotibial tract

| Figure 3-149 | Separation of muscle |

The gluteus maximus muscle should be bluntly dissected along its muscular fibers and cut off at its attachment on the iliotibial tract.

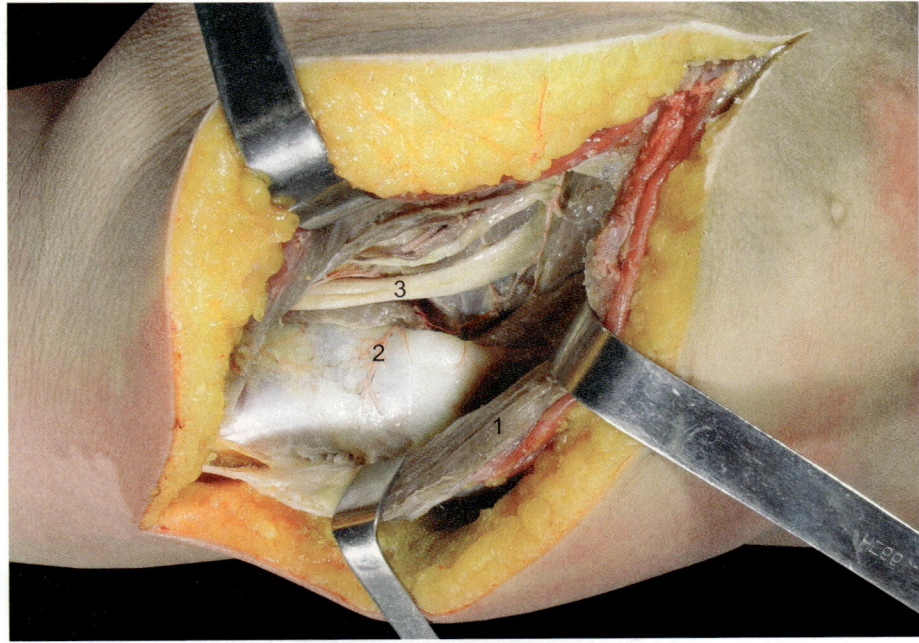

1. Gluteus maximus muscle
2. Trochiterian branch
3. Sciatic nerve

| Figure 3-150 | Exposure for vessels |

Part of the attachment on the femoral bone should be incised and the gluteus maximus muscle pulled bilaterally to expose the external rotator muscle groups. The diseased limb should be rotated inward, and the terminal point of the gluteus medius muscle on the trochiterian point incised and pulled laterally to expose thoroughly the posterior tissue on the femoral neck and the greater trochanter. The trochiterian branches that are distributed in a claw-like shape on the lateral trochiterian osseous surface should be traced carefully in the posterior trochiterian connective tissue. The quadratus femoris muscle should be dissected along the trochiterian branch to expose the deep branch of the medial femoral circumflex artery.

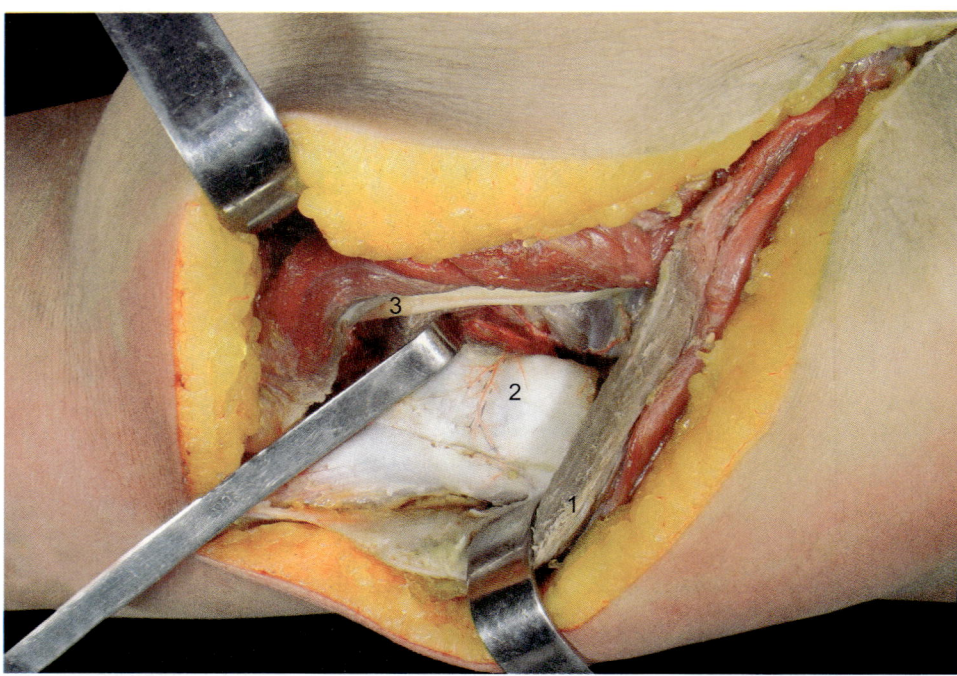

1. Gluteus maximus muscle
2. Trochiterian bone flap
3. Sciatic nerve

| Figure 3-151 | Incision of the bone flap |

A stripe-shaped bone block should be chiseled on the posterior greater trochanter as is needed. The nutrient vessel of the bone flap should not be damaged.

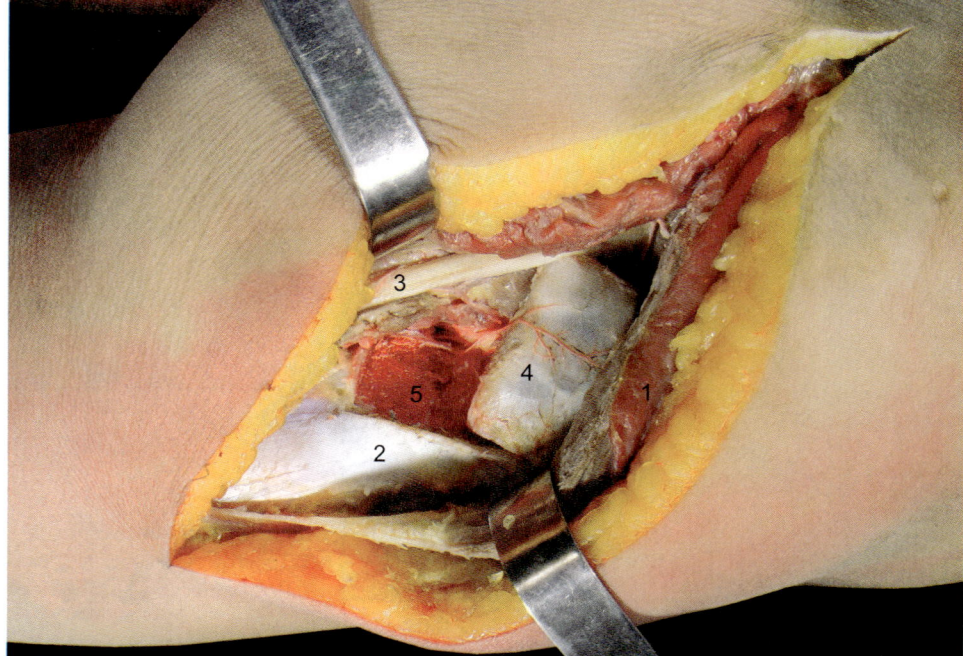

1. Gluteus maximus muscle
2. Greater trochanter
3. Sciatic nerve
4. Bone flap
5. Donor site

| Figure 3-152 | Transposition of the bone flap |

The hip capsule should be incised in an inverse T-shape, restored and internally fixed. The transferred osseous bed should be chipped with an osseous chisel on the cortical bone of the posterior femoral neck. An osseous hole (1-1.5cm in depth) should be chiseled in the femoral head so that the trochiterian part of the bone flap could be rotated and implanted into the osseous slot inside the femoral head and so that the bone flap could be attached tightly with the transferred osseous bed in the posterior femoral neck.

B. Trochiterian bone flap pedicled with anastomotic branch of inferior gluteal artery

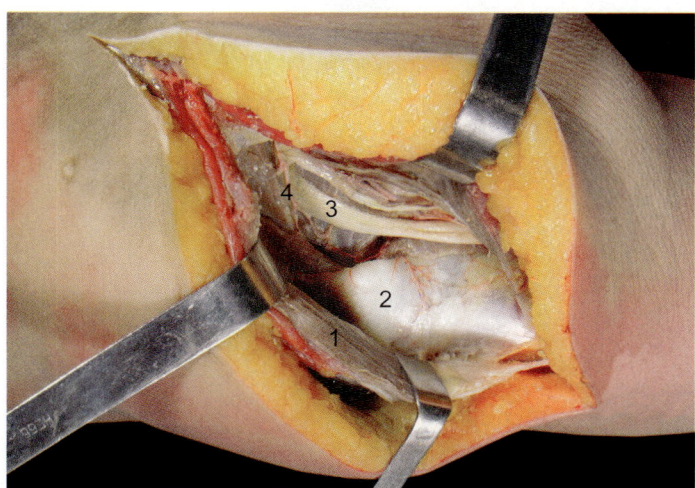

1. Gluteus maximus muscle
2. Greater trochanter
3. Sciatic nerve
4. Anastomotic branch

| Figure 3-153 | Exposure of the vessel |

The design of the incision, the exposure and dissection of the muscle might be illustrated in Fig. 3-147, 3-148, and 3-149. The gluteus maximus muscle should be pulled inwards and outwards to expose the greater trochanter, the external rotator muscle group and the sciatic nerve. The sciatic nerve and the anastomotic branch of the inferior gluteal artery that transverses the sciatic nerve should be identified clearly. The incision should trace laterally downwards along the anastomotic branch and continue through the septum between the quadratus femoris muscle and the inferior gemellus muscle to the intertrochanteric crest. The terminal part of the quadratus femoris muscle should be subsequently incised to expose the deep branch of the medial femoral circumflex artery and its trochiterian branches. The anastomotic part between the anastomotic branch and the deep branch should be kept intact. Then the main trunk of the deep branch of the medial femoral circumflex artery and its distal terminal branch should be ligated and cut off.

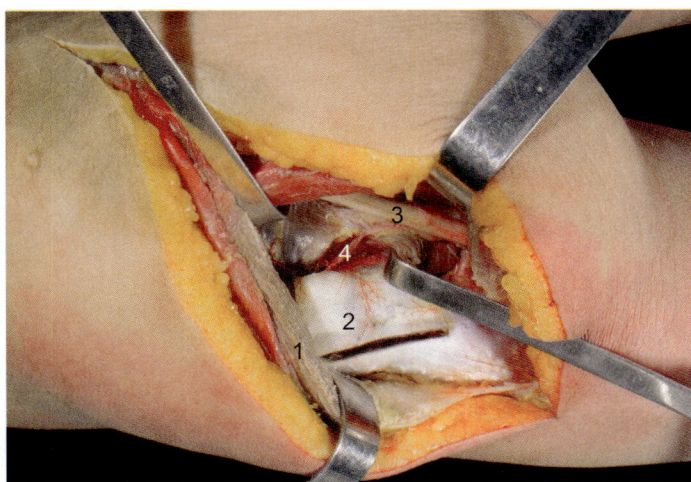

1. Gluteus maximus muscle
2. Trochiterian bone flap
3. Sciatic nerve
4. Anastomotic branch

| Figure 3-154 | Chisel of the bone flap |

The main trunk of the deep branch of the medial femoral circumflex artery and its distal terminal branch should be ligated and cut off at the proximal anastomotic part. Partial initiation of the vastus lateralis muscle should be pushed downwards. A bone flap should be chiseled on the posterolateral greater trochanter with its longitudinal axis falling in the same direction of the main trunk of the trochiterian branch.

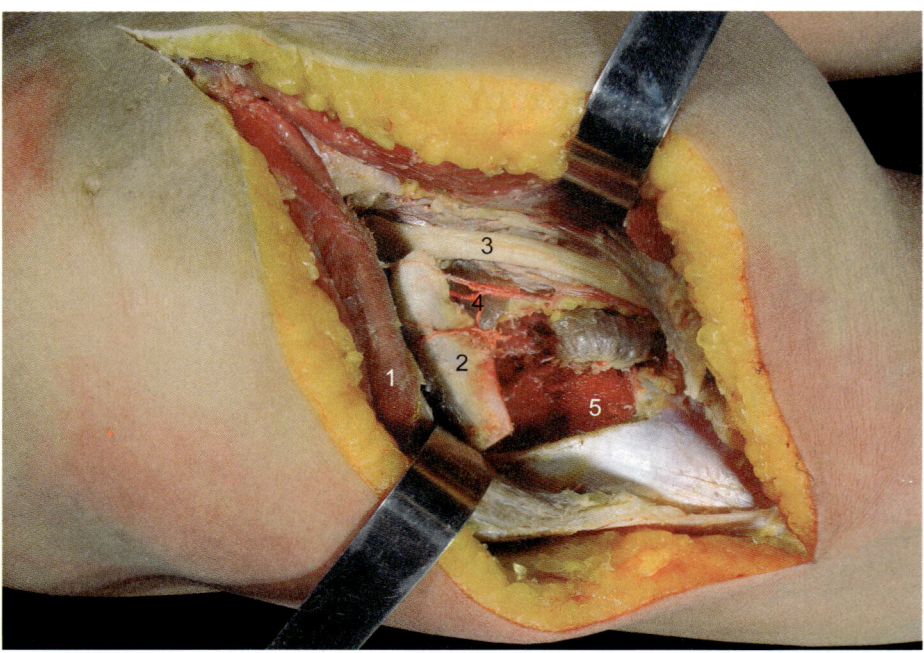

| Figure 3-155 | Transposition of the bone flap |

The hip capsule should be incised in a reverse T-shape to bring the femoral head out of it. The diseased osseous tissue should be removed and the chipped bone flap transferred to the stump of the femoral head and fixed with a kirschner wire.

1. Gluteus maximus muscle
2. Trochiterian bone flap
3. Sciatic nerve
4. Anastomotic branch
5. Donor site

Key points in applied anatomy

Firstly, the anastomotic branch of the inferior gluteal artery that anastomoses with the deep branch of the medial femoral circumflex artery should be traced and confirmed carefully in the septum between the quadratus femoris muscle and the inferior gemellus muscle. If it does exist, the main vessel that forms the arterial loop or both of the two arteries should be adopted as a pedicle. Secondly, the vascular pedicle should be examined carefully to confirm whether it has been pressed at its perforating point through the hip capsule. Thirdly, the limb of the avascular necrosis of the femoral head should be treated postoperatively with skin traction for two weeks and freed from bearing weight for 3-6 months. The duration should be lengthened in cases of the reconstruction of the femoral head. Fourthly, the terminal tendon of the gluteus maximus muscle should be incised at a part as close to the glutaeal crest as possible. Fifthly, the trochiterian bone flap based on the anastomotic branch of inferior gluteal artery might be transferred with the adductor muscle routinely relieved and the diseased tissue of the femoral head thoroughly removed. Sixthly, the bone flap should be aligned tightly with the stump of the femoral head without a vacant space, and fixed with two Kirschner wires to prevent the bone flap from dislocated. Seventhly, the remained space should be thoroughly hemostased to prevent a haematoma formation.

Trochiterian Bone Flap Pedicled with Ascending Branch of 1st Perforating Vessel

26

The 1st perforating artery might have such advantages as a constant anatomical location and an abundant blood supply. A bone flap based on it might be transferred mainly to repair the bone fracture and the defect on the femoral superior segment.

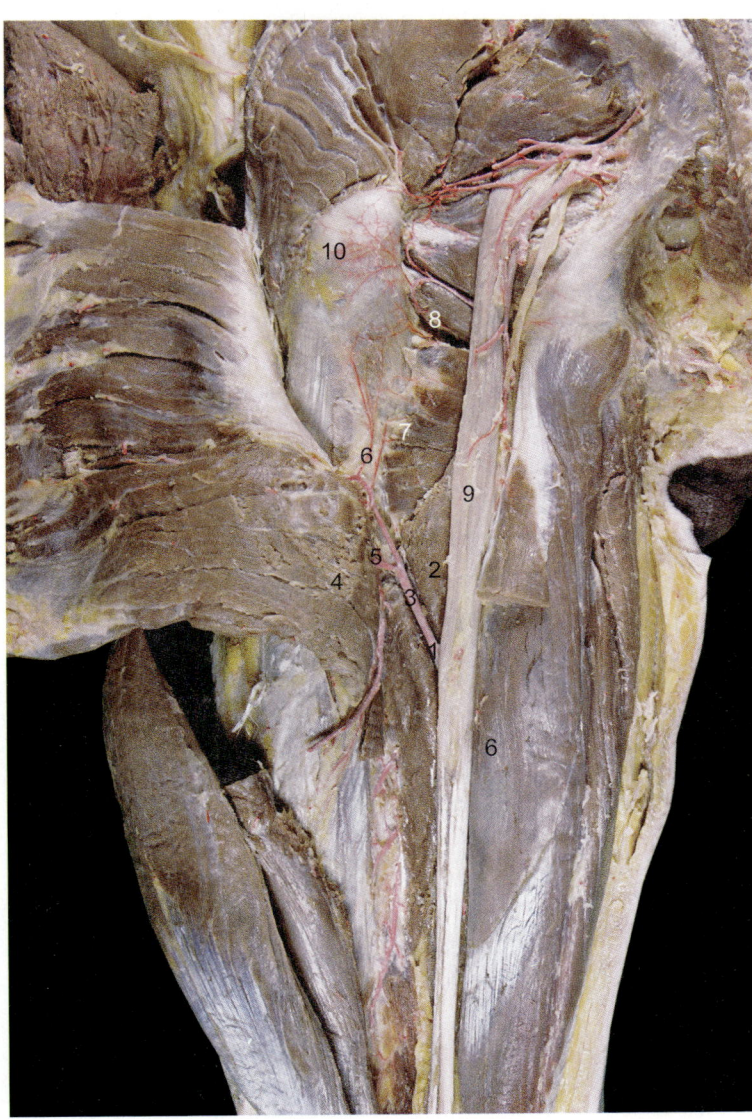

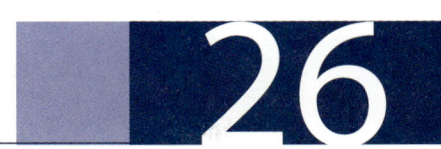

Figure 3-156   Applied anatomy

The 1st perforating artery perforates through the great adductor muscle at about 4.6cm beneath the tip of the femoral lesser trochanter, attaching tightly to the medial femoral shaft. It immediately bifurcates into ascending and descending branches. The ascending branch runs closely to the medial terminal tendon of the gluteus maximus muscle at about 3mm laterosuperior to the gluteal tuberosity, and along its course it gives 1-4 gluteus muscular branches. There is a prevalent muscular branch that enters the gluteus maximus muscle at the inferior margin of the trochanter. The terminal part of the ascending branch turns into the trochiterian branch and ascends to the posteroinferior greater trochanter to fan out in a claw-shape over the terminal point of the quadratus femoris muscle and its lateral posteroinferior greater trochanter. The trochiterian branch of the ascending branch of the 1st perforating artery anastomoses constantly with the deep branch of the medial femoral circumflex artery in the trochiterian periosteum around the terminal point of the quadratus femoris muscle.

1. 1st perforating artery
2. Great adductor muscle
3. Ascending branch
4. Gluteus maximus muscle
5. Gluteus muscular branch
6. Trochiterian branch
7. Quadratus femoris muscle
8. Deep branch of medial femoral circumflex artery
9. Sciatic nerve
10. Greater trochanter

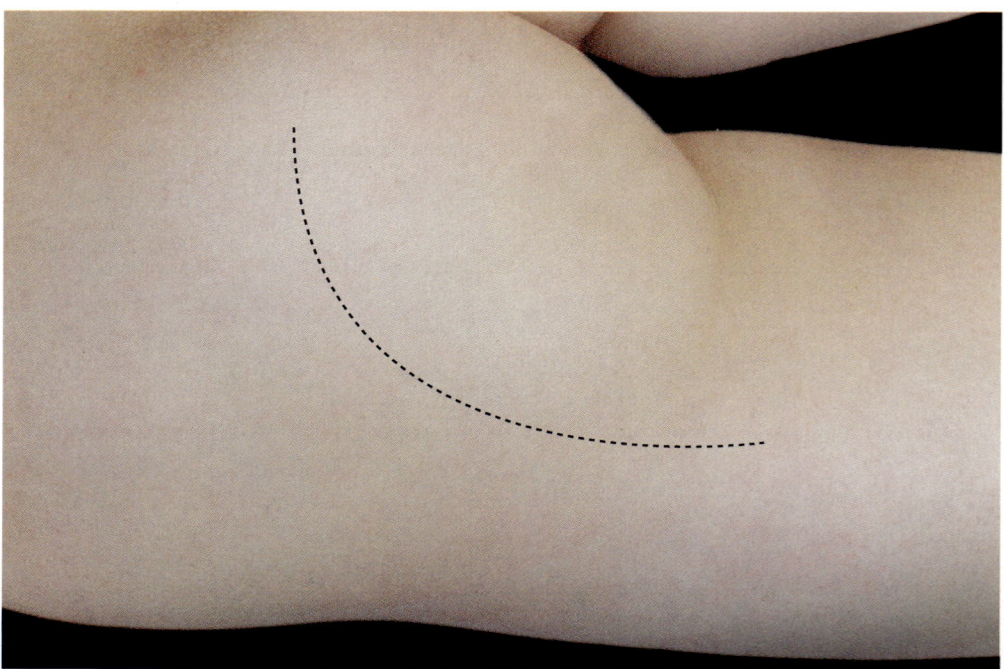

| Figure 3-157 | Design of the incision |

The incision should be drawn laterally downwards at 3 cm to the posterior superior iliac spine, and extend along the gluteus maximus muscular fibers to the great trochanter until it reaches the distal diseased part.

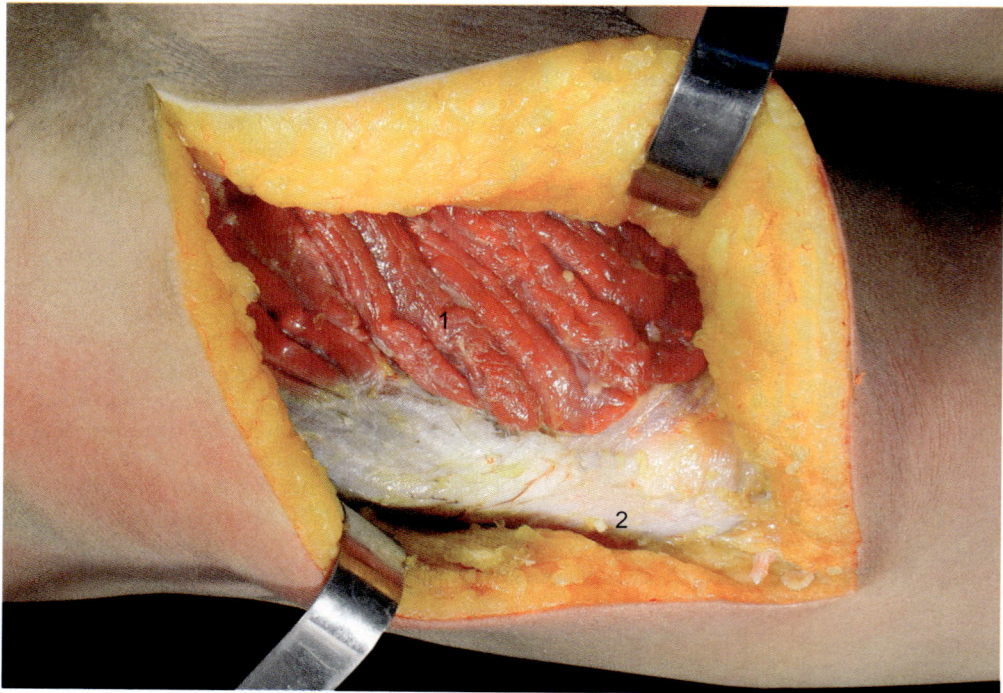

| Figure 3-158 | Exposure of the muscle |

The skin and the subcutaneous tissue should be incised to expose the gluteus maximus muscle.

1. Gluteus maximus muscle
2. Iliotibial tract

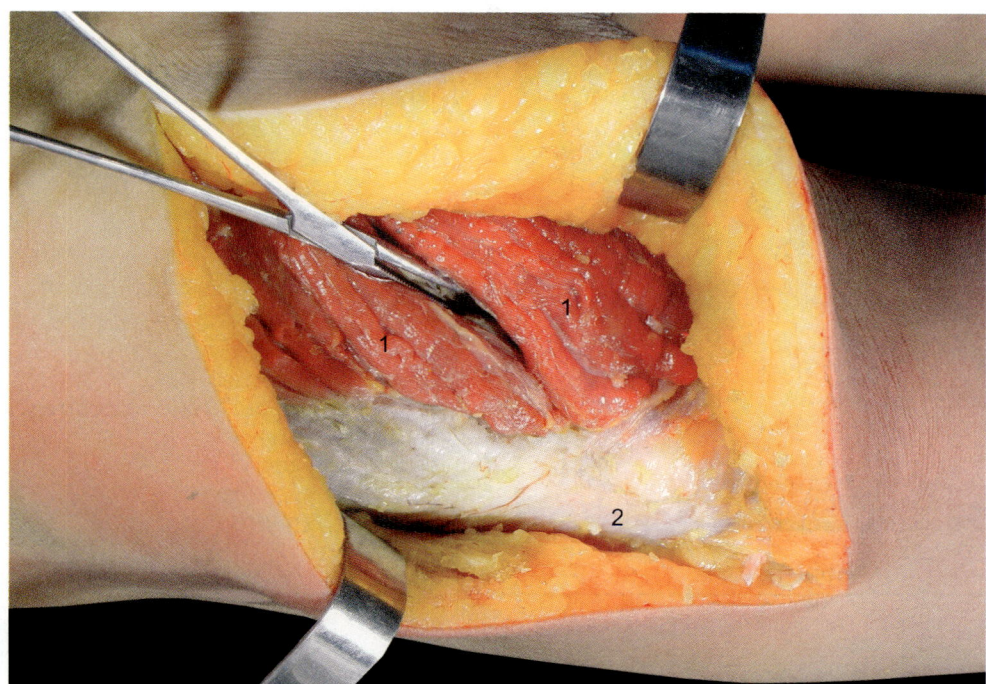

1. Gluteus maximus muscle
2. Iliotibial tract

Figure 3-159   Dissection of the muscle

The gluteus maximus muscle should be dissected bluntly in the direction of the muscular fibres.

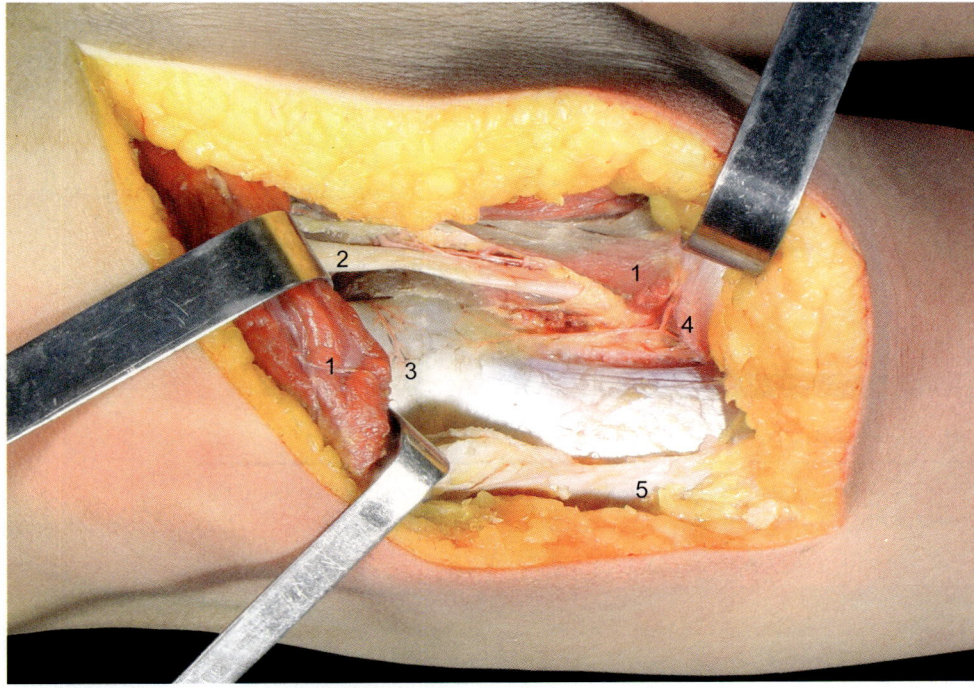

1. Gluteus maximus muscle
2. Sciatic nerve
3. Greater trochanter
4. Ascending branch of 1st perforating artery
5. Iliotibial tract

Figure 3-160   Exposure of the vessel

The iliotibial tract should be incised longitudinally downwards, and the terminal tendon of the gluteus maximus muscle on the gluteal tuberosity should be incised. The medial part of the gluteus maximus muscle, the long head of biceps muscle and the sciatic nerve should be pulled medially and the lateral gluteus maximus muscle laterally to expose the femoral greater trochanter and the main trunk of the ascending branch of the 1st perforating artery.

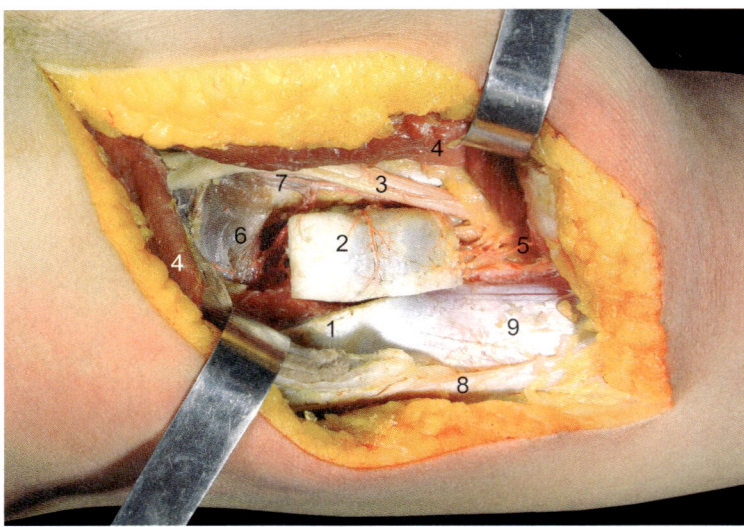

1. Greater trochanter
2. Bone flap
3. Sciatic nerve
4. Gluteus maximus muscle
5. Ascending branch of 1st perforating artery
6. Inferior gemellus muscle
7. Inferior gluteal artery
8. Iliotibial tract
9. Vastus lateralis muscle

Figure 3-161	Incision of the bone flap

A stripe-shaped bone flap should be chiseled on the posterior greater trochanter as large as is needed. It should be about 6×3×2cm in volume and about 6×5cm in size.

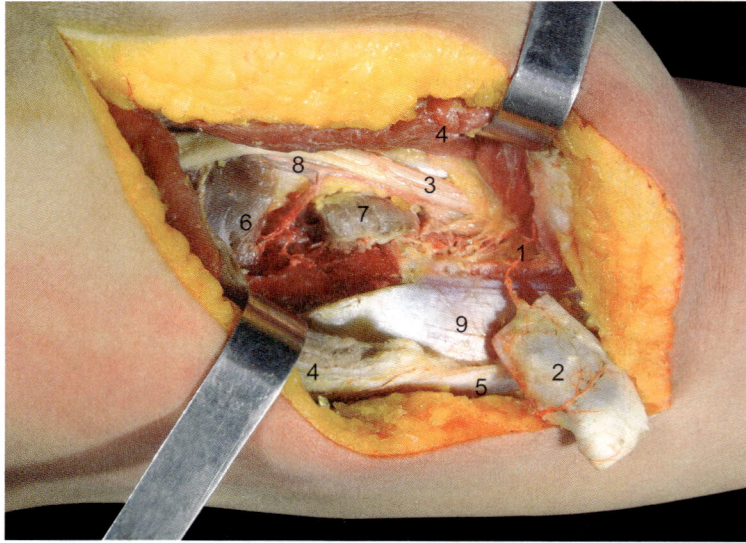

1. Ascending branch of 1st perforating artery
2. Bone flap 3. Sciatic nerve
4. Gluteus maximus muscle
5. Iliotibial tract
6. Inferior gemellus muscle
7. Quadratus femoris muscle
8. Inferior gluteal artery
9. Vastus lateralis muscle

Figure 3-162	Transposition of the bone flap

The bone fracture should be restored and fixed internally before the pedicled trochiterian bone flap or the periosteal bone is transferred to the donor site.

Key points in applied anatomy

Firstly, the routine posterior approach to the hip is preferred. The incision should be distally extended. Secondly, the 1st perforating artery might be traced along the inferior margin of the quadratus femoris muscle when the long head of the biceps femoris and the sciatic nerve are pulled inwards and the lateral gluteus maximus muscle outwards. Thirdly, the branches of the 1st perforating artery should be ligated one by one along its course. Fourthly, the 1st perforating vessel might be damaged or even broken when the bone fracture of the femoral greater trochanter occurs. If so, a wide pedicle (1.5-2cm) of the deep fascial should be dissected upwards together with the main trunk of the ascending branch from the proximal segment of the bone fracture to the posteroinferior greater trochanter.

Trochiterian Bone Flap Pedicled with Transverse Branch of Lateral Femoral Circumflex Vessel

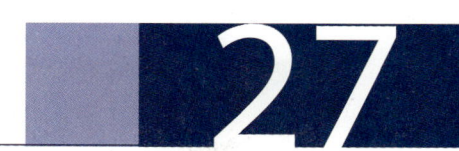

The anterolateral greater trochanter might obtain its blood supply from the transverse branch of the lateral femoral circumflex artery. Its bone flap might have such advantages as an abundant blood supply, a constant vascular course and a relatively long vascular pedicle. A bone flap based on it might be transferred upwards to repair the bone fracture or the osseous nonunion in the femoral head and neck. It might also be transferred downwards to repair the bone fracture or the osseous nonunion in the middle-superior segments of the femur.

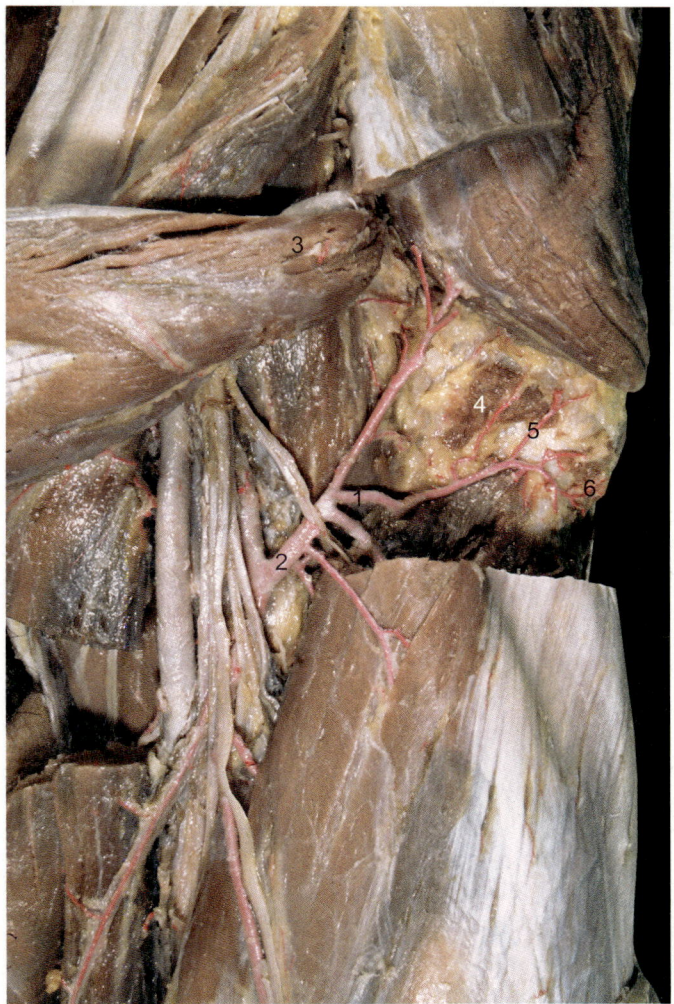

| Figure 3-163 | Applied anatomy |

The transverse branch of the lateral femoral circumflex artery is one of the branches of the lateral femoral circumflex artery. It runs outwards to the muscular porta of the tensor muscle of the fascia lata via the deep surface of the rectus femoris muscle. Its main trunk gives muscular branches to the vastus lateralis muscle and continues laterally upwards to the inferior greater trochanter via the deep layer of the vastus lateralis muscle. It gives 2-4 anterior and lateral branches on the deep surface to form a vascular net on the anterolateral greater trochanter.

1. Transverse branch of lateral femoral circumflex artery
2. Lateral femoral circumflex artery
3. Rectus femoris muscle
4. Greater trochanter
5. Anterior branch
6. Lateral branch

293

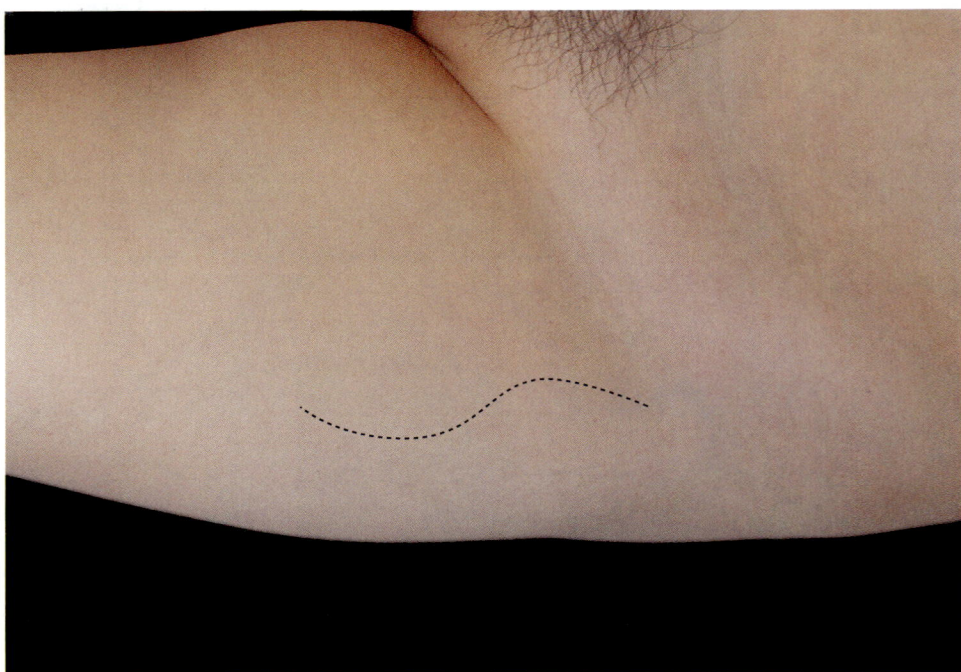

| Figure 3-164 | Design of the incision |

An incision in the S-shape should be drawn and fall on the connecting line between the anterior superior iliac spine and the lateral patellar margin.

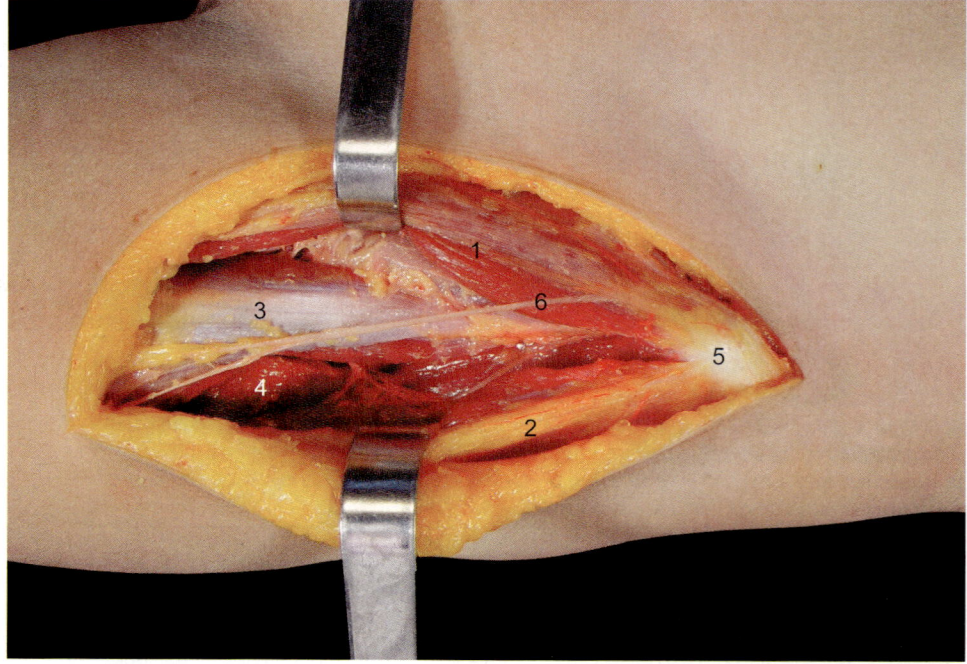

1. Sartorius muscle
2. Tensor muscle of fascia lata
3. Rectus femoris muscle
4. Vastus lateralis muscle
5. Anterior superior iliac spine
6. Lateral femoral cutaneous nerve

| Figure 3-165 | Exposure of the muscle |

A curved incision might be made downwards from the anterior superior iliac spine and the flap dissected and lifted bilaterally under the deep fascia. The sartorius muscle should be pulled inwards, and the tensor muscle of the fascia lata outwards to expose the rectus femoris muscle and the vastus lateralis muscle.

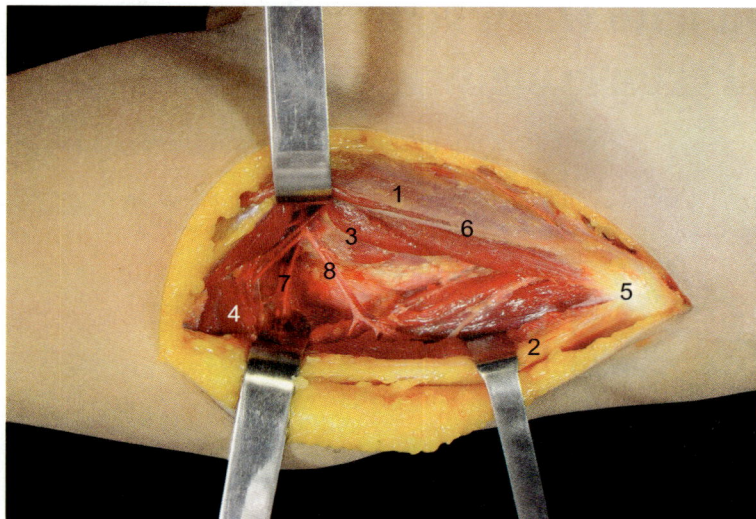

1. Sartorius muscle
2. Tensor muscle of fascia lata
3. Rectus femoris muscle
4. Vastus lateralis muscle
5. Anterior superior iliac spine
6. Lateral femoral cutaneous nerve
7. Transverse branch of lateral femoral circumflex artery
8. Ascending branch of lateral femoral circumflex artery

Figure 3-166   Exposure of the vessel

The rectus femoris muscle should be pulled inwards to expose the transverse branch of the lateral femoral circumflex artery on the deep surface of the rectus femoris muscle. The vessel should be separated in the vascular direction and the muscle incised under the direct visus to expose the transverse branch and the femoral greater trochanter at 2cm inferior to the origin of the vastus lateralis muscle.

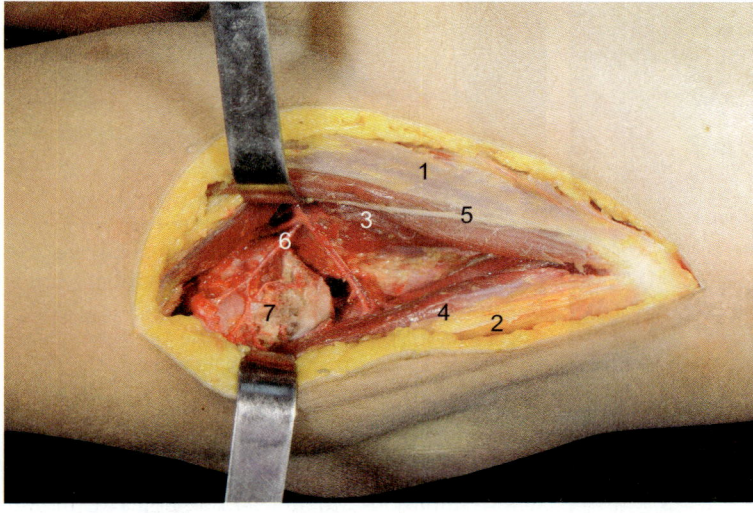

1. Sartorius muscle
2. Tensor muscle of fascia lata muscle
3. Rectus femoris muscle
4. Vastus lateralis muscle
5. Lateral femoral cutaneous nerve
6. Transverse branch of lateral femoral circumflex artery
7. Bone flap

Figure 3-167   Incision of the bone flap

A bone flap about 3.5×3.5×2.0 cm in size should be chiseled on the anterolateral greater trochanter. It could also carry simultaneously a periosteal flap that is larger than it. It might be transferred upwards to repair the femoral neck fracture or downwards to treat the osseous nonunion in the middle-superior segment of the femur.

Key points in applied anatomy

Firstly, the transverse branch of the lateral femoral circumflex artery runs behind the branch of the femoral nerve, which should be separated and kept intact when the vascular pedicle of the bone flap is being dissected. Secondly, the vascular pedicle should be long enough to reach the middle-superior segment of the femoral bone in most cases. The main trunk of the lateral femoral circumflex artery might be ligated when a longer vascular pedicle is necessary. In this way the bone flap might obtain its blood supply retrogradely from its ascending branch.

Femoral Periosteal (bone) Flap Pedicled with Deep Femoral Vessel and its Perforating Branches

The deep femoral vessel and the branches of its perforators might serve as the main source to nourish the posterior shaft of the femur. The vessels might have such advantages as a constant anatomical position and a multiple vessel sources available. A periosteal (bone) flap based on it might be large enough to treat bone fractures and osseous nonunion in any femoral segments, and those in the femoral head and neck.

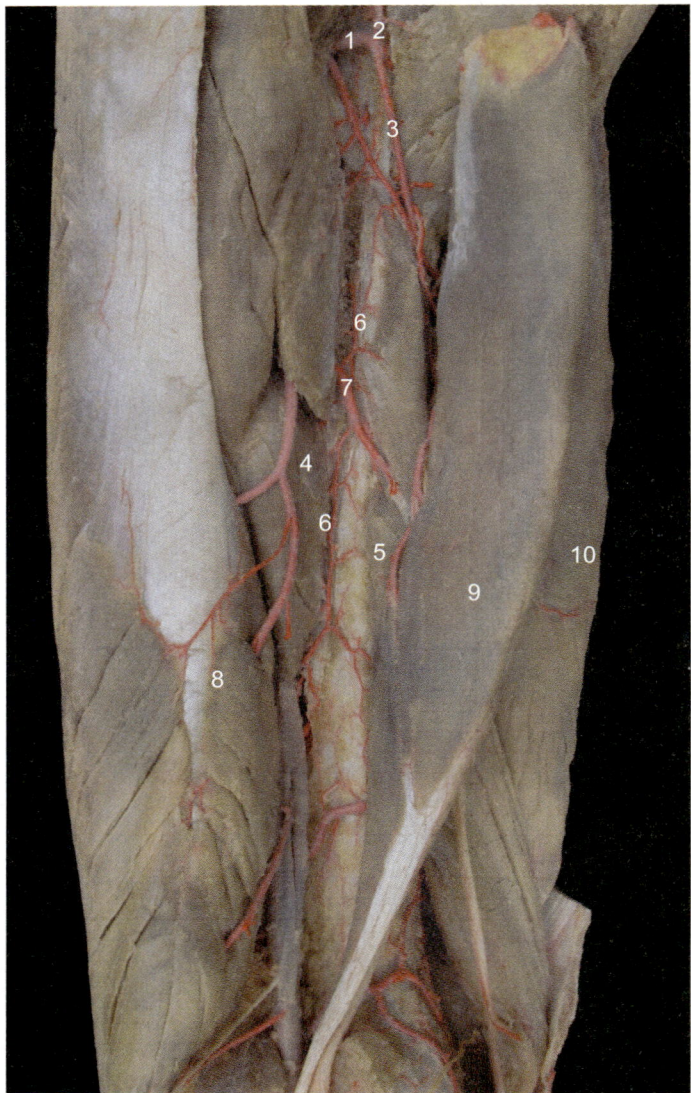

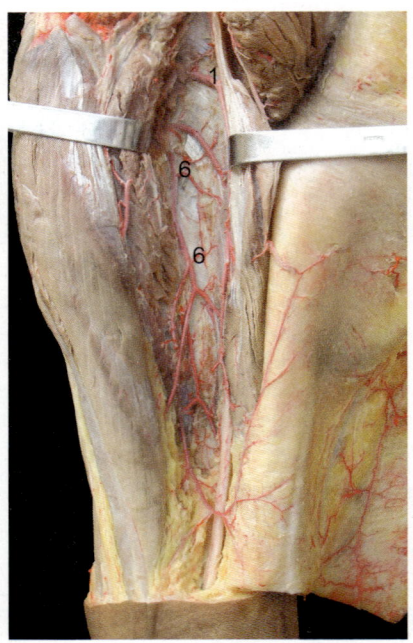

| Figure 3-168 | Applied anatomy |

The deep femoral artery descends along the posterolateral femoral artery to reach the posterior femur via the adductor muscle. Its main trunk descends gradually close to the posteromedial femur via the septum among the great, the short and the long adductor muscles. It runs along the posteromedial femoral crest between the great adductor muscle and the adductor muscular terminal tendon to give 3-4 perforating branches, whose initiations are at 4.5cm, 9.3cm, 14.6cm and 16cm respectively beneath the trochanter tip. Of all the branches, the 1st one might be the largest. It divided into two branches. The ascending branch reaches the greater trochanter and the descending branch runs medially downwards. The 2nd and the 3rd ones perforate obliquely through the great adductor muscle and extend in the septum between the great adductor muscle and the biceps femoris muscle. The 4th one is actually a small terminal branch of the deep femoral artery. All the perforating branches give musculoperiosteal branches to anastomose with one another and fan out over the femoral crest and its bilateral surfaces. The distal deep femoral artery gives an anastomotic branch to anastomose with the popliteal artery.

1. 1st perforating branch
2. Ascending branch
3. Descending branch
4. Great adductor muscle
5. Short head of biceps femoris muscle
6. Musculoperiosteal branch
7. 2nd perforating artery
8. Semimembranous muscle
9. Semitendinosus muscle
10. Long head of biceps femoris muscle

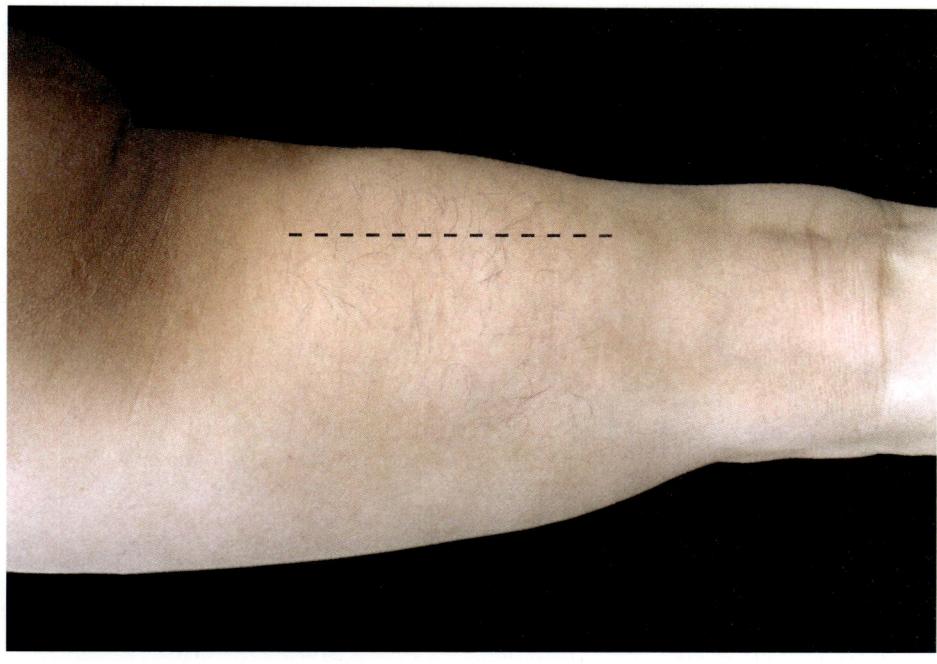

| Figure 3-169 | Design of the incision |

A longitudinal incision is preferred on the middle part of the posterior femur.

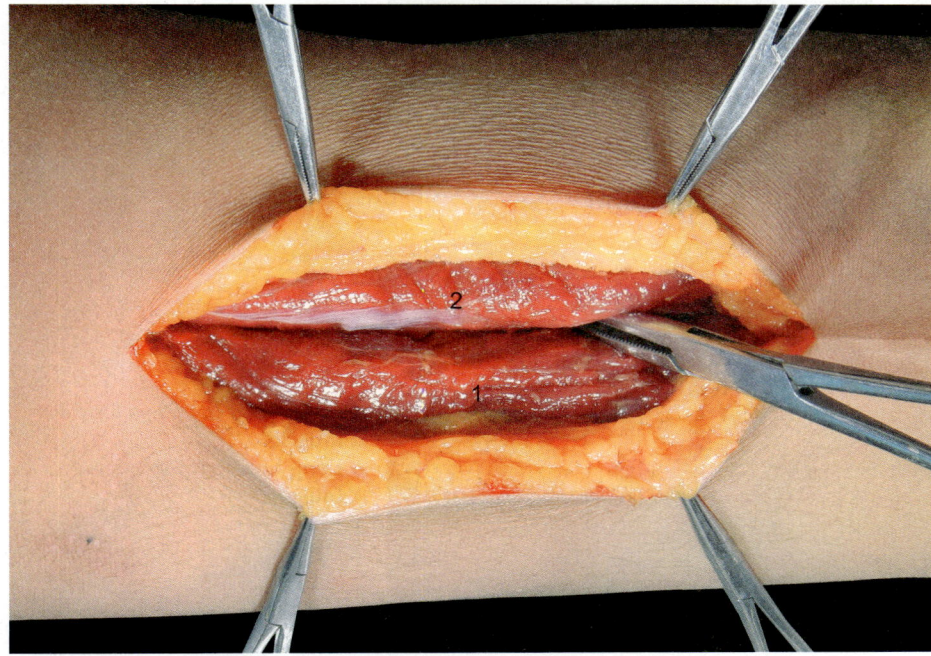

1. Long head of biceps femoris muscle
2. Short head of biceps femoris muscle

| Figure 3-170 | Exposure of the muscle |

The skin, the deep and the superficial fascia should be incised longitudinally to expose the long head of the biceps femoris muscle, the semitendinosus muscle and the semimembranous muscle. The long head and the short head of the biceps femoris muscle as well as the vastus lateralis muscle should be bluntly dissected.

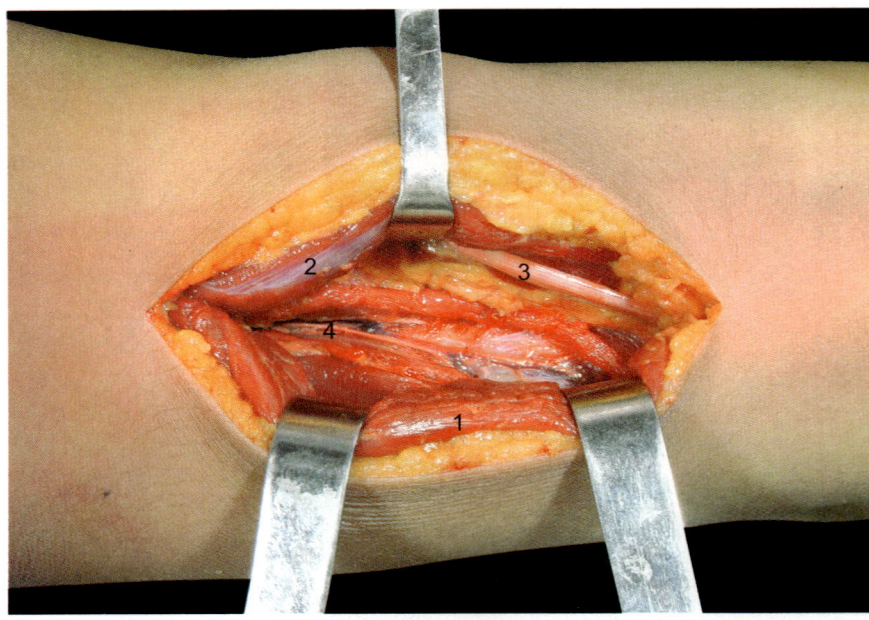

1. Short head of biceps femoris muscle
2. Long head of biceps femoris muscle
3. Sciatic nerve
4. Deep femoral vessel

| Figure 3-171 | Exposure of the vessel |

The short head of the biceps femoris muscle, the vastus lateralis muscle and the posterior femoral cutaneous nerve should be pulled outwards; the long head of the biceps femoris muscle, the sciatic nerve, the semitendinosus muscle and the semimembranous muscle pulled inwards; and the septum between the biceps femoris muscle and vastus lateralis muscle enlarged along the lateral margin of the biceps femoris muscle to expose the muscle, the deep femoral vessel and its branches.

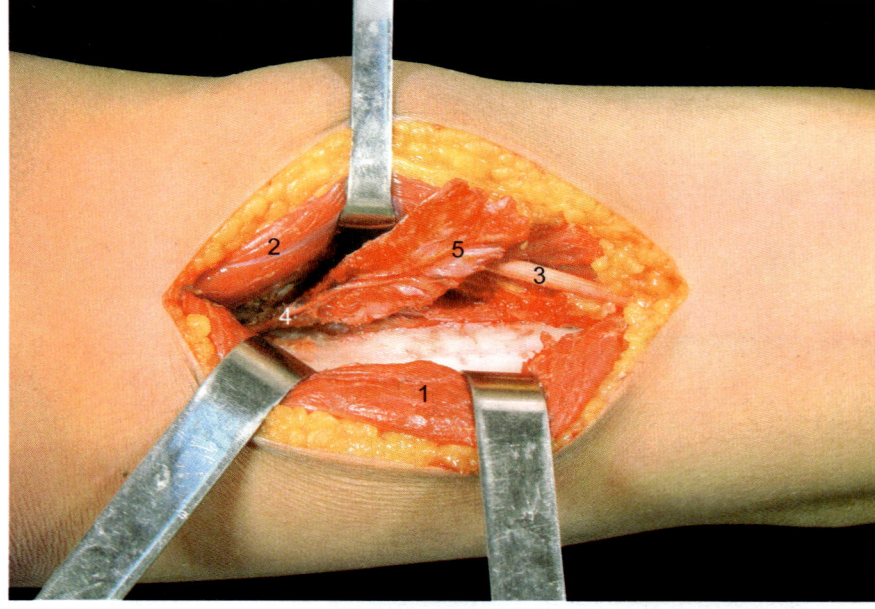

1. Short head of biceps femoris muscle
2. Long head of biceps femoris muscle
3. Sciatic nerve
4. Deep femoral blood vessel
5. Periosteal flap

| Figure 3-172 | Incision of the periosteal flap |

The vascular pedicle might be chosen and traced to the periosteal branch according to the donor site. There are three design options. The femoral periosteal flap might be pedicled with the deep femoral vascular perforating branch, with the deep femoral vessel or with the distal anastomotic branch of the deep femoral vessel. The incised periosteal flap should be lifted so that its vascular pedicle could be dissected for a transposition to the donor site.

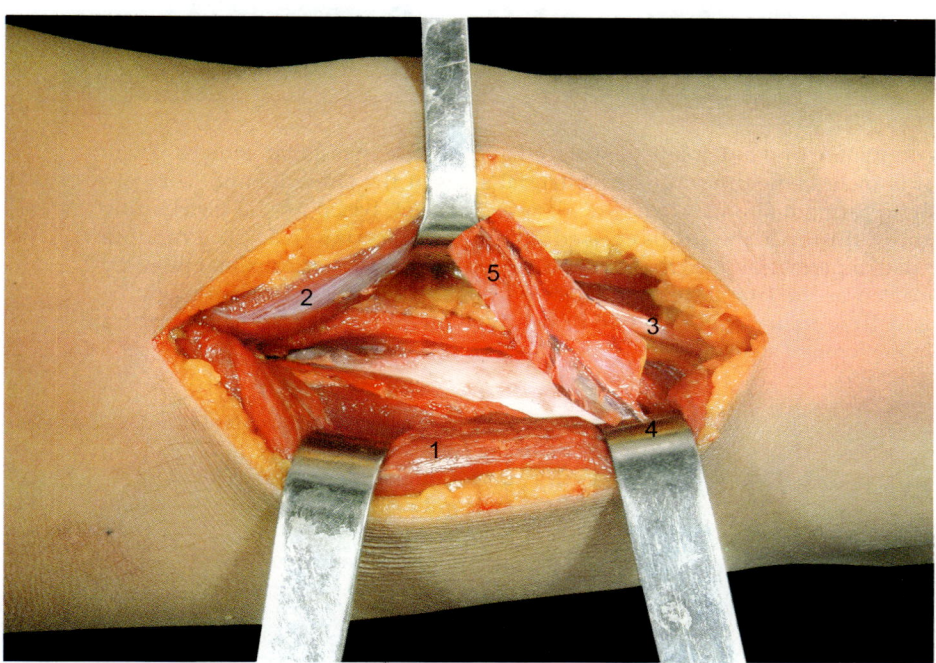

| Figure 3-173 | Retrograde transposition of the flap |

The periosteal flap could be designed with the distal anastomotic branch of the deep femoral vessel as its pedicle and transferred retrogradely for the repair of a diseased part. The chiseled periosteal flap should be lifted so that vascular pedicle could be dissected and transferred to the donor site.

1. Short head of biceps femoris muscle
2. Long head of biceps femoris muscle
3. Sciatic nerve
4. Anastomotic branch
5. Periosteal flap

Key points in applied anatomy

Firstly, there are three types of periosteal flap that might be designed and incised, taking the deep femoral vascular perforating artery as its pedicle. Type A refers to the femoral periosteal flap pedicled with the deep femoral vascular perforator, type B the femoral periosteal flap pedicled with the perforating branch of the deep femoral vessel, and type C pedicled with the distal anastomotic branch of the deep femoral vessel. Secondly, the sciatic nerve mainly gives its branches inwards along its course on the posterior femur and so the sciatic nervous lateral approach might be safe in the operation. Thirdly, the nerve should be properly protected. Fourthly, a thin layer of the muscular sleeve should be retained on the surface of the periosteal flap. Fifthly, the muscle should be dissected bluntly to enlarge the operative visual field, and the long head of the biceps femoris muscle should not be separated unless it is necessary. Sixthly, the periosteal flap could be designed with the distal anastomotic branch as an alternative when the main trunk of the deep femoral vessel is damaged.

29 Periosteal Flap of Femur Anterolateral Surface with Blood Supply

The periosteal vessels on the femoral anterolateral surface have abundant vascular sources. There are 11 direct periosteal branches emerging from the bilateral sides of the femoral bone. They are distributed segmentally to form an abundant and regular vascular net. Based on the distributing feature, the periosteum in this area should be incised adjusted to a certain rule. The random periosteal (bone) flap with a periosteal pedicle should be incised at the distal or proximal diseased area with its pedicle located at the lateral of the periosteal (bone) flap. The operation might be performed with ease and 1ittle injury, and so a flap of this type might be transferred to repair a defect at any position in the femoral shaft.

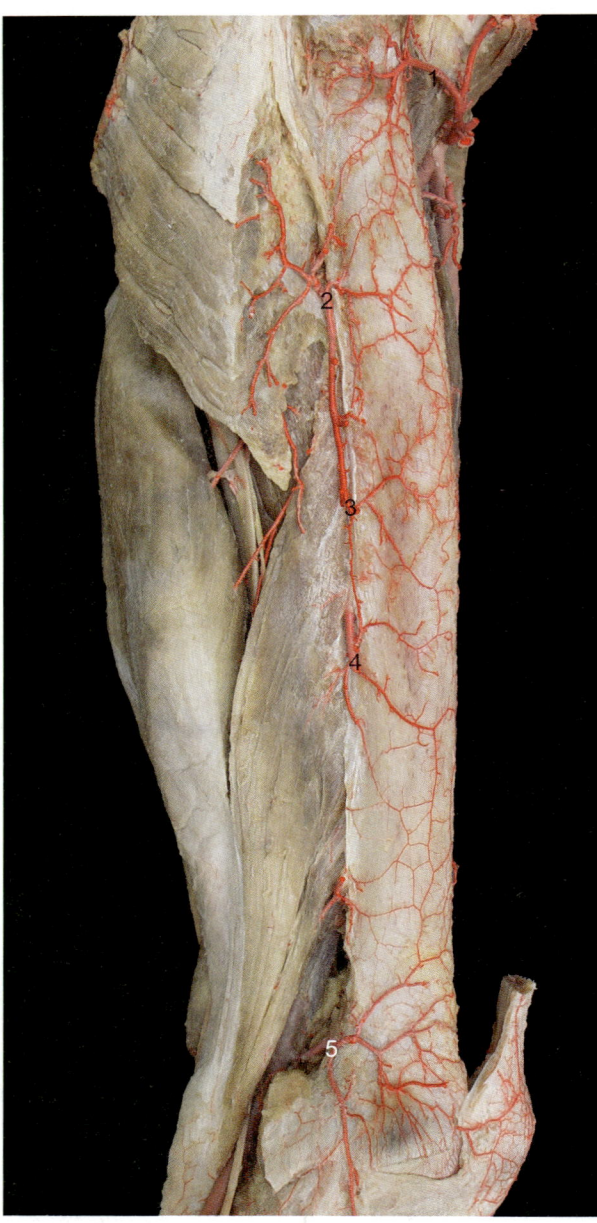

1. Transverse branch of lateral femoral circumflex artery
2. 1st perforating artery
3. 2nd perforating artery
4. 3rd perforating artery
5. Lateral superior genicular artery

Figure 3-174   Applied anatomy

The vascular distribution on the anterior femoral bone might be described as follows: Firstly, the transverse branch of the lateral femoral circumflex artery runs outwards to give a periosteal branch (15cm long) that descends gradually to form an arborized distribution. Secondly, the ascending branch of the lateral femoral circumflex artery runs outwards to the muscular porta of the tensor muscle of the fascia lata and gives the vastus lateralis muscular branch. Thirdly, the proximal muscular artery of the intermediate great muscle has a constant periosteal branch. The 1st perforating artery perforates through the lateral intermuscular septum and gives a direct periosteal branch to fan out obliquely. Fourthly, the periosteal branch emerges from the intermuscular septal branch of the 2nd perforating artery. Fifthly, the periosteal branch emerges from the intermuscular septal branch of the 3rd perforating artery Sixthly, the direct periosteal branch of the femoral artery passes by the medial femoral bone to the anterior femoral bone. The periosteal branch emerges from the intermuscular septal branch of the 4th perforating artery and distributes in a limited area. Seventhly, the periosteal branch emerges from the articular branch of the decending genicular artery. Eighthly, the vastus lateralis muscular branch enters the vastus lateralis muscle at 7 cm above the vastus lateralis muscle to give periosteal branches. The lateral superior genicular artery perforates through the muscular septum between the biceps femoris muscle and the vastus lateralis muscle at 2.5 cm above the lateral muscle and gives a periosteal branch into the anterior articular genu to anastomose with the genicular rete. There are in total 11 direct periosteal branches from the vessels mentioned above. They are 0.5-1.4mm in diameter. The periosteal branches on the anterolateral surface of the femoral bone enter the periosteum via the medial and the lateral femoral bones to give numerous smaller branches: the horizontal branches, the ascending branches and the descending branches. These affiliated branches anastomose with one another on the anterolateral surface of the femoral bone to form an abundant periosteal vascular net.

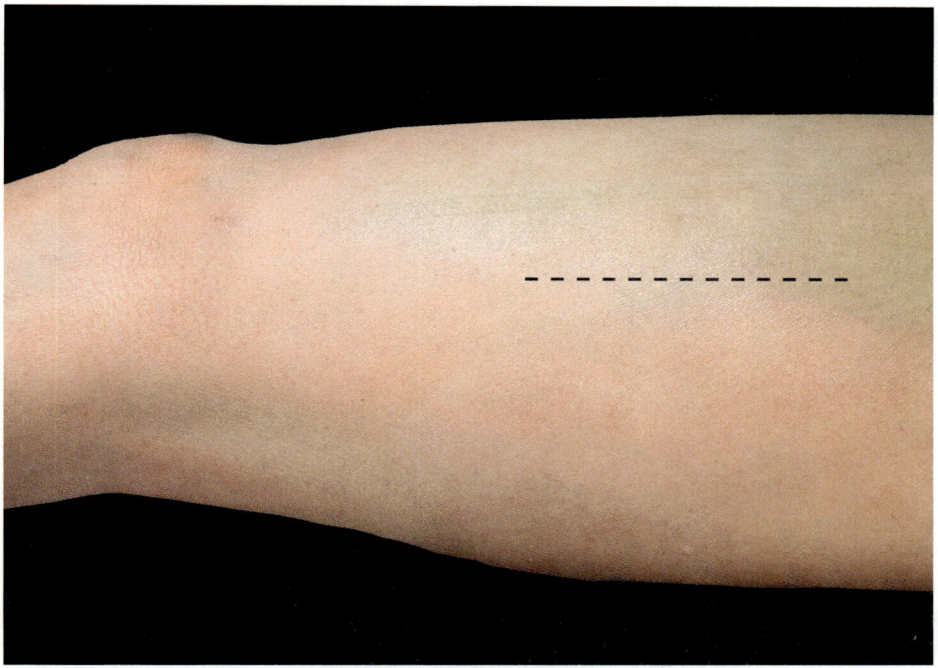

Figure 3-175	Design of the incision

The patient should be positioned with a pillow behind the posterior hip or on its lateral side. An anterolateral or a lateral approach to the femoral bone should be performed.

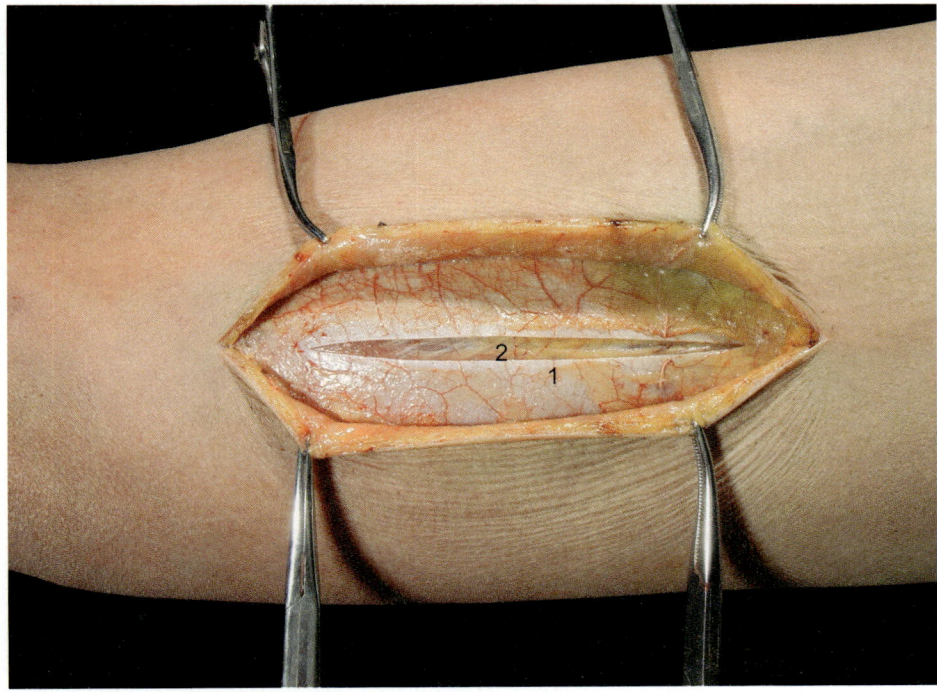

1. Femoral fascia
2. Vastus lateralis muscle

Figure 3-176	Exposure of the vastus lateralis muscle

The skin, the subcutaneous tissue and the femoral fascia should be incised to expose the vastus lateralis muscle.

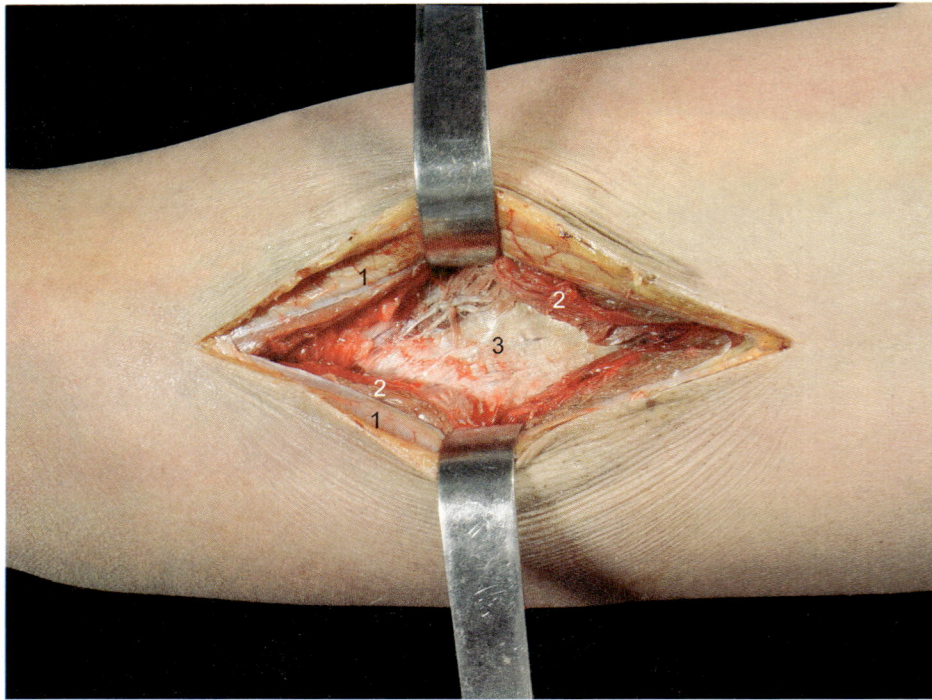

1. Femoral fascia
2. Vastus lateralis muscle
3. Vastus intermedius muscle

| Figure 3-177 | Exposure of the intermediate great muscle |

The vastus lateralis muscle should be directly splitted or the septum between the vastus lateralis muscle and the rectus femoris muscle should be separated to expose the intermediate femur muscle.

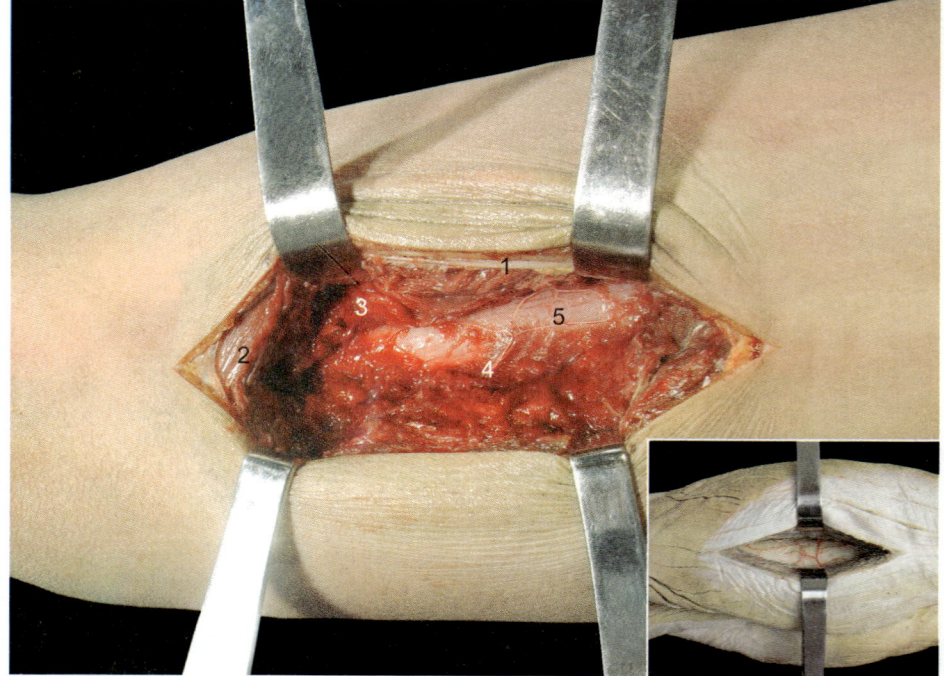

1. Femoral fascia
2. Vastus lateralis muscle
3. Vastus intermedius muscle
4. Periosteal branch
5. Femoral bone

| Figure 3-178 | Exposure of the vessel |

The vastus intermedius muscle should be dissected carefully and a thin layer of muscular sleeve retained to protect the periosteal branch.

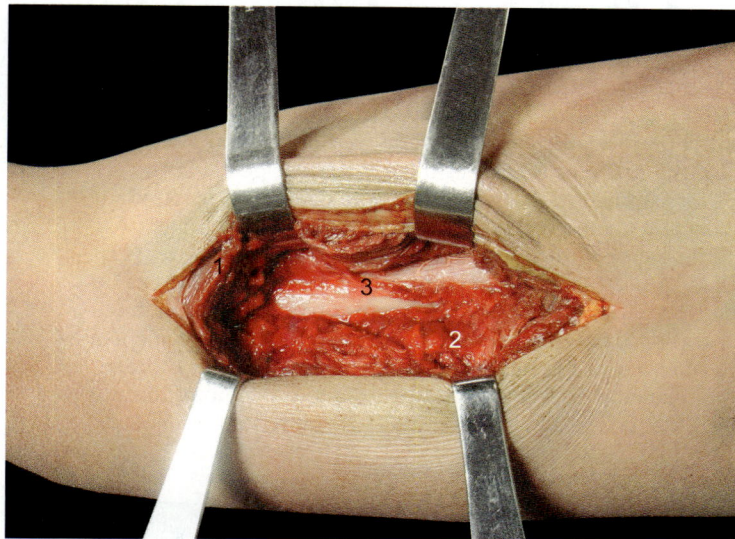

1. Vastus lateralis muscle
2. Vastus intermedius muscle
3. Periosteal flap

Figure 3-179   Dissection of the periosteal (bone) flap

The periosteal (bone) flap should be dissected at the proximal or the distal end of the diseased area.

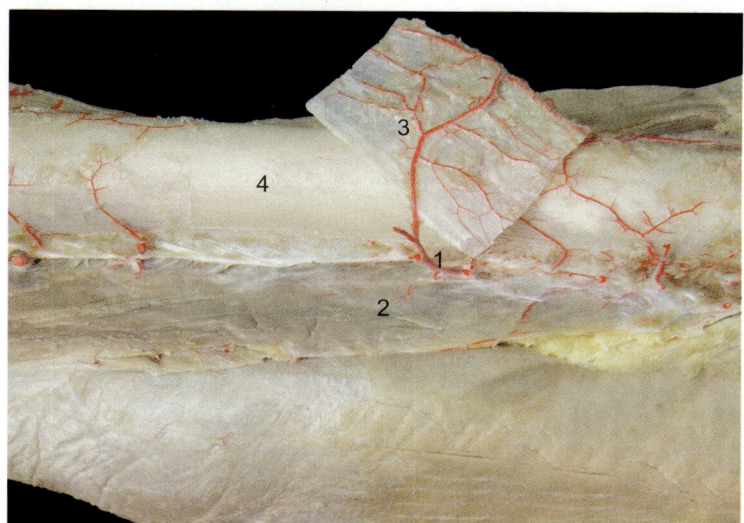

1. Periosteal branch of perforating artery
2. Great adductor muscle
3. Periosteal flap
4. Donor site

Figure 3-180   Transposition of the periosteal (bone) flap

The periosteal flap should not be transferred upwards to wrap around the fractured bone segment until the diseased parts are debrided and fixed both internally and externally.

Key points in applied anatomy

Firstly, the periosteal branch on the anterior femoral bone tends to be relatively large with some exceptions, in which the branch might be thin and small. In that case, part of the periosteum should be incised and used as a pedicle to form a periosteal flap. The length of the periosteal flap and the width of the pedicle should be in the ratio of three to one. Secondly, the septum between the intermediate great muscle and the vastus medialis muscle might serve as the approach to trace the vascular pedicle. Thirdly, the periosteal flap should be designed at the distal periosteal branch, the more distal the better. Fourthly, the adjacent anastomotic branch and the muscular branch should be ligated. Fifthly, some muscular sleeve should be retained with the periosteal flap to protect the periosteal vessels. Sixthly, the distal anastomosis should be confirmed before it is used as the rotating point if the periosteal flap is to be retrogradely transferred. Seventhly, the periosteal flap might carry with it some stripe-shape bone blocks.

30 Pedicled Periosteal (bone) Flap of Lateral Condyle of Femur

The direct periosteal branch of the lateral superior genicular artery and that of the femoral artery anastomoses with the transverse branch of the articular branch of the descending genicular artery to form a constant anastomosis at the inferior segment of the femoral bone to construct an abundant periosteal vascular net. The vessel has a constant anatomical position. The trauma might range from the superior condyles of femur to the middle segment of femur. The lateral approach to the femoral bone is recommended for orthopedics. It is unnecessary that the important vessels and nerves be damaged in this area. But it is necessary that various internal and external fixations be available in this area. The inferior femoral periosteal (bone) flap pedicled with the lateral superior genicular vessels might be transferred to repair the condyles of the femur. For example, the periosteal (bone) flap pedicled with the direct periosteal branch could be transferred upwards to the femoral middle segment via the periosteal vascular network that is located at the femoral anteroinferior segment.

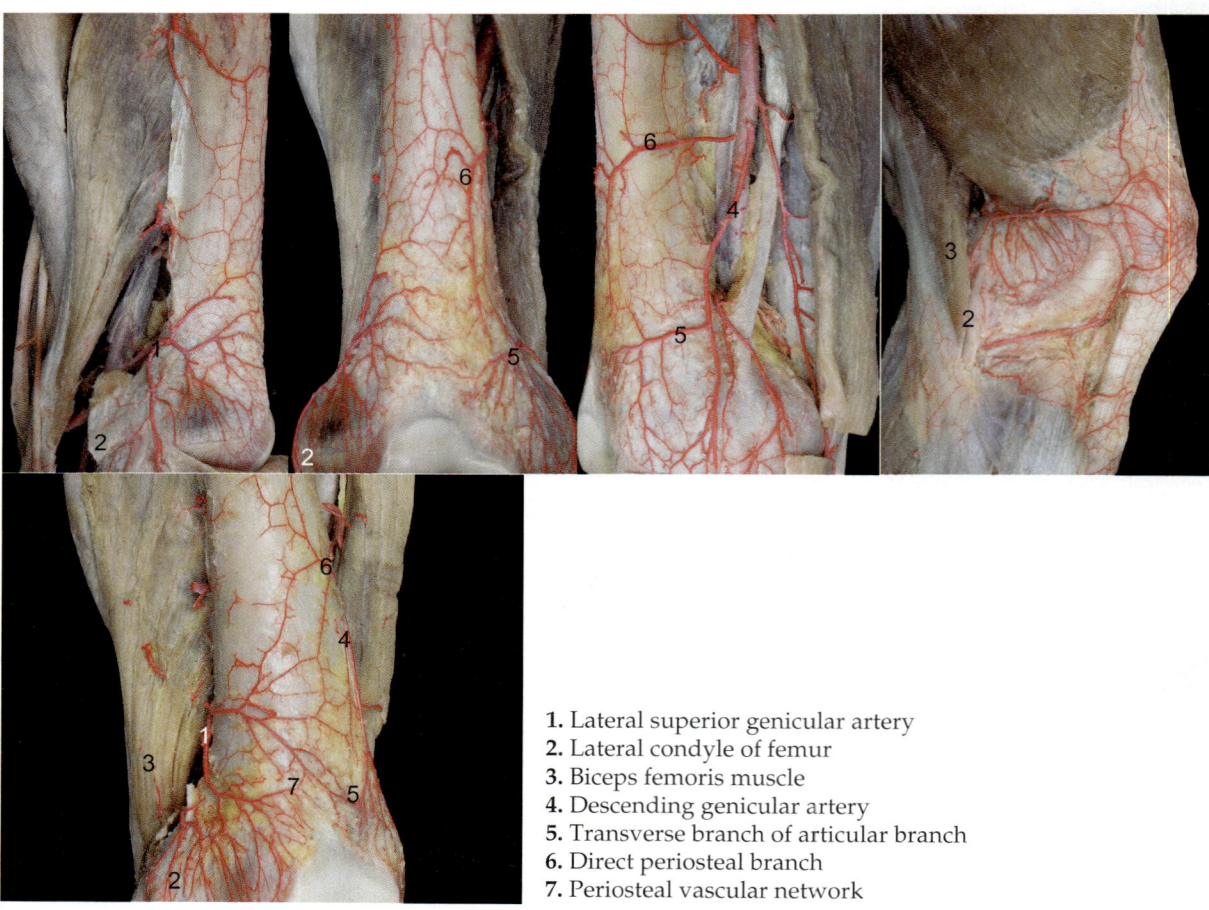

1. Lateral superior genicular artery
2. Lateral condyle of femur
3. Biceps femoris muscle
4. Descending genicular artery
5. Transverse branch of articular branch
6. Direct periosteal branch
7. Periosteal vascular network

Figure 3-181　Applied anatomy

The Lateral superior genicular artery emerges from the popliteal artery at 2.5 cm above the most prominent lateral point of the lateral condyle of the femur. Its origin is 1.5mm in diameter. It runs inwards to transverse over the superior lateral condyle after it emerges, and perforates through the biceps femoris tendon and the lateral femoral intermuscular septum to reach the bone face. The main trunk in this segment is 4.4 cm in length and 1.1 mm in diameter. The vascular stem immediately gives branches to fan out in a claw shape over the lateral surface of the lateral condyle and anastomose with the transverse branch of the descending genicular arterial articular branch and the direct branch of the femoral artery to construct the periosteal vascular net on the inferior femoral bone altogether.

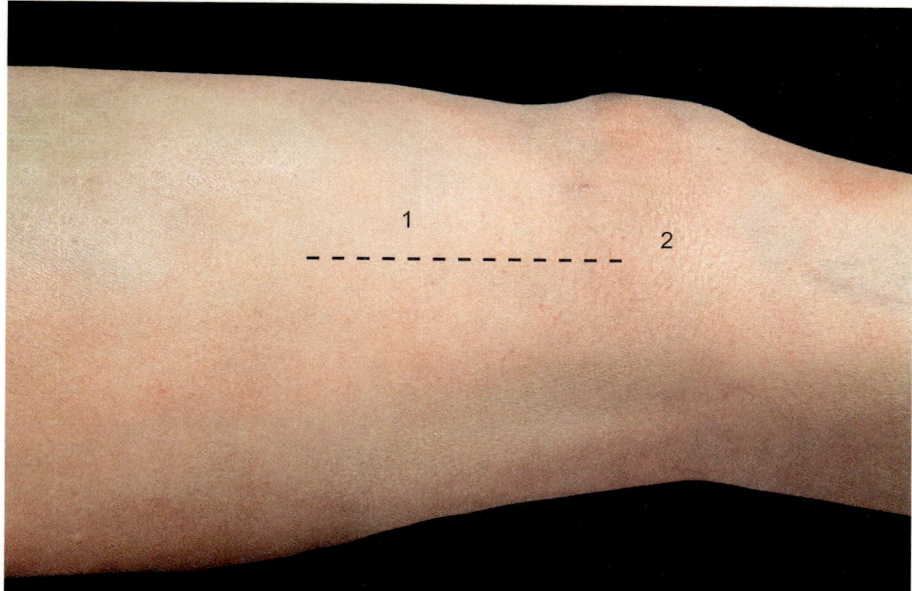

1. Vastus lateralis muscle
2. Lateral condyle

Figure 3-182   Design of the incision

The patient should be placed in supine position, the diseased hip and knee padded up with cushions. The lateral approach to femoral bone might be preferred. An incision might be drawn from the diseased superior osseous area to the most prominent point of the lateral condyle along the lateral margin of the vastus lateralis muscle.

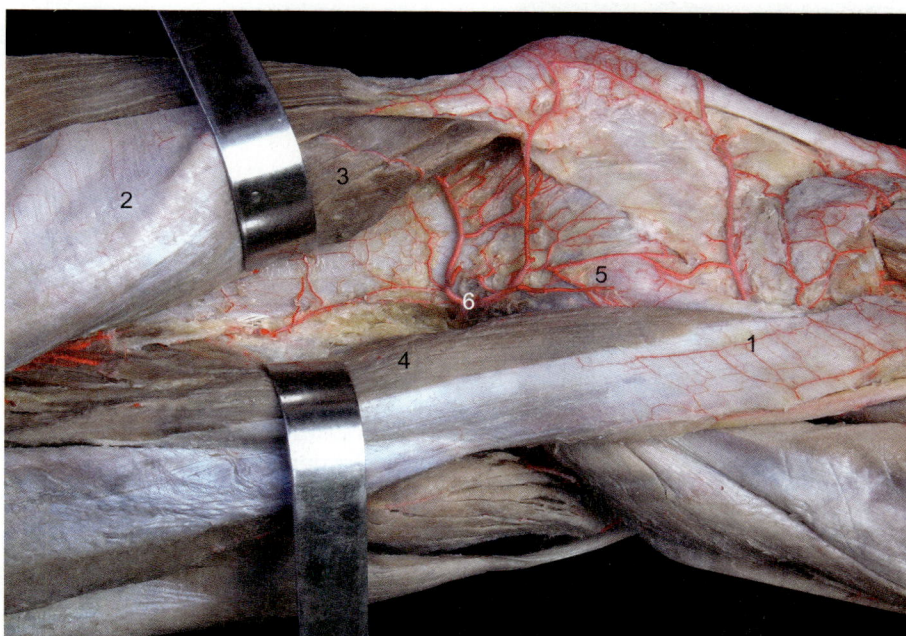

1. Biceps femoris tendon
2. Iliotibial tract
3. Vastus lateralis muscle
4. Biceps femoris muscle
5. Lateral condyle of femur
6. Lateral superior genicular artery

Figure 3-183   Exposure of the vessel

The skin and the superficial fascia should be incised longitudinally along the arch that is from the superior margin of the biceps femoris tendon to the inferior segment, and the iliotibial tract cut off in a Z shape. The septum between the vastus lateralis muscle and the biceps femoris muscle should be dissected and pulled bilaterally to expose the anterior surface of the inferior femoral bone and the lateral surface of the lateral condyle. The lateral superior genicular artery, the direct periosteal branch of the femoral artery, the transverse branch of articular branch and the periosteal vascular net on anterior surface of the inferior segment of the femur could be subsequently exposed. It is recommended that the demanded vascular pedicle be selected adjusted to the traumatic position.

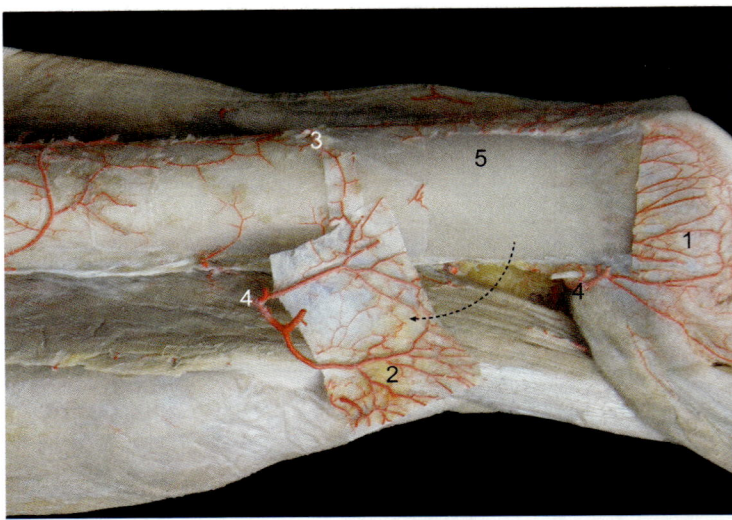

1. Lateral condyle of femur
2. Periosteal flap
3. Direct periosteal branch
4. Lateral superior genicular artery
5. Donor site

| Figure 3-184 | Harvest of the periosteal (bone) flap |

The vascular pedicle exposed, the periosteum on the lateral condyle should be incised at 1 cm above the inferior marginal plane of the lateral condyle of the femur. A cortical bone block should be included if necessary. The periosteum on the femoral shaft should be decohesed upwards along the anterolateral surface of the femoral bone. The periosteal (bone) flap pedicled with the direct periosteal branch of the femoral artery might be transferred upwards to the middle segment of the femoral bone via the periosteal vascular net on the anterior surface of the inferior segment of the femur.

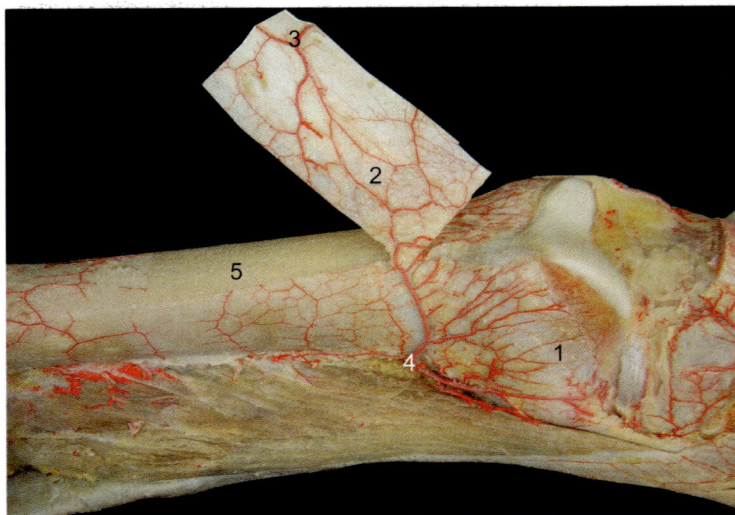

1. Lateral condyle of femur
2. Periosteal flap
3. Direct periosteal branch
4. Lateral superior genicular artery
5. Donor site

| Figure 3-185 | Transposition of the periosteal flap |

The inferior femoral periosteal (bone) flap pedicled with the lateral superior genicular vessels might be transferred to repair the condyles of the femur.

Key points in applied anatomy

Firstly, the periosteal (bone) flap pedicled with the direct branch of the femoral artery should carry bilaterally with it part of the periosteum (1-1.5cm wide) to guarantee that its vascular pedicle could be safely being dissected. Secondly, the articular capsule should not be incised open in the operation. Thirdly, the superior margin of the periosteal flap should be located at 1cm above the inferior margin of the lateral condyle of the femur to prevent the articular surface from being damaged. Fourthly, a periosteum should be larger than the bone flap if the flap has to carry a piece of the periosteum.

Periosteal Flap Pedicled with Direct Periosteal Branch of Femoral Artery in Inferior Segment of Femur Shaft

31

The periosteal flap based on the direct inferior periosteal branch of the femoral artery has such advantages as a constant vascular anatomical position in the donor site, a large size of the bone flap, an easy operation and generalization. Moreover, due to the adoption of the medial approach in the inferior segment of the femoral shaft, the operation in the donor or recipient area could be done in the same incision. A flap of this type might be suitable for repairing a nonunion and a small bone defect in the middle-shaft of the femur.

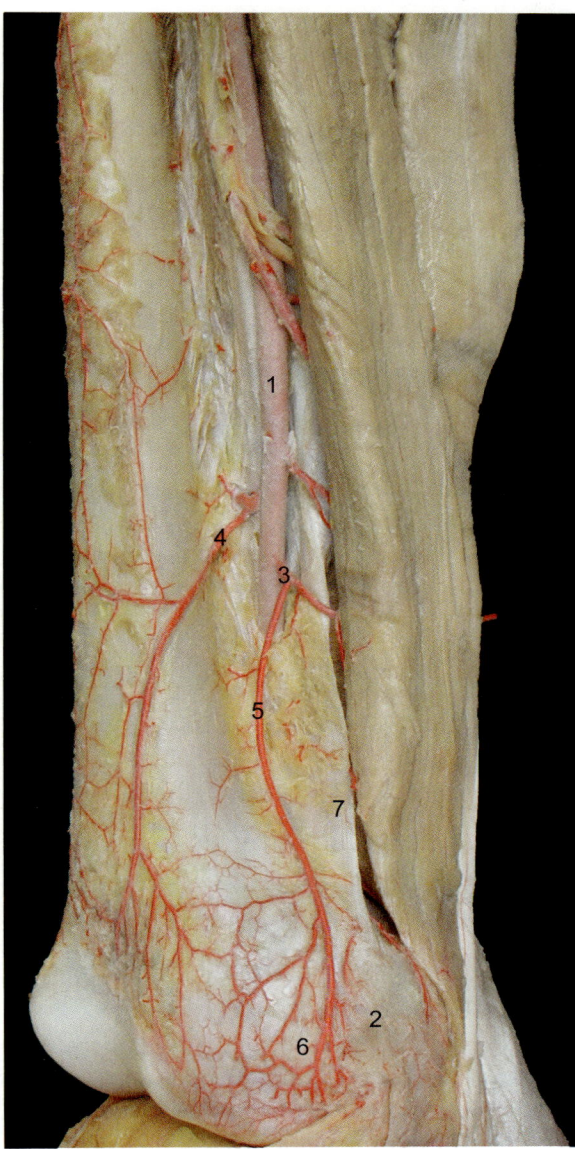

Figure 3-186	Applied anatomy

At about 9.4 cm above the adductor tubercle of the femur, the femoral artery gives a direct periosteal branch to supply the anteromedial area in the inferior segment of the femur (most of it lying at 2-3cm above the origin of the descending genicular artery). The direct periosteal branch descends obliquely for 2.8 cm in the septum between the vastus medialis and the adductor magnus and crosses the medial surface of the femur, attaching tightly to the periosteum. It then turns to the anterior surface of the femur and descends vertically along the femoral antemedial line to form the constant anastomosis with the transverse branch of the articular branch from the descending genicular artery at about 3.1cm above the adductor tubercle. Upon entering the femoral periosteum, this direct branch gives numerous branches to distribute on the anterior and medial area of the inferior segment of the femur and form a rich vascular net with the articular branches of the descending genicular artery.

1. Femoral artery
2. Adductor tubercle
3. Descending genicular artery
4. Direct periosteal branch
5. Articular branch
6. Medial condyle
7. Adductor magnus tendon

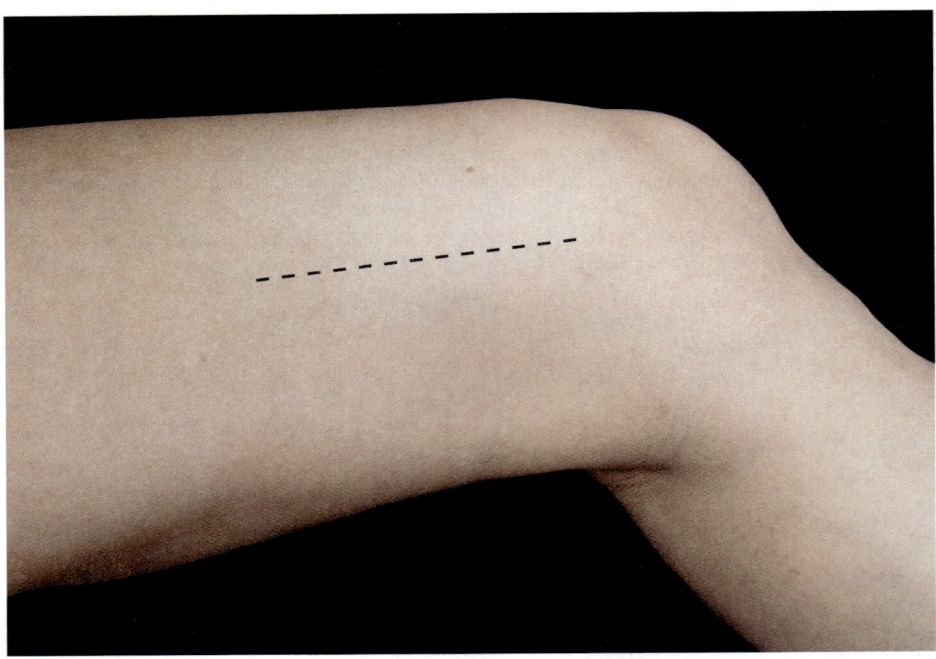

| Figure 3-187 | Design of the incision |

The medial approach in the inferior segment of the femoral shaft should be adopted.

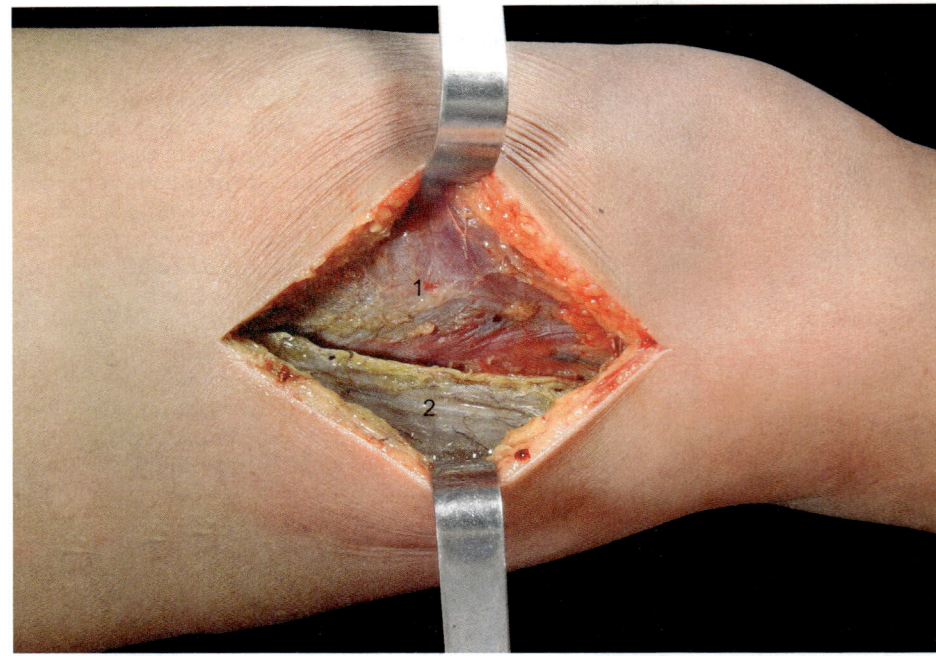

1. Medial vastus muscle
2. Sartorius muscle

| Figure 3-188 | Exposure of the muscle |

The skin and the superficial fascia should be incised open longitudinally to expose the medial vastus muscle and the sartorius muscle.

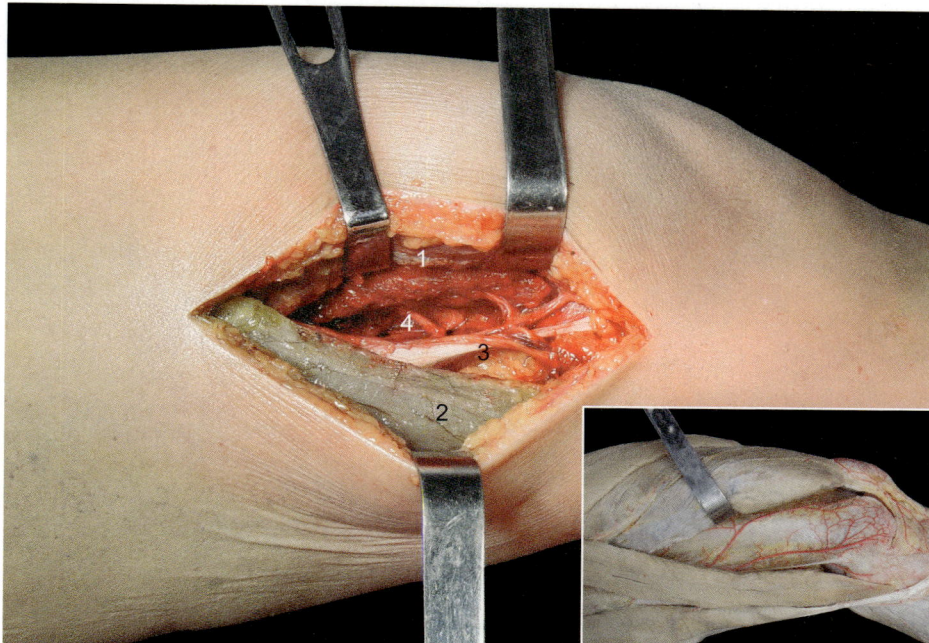

1. Vastus medialis muscle
2. Sartorius muscle
3. Adductor magnus tendon
4. Direct periosteal branch

| Figure 3-189 | Exposure of the vessels |

The medial patellar retinaculum should be opened curvely along the medial margin of the medial vastus muscle, and the vastus medialis and the sartorius pulled bilaterally. The incision should then trace upwards along the adductor magnus to the aponeurotic plate of the adductor magnus to find out the direct periosteal branch diverging from the lateral wall of the femoral artery at about 9.5 cm above the internal adductor tubercle.

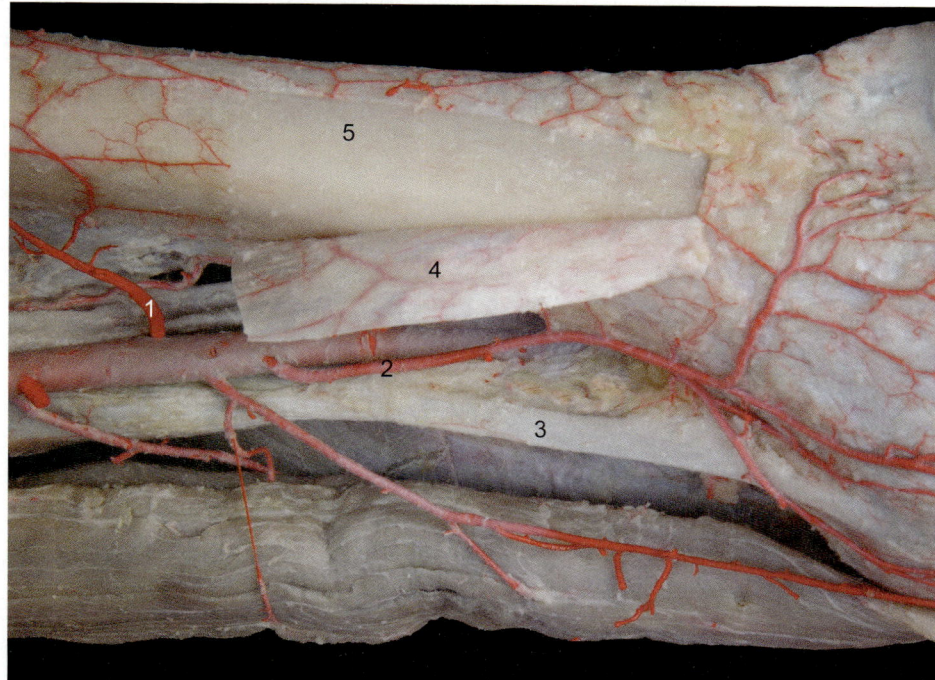

1. Direct periosteal branch
2. Articular branch of descending genicular artery
3. Vastus adductor aponeurotic plate
4. Periosteal flap
5. Donor site

| Figure 3-190 | Incision of the periosteal flap |

The main periosteal branch should be separated, and the periosteal flap dissected as is needed for the operation.

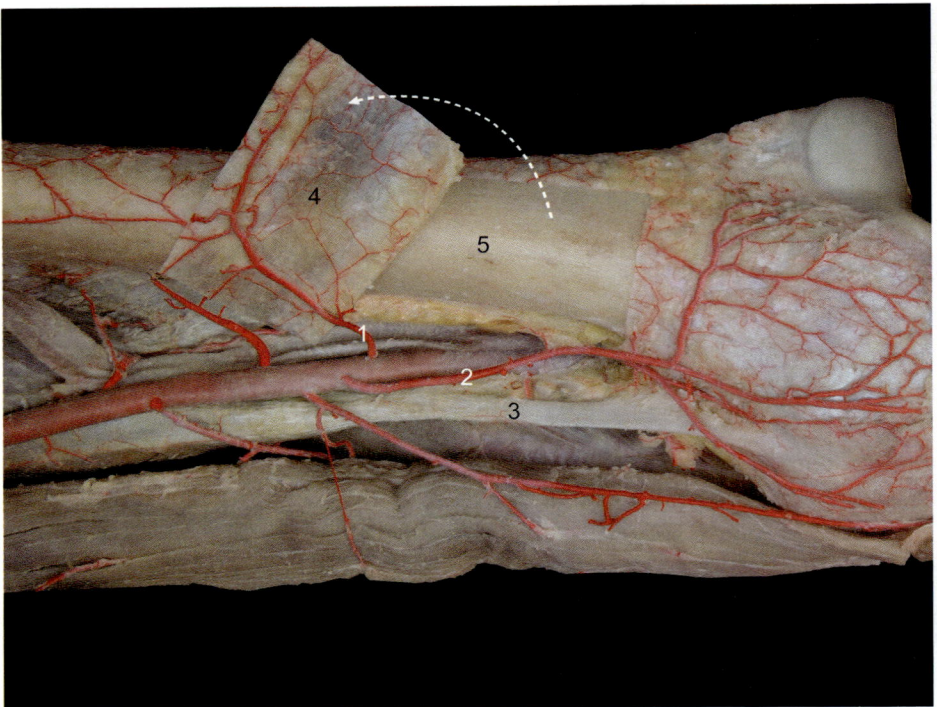

| Figure 3-191 | Transposition of the periosteal flap |

The lesion should be debrided and the internal fixation or external fixators completed before the periosteal flap could be transferred upwards to surround the fracture position.

1. Direct periosteal branch
2. Articular branch of descending genicular artery
3. Vastus adductor aponeurotic plate
4. Periosteal flap
5. Donor site

Key points in applied anatomy

Firstly, the available periosteal flap that takes the direct periosteal branch of the femoral artery as a pedicle should include the inferior 1/3 segment of the femoral periosteum and the medial femoral condyle. The flap area might amount to about 12×5cm. In the medial femoral condyle site, the direct branch might also be taken together with a 4×2×1.5cm volume bone flap to make a periosteal bone flap. This flap might be transferred upwards to above the midpoint of the femur. Secondly, when the direct periosteal branch emerges from under the origin of the descending genicular artery or shares the trunk with the latter, the descending genicular artery should be retained to form a double-pedicle periosteal flap. Thirdly, the adductor magnus tendon and the vastus adductor aponeurotic plate might serve as an indication in the search for the direct periosteal branch.

Periosteal Flap of Medial Femoral Condyle Pedicled with Descending Genicular Vessel

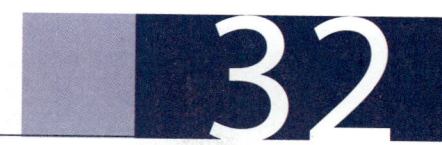

32

The periosteal flap of the medial femoral condyle is based on the descending genicular artery with its pivot point located at the original point of the artery. It also carries part of the articular branch. Generally it might be transferred to the midpoint of the femur to restore a nonunion or a bone defect in the middle-inferior segment of femur. There are many advantages of this operation such as a constant vascular anatomical position, a long and wide vascular pedicle and a large periosteal flap.

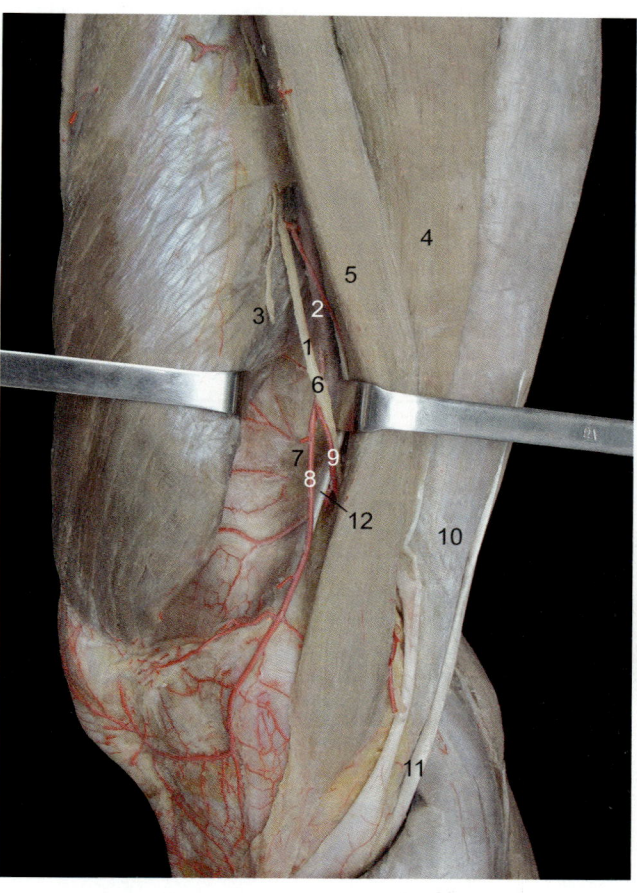

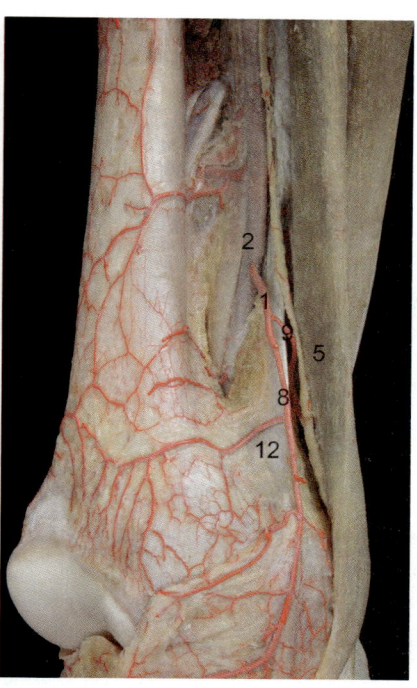

| Figure 3-192 | Applied anatomy |

The desending genicular artery emerges from the femoral artery at about 12.8cm above the medial femoral epicondyle, where it is 2.3mm in diameter. It then descends along the deep layer of the sartorius muscle between the vastus medialis and the gracilis, accompanying the saphenous nerve. It divides into the vastus medialis branch, the articular branch and the saphenous artery at 11.6cm above the medial femoral condyle. The articular branch distributes on the medial femoral condyle and the nearby periosteum. The saphenous artery descends along the deep layer of the sartorius and comes superficially out at 3.5cm below the medial femoral condyle through the posteroinferior border of the sartorius. It continues downwards with the saphenous nerve and the great saphenous vein to anastomose with the medial inferior genicular artery and then to send the periosteal branch.

1. Desending genicular artery
2. Femoral artery
3. Vastus medialis muscle
4. Gracilis muscle
5. Sartorius muscle
6. Saphenous nerve
7. Vastus medialis branch
8. Articular branch
9. Saphenous artery
10. Semimembranosus muscle
11. Semitendinosus muscle
12. Adductor magnus muscle

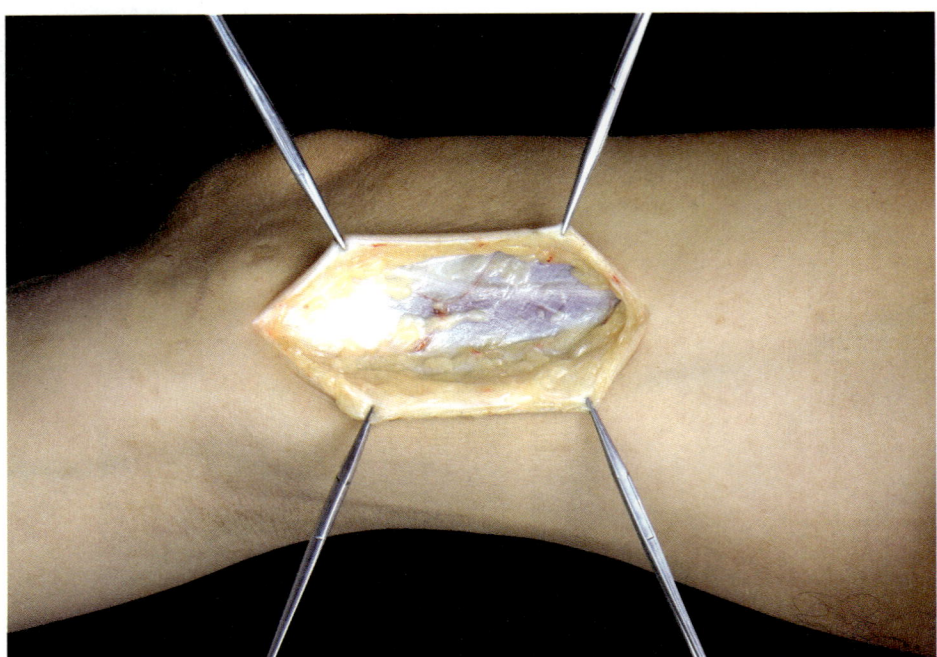

Figure 3-193   Design of the incision

The incision should begin from the anteromedial knee.

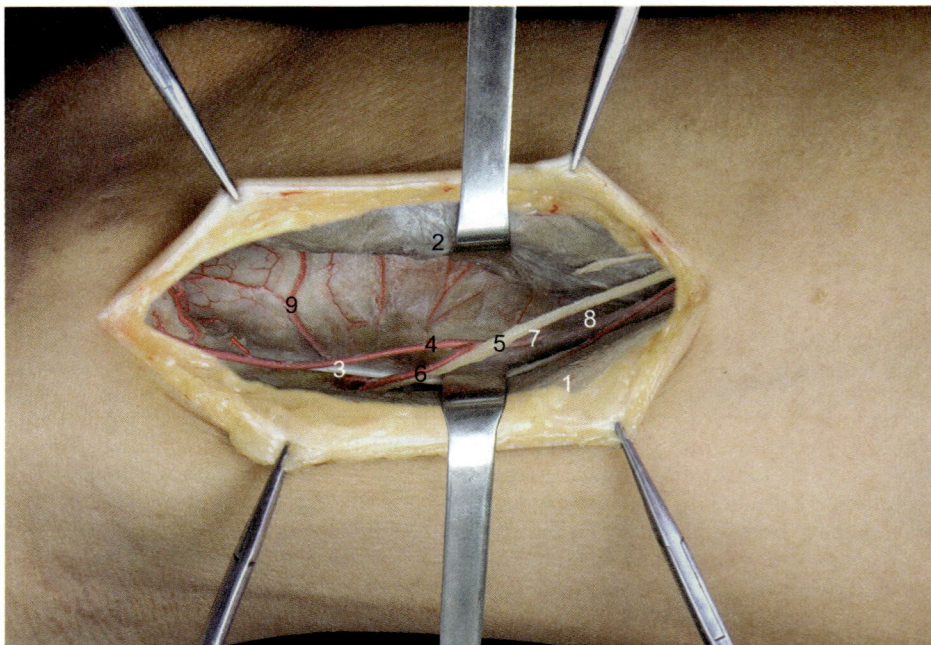

1. Sartorius muscle
2. Vastus medialis muscle
3. Adductor magnus tendon
4. Articular branch
5. Saphenous nerve
6. Saphenous artery
7. Desending genicular
   artery
8. Femoral artery
9. Transverse branch

Figure 3-194   Exposure of the vessels

The skin and the superficial fascia should be incised longitudinally, and the sartorius pulled posteriorly inwards. The medial patellar retinaculum should be incised open along the posteromedial border of the vastus medialis, and the vastus medialis separated bluntly from the vastus adductor aponeurotic plate and the adductor magnus tendon. The vastus medialis should be pulled laterally to expose the articular branch of the desending genicular artery on the surface of the vastus adductor aponeurotic plate.

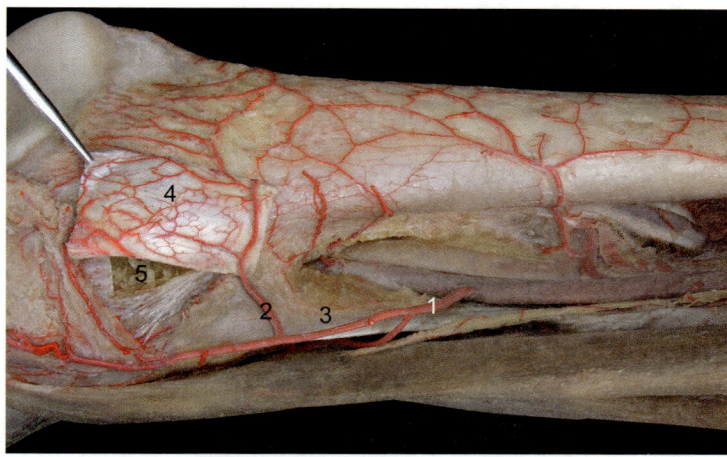

1. Desending genicular artery
2. Articular branch
3. Vastus adductor aponeurotic plate
4. Periosteal flap
5. Donor site

Figure 3-195   Harvest of the periosteal flap

After that, the medial condyle periosteum should be incised transversely at 1cm above the plane of the inferior border on the medial femoral condyle (with a bone block if necessary) and then the periosteum of the femoral shaft stripped upwards along the front and medial surface of the femur.

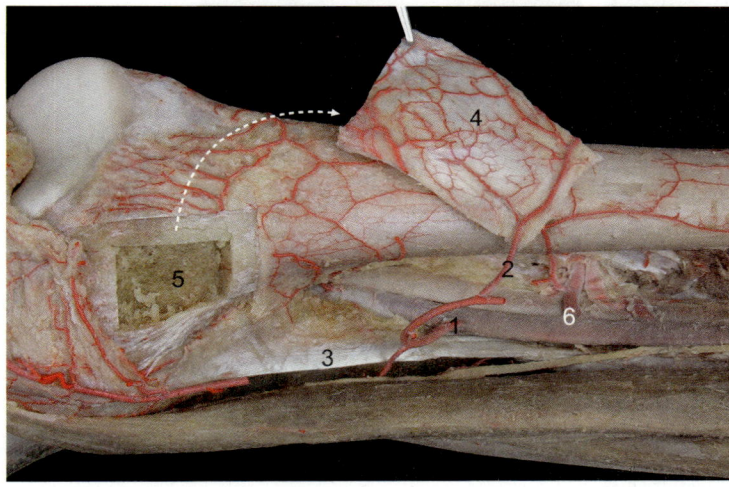

1. Desending genicular artery
2. Articular branch
3. Vastus adductor aponeurotic plate
4. Periosteal flap
5. Donor site
6. Femoral artery

Figure 3-196   Transposition of the periosteal flap

After the impairment is debrided and the internal or external fixation completed, part of the cancellus should be taken from the medial condyle to fill in the gap between the two ends of the fractures, and the periosteal flap transferred upwards to wrap the ends of the fractures.

Key points in applied anatomy

Firstly, when the vastus medialis stick to the front segment of the medial intermuscular septum is being separated, the medial intermuscular septum should be retained on the surface of the vastus adductor aponeurotic plate to avoid damaging the desending genicular vessel and its articular branches. Secondly, the articular capsule should not be incised open in the operation. Thirdly, the inferior border of the periosteal flap should be located at 1 cm above the inferior border of the medial femoral condyle to protect the articular surface from being damaged. Fourthly, when the flap carries part of the periosteum, the size of the periosteum should be larger than that of the bone. Fifthly, the periosteal flap might be harvested with its superior border extending to 7 cm above the inferior border of the medial femoral condyle, its inferior border to 1 cm above the inferior border of the medial femoral condyle, its anterior border to the anterior midline and its posterior border to the adductor tubercle. The area of the flap might amount to about 6×3cm.

33

Periosteal Flap of Lateral Tibia Pedicled with Periosteal Branch of Anterior Tibial Vessel

The lateral surface of the tibia is quite flat and broad with thick periosteum and might be chosen as a large donor site, distributed with many segments of vascularity. The periosteal flap might be designed carrying a strip bone block. A flap of this type might be suitable for the repair of fractures and nonunion of any tibial segment.

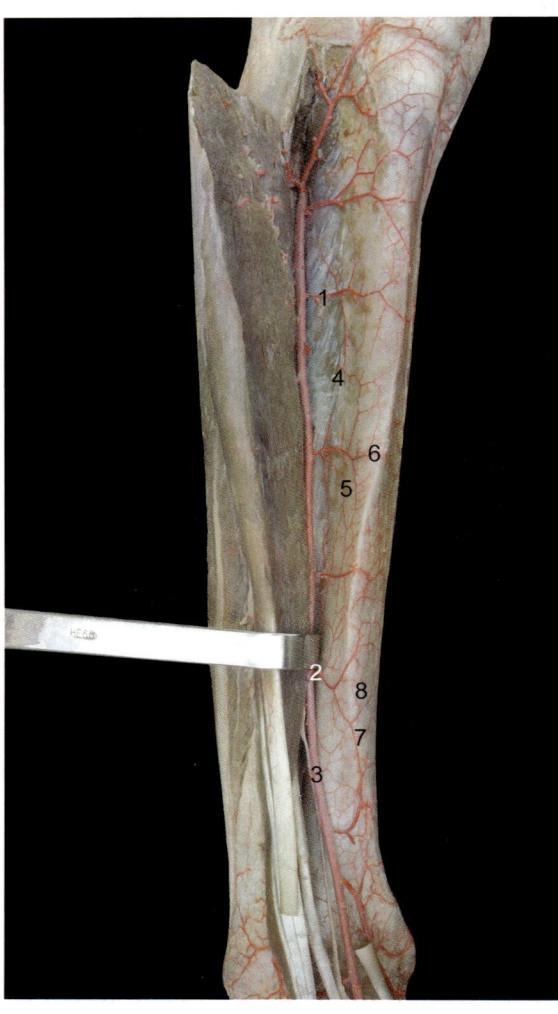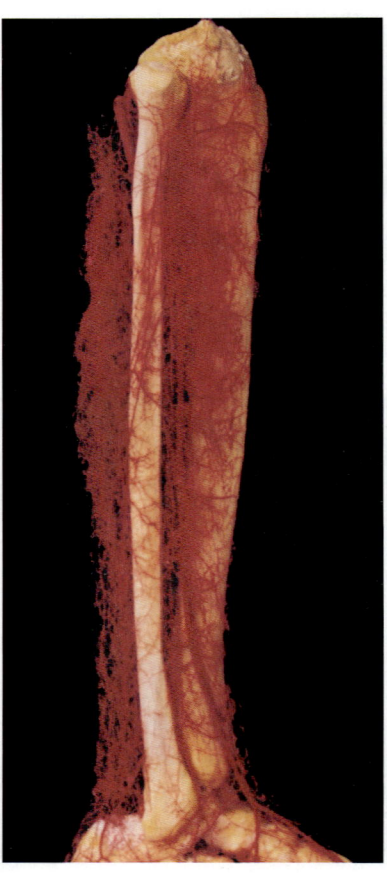

Figure 3-197	Applied anatomy

There are musculoperiosteal branches and periosteal branches distributed on the superior, the middle and the inferior segments of the lateral tibia. There are 4 - 8 branches in the middle-inferior segments that emerge from the anterior tibial artery and extend either superiorly or horizontally to the anterior border of the tibia. There they send ascending branches, descending branches and horizontal branches to form a vascular chain and a periosteal vascular net.

1. Musculoperiosteal branch
2. Periosteal branch
3. Anterior tibial artery
4. Ascending branch
5. Descending branch
6. Horizontal branch
7. Chain link of vessels
8. Periosteal vascular net

314

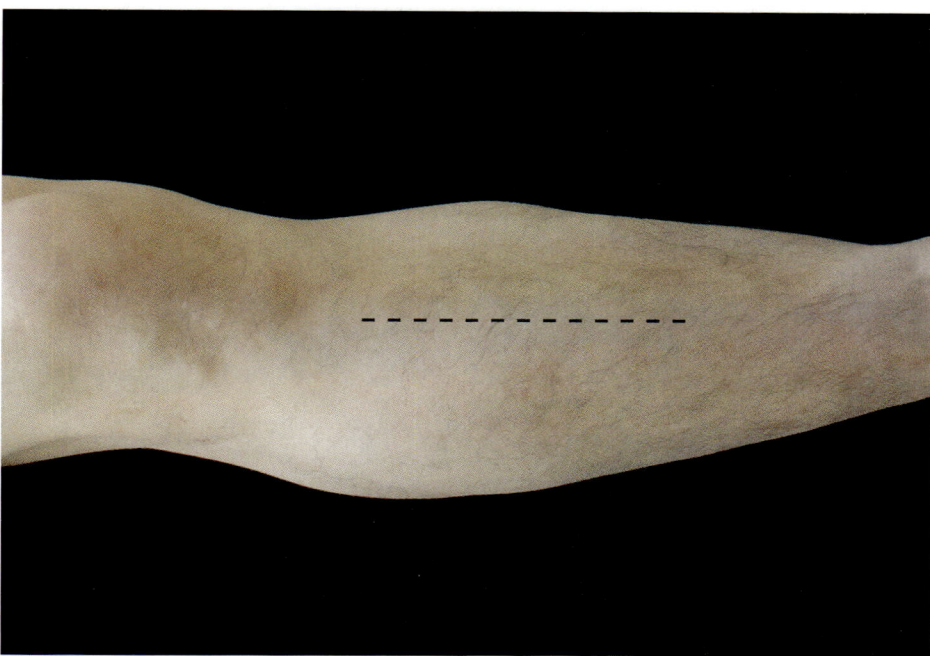

Figure 3-198   Design of the incision

The patient should be placed in supine position, and a vertical incision (about 1 cm long) made on the anterolateral border of the tibia.

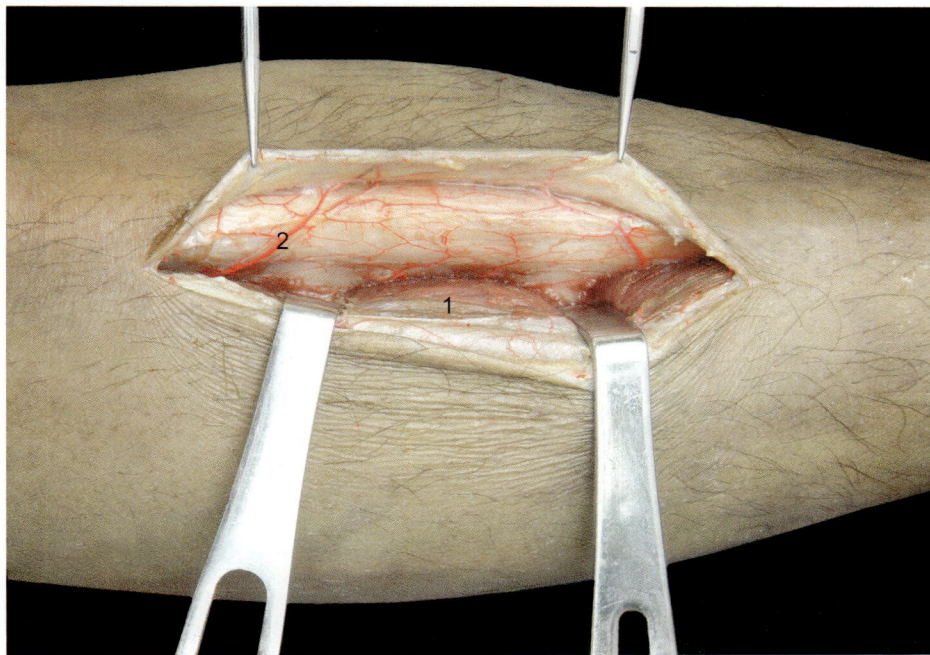

1. Tibialis anterior muscle
2. Periosteal branch

Figure 3-199   Exposure of the vessels

Then the skin, the subcutaneous tissue and the deep fascia should be incised open, and the tibialis anterior muscle pulled laterally to expose the periosteal branch that emerges from the anterior tibial artery and extends inferiorly or horizontally to the tibia.

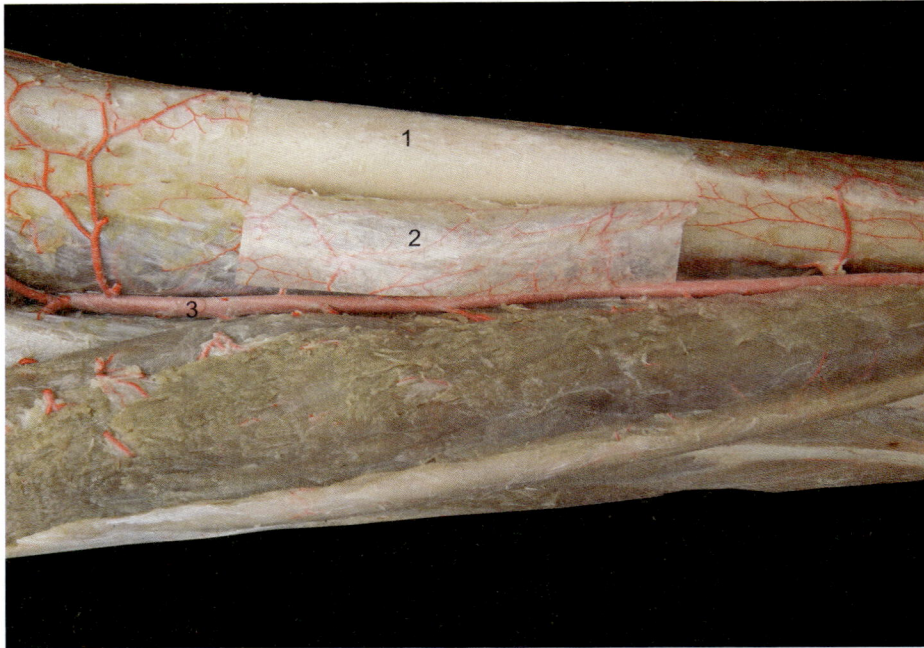

1. Tibia
2. Periosteal flap
3. Anterior tibial artery

| Figure 3-200 | Harvest of the periosteal flap |

The tibia periosteum should be incised open at l cm from the anterior border and on the medial surface of the tibia. The flap should be stripped under the periosteum with a sharp osteotome to form a rectangle island pedicled with 1-2 periosteal branches. The periosteal flap should be designed and chiseled near the end of the fracture and the fractures repositioned and fixed interally before it is transferred.

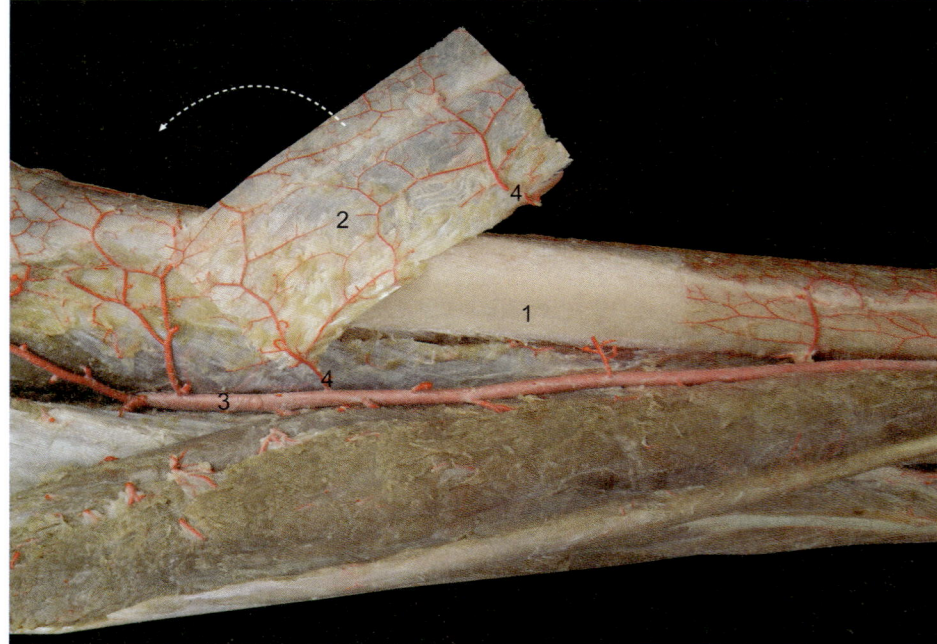

1. Donor site
2. Periosteal flap
3. Anterior tibial artery
4. Periosteal branch

| Figure 3-201 | Transposition of the periosteal flap |

A periosteal flap could be designed based on the branches distal to the fracture and circumrotated upwards to cover the fracture on the tibia.

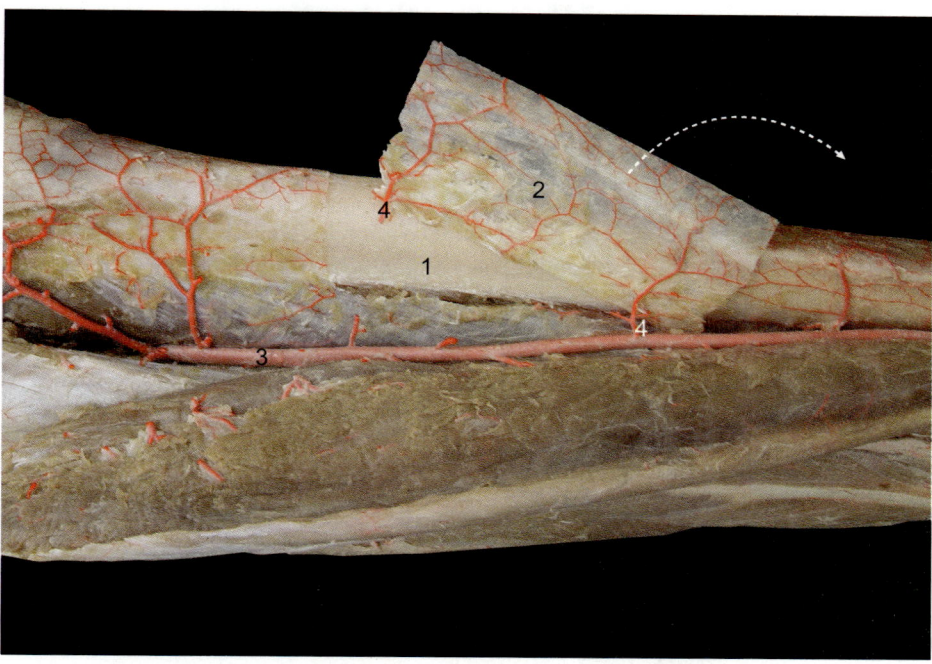

| Figure 3-202 | Retrograde transposition of the periosteum flap |

A periosteal flap could be designed based on the branches proximal to the fracture and then circumrotated downwards to cover the fractured part of the tibia.

1. Donor site
2. Periosteal flap
3. Anterior tibial artery
4. Periosteal branch

Key points in applied anatomy

Firstly, in the operation, a periosteal flap should be made firstly and then the fractures fixed. Secondly, the anterior periosteum should be incised quite long and part of the posterior periosteal flap retained to protect the vascular pedicle. Thirdly, When there are fractures on the middle-inferior segment, the pedicle of the periosteal flap should be designed as close to the proximal part of the fracture as possible. Fourthly, when the flap carries part of the bone substance, only the strip-shape bone should be retrieved to prevent a disconnection of the bone block and the periosteum. Fifthly, the vascular pedicle should be dissected with bilateral deep fascia cuffs (1-1.5 cm wide) to protect the vessel.

The inferolateral segment of the tibia is flat and broad with thick periosteum. It obtains its blood supply mainly from the superior ankle branch of the anterior tibial artery. Here, the anterior tibial vessel runs superficially and the anterior group of muscles of the leg have migrated into the tendons, which makes it convenient to expose the blood vessel. Given the relation between the superior ankle branch and the musculoperiosteal branch of anterior tibial artery, or the relation between the superior ankle branch and the medial anterior malleolar artery, the flap should be designed at the inferolateral segment of the tibia with an area about (8-10)×(4-5) cm. It might be used to repair the nonunion on the middle-inferior segment of the tibia, the talus fracture or the fusion of the ankle.

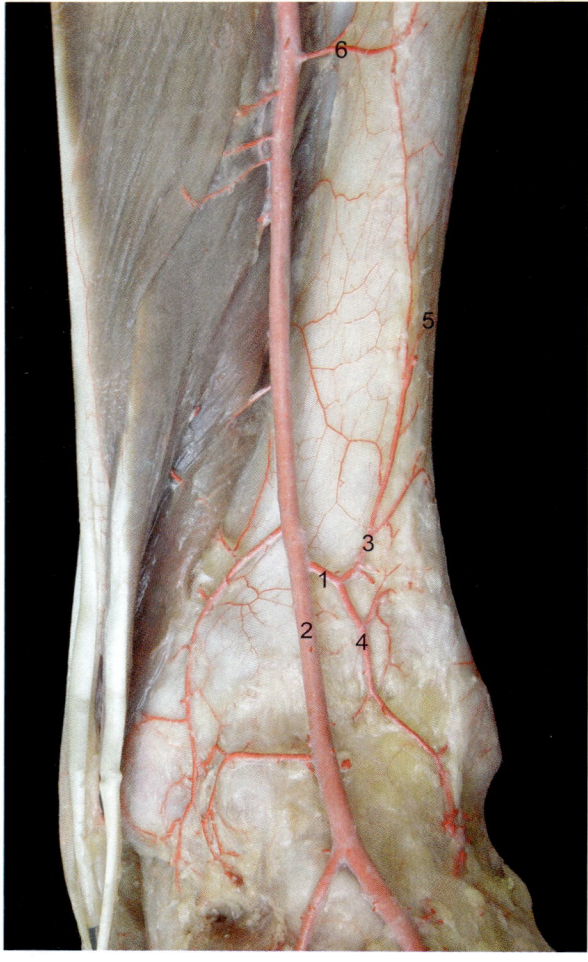
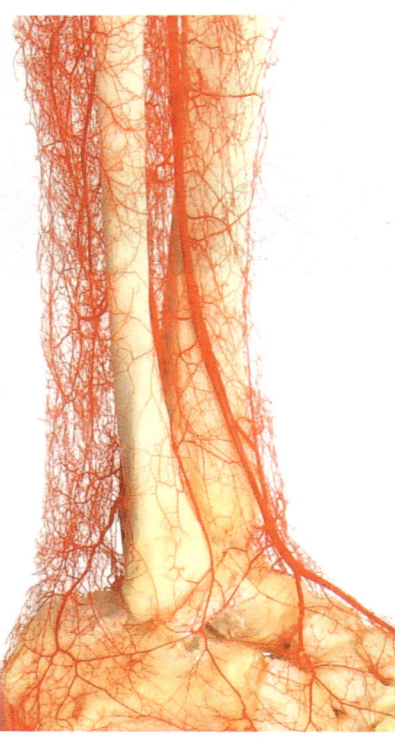

| Figure 3-203 | Applied anatomy |

The superior ankle branch of the anterior tibial artery originates from the anterior tibial artery at 3.1cm above the ankle line. It runs forward to the anterior tibial border clinging to the bone surface, and sends an ascending branch and a descending branch. The ascending branch ascends along the anterior tibial border to anastomose with the musculoperiosteal branch of the anterior tibial artery at 6.3cm above the ankle line. The descending branch descends to anastomose with the medial anterior malleolar artery. The superior ankle branch is 2.2cm in length and 1.1mm in diameter. It has two accompanying veins.

1. Superior ankle branch   **2.** Anterior tibial artery
3. Ascending branch   **4.** Descending branch
5. Anterior tibial border   **6.** Musculoperiosteal branch

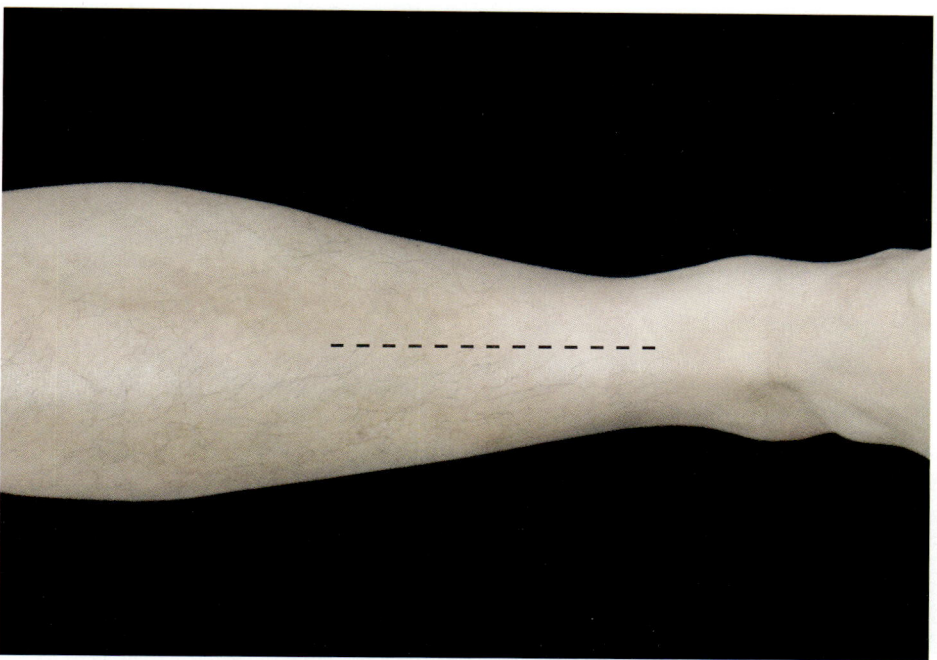

Figure 3-204 Design of the incision

The patient should be placed in supine position, and the incision begins with the midpoint of the ankle.

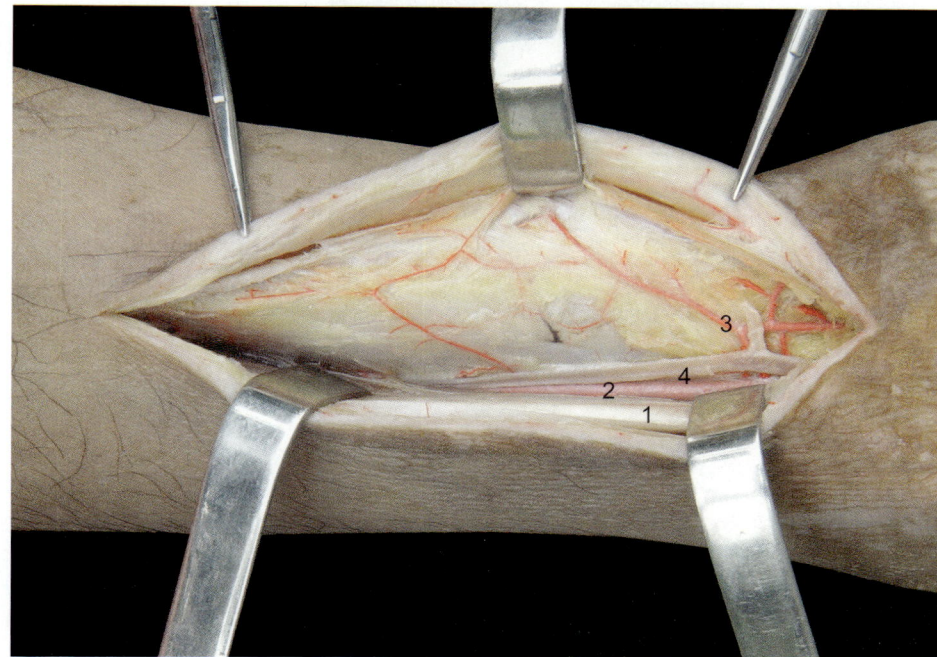

1. Tibialis anterior tendon
2. Anterior tibial artery
3. Superior ankle branch
4. Anterior tibial veins

Figure 3-205 Exposure of the vessels

The skin, the subcutaneous tissue and the extensor retinaculum should be incised open along the septum between the tendons of the tibialis anterior and the extensor hallucis longus. The two tendons should be pulled laterally to expose the anterior tibial artery and the superior ankle branch.

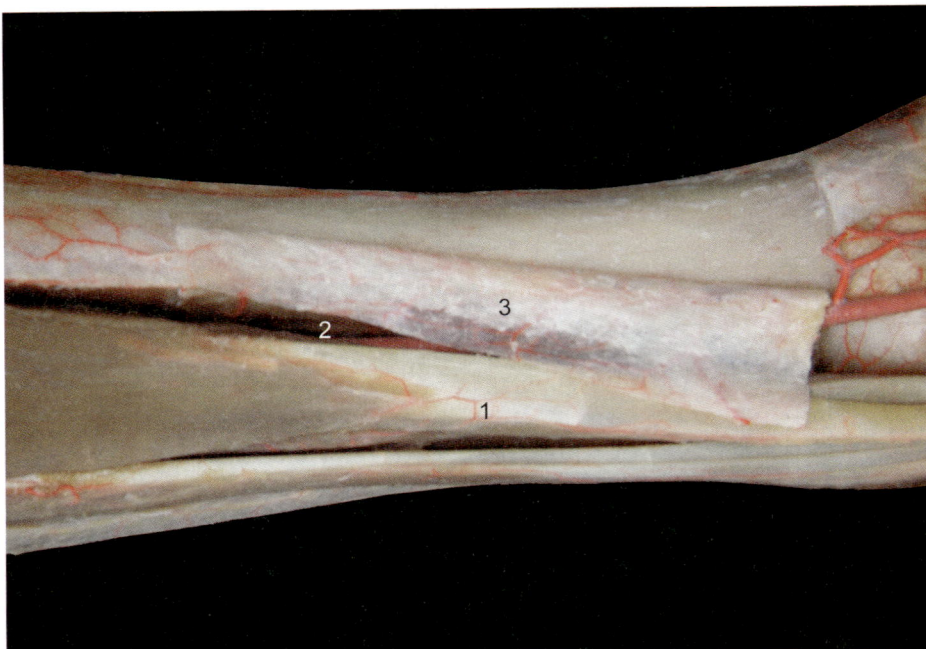

1. Tibialis anterior tendon
2. Anterior tibial artery
3. Periosteal flap

| Figure 3-206 | Harvest of the periosteal flap |

As is needed for the recipient site, the vascular pedicle should be chosen and the periosteal flap (about [8-10]×[4-5] cm) chiseled from the inferolateral segment of the tibia. The flap should be first dissected from the anterior tibial border, its superior border or its inferior border and then stripped under the periosteum down to the pedicle with a sharp osteotome. Finally, the border close to the interosseous membrane should be cut off.

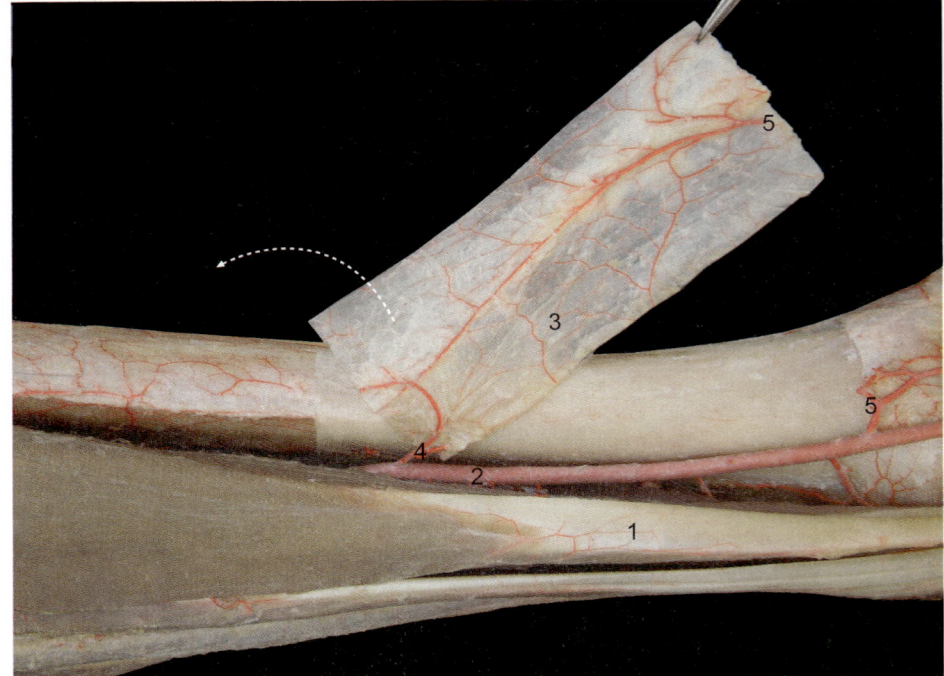

1. Tibialis anterior tendon
2. Anterior tibial artery
3. Periosteal flap
4. Musculoperiosteal branch
5. Superior ankle branch

| Figure 3-207 | Transposition of the periosteal flap |

The periosteal flap could be designed based on the musculoperiosteal branch of the anterior tibial artery. A flap of this type might be transferred upwards to repair the nonunion of the middle-inferior segment of the tibia.

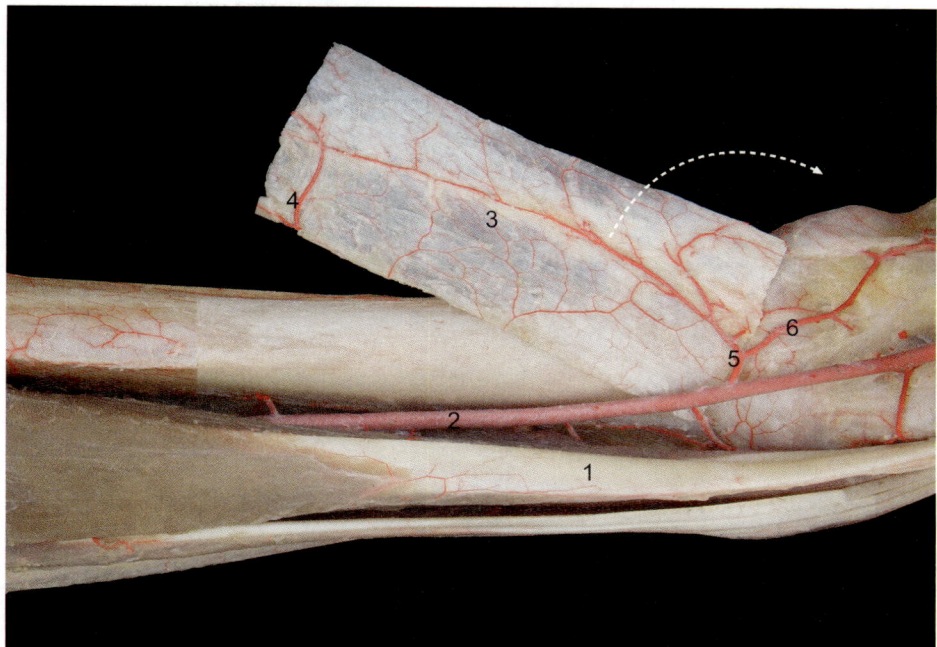

Figure 3-208   Retrograde transposition

The periosteal flap should be designed based on the superior ankle branch or the descending branch of the superior ankle branch. A flap of this type might be transferred downwards to repair a talus fracture or be used in an ankle fusion.

1. Tibialis anterior tendon
2. Anterior tibial artery
3. Periosteal flap
4. Muscular periosteal branch
5. Superior ankle branch
6. Descending branch of superior ankle branch

Key points in applied anatomy

Firstly, the tibialis anterior muscle tendon should be pulled laterally to expose adequately the anterior tibial vessel. The deep peroneal nerve at the anterolateral of the vessel should be protected. Secondly, the superior ankle branch anastomoses with the nearby vessels directly and sends periosteal branches to form a vascular network. The periosteal flap should be chiseled as distal to the pedicle vessel as possible to enlarge the transferring range of the flap. Thirdly, when the periosteal flap based on the descending branch of superior ankle branch should be chiseled, the origin of the superior ankle branch should be tentatively blocked to observe the retrograde blood supply before it is ligated and cut off. Fourthly, a periosteal flap should be made to avoid a disconnection of the periosteum and the bone block. Fifthly, the flap should be harvested and transferred upwards or downwards. The former incision might be extended and the fracture repositioned and fixed internally. Sixthly, these procedures should be completed before the extensor retinaculum is sutured.

Periosteal Flap on Medial Surface of Superior Tibia

There are many non-trunk vessels on the medial surface of the tibial periosteum. Among them is the direct periosteal branch that could be chosen as a pedicle for the periosteal flap. The pedicle might be located proximally or distally to the fracture. The flap could be harvested, the fracture repositioned and the flap with blood supply implanted in the same incision. A flap of this type might be transferred to treat an adjacent fracture and nonunion of the bone.

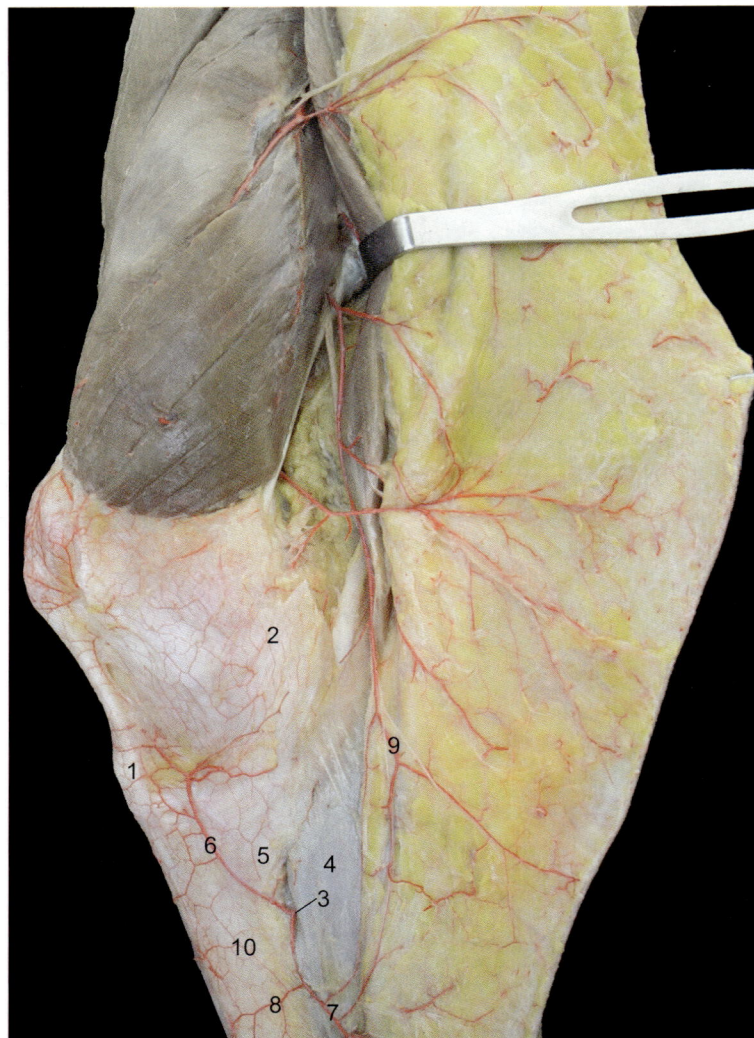

1. Tibial tuberosity
2. Medial condyle of tibia
3. Osseous-fascial branch
4. Medial head of gastrocnemius muscle
5. Tibia
6. Ascending branch
7. Descending branch
8. Horizontal branch
9. Cutaneous branch of saphenous artery
10. Periosteal arterial net

| Figure 3-209 | Applied anatomy |

The medial inferior genicular artery originates constantly from the popliteal artery. Its origin is situated at 5.8±2.1cm above the tibial tuberosity and is 1.7±0.4mm in diameter. Its trunk turns around the medial condyle of the tibia and extends forwards through the fascia of the superior border of the popliteal muscle to bifurcate into the articular branch and the osseous-fascial branch. The articular branch anastomoses with the anterior tibial recurrent artery and the articular branch of the saphenous artery. The osseous-fascial branch (the terminal branch) turns forwards to the medial surface of the tibia and runs superficially out through the space between the medial head of the gastrocnemius muscle and the tibia. It then divides into an ascending branch, a descending branch and a horizontal branch to anastomose with the intermuscular artery, the cutaneous branch of the saphenous artery. The articular branch and the osseous-fascial branch send periosteal branches and subbranches once and again to anastomose with each other and form a periosteal arterial net.

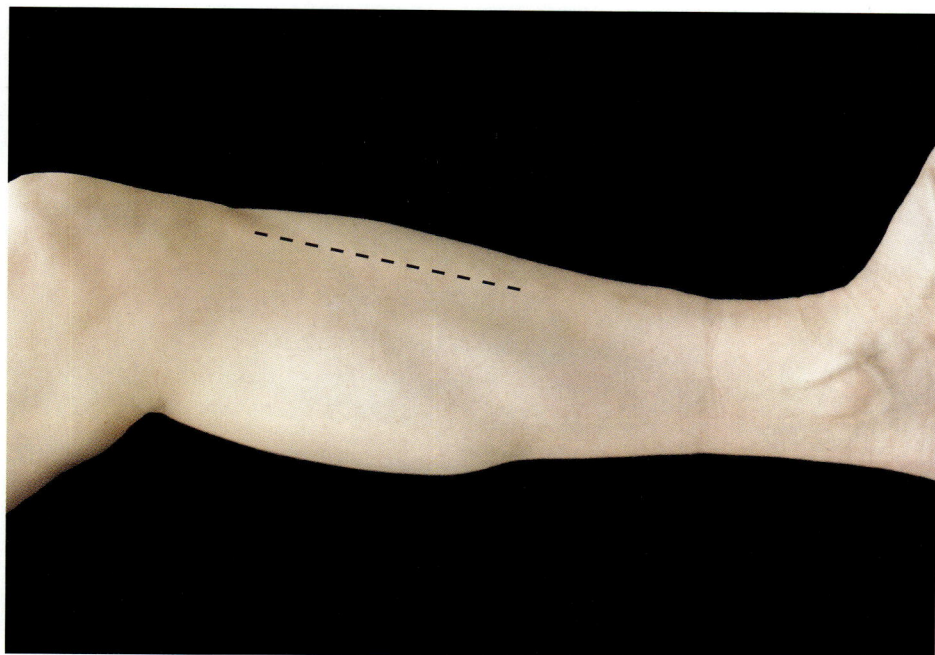

Figure 3-210   Design of the incision

The patient should be placed in supine position, and a longitudinal incision made at 1.5cm from the medial border of the superior tibia.

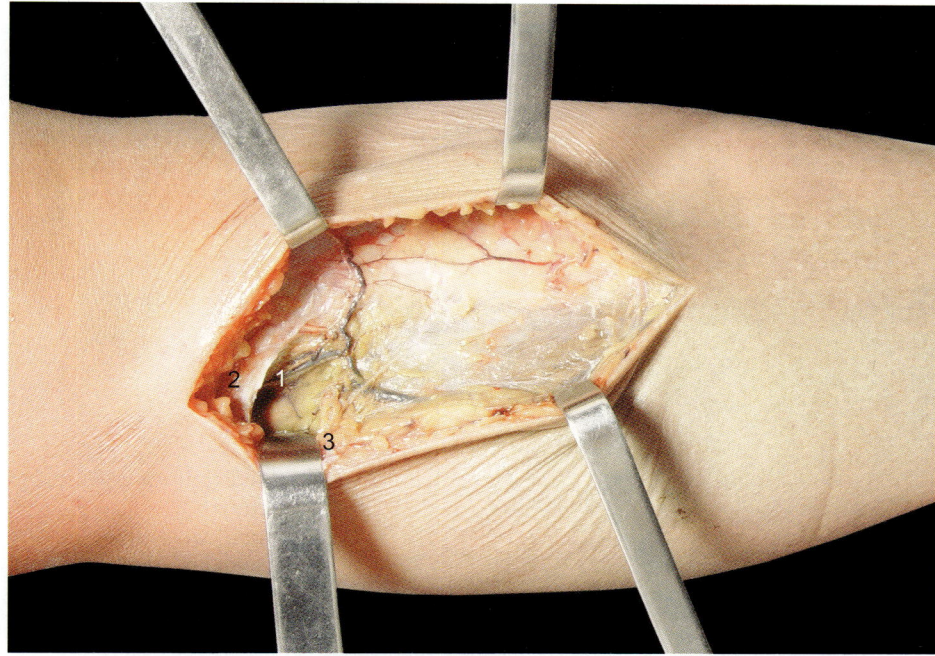

1. Medial inferior genicular artery

2. Popliteal muscle
3. Medial head of gastrocnemius muscle

Figure 3-211   Exposure of the vessels

The skin should be incised down to the deep fascia to expose the medial head of the gastrocnemius muscle, which should be pulled to the lateral side. The medial inferior genicular artery should be dissected in the space between the inferior border of the tibial medial condyle and the superior border of the popliteal muscle.

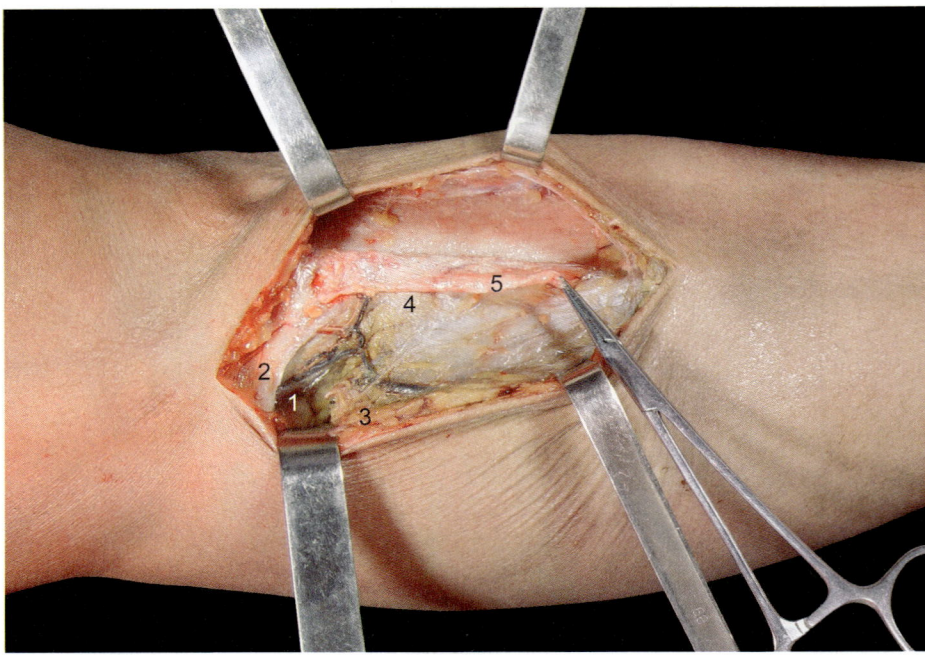

| Figure 3-212 | Harvest of the periosteal flap |

1. Medial inferior genicular artery
2. Popliteal muscle
3. Medial head of gastrocnemius muscle
4. Donor site
5. Periosteal flap

The periosteal flap should be retrieved at 8cm beneath the tibial plateau, namely, beneath the pes anserinus.

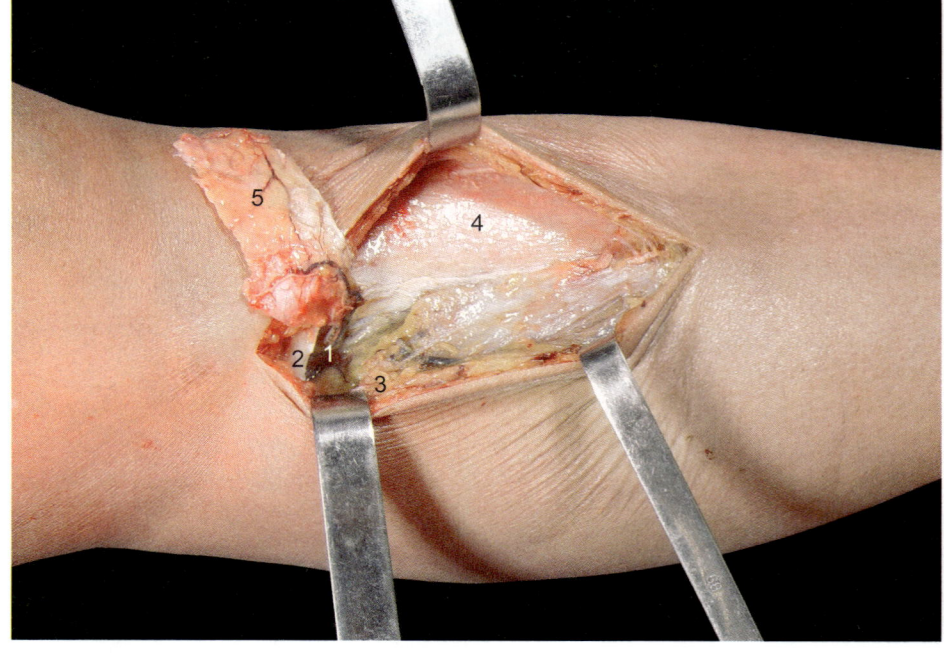

| Figure 3-213 | Transposition of the periosteal flap |

1. Medial inferior genicular artery
2. Popliteal muscle
3. Medial head of gastrocnemius muscle
4. Donor site
5. Periosteal flap

The medial inferior genicular artery should be taken as a pedicle and the anastomosis between the artery and the intermuscular branch of the posterior tibial artery retained. The periosteal flap might be dissected distributed with the intermuscular branches of the posterior tibial artery. A flap of this type is suitable for the repairs of fractures of the tibia or the tibia medial condyle.

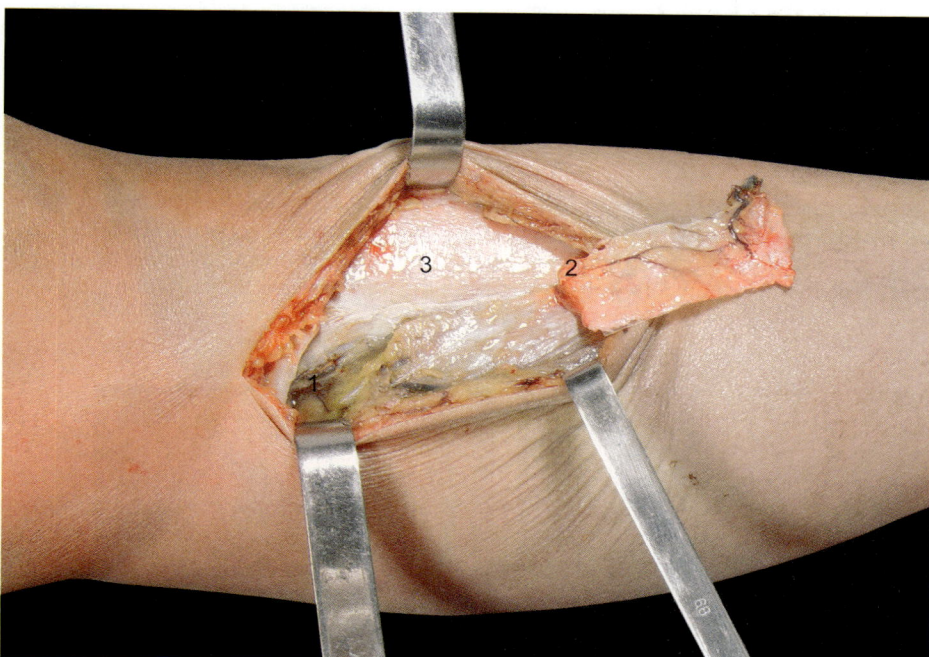

| Figure 3-214 | Retrograde transposition of the periosteal flap |

The intermuscular branch of the posterior tibial artery should be taken as a pedicle and its anastomosis with the descending branch of the medial inferior genicular artery retained. The periosteal flap might be harvested distributed with the horizontal branch and the ascending branch of the medial inferior genicular artery. A flap of this type is suitable for the repair of a fracture on the middle segment of the tibia.

1. Medial inferior genicular blood vessel
2. The intermuscular branch
3. Donor site

Key points in applied anatomy

Firstly, most of the periosteal branches are distributed on the middle-superior segment of the tibia. They are large in diameter. They could be taken individually as the vascular pedicle of a periosteal flap for grafting. In some cases the periosteal branches are small, and so part of the periosteum with several periosteal branches in it should serve as periosteal pedicle to guarantee the blood supply. Secondly, the tough tibia is the important weight-bearing bone of the lower limb. The flap should be designed and dissected neither too large nor too thick to avoid affecting the physiological function of the tibia.

The periosteum on the medial surface of the tibia is thick and rich in vessels. Its available area is so broad and its position so superficial without muscular attachment that it is easy to retrieve the needed materials. The composite periosteal flap could carry strip-shape bone so that it is suitable for the repair of fractures. There are so many vascular branches in the medial surface of the tibia so that the flap might be designed at different segment, adjusted to the recipient site and that the operation could be flexibly done. A flap of this type might be transferred for the repair of the tibial fracture and nonunion.

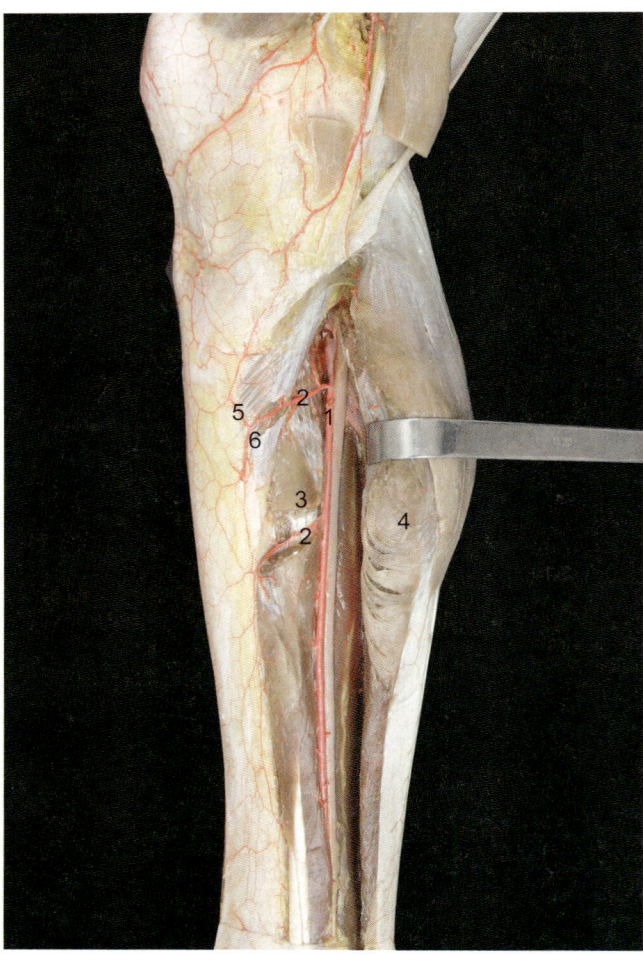
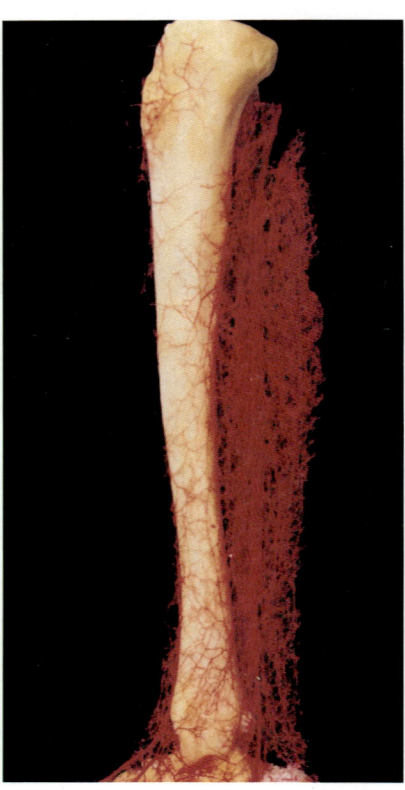

| Figure 3-215 | Applied anatomy |

On the medial surface of the tibia, from the tibial tuberosity to the protruding tip of the medial malleolus, there are 2-7 intermuscular branches that emerge from the posterior tibial artery. They run along the surface of the flexor digitorum longus muscle, descend obliquely forward or extend almost horizontally through the septum between the soleus muscle and the flexor digitorum longus muscle to the medial tibial border and divide into the ascending branch, the descending branch and the horizontal branch. The ascending and the descending branches anastomose with the adjacent intermuscular branches to form a vascular chain. The chain and the horizontal branch send periosteal branches and anastomose with each other to form a periosteal arterial net.

1. Posterior tibial artery
2. Intermuscular branch
3. Flexor digitorum longus muscle
4. Soleus muscle
5. Ascending branch
6. Descending branch

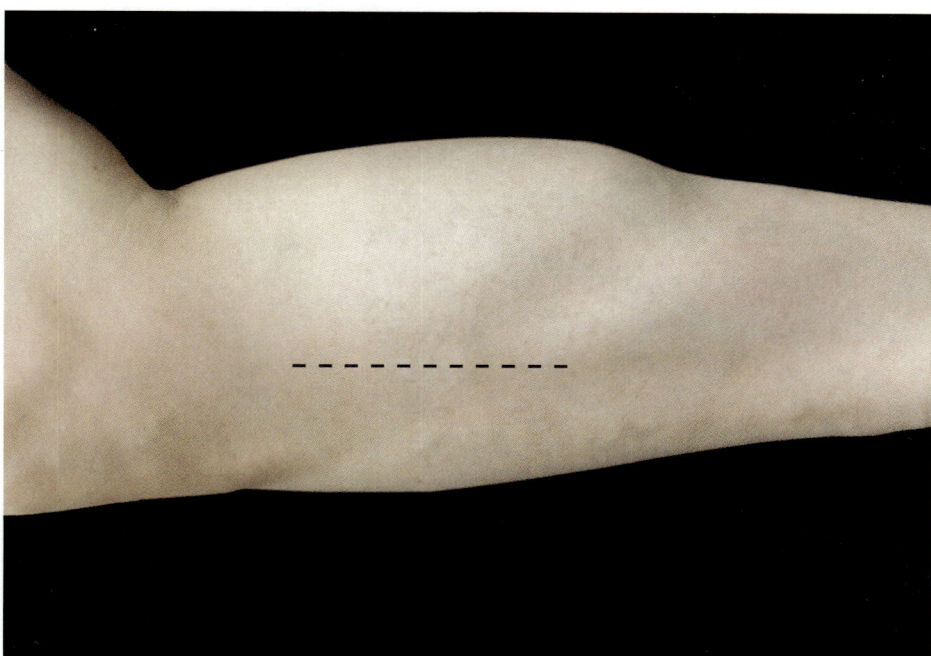

Figure 3-216   Design of the incision

The patient should be placed in supine position, and a vertical incision made from the medial border of the tibia.

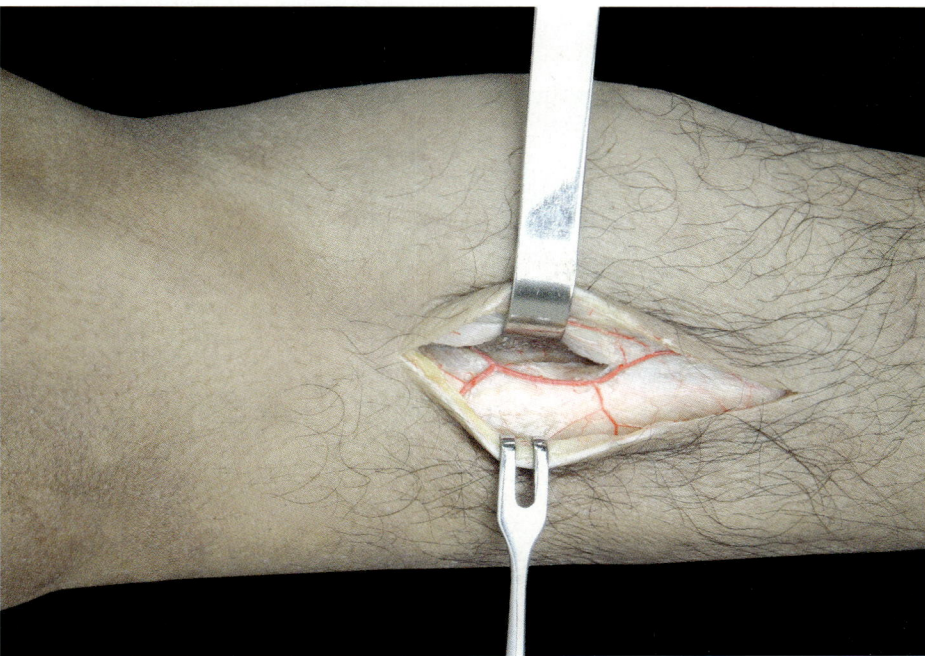

Figure 3-217   Exposure of the vessels

The incision should be designed as usual for reposition of the fracture. The soleus muscle should be first pulled apart to expose the posterior tibial artery and its intermuscular branch. The septum between the soleus muscle and the flexor digitorum longus muscle should be separated to trace the intermuscular branch to the medial tibial border.

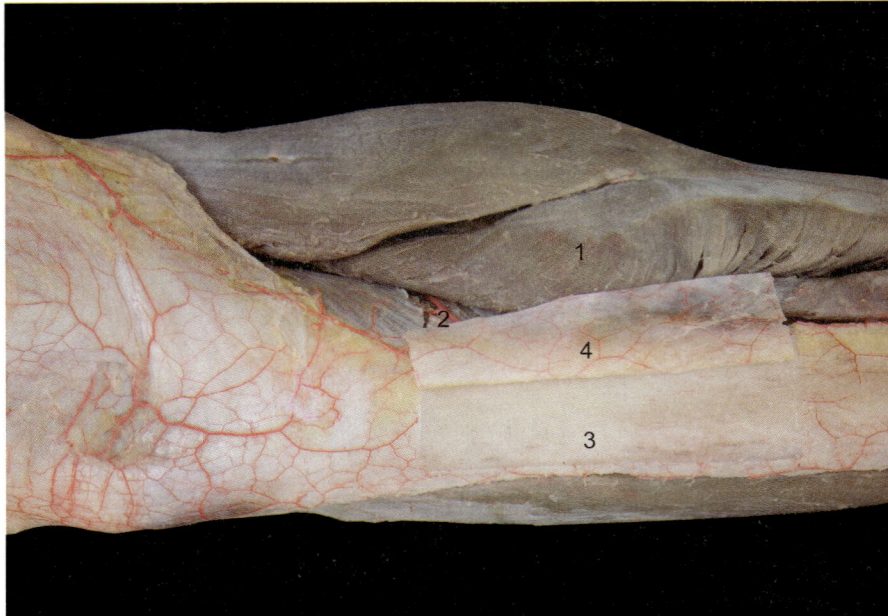

1. Soleus muscle
2. The intermuscular branch
3. Tibia
4. Periosteal flap

Figure 3-218	Harvest of the periosteal flap

The vascular pedicle should be chosen according to the fracture level before the periosteal flap is dissected at the anterior border of the tibia and at the superior or inferior border of the periosteal flap. Then the flap should be stripped to the vascular pedicle with a sharp osteotome and finally cut off at the border of the interosseous membrane. When the flap is chiseled, the vascular pedicle should be loosened a little before the fracture is repositioned and fixed internally. All this done, the periosteal flap might be transferred and implanted into the recipient site.

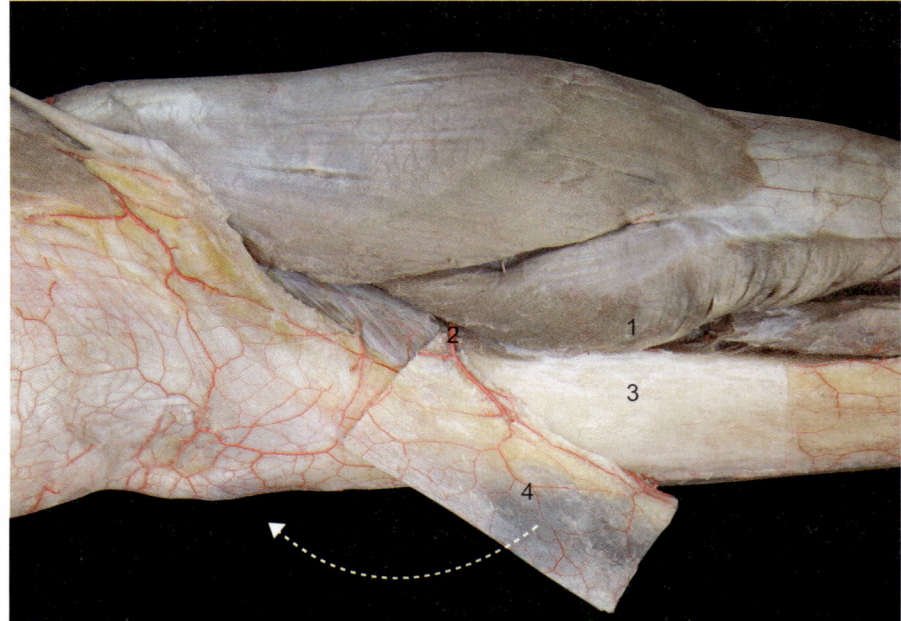

1. Soleus muscle
2. Intermuscular branch
3. Tibia
4. Periosteal flap

Figure 3-219	Transposition of the periosteal flap

The periosteal flap should be designed carrying the intermuscular branch of the posterior tibial artery as its pedicle and then circumrotated upwards to repair the tibial fracture above the pedicle.

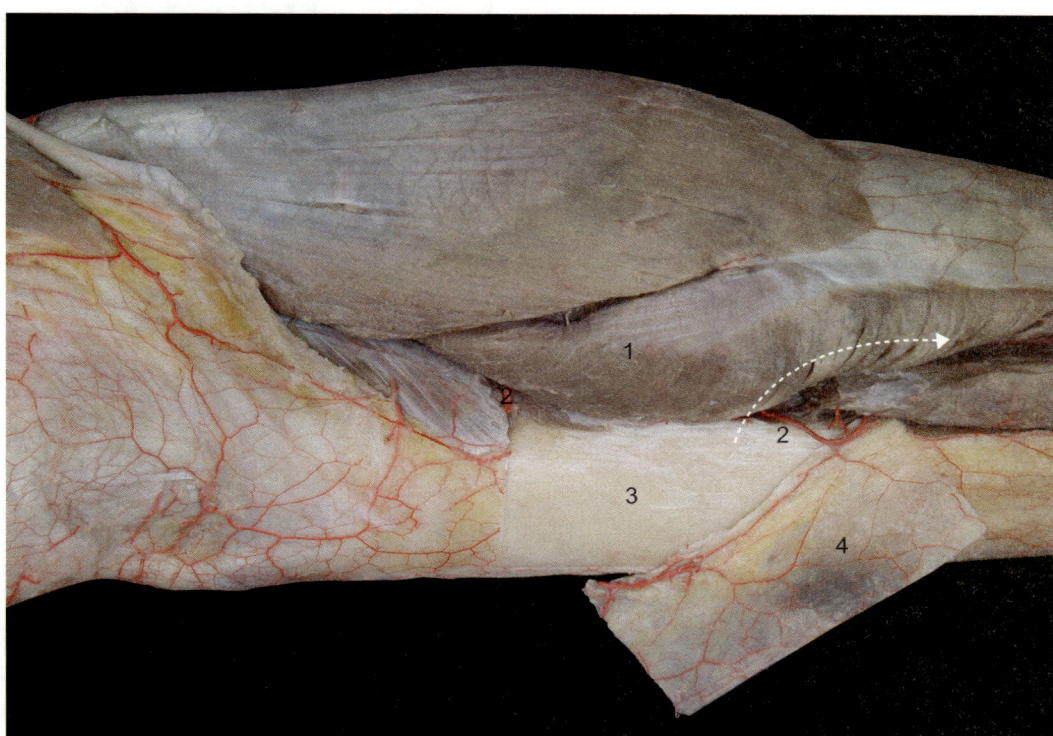

| Figure 3-220 | Retrograde transposition |

The periosteal flap should be designed carrying the intermuscular branch of the posterior tibial artery as a pedicle and circumrotated downwards to repair the tibial fracture beneath the pedicle.

1. Soleus muscle
2. Intermuscular branch
3. Tibia
4. Periosteal flap

Key points in applied anatomy

Firstly, when the periosteal flap on medial surface of the tibia is made carrying the intermuscular branch of the posterior tibial blood as its pedicle, the vascular pedicle should be firstly chosen according to the fracture level, the periosteal flap chiseled, and the fracture fixed. Secondly, the flap should be stripped beneath the periosteum of the tibia to avoid disconnecting the deep fascia with the periosteum and damaging the blood supply. Thirdly, the periosteal flap should be designed away from the vascular pedicle, and the pedicle in the intermuscular septum loosened so that the flap could be transferred smoothly. Fourthly, when the periosteal flap is transferred to the fractured part, it should be sutured and fixed with the nearby tissues. Fifthly, parts (about 2cm) of the deep fascia and the periosteum should be retained at the medial border of the tibia to guarantee the blood supply of the tibia.

37

Periosteal Flap on Distal Anterior Surface of Tibia and Fibula

The pedicled periosteal flap on the distal anterior tibia and the distal anterior fibula refers to a periosteal (bone) flap that takes the deep fascia as its pedicle and the superficial peroneal vessels as its axis. It has such advantages as a superficial position, long pedicles, easy anatomization and easy transposition. It could carry stripped bones and be made into composite flaps. The periosteal flap might be transferred anterogradely to repair the nonunion at any segments of the tibia or transferred retrogradely to repair a wound on the tarsalis.

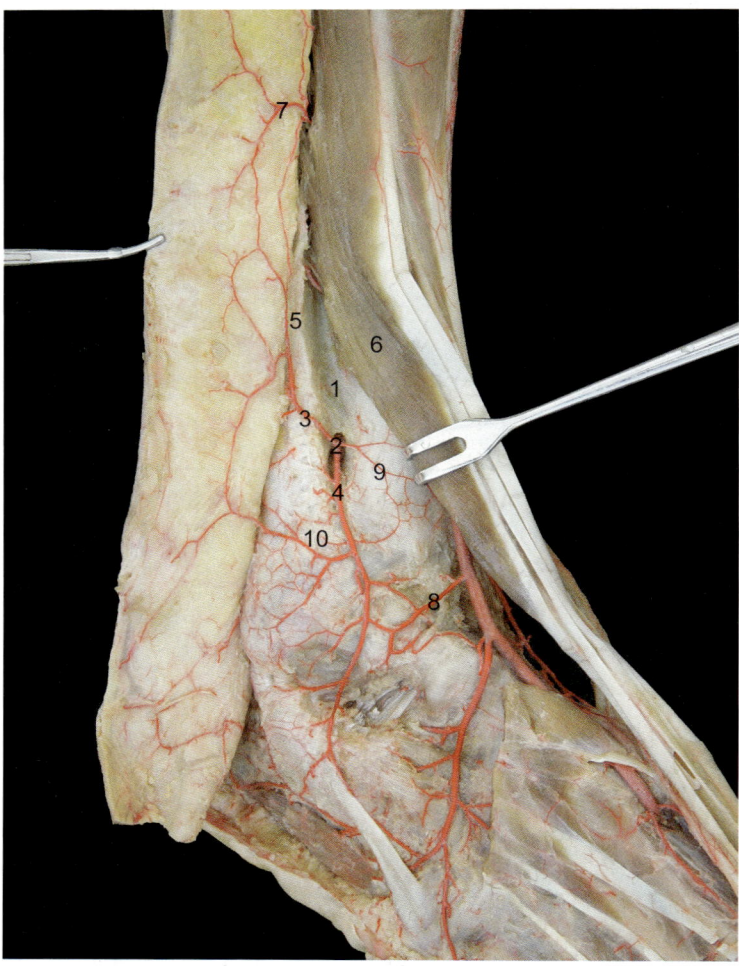

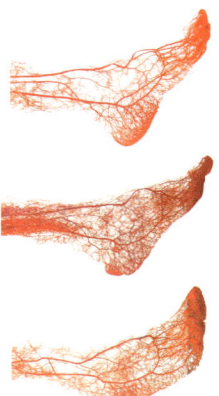

Figure 3-221	Applied anatomy

The peroneal artery perforates through the interosseous membrane at 5.7cm above the tip of the lateral malleolus, and is renamed the perforating branch. The perforator further bifurcates into the ascending branch and the descending branch. The ascending branch extends in the septum between the peroneus longus muscle and the extensor digitorum longus muscle and perforates through the deep fascia to enter the subcutaneous tissue. It then ascends to anastomose with the superficial peroneal artery (The direct anastomosis of the two accounts for 20%. The indirect anastomosis between the two through the interseptus arteries at different level of leg accounts for 80%.). The descending branch descends along the anterolateral border of the lateral malleolus and anastomoses with the lateral anterior malleolar artery close to the malleolar sulcus. The ascending and the descending branches send 2-5 tibial periosteal branches and 2-7 lateral malleolar periosteal branches to nourish the periosteum at the inferior segments of tibia and fibula. In general, the perforating branch of peroneal artery is 1.6mm in diameter at its initiation, the descending branch 1.0mm, the superficial peroneal artery 1.0-1.5mm and the 2 concomitant veins 1.4-1.5mm.

1. Interosseous membrane
2. Perforating branch
3. Ascending branch
4. Descending branch
5. Peroneus longus muscle
6. Extensor digitorum longus muscle
7. Interseptus artery
8. Lateral anterior malleolar artery
9. Tibial periosteal branches
10. Lateral malleolar periosteal branches

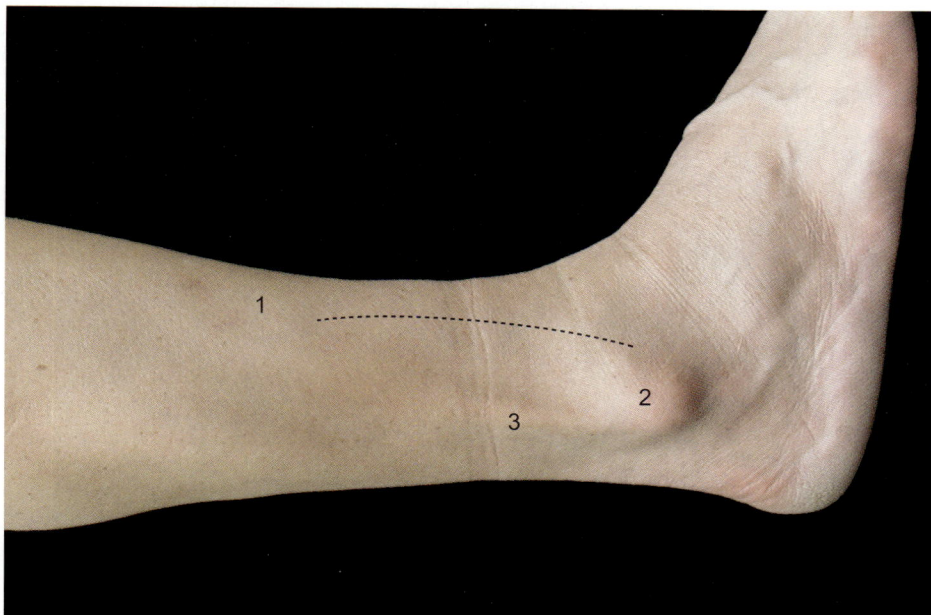

1. Anterior border of tibia
2. Lateral malleolus
3. Peroneus longus tendon

Figure 3-222   Design of the incision

The incision should begin from above the lesion part and at 1cm laterally from the anterior border of the tibia and extend longitudinally downwards to pass the lesion site. It should continue laterally downwards along the anterolateral septum of the leg to reach the anteroinferior border of the lateral malleolus.

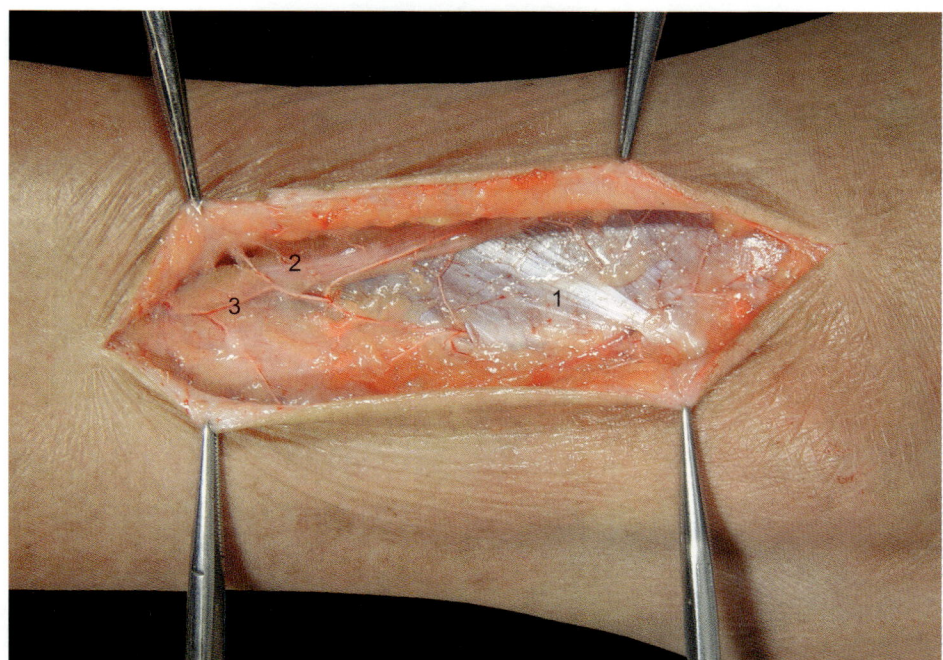

1. Superior extensor retinaculum
2. Superficial peroneal nerve
3. Superficial peroneal vessels

Figure 3-223   **Exposure of the nerve**

The skin and the subcutaneous tissue should be incised open to expose the deep fascia and the superior extensor retinaculum, which is formed due to the thickened deep fascia above the ankle joint. The skin should be drawn bilaterally to expose the superficial peroneal nerve and its concomitant superficial peroneal vessels at the middle-inferior segments of the leg.

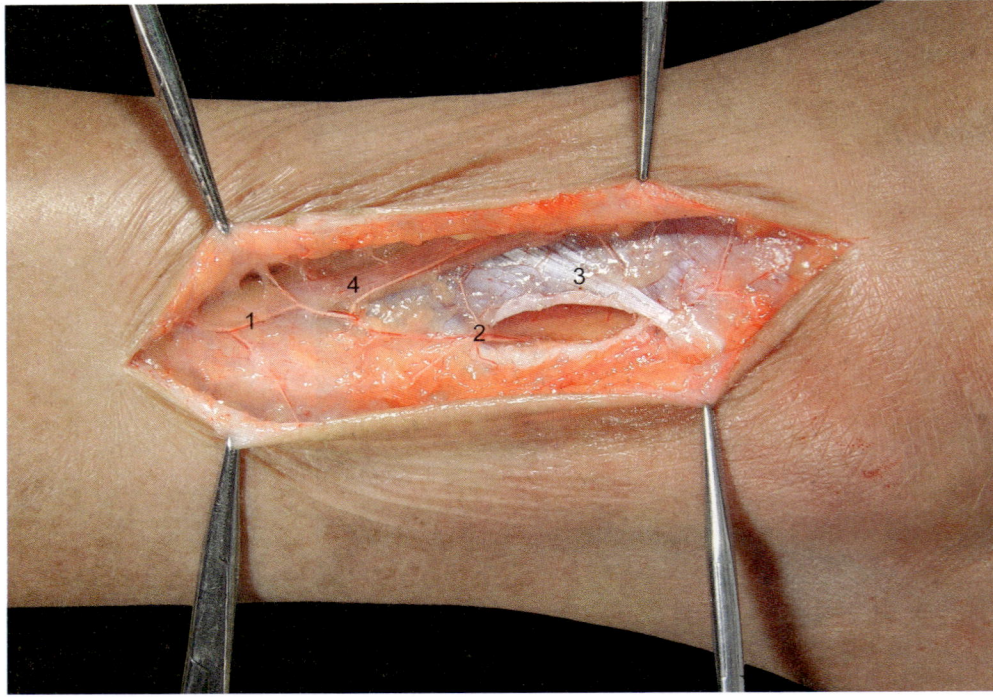

1. Superficial peroneal vessels
2. Ascending branch of the perforating branch of peroneal artery
3. Superior extensor retinaculum
4. Superficial peroneal nerve

Figure 3-224   Incision of the deep fascia

The incision should continue along the superficial peroneal vessels to expose the ascending branch of the perforator before the superior extensor retinaculum is incised open.

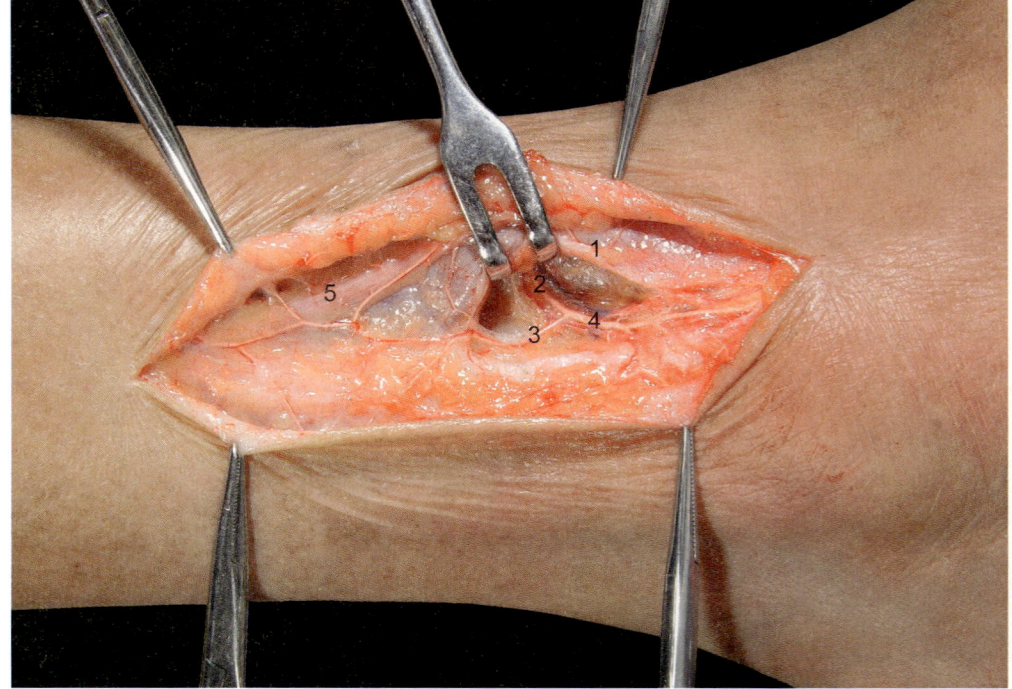

1. Extensor digitorum longus muscle
2. Perforating branch of the peroneal artery
3. Ascending branch
4. Descending branch
5. Superficial peroneal nerve

Figure 3-225   Exposure of the vessels

The extensor digitorum longus should be pulled medially to expose the periosteum in front of the tibia, the perforating branch of the peroneal artery and its ascending and descending and periosteal branches.

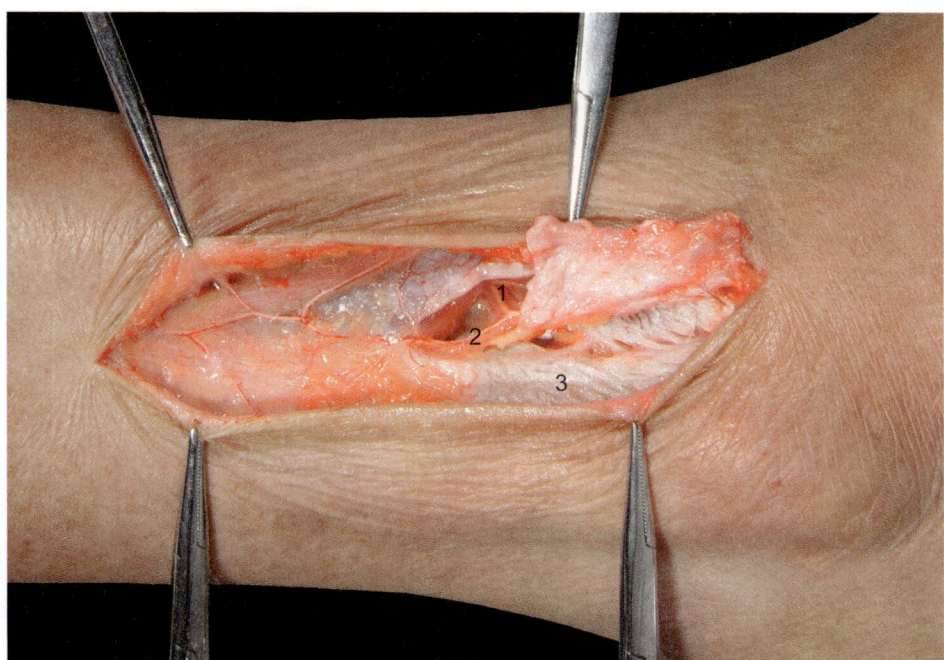

1. Perforating branch of peroneal artery
2. Ascending branch
3. Periosteal flap

Figure 3-226   Harvest of the fibular periosteal flap

The deep fascia should be incised directly down to the bone along the posterior border of the fibula. A slice of the bone on the surface of the lateral malleolus should be chiseled and cut off with an osteotome above the superior border of the protrudent tip of the lateral malleolus. The dissection should continue upwards to retrieve a fibula periosteum about 2 cm wide.

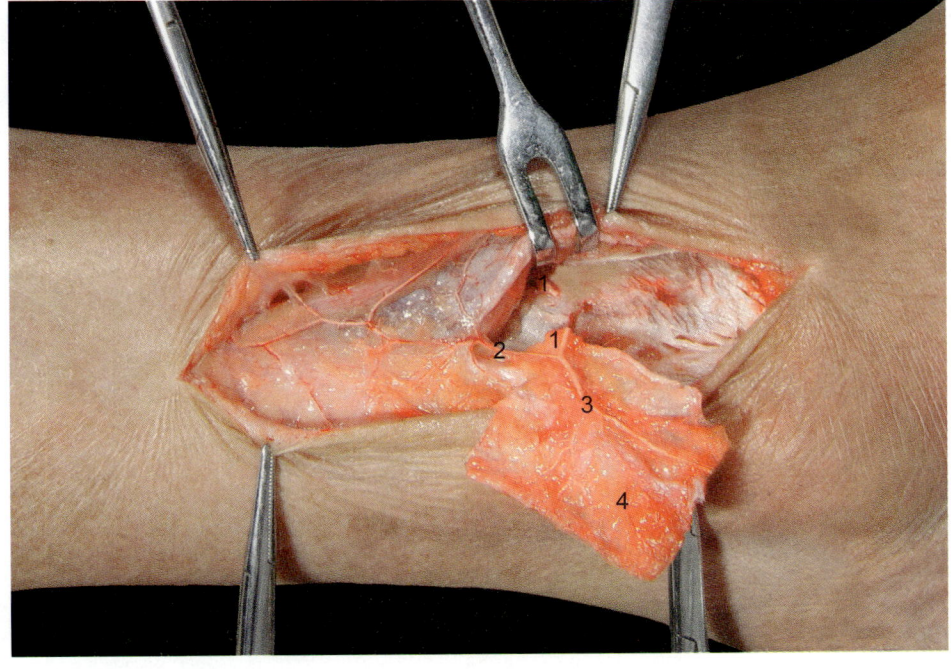

1. Perforating branch of peroneal artery
2. Ascending branch
3. Descending branch
4. Periosteal flap

Figure 3-227   Harvest of the tibial periosteal flap

After that, the tibial periosteum should be dissected transversely at the superior level of the protrudent tip of the medial malleolus and the dissection continue upwards along the tibial medial border to retrieve a tibial periosteum about 3-4cm wide.

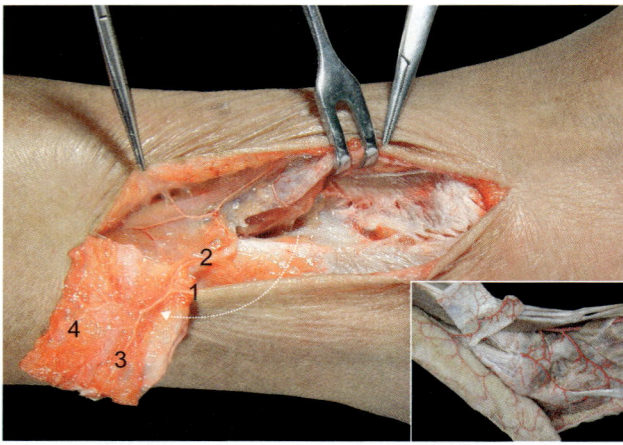

1. Perforating branch of peroneal artery
2. Ascending branch
3. Descending branch
4. Periosteal flap

| Figure 3-228 | Transposition of the periosteal flap |

The lengths of the separated superficial peroneal vessels and the deep fascia should be adjusted to the position of the lesion. The fracture should be repositioned and fixed internally before the periosteal flap could be implanted into the recipient site.

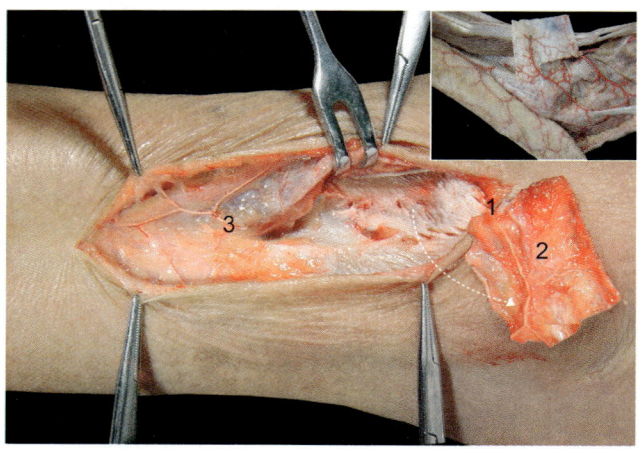

1. Descending branch of the perforating branch of the peroneal artery
2. Periosteal flap
3. Ascending branch

| Figure 3-229 | Retrograde transposition of the periosteal flap |

The periosteal flap should be made with the descending branch of the perforating branch of the peroneal artery as its pedicle and transferred retrogradely to repair the tarsalia.

Key points in applied anatomy

Firstly, the connecting line between the midpoint of the tibial tuberosity and the fibula head and the anterior border of the lateral malleolus might be regarded as the body surface projection of the superficial peroneal artery. Secondly, the superficial peroneal nerve that accompanies the superficial peroneal blood vessels might serve as an indication to look for the blood vessels in the operation, and the nerve should be dissected and protected carefully. Thirdly, the deep fascia around the lateral malleolus attaches tightly to the periosteum. It is preferable that the periosteal branch of the ascending branch be retrieved together with the deep fascia and that both not be separated too much to avoid damaging the periosteum blood vessels. Fourthly, the superficial peroneal artery tends to be rather thin. It is unnecessary that the perivascular tissue be dissected too much. When the vascular pedicle is being dissected, the superficial peroneal vessels, the fascia and the intermuscular septum should be integrated to form a deep fascia-intermuscular septum periosteal flap. Fifthly, the periosteal flap should have such a size as follows: its inferior border generally falls on the superior border of the line between the protrudent tip of the malleolus, its medial and lateral borders on the medial tibia and the posterior fibula, respectively, and its superior border at 7cm above the inferior border. But the inferior border often departs from the epiphyseal plate in child cases. It should be positioned with X-ray preoperatively.

Posterolateral Tibia and Fibular Periosteal Flap Pedicled with Peroneal Blood Vessels

38

The inferior segment of the posterior tibia is flat, broad and easy to be exposed. The donor site is large in size and the peroneal blood vessels large in diameter. The dissecting position is constant and easy to determine in the operation. The periosteal flap taking the peroneal blood vessels as its pedicle might be located at the distal end of the posterior part of the tibia and the fibula. A flap of this type might be suitable for the repair of the osseous nonunion of the middle-inferior segments of the tibia. The periosteal flap should be dissected from the backside with the terminal branch of the peroneal artery as the pedicle if the patient has undertaken some operations and this soft tissue of the anterior lateral tibia is in poor conditions. A flap made in this way might be transferred retrogradely to repair a wound on the malleolus articulation.

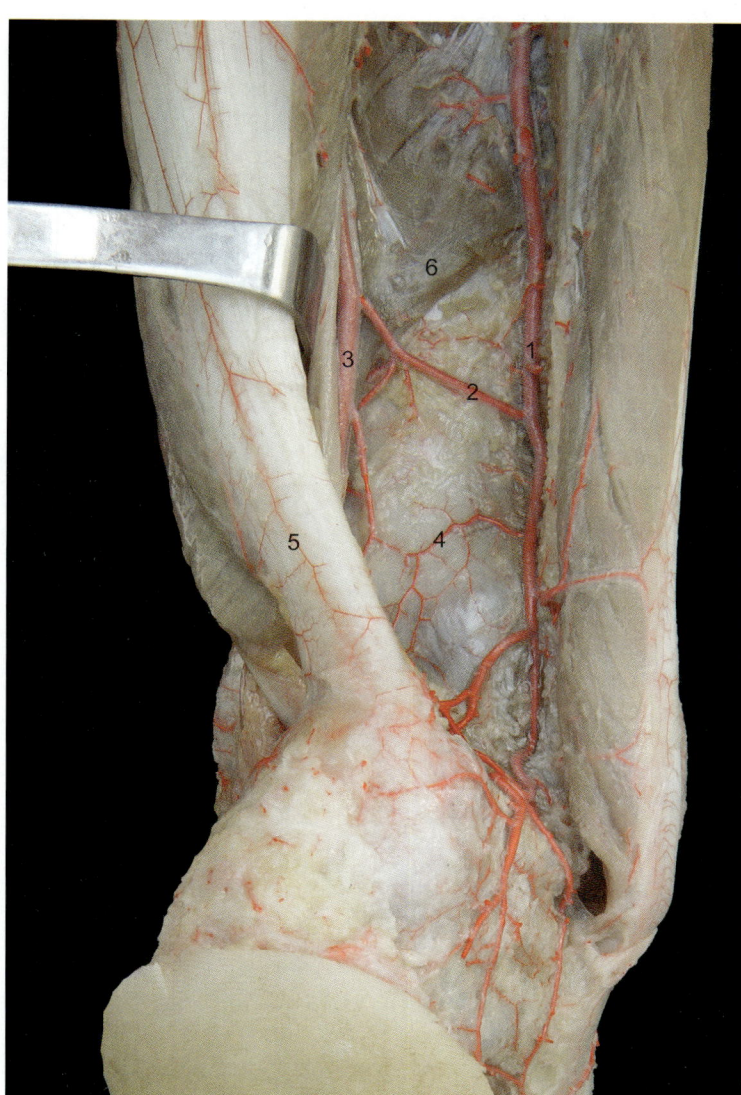

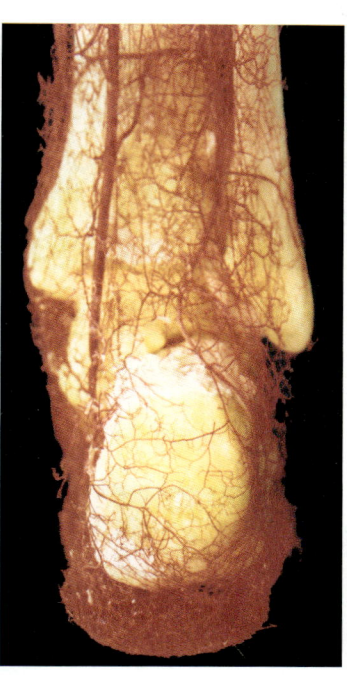

Figure 3-230	Applied anatomy

The peroneal artery gives anastomotic branches at 4.7cm (on average) above the posterior ankle of the inferior extremity of the tibia and runs transversely downwards or inwards clinging to the posterior tibia. Its terminal anastomoses with the posterior tibial artery and gives ascending and decending periosteal branches to distribute in a tree-like shape on the posterior segment of the tibia. The peroneal artery gives periosteal branches to distribute on the inferior segment of the fibula.

1. Peroneal artery
2. Anastomosis branch
3. Posterior tibial artery
4. Periosteal branch
5. Calcaneal tendon
6. Musculus flexor pollicis longus

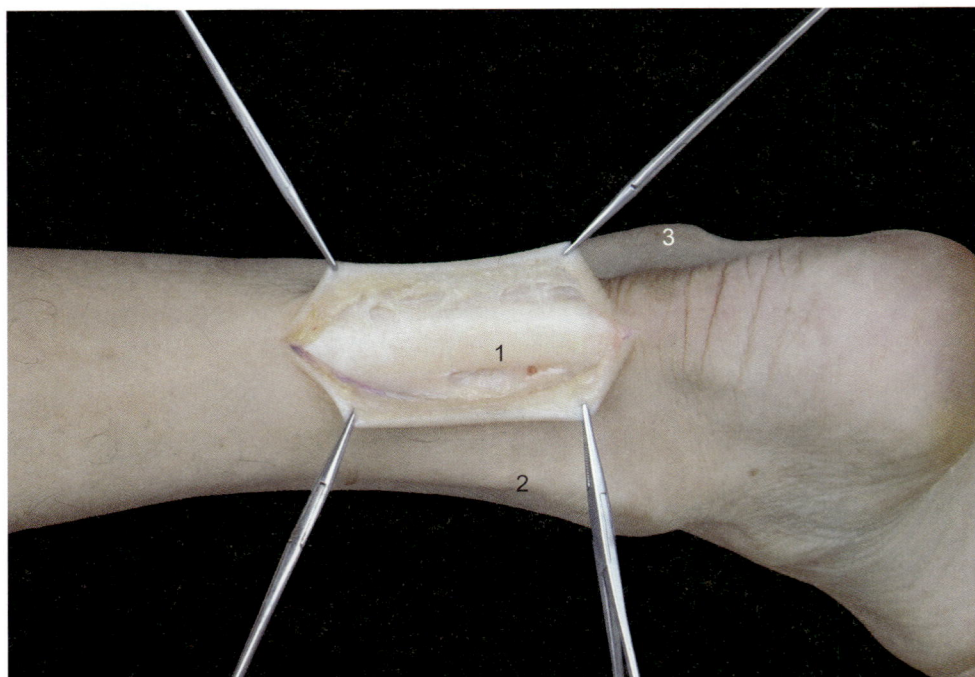

1. Calcaneal tendon
2. Medial border of the tibia
3. Lateral malleolus

Figure 3-231   **Design of the incision**

The incision should begin with the medial calcaneal tendon and continue longitudinally upwards at 1cm from the posteromedial border of the tibia to 3-5cm near the osseous nonunion.

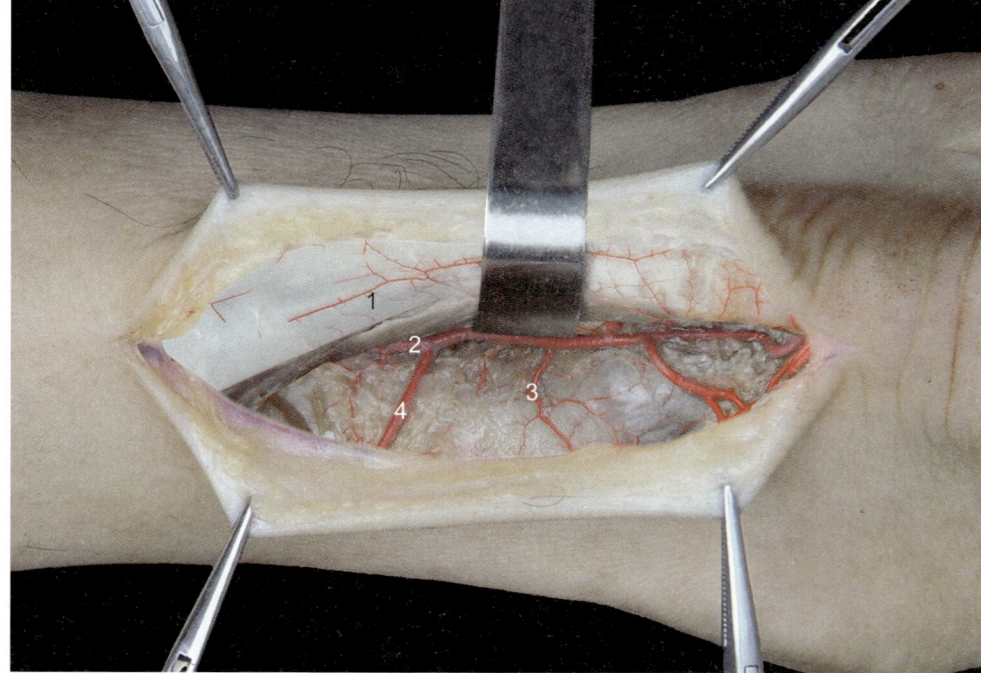

1. Calcaneal tendon
2. Peroneal artery
3. Periosteal branch
4. Anastomotic branch

Figure 3-232   **Exposure of the vessels**

The calcaneal tendon, the muscular fibularis longus and the muscular fibularis brevis should be pulled outwards whereas the other tissues at the posterior calf should be pulled inwards to expose the distal segment of the peroneal artery and the donor area.

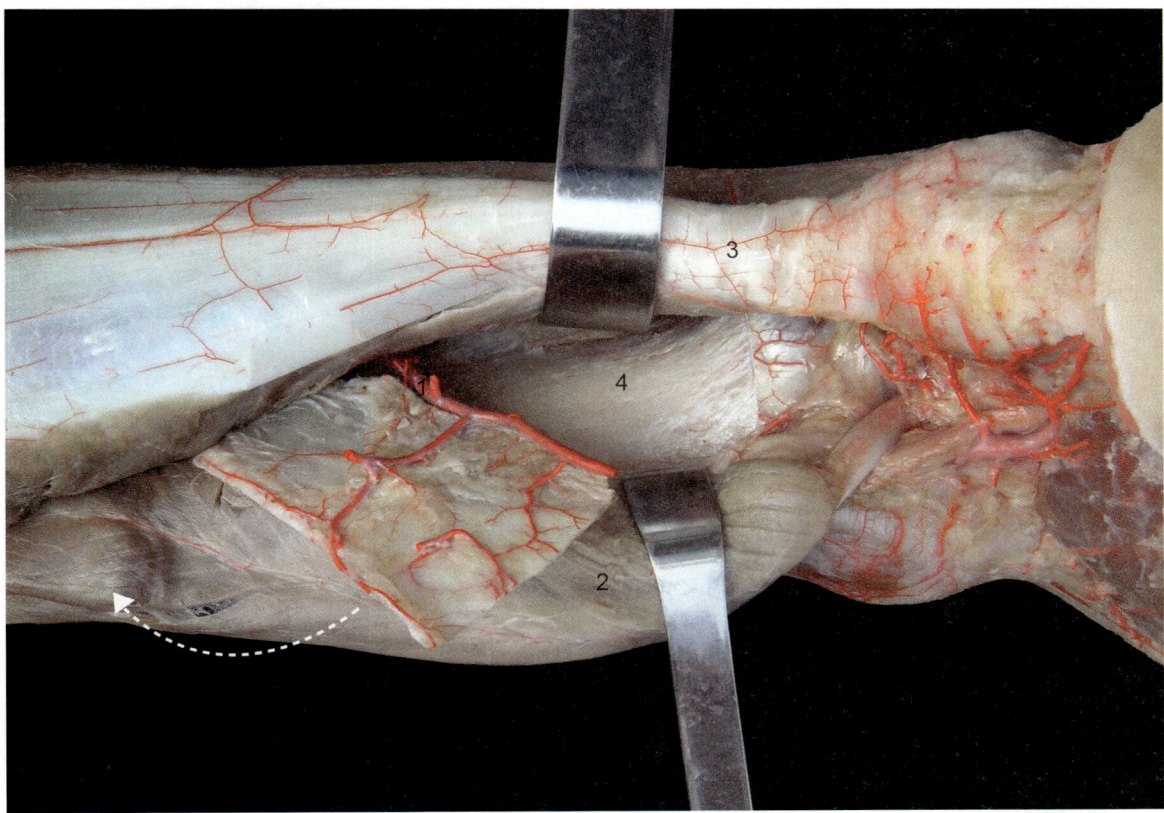

Figure 3-233   **Harvest and transposition of the periosteal flap**

The peroneal artery should be ligated at the level of the posterior ankle. The posterior tibia (5×
2.5cm) and the inferior segment of the fibula (5cm ×1/2 of the fibula) should be retrieved to make a
double-lobe periosteal flap. A flap of this type might be used to repair the tibial fracture or osseous
nonunion. The proximal incision might be extended so the vascular pedicle could be lengthened
appropriately before the flap could be implanted into the recipient site. When the flap is used to
repair the malleolus articulation, the initiation of the anastomosis branch should be ligated, the
peroneal artery cut off, and the flap transferred retrogradely to the ankle joint.

1. Peroneal artery
2. Musculus flexor pollicis longus
3. Calcaneal tendon
4. Donor site

Key points in applied anatomy

Firstly, when the perforating branch of the peroneal artery is being ligated and cut off, the peroneal
artery should be given great attention to avoid getting it damaged. Secondly, when the periosteal flap
based on the inferior segment of the fibula is being retrieved, a thin layer intramuscular cuff should
be retained on the surface of the fibula to protect the arch blood vessels that provide nutrition for the
fibula. Thirdly, in the operation, the end of the anastomosis branch of the posterior tibial artery should
be ligated and cut off to avoid vascular laceration caused by pulling the periosteal flap. Fourthly, the
dissection should continue upwards with a thin layer interosseous membrane to keep the tibia and the
fibular flaps conjoined with each other. Fifthly, in child case, the epiphyseal plate should be excluded
and the position determined preoperatively with X-ray.

39 Periosteal Flap Pedicled with Peroneal Artery

The fibular periosteal flap based on the peroneal artery has such advantages as a large size and a convenient transposition. It might be transferred antegradely to repair bone defects of the middle-superior segments of the tibia, the inferior segment of the knee or the femur. It might be transferred retrogradely to repair bone defects of the inferior segment of the tibia and the calcaneus, or to fuse the ankle joint. It might be dissected and transferred to repair defects of the long bones, too.

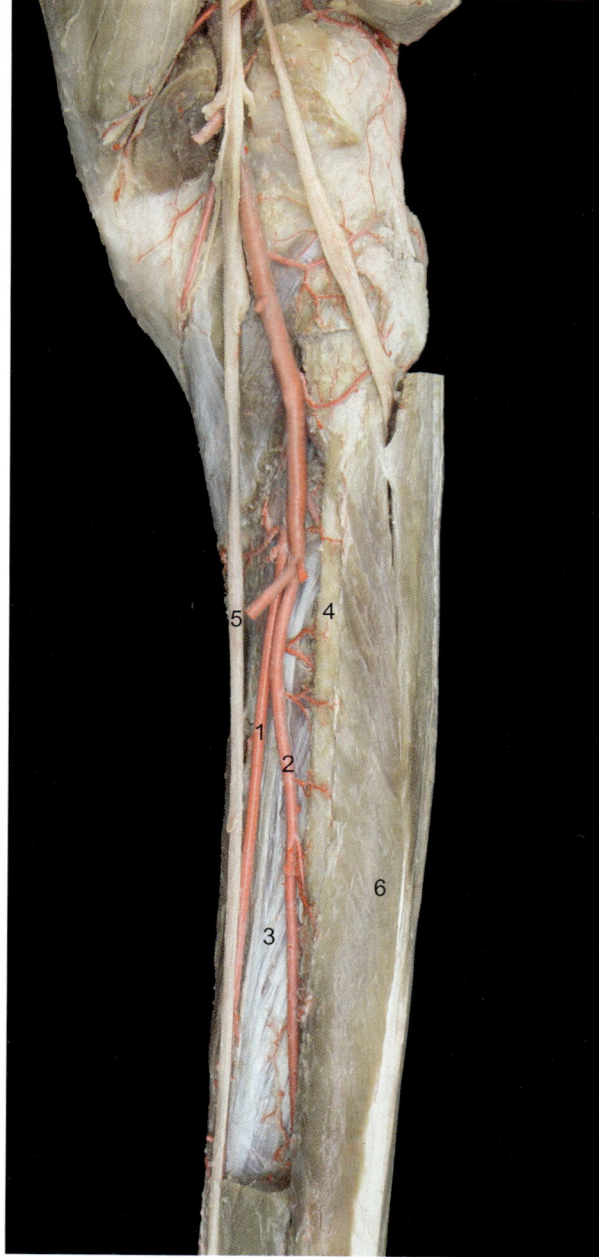

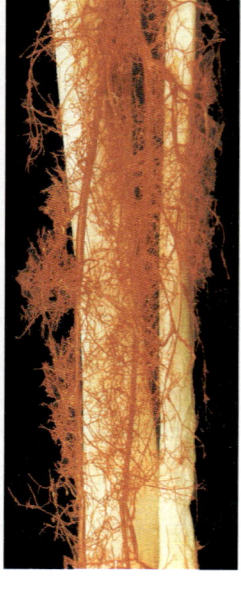

Figure 3-234	Applied anatomy

The nutrient vessel of the fibular shaft emerges from the peroneal artery. This artery is situated at 3.0cm (on average) to the midpoint of the inferior border of the popliteal muscle (i.e. 6.6cm or so below the apex of the fibular head) among the soleus, the tibialis posterior and the musculus flexor pollicis longus. Its initiation is 4.0mm in diameter. The artery descends inferiorly outwards between the posterior surface of the fibula and the musculus flexor pollicis longus, and terminates at the lateral calcaneal artery. At the proximal beginning it is away from the fibula. But the farther it goes down, the closer it runs to the fibula until it enters the deep side of the musculus flexor pollicis longus at about 8.9cm to the fibular head. The total artery might be covered in some cases under the muscle. Along the course, the artery gives the fibular nutrient branch to enter the middle-superior segments of the fibula. It covers on average 8.6 cm from the fibular nutrient foramen to the beginning point of the peroneal artery.

1. Posterior tibial artery   **2.** Peroneal artery
3. Tibialis posterior   **4.** Fibula
5. Tibial nerve   **6.** Peroneus longus

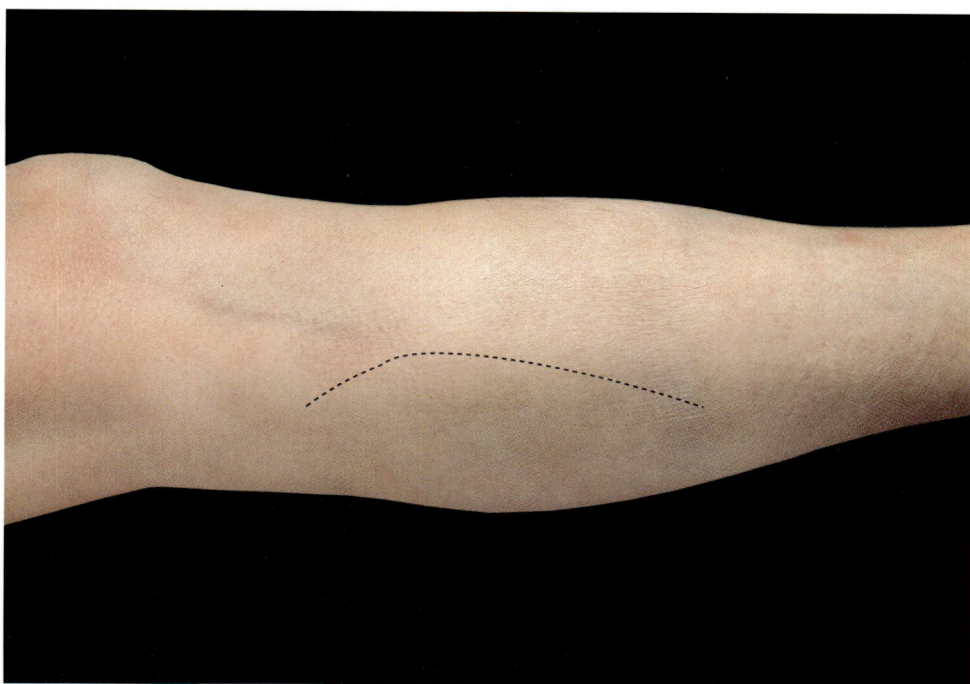

Figure 3-235	Design of the incision

A longitude incision should be made along the posterior border of the fibula, with the midpoint located at the intersection of the proximal 2/5 segment and the distal 3/5 segment of the fibula as its central part. The proximal end should be curved toward the popliteal fossa. The length of the incision depends on that of the fibular section.

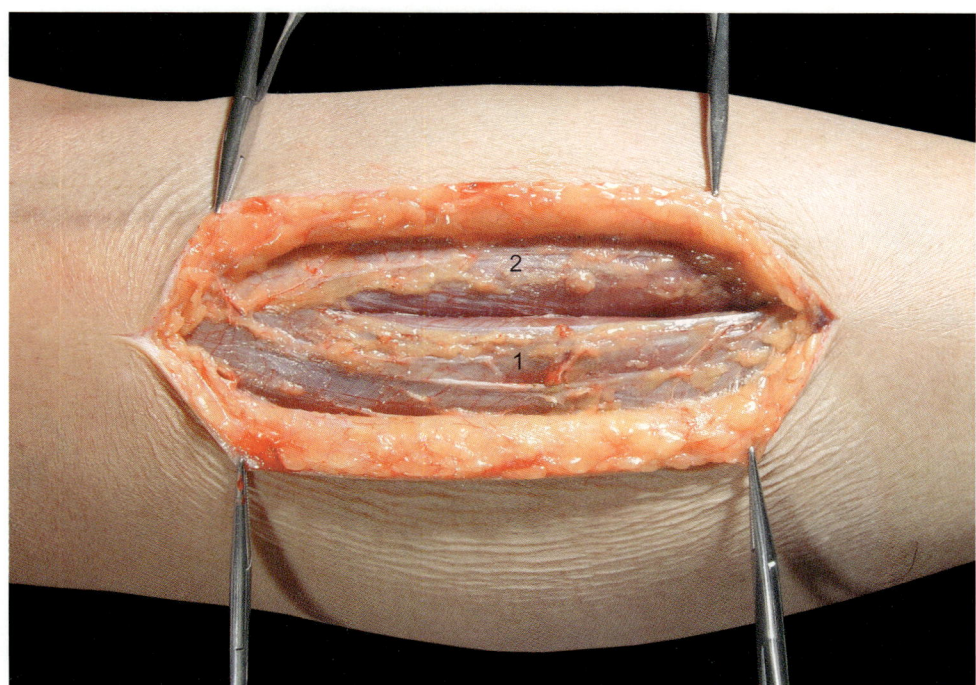

1. Soleus
2. Peroneus longus

Figure 3-236	Exposure of the muscle

Then the skin and the subcutaneous tissue should be incised open to expose the septum between the soleus and the peroneus longus.

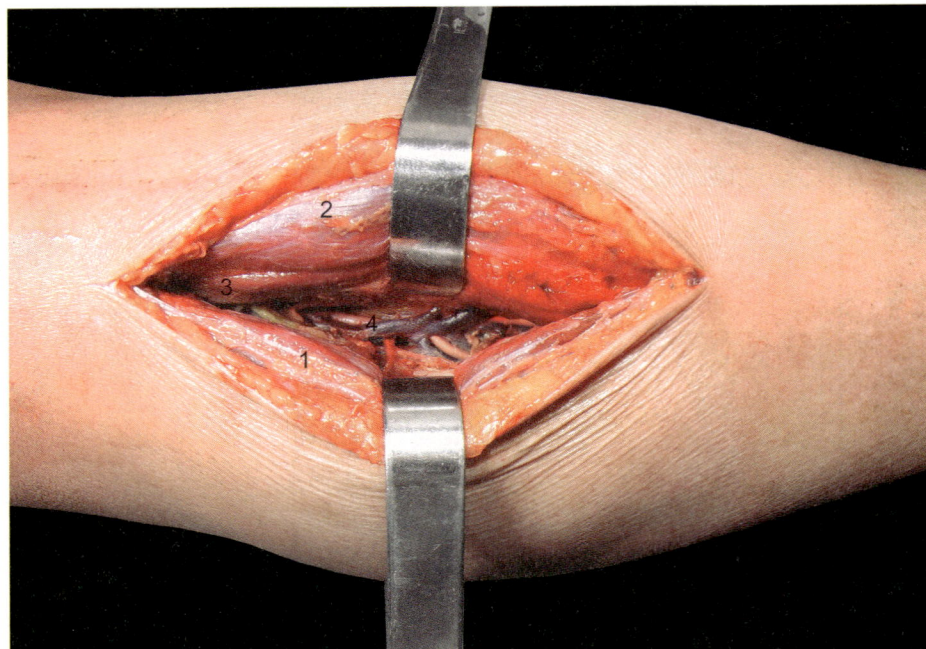

1. Soleus
2. Peroneus longus
3. Peroneus brevis
4. Peroneal artery and vein

| **Figure 3-237** | **Exposure of the vessels** |

The interstice of the soleus and the peroneus longus should be separated to expose the peroneal artery and vein behind the tibialis posterior and at the medial side of the musculus flexor pollicis longus.

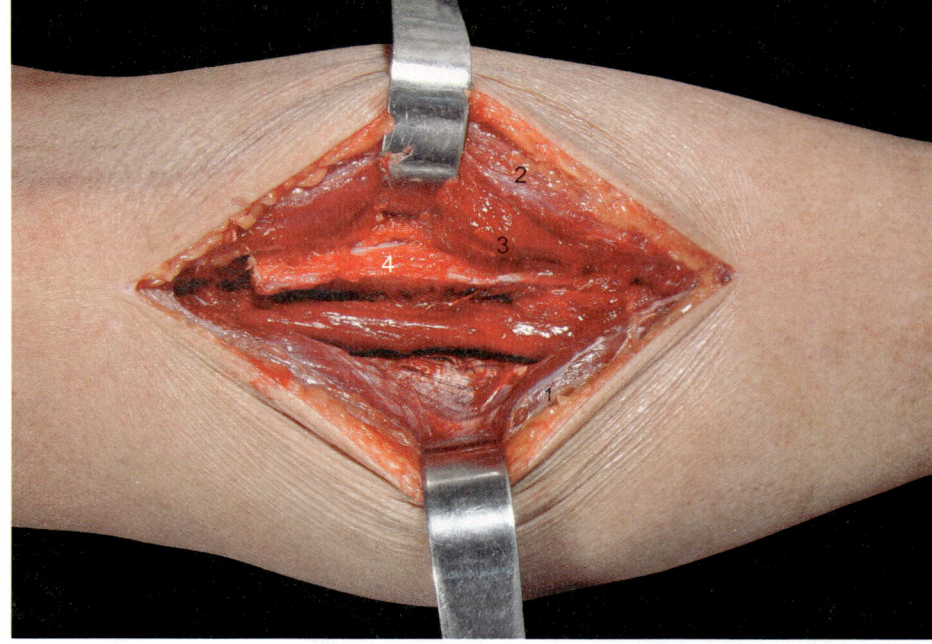

1. Soleus
2. Peroneus longus
3. Peroneus brevis
4. Fibular periosteal flap

| **Figure 3-238** | **Truncation of the fibula** |

The peroneus longus and the peroneus brevis should be dissected and the lamina of intramuscular cuff retained on the fibula to expose the posterior and lateral surface of the fibula. The periosteum should be incised at the superior and the inferior ends and the fibula osteotomied with a wire saw.

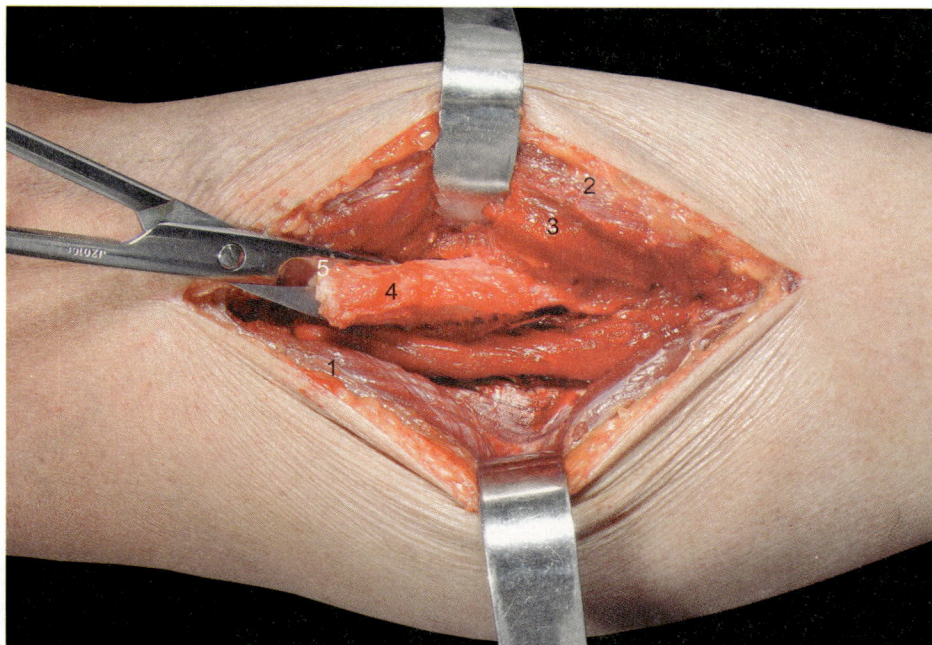

1. Soleus
2. Peroneus longus
3. Peroneus brevis
4. Fibular periosteal flap
5. Interosseous membrane

Figure 3-239   Incision of the interosseous membrane

Finally, the fibular segment should be turned forward, and the link between the interosseous membrane and the tibia cut open.

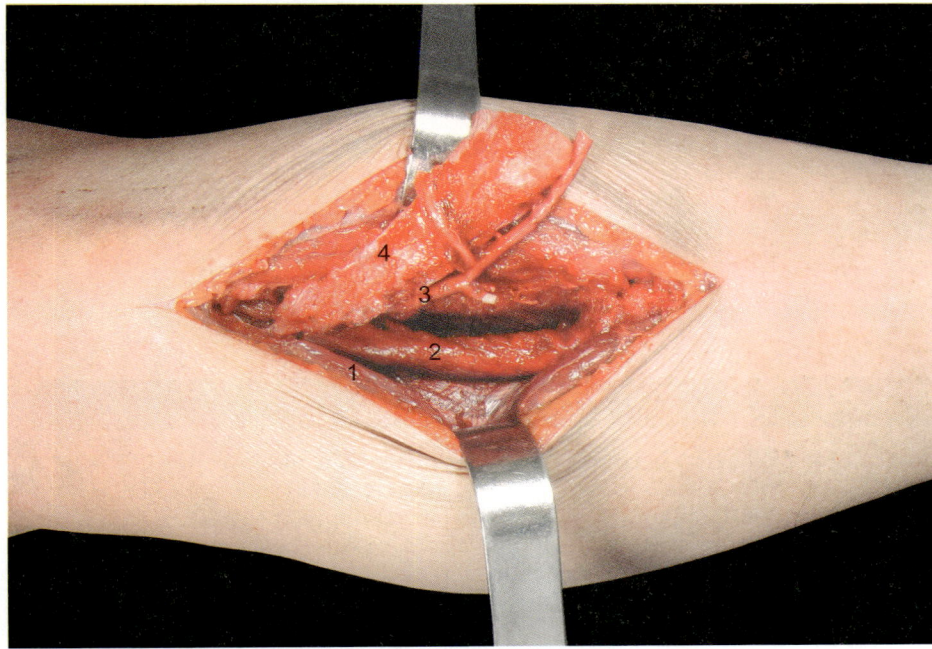

1. Soleus
2. Tibialis posterior
3. Peroneal artery
4. Fibular periosteal flap

Figure 3-240   Antegrade transposition

The tibialis posterior and the long flexor (about 1cm) should be retained on the fibular segment at the initiation of the fibula to protect the peroneal artery musculoperiosteal branch. The periosteal flap should be lifted before it is transferred.

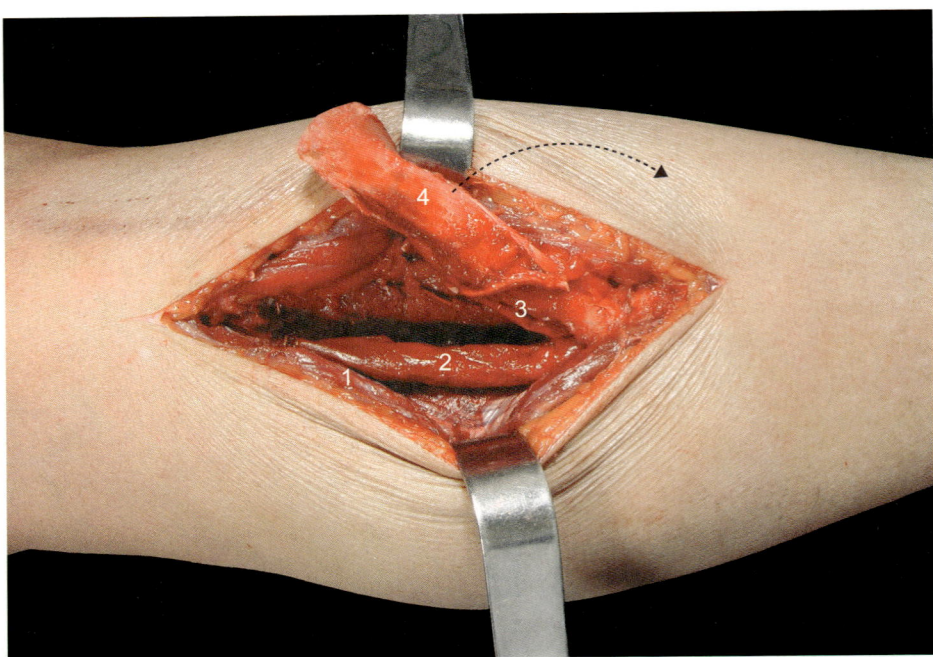

| **Figure 3-241** | **Retrograde transposition** |

The periosteal flap should be lifted upwards and then transferred distally.

1. Soleus   **2.** Tibialis posterior
3. Peroneal artery   **4.** Fibular periosteal flap

Key points in applied anatomy

Firstly, the superior extremity of the fibula is a nonparticipator of the knee joint and its superior 3/4 segment serves as the appendiculate point of the muscles. Therefore, this segment including the fibular head, especially the middle segment of the fibula, is abundant in blood supply. It is suitable to be chosen as a bone donor site. Secondly, the distal fibula is a part of the ankle joint. Therefore, it requires careful consideration how long the fibular periosteal flap should be cut off to maintain the stability of the ankle joint. Thirdly, the common peroneal nerve runs across the fibular neck. It should be separated carefully to keep it intact when the fibula is being cut off under the neck. The superficial peroneal nerve and its muscle branch should be given great attention to avoid getting them damaged when the peroneus longus and the peroneus brevis are being cut off. The deep peroneal nerve and its branches should also be given great attention to avoid getting them damaged when the extensor digitorum longus and the musculus extensor pollicis longus are being cut off. Fourthly, the anterior tibial vessel should be kept intact when the tibiofibular joint is being broken off and the fibular periosteal flap transferred with the fibular head. The vessel extends through the interosseous membrane foramen a little beneath tibiofibular joint to reach the extending border of the calf. It, in the operation, should be exposed before the tibiofibular joint is cut open.

Lateral Tarsal Blood Vessel Cuboid Bone Flap

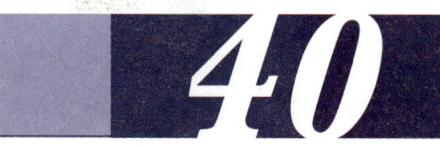

The cuboid bone flap based on the lateral tarsal blood vessels has an adequate blood supply. Its vascular pedicle is large, long and constant in position. The pedicle is elastic for a transposition and needs no vascular sutures. Most of its donor bones are cancellous. The flap is suitable for the repair of a fracture on the talus neck or an ischemic necrosis of the talus body, for the fusion of a transplanted bone on the articulation or for the repair of a fracture, osseous nonunion and defects of the lateral malleolus.

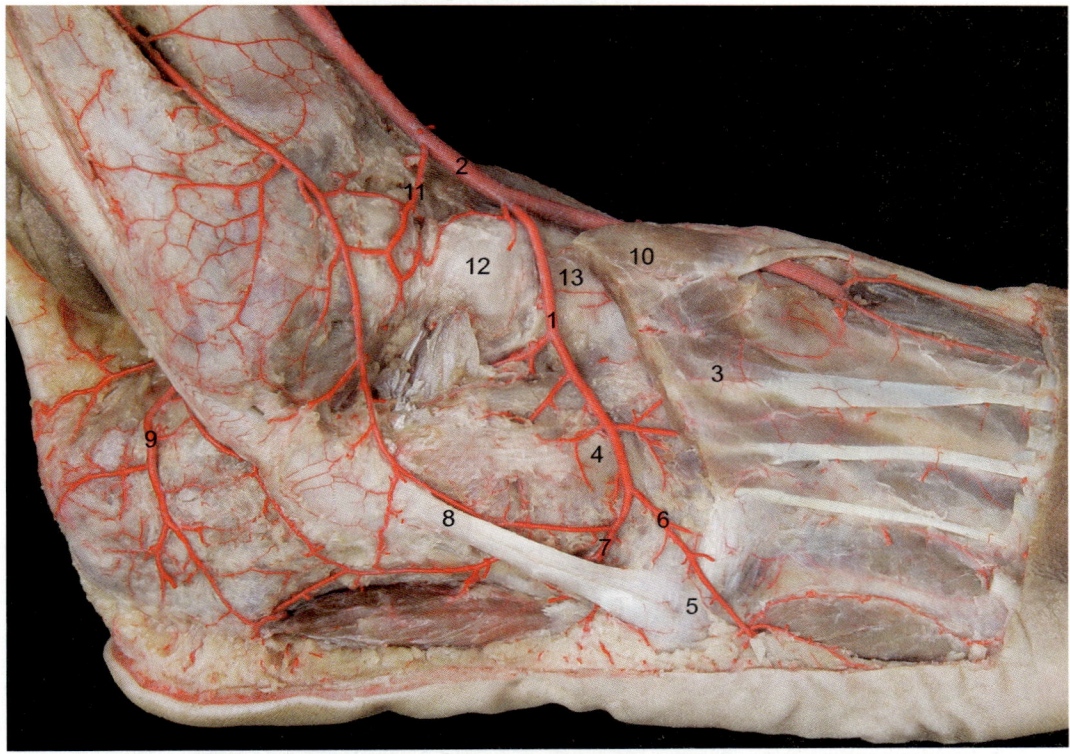

Figure 3-242	**Applied anatomy**

The blood supply of the dorsal cuboid bone comes from the lateral tarsal artery. The initiation of the artery is situated near the talonavicular joint. The artery emerges from the lateral dorsal pedal artery, perforates through the deep layer between the musculus extensor pollicis brevis and the extensor digitorum brevis, attaching tightly to the dorsal surface of the cuboid bone until it comes close to the 5th plantar metatarsal bone, where it gives two terminal branches: the anterior branch and the posterior branch. The posterior branch runs backwards and perforates through the deep layer of the peroneus longus tendon and the peroneus brevis tendon to anastomose with the lateral calcaneal artery. The anterior branch anastomoses with the arcuate artery. It migrates to the 4th and the 3rd dorsal digital arteries when the arcuate artery is congenital absence. It passes across the surface of the bone and gives the cuboid osseous branch to penetrate through the osseous substance. The lateral tarsal artery is 1.9 mm in diameter at its initiation. It runs for 4.6 cm from its root to the point just before it bifurcates into the anterior and the posterior branches.

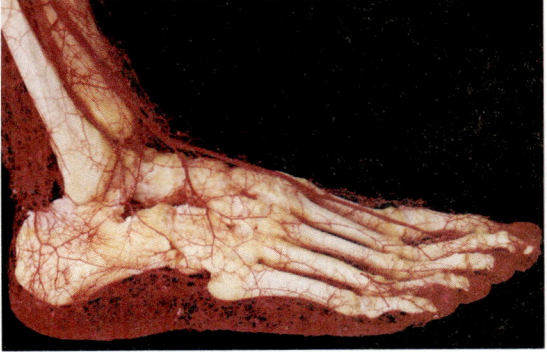

1. Lateral tarsal artery
4. Cuboid bone
7. Posterior branch
10. Musculus extensor pollicis brevis
13. Scaphoid bone

2. Dorsal pedal artery
5. 5th metatarsal tuberosity
8. Peroneus brevis tendon
11. Lateral anterior malleolar artery

3. Extensor digitorum brevis
6. Anterior branch
9. Lateral calcaneal artery
12. Talus

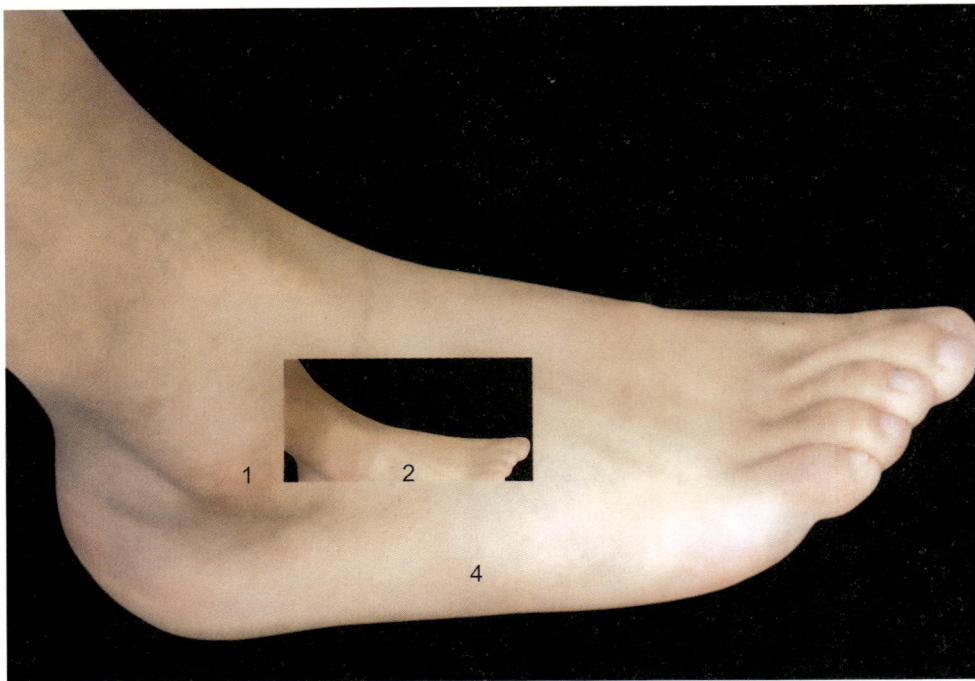

| **Figure 3-243** | **Design of the incision** |

1. Lateral malleolus
2. Extensor digitorum brevis
3. Extensor digitorum longus
4. 5th metatarsal tuberosity

The patient in supine position, the incision should begin from the supra-lateral side of the ankle joint, continue obliquely downwards to transverse the anterior lateral side of the talus body, and extend along the 4th metatarsal bone until it reaches the posterior side of the cuboid bone.

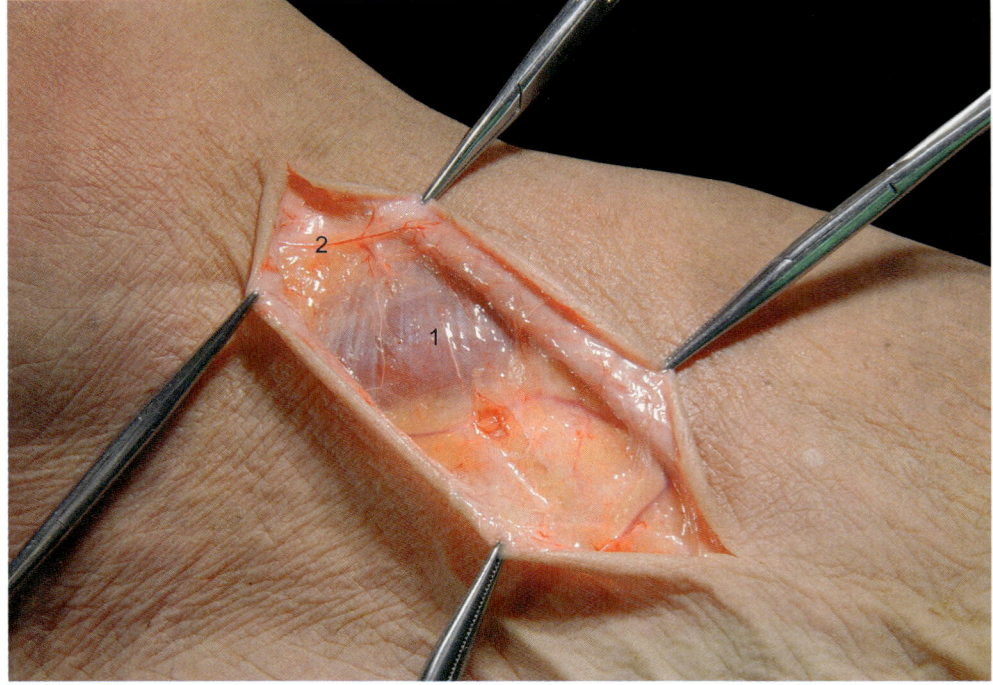

| **Figure 3-244** | **Exposure of the muscle** |

The skin and the subcutaneous tissue should be incised to expose the extensor digitorum brevis.

1. Extensor digitorum brevis   **2.** Cutaneous branches of lateral tarsal artery

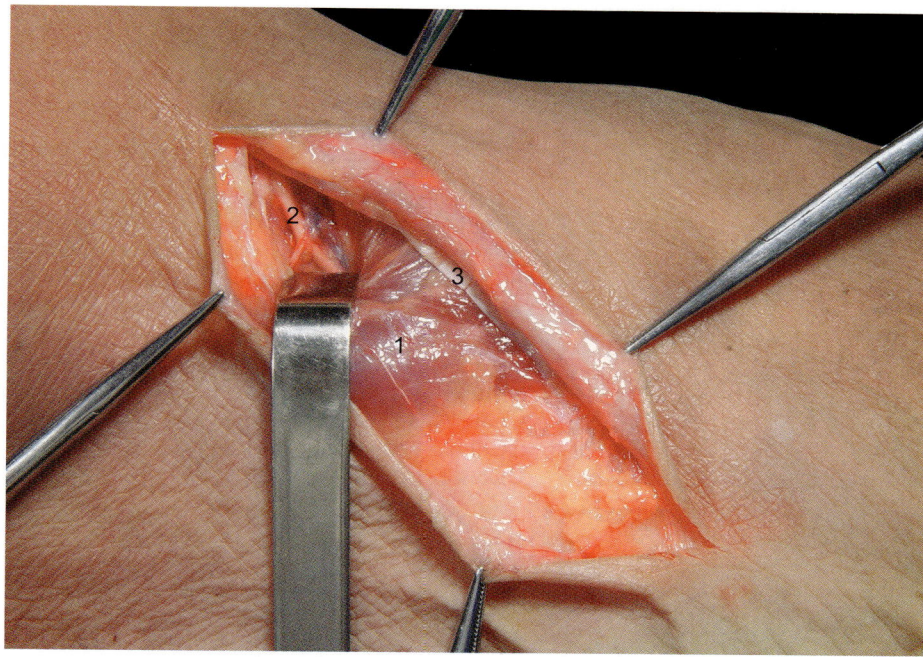

1. Extensor digitorum brevis
2. Lateral tarsal artery
3. Extensor digitorum longus tendon

Figure 3-245   **Exposure of the vessels**

The musculus extensor pollicis longus and the extensor digitorum longus should be pulled inwards and the incision traced along the lateral dorsal pedal artery to expose the initiation of the blood vessel of the ankle in the neighborhood of the talonavicular joint.

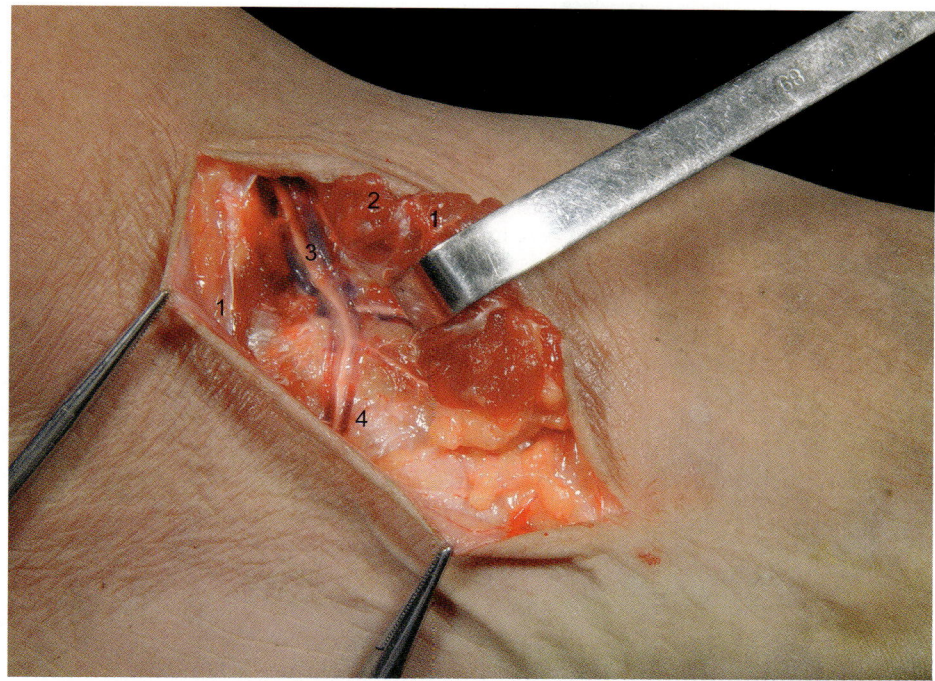

1. Extensor digitorum brevis
2. Musculus extensor pollicis brevis
3. Lateral tarsal artery
4. Cuboid bone

Figure 3-246   **Dissection of the muscle**

The musculus extensor pollicis brevis and the extensor digitorum brevis should be cut off in front of the calcaneus and turned distally to expose the branches of the lateral tarsal blood vessels on the surface of the cuboid bone. Then these vessels should be retrogradely dissected.

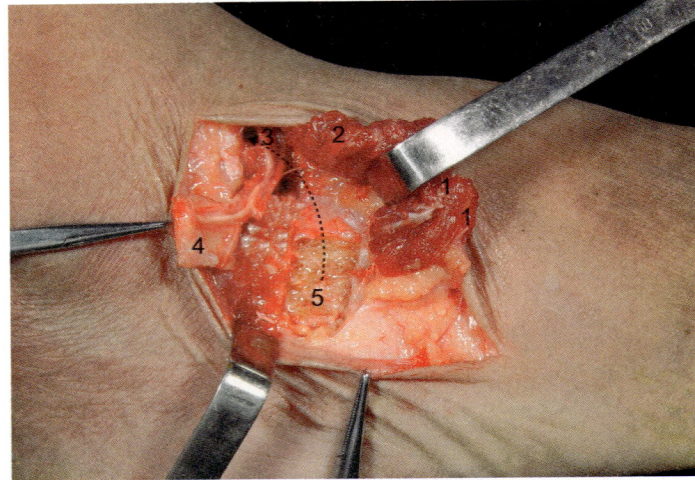

Figure 3-247   Harvest of the bone flap

A periosteal flap, about 2×1.5×0.5cm in size, should be chiseled with the blood vessels across the surface of the bone as its axis. The flap should be elevated with its vascular pedicle and separated proximally onto the initiation of the vascular bundle.
1. Extensor digitorum brevis
2. Musculus extensor pollicis brevis
3. Lateral tarsal artery
4. Cuboid bone periosteal flap
5. Donor site

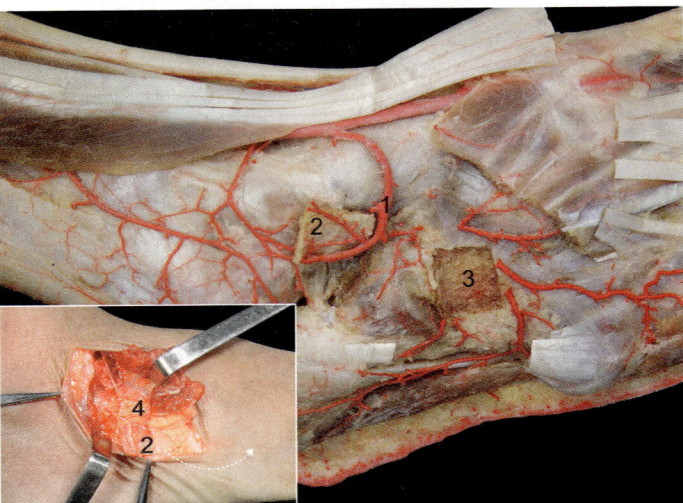

1. Lateral tarsal artery
2. Periosteal flap
3. Donor site
4. Anterior branch

Figure 3-248   Transposition of the periosteal flap

In case of the talar neck fracture, the articular capsule should be incised open to expose the talus. The fracture should be repositioned and internally fixed before the cuboid periosteal flap is implanted into the osseous slot of the neck and in vitro. A composite flap consisting of a skin flap pedicled with the anterior branch and a periosteal flap might be transferred to repair the 5th metatarsal bone.

Key points in applied anatomy

Firstly, the incision should begin from the lateral anterior ankle, curve to the cuboid bone gradually and extend along the 4th metatarsal bone to expose completely the donor site and the recipient site. Secondly, the periosteal flap should be chiseled with its axial line falling along the blood vessel on the dorsal cuboid bone, almost parallel to the calcaneocuboid joint line. It might be about 2.0×1.0×0.5cm in size. Thirdly, the talus should be repositioned and internally fixed, and the bone sulcus in the recipient site chiseled in the space outside the talar neck and in vitro. Fourthly, the periosteal flap should be cut off, and the residual cavity filled in with the extensor digitorum brevis. Fifthly, the lateral tarsal artery might serve as the nutrient vessel of the extensor digitorum brevis, and so the blood vessels outside the ankle should be adopted as a pedicle to form a cuboid bone-extensor digitorum-brevis composite flap. The cuboid periosteal flap tends to be small, and should be given great attention to avoid degloving it with the muscle flap.

Calcaneus Periosteal Flap Pedicled with Calcaneus Lateral Blood Vessels

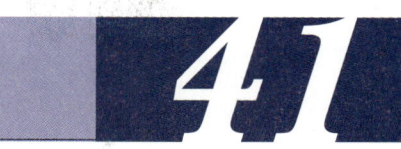

The lateral calcaneal arteries have constant initiations, courses and anastomoses, and they are large and long. They could be adopted as vascular pedicles. A flap pedicled with the lateral calcaneal artery might be transferred smoothly to the recipient site. The calcaneus periosteal flap with a vascular pedicle might be transferred to repair the fractures on the talar neck and the ischemic necrosis of the talar body, to fuse the grate bone with the joint, or to repair the fracture, osseous nonunion and bone-defect of the lateral malleolus.

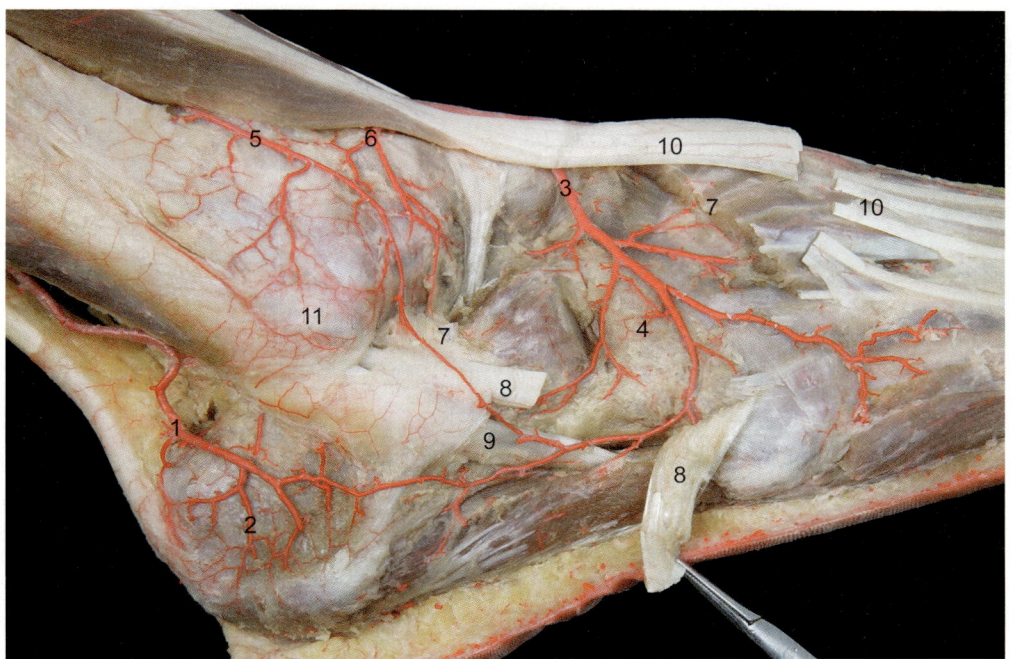

| **Figure 3-249** | **Applied anatomy** |

The lateral calcaneus has multiple blood supplies and the blood vessels are distributed as follows. The lateral calcaneal artery runs anteriorly close to the plane of the bone and reach the part near the 5th metatarsal tuberosity. Along the course it gives 6-12 calcaneal periosteal branches (0.33-1.1mm in diameter) to distribute on the lateral calcaneus. The lateral tarsal artery reaches the dorsal cuboid bone and gives backwards 3-4 muscular periosteal branches (0.8-1.1mm in diameter) to distribute on the anterolateral calcaneus. The descending branch of the perforator from the peroneal artery descends anteriorly outwards along the lateral malleolus to anastomose with the anterolateral malleolar artery near the malleolar sulcus. The anastomosed artery extends across the surface of the extensor digitorum brevis and the anterior border of the peroneus brevis tendon. Along the course, it gives 1-2 musculoperiosteal branches (0.2-0.7mm in diameter) to distribute on the anterolateral calcaneus. These arteries anastomose with each other directly and invariably.

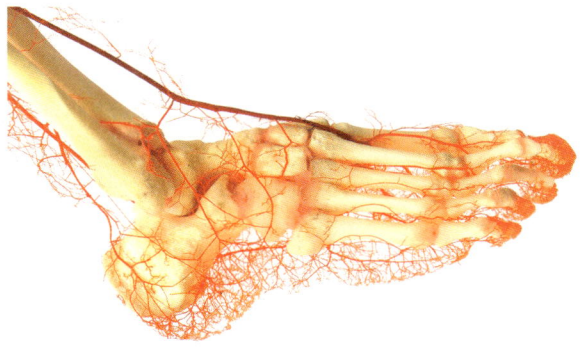

1. Laterior calcaneal artery
2. Calcaneal periosteal branch
3. Lateral tarsal artery
4. Cuboid bone
5. Descending branch of peroneal arterial perforator
6. Lateral anterior malleolar artery
7. Extensor digitorum brevis
8. Peroneus brevis tendon
9. Peroneus longus tendon
10. Extensor digitorum longus
11. Lateral malleolus

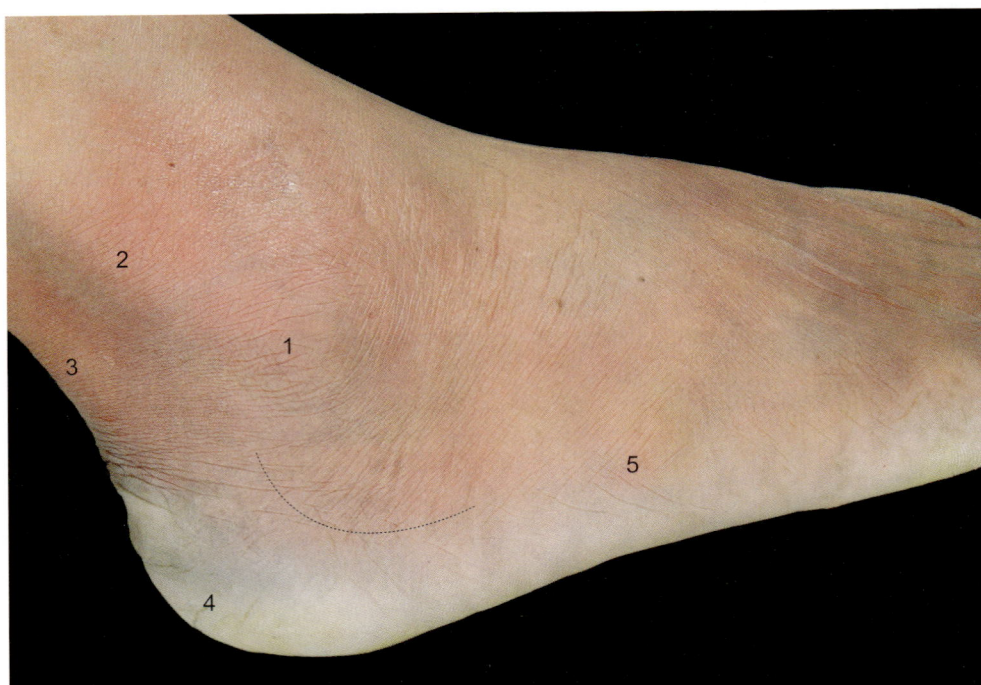

1. Lateral malleolus
2. Peroneus muscle
3. Calcaneal tendon
4. Calcaneal nodule
5. 5th metatarsal
   tuberosity

| **Figure 3-250** | **Design of the incision** |

The patient should be placed in the lateral recumbent position, and the incision begin with the posteolateral or the anterolateral surface of the ankle joint.

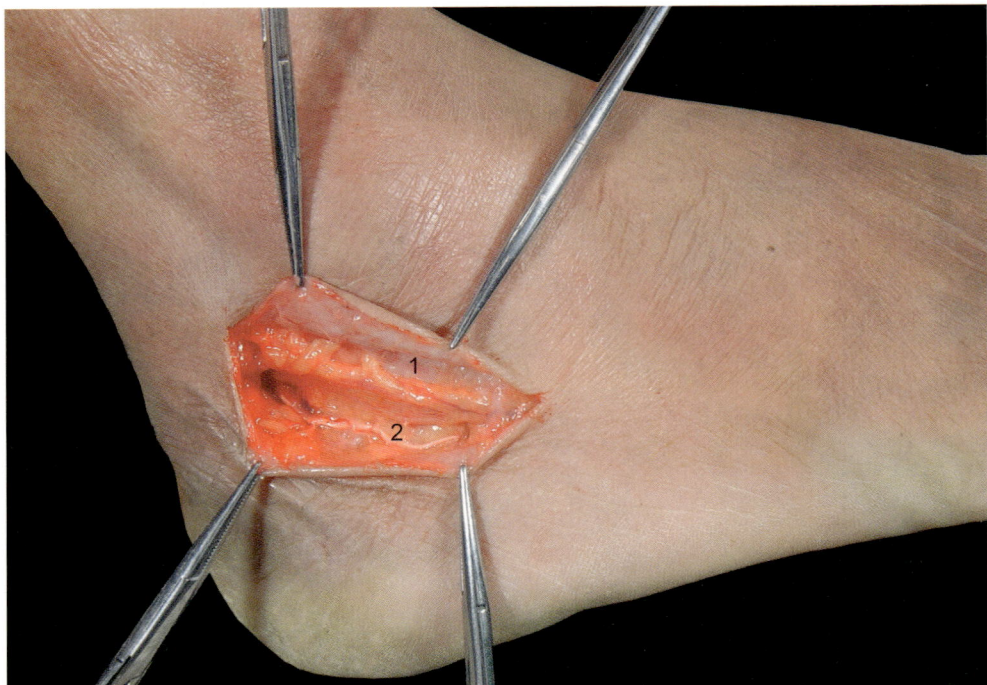

| **Figure 3-251** | **Exposure of the vessels** |

The skin should be incised down to the deep fascia to expose the vascular bundle and the lateral calcaneal vessels.
1. Peroneus longus tendon
2. Laterior calcaneal artery

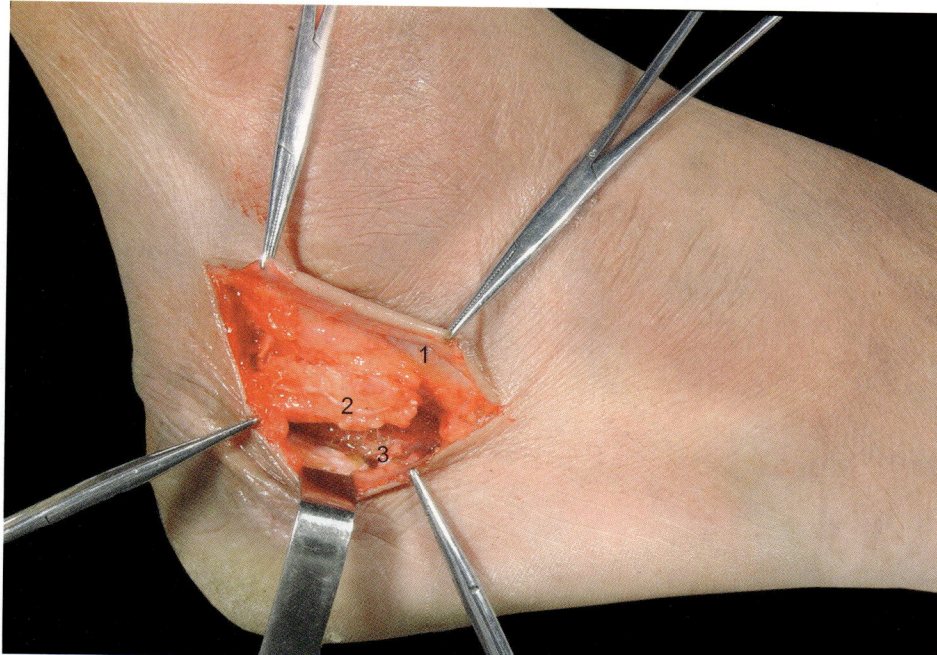

1. Peroneus longus tendon
2. Laterior calcaneal artery
3. Donor site

Figure 3-252   **Harvest of the bone flap**

The periosteal flap should be chiseled with the lateral calcaneal vessels that pass across the bone surface as its axis. The flap might be 2×1.5×0.5cm in size. It should be elevated with the vascular pedicle, and then the vascular bundle separated proximally until it is long enough to meet the need.

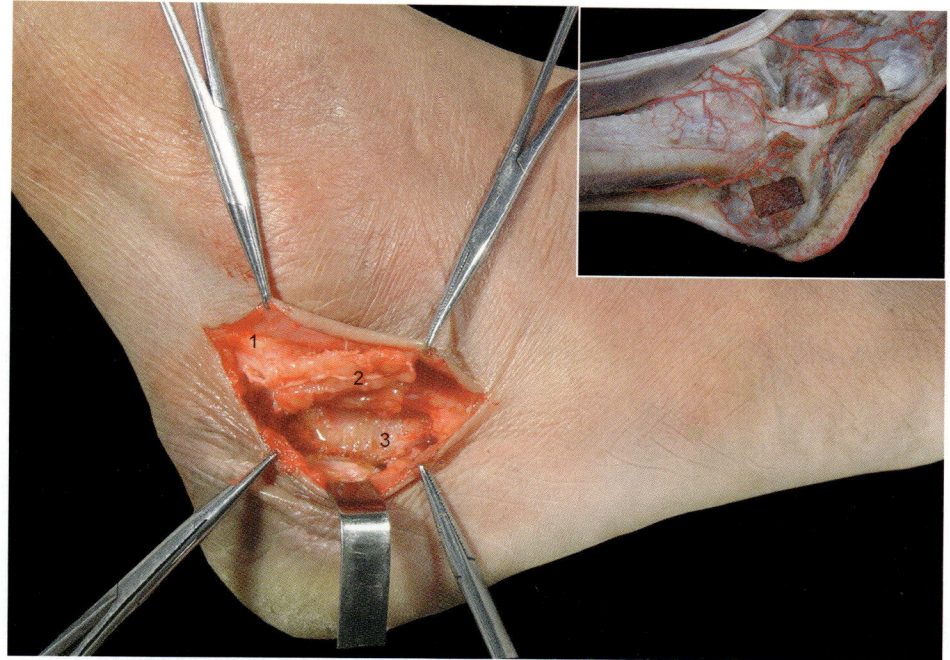

1. Peroneus longus tendon
2. Laterior calcaneal artery
3. Donor site

Figure 3-253   **Transposition of the periosteal flap**

In case of the talar neck fracture, the articular capsule should be incised open to expose the talus. The fracture should be repositioned and internally fixed before the calcaneus periosteal flap is implanted into the slot lateral to the talar neck and the corpus tali. In the case of the fracture and osseous nonunion or bone-defects of the lateral malleolus, the fractured bone should be repaired and repositioned before the periosteal flap is implanted into it.

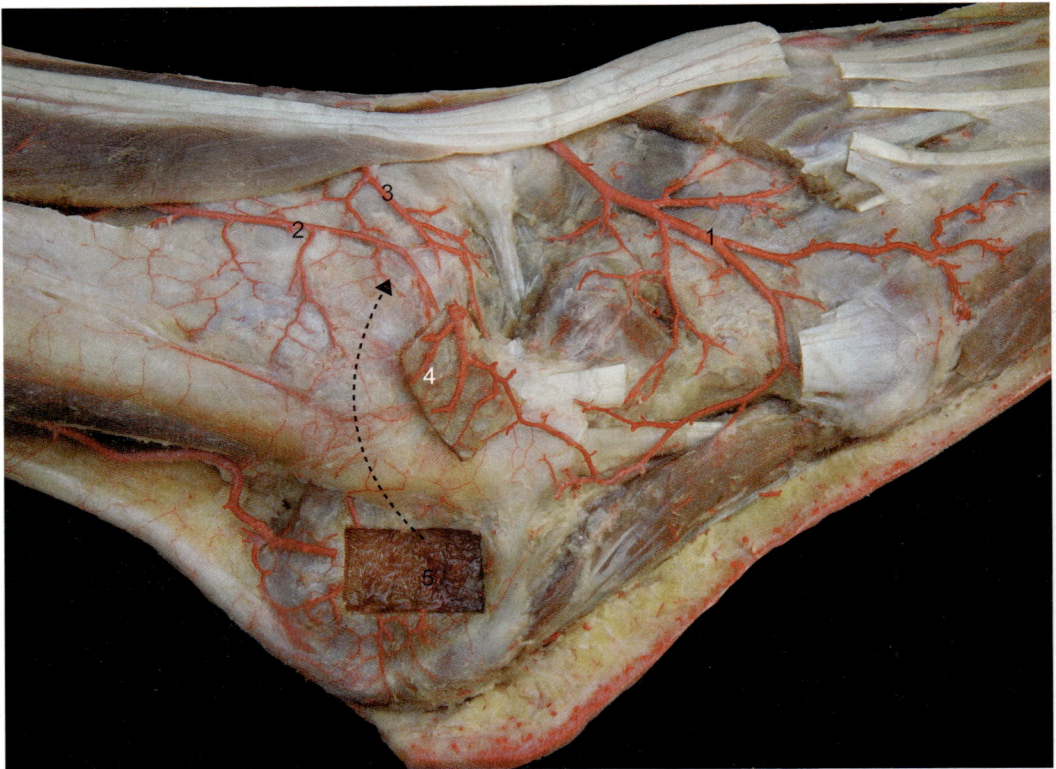

| **Figure 3-254** | **Retrograde transposition** |

The flap based on the lateral tarsal artery, the descending branch of the perforator of the peroneal artery or the anterior lateral malleolar artery might be used with the calcaneus periosteal flap to repair the fracture and osseous nonunion or the bone-defect of the lateral malleolus.

1. Lateral tarsal artery
2. Descending branch of peroneal arterial perforator
3. Lateral anterior malleolar artery
4. Calcaneus periosteal flap
5. Donor site

Key points in applied anatomy

Firstly, the periosteal flap should be dissected from the anterior or the posterior lateral malleolus and extend to the 4th or the 5th plantar metatarsal bone. Secondly, the flap should be designed at the distal part of the vascular pedicle so that it could be easily transferred. Thirdly, when the periosteal flap is being chiseled, part of the intramuscular cuff should be retained to protect the intramuscular periosteal vascular branches. Fourthly, when the composite flap is being chiseled, part of the extensor digitorum brevis should be retained to protect the musculo-cutaneous artery in the vascular pedicle.

Medial Cuneiform Flap with Vascular Pedicle

The medial cuneiform vessels have constant origins, courses and anastomoses and they are large and long. They could serve as vascular pedicle. A flap based on these vessels might be transferred smoothly to the recipient site to repair the fracture of the talar neck, the ischemic necrosis of the talar body or to fuse the grafted bone with the joint.

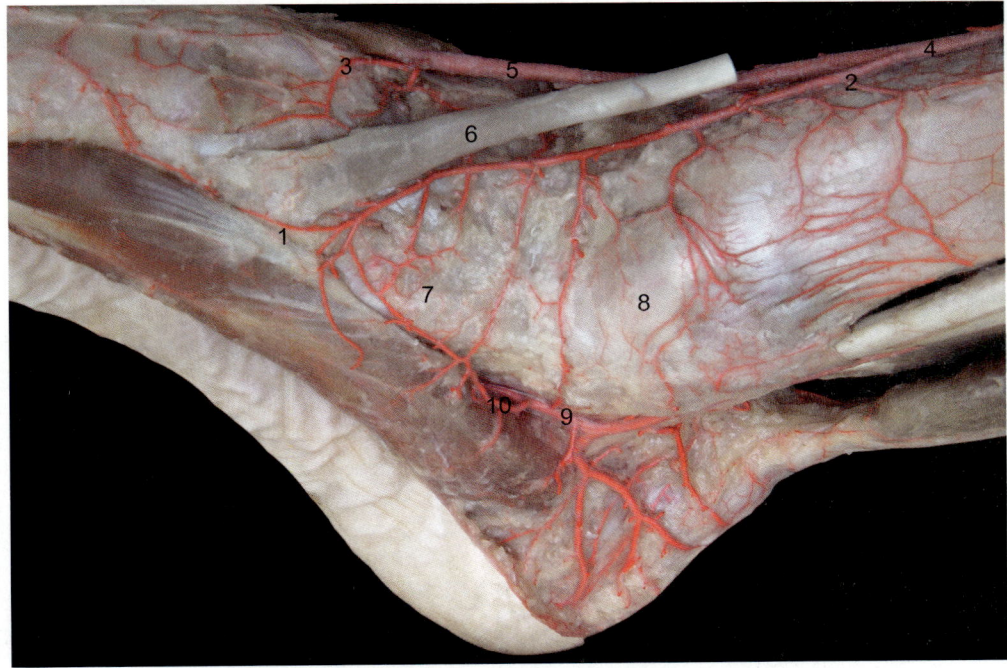

Figure 3-255	Applied anatomy

The medial cuneiform bone has multiple blood supplies. The medial anterior malleolar artery and the medial tarsal artery are its main nutrient vessels. The medial anterior malleolar artery emerges from the anterior tibial artery or the dorsal pedal artery near the connection between the ankles. It is 1.6mm in diameter. Its trunk attaches tightly to the medial border of the tibialis anterior tendon and runs across the talus and the navicular bones to reach the medial margin of the medial cuneiform bone. The medial tarsal artery emerges from the dorsal pedal artery near the talus and the navicular joint. It is 1.3mm in diameter. Its trunk attaches tightly to the lateral border of the tibialis anterior tendon and extends to the medial cuneiform bone. These blood vessels each give 2-8 periosteal branches (0.2-0.8mm in diameter) to distribute on the lateral surface of the medial cuneiform bone.

1. Medial cuneiform bone
2. Medial anterior malleolar artery
3. Medial tarsal artery
4. Anterior tibial artery
5. Dorsal pedal artery
6. Tibialis anterior tendon
7. Tuberosity of navicular bone
8. Medial malleolus
9. Medial plantar artery
10. Superficial branch of medial plantar artery

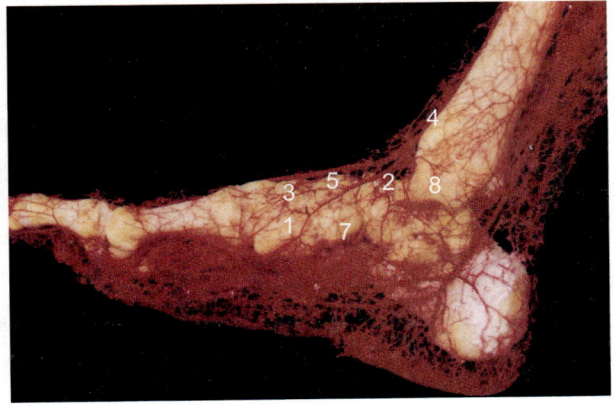

351

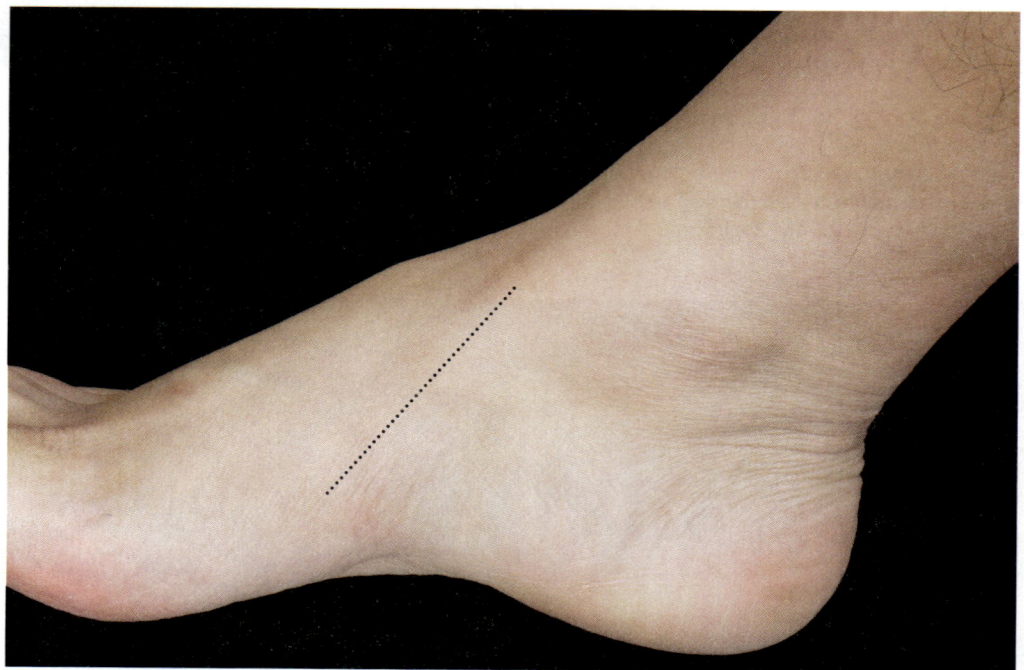

| **Figure 3-256** | **Design of the incision** |

An anterior-medial approach to the ankle taken, the incision should begin from above the medial ankle and extend distally along the tibialis anterior tendon onto the cuneiform-metatarsal joint.

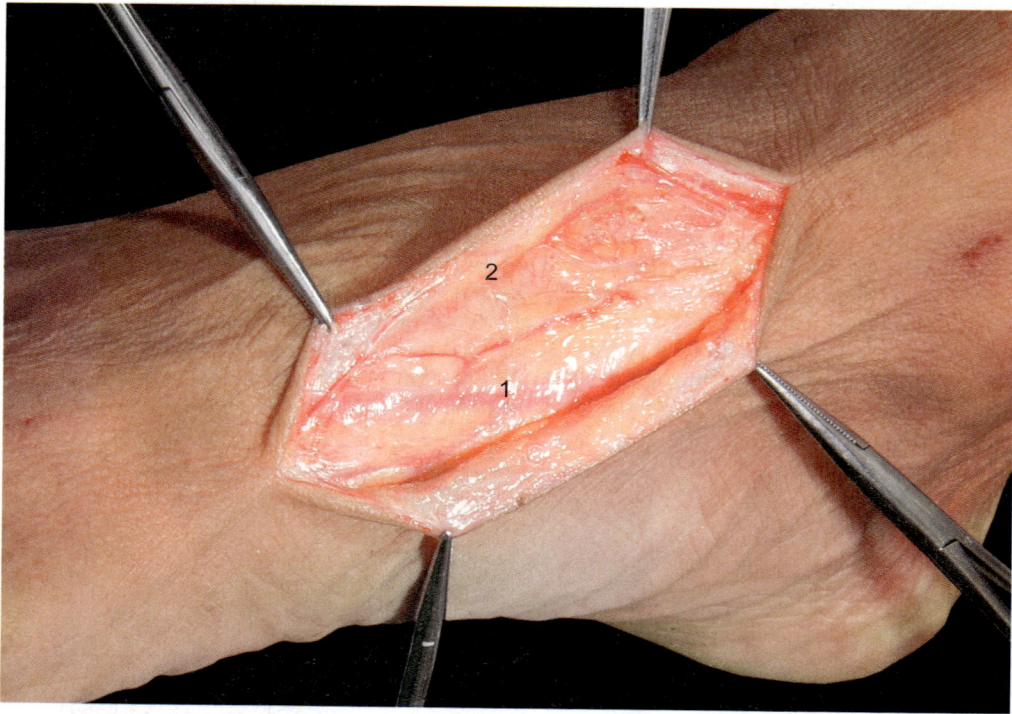

| **Figure 3-257** | **Exposure of the incision** |

The skin and the subcutaneous tissue should be incised open to expose the medial pedal venous rete and the medial dorsal cutaneous nerve of the foot.

1. Venous rete   **2.** Cutaneous nerve

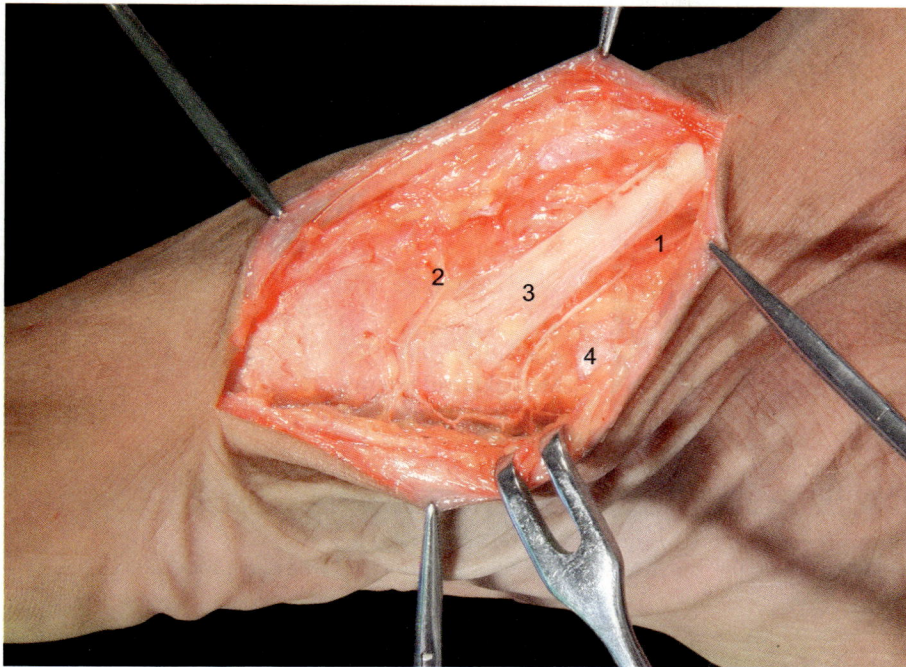

1. Medial anterior malleolar artery
2. Medial tarsal arteries
3. Tibialis anterior tendon
4. Tuberosity of navicular bone

Figure 3-258   **Exposure of the vessels**

The tibialis anterior tendon and the musculus extensor pollicis longus tendon should be incised to expose the trunk of the medial anterior malleolar artery near the medial border of the tibialis anterior tendon. If the medial tarsal artery is taken as a pedicle, the dorsal pedal artery should be first exposed to spot the medial tarsal arteries at the lateral border of the tibialis anterior tendon, i.e. the talonavicular joint.

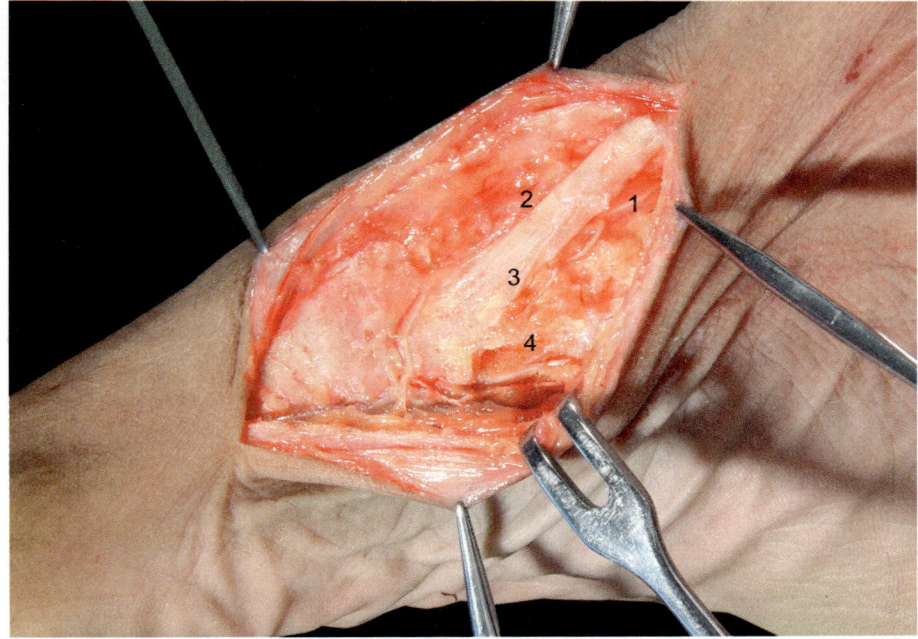

1. Medial anterior malleolar artery
2. Medial tarsal arteries
3. Tibialis anterior tendon
4. Periosteal flap

Figure 3-259   **Harvest of the bone flap**

The border of the cuneiform bone should be identified before the periosteal flap is chiseled. Then the flap with the vascular bundle should be elevated and the vascular bundle separated proximally.

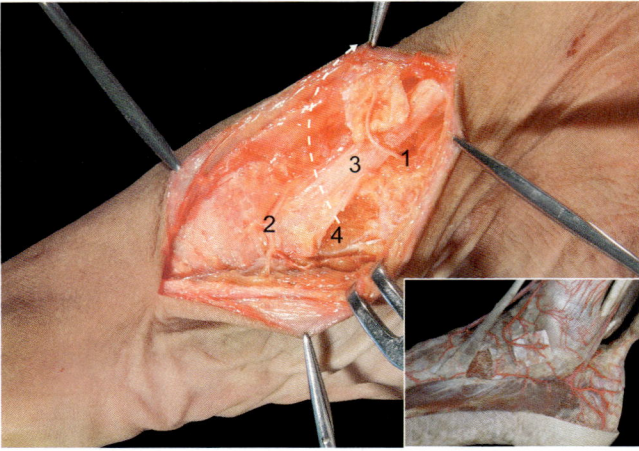

1. Medial anterior
   malleolar artery
2. Medial tarsal arteries
3. Tibialis anterior tendon
4. Donor site

Figure 3-260   **Transposition of the periosteal flap**

The ankle capsule should be incised to expose the talus and an accurate reposition and an internal fixation performed. A bone osseous slot across the fracture surface should be chiseled in the medial body of the talar neck before the periosteal flap is transferred and implanted into it.

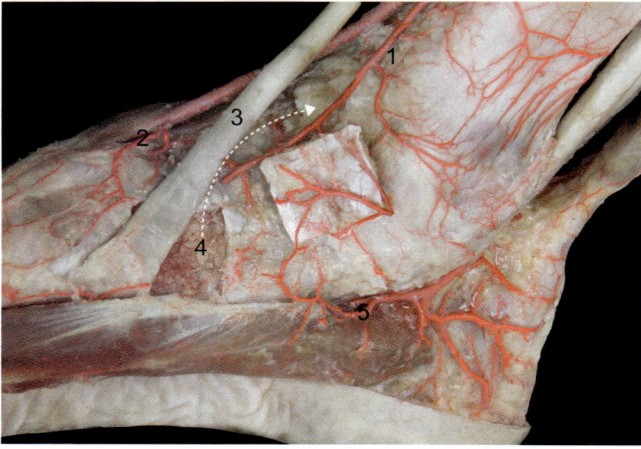

1. Medial anterior malleolar
   artery
2. Medial tarsal arteries
3. Tibialis anterior tendon
4. Donor site
5. Superficial branch of
   medial plantar artery

Figure 3-261   **Transposition of the periosteal flap**

The cuneiform periosteal flap based on the superficial or the deep branch of the medial plantar artery branch might be transferred to repair the fracture of the talus or/and the medial malleolus.

Key points in applied anatomy

Firstly, the medial cuneiform periosteal flap has abundant blood supplies. The medial anterior malleolar artery, the deep and the superficial branches of the medial tarsal arteries and the medial plantar artery all give many periosteal branches (0.2-1.0mm in diameter) to anastomose with one another and penetrate through the bone. In clinical application, anyone of them might be adopted according to the need of the recipient site. The medial anterior malleolar artery might be recommended if the flap is to repair the fracture of the talus. The artery emerges just from near the graft bone so that the vascular pedicle could be long enough to guarantee a flexible transposition. The distal extremity of the incision extends beyond the distal plantar joint along the space between the tendons to expose the medial cuneiform bone completely. Secondly, when the periosteal flap is being retrieved, the tibialis anterior tendon should be lifted and pulled medially, and the periosteal flap with vascular pedicle circumrotated medially downwards from the position under the tendon to the graft position. Thirdly, when the operation is completely done, the cuneiform residual cavity should be managed properly. Fourthly, when the vascular pedicle is being dissected, the anastomosis branches of the adjacent blood vessels should be ligated.

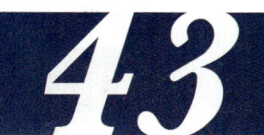
The medial anterior malleolar artery, the medial tarsal artery and the superficial branch of the medial plantar artery are distributed on the dorsal navicular bone. They have constant origins, courses and anastomoses. They could form large and long pedicles so that the flap based on them might be transferred smoothly to the recipient site. A flap of this type might be used to repair the fracture and osseous nonunion of the talar neck, and the ischemic necrosis of the talar body.

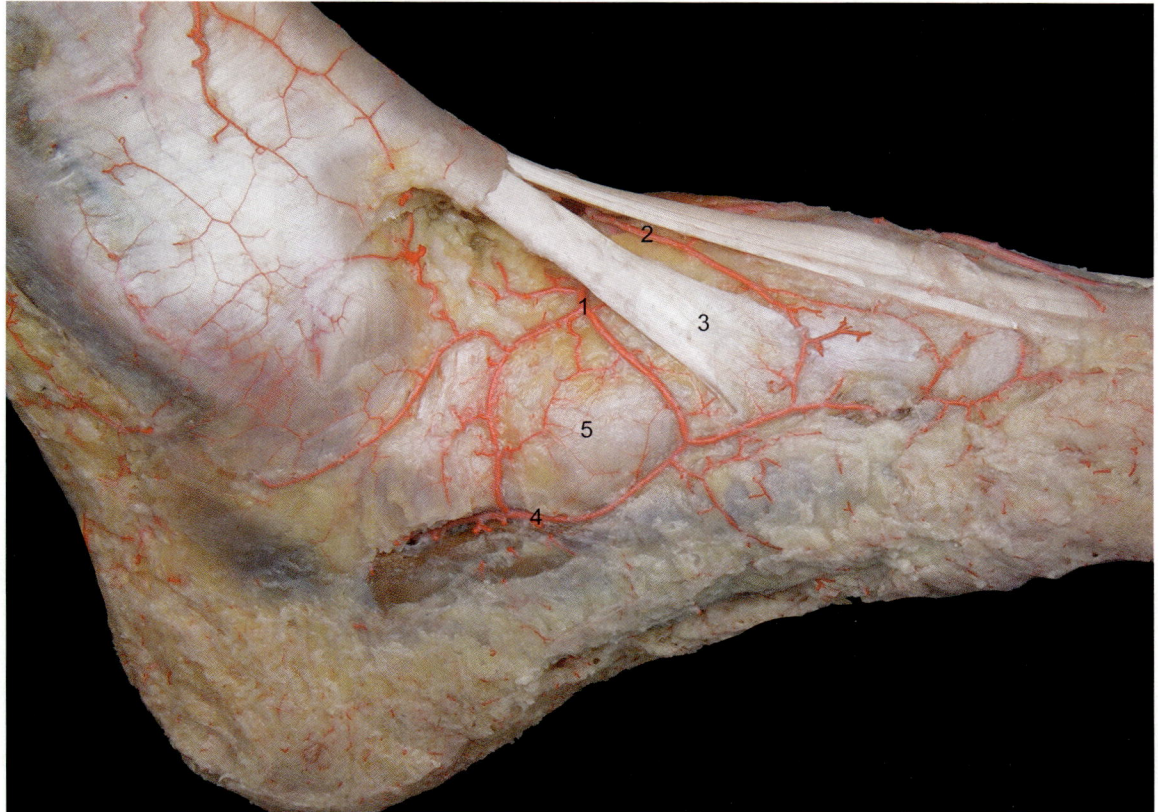

Figure 3-262	Applied anatomy

There are the medial anterior malleolar artery, the medial tarsal artery and the superficial branch of the medial plantar artery that are distributed on the dorsal navicular bone. The medial anterior malleolar artery emerges from either the anterior tibial artery or the dorsal pedal artery. The medial tarsal artery emerges from the dorsal pedal artery. Each of the two gives 5-8 periosteal branches, among which, 3-5 ones are 0.3-1.0 mm in diameter, and 2-3 ones 0.3-0.8mm in diameter. They are mainly distributed on the posterior and the anterior dorsal navicular bone. The medial plantar artery is one of the terminal branches of the posterior tibial artery. It extends along the deep layer of the musculus abductor hallucis to the posterior navicular tuberosity and bifurcates into the superficial and the deep branches. The superficial branch perforates through the musculus abductor hallucis and comes superficial near the navicular tuberosity. It runs forwards beneath the fascia between the musculus abductor hallucis and the tarsal bones and gives 1-3 periosteal branches (0.2-0.6mm in diameter) to distribute on the navicular tuberosity.

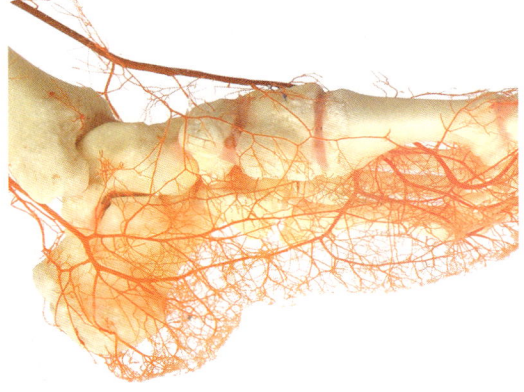

1. Medial anterior malleolar artery
2. Medial tarsal artery
3. Tibialis anterior tendon
4. Superficial branch of medial plantar artery
5. Tuberosity of navicular bone

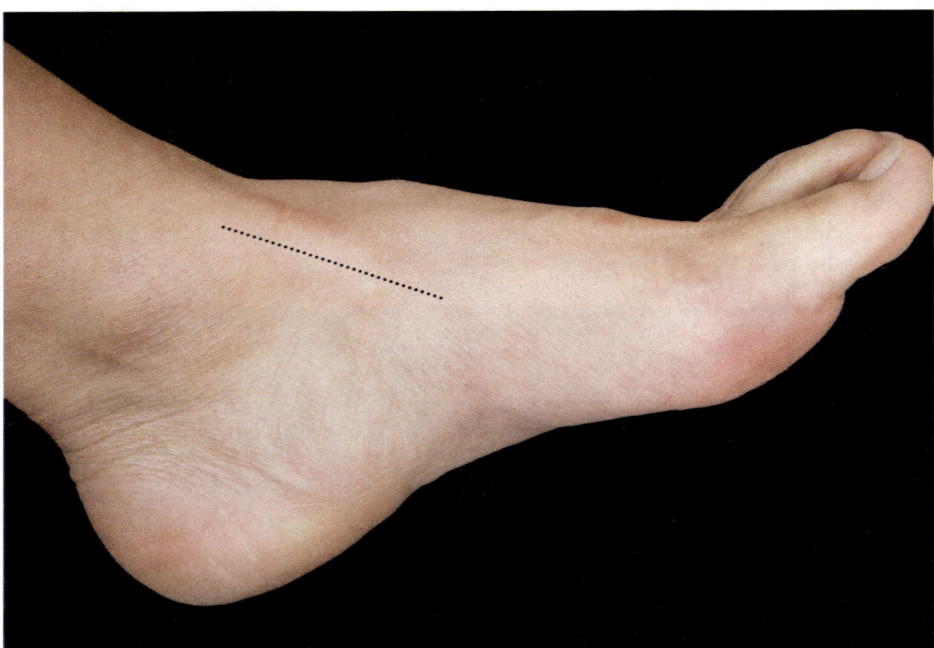

| **Figure 3-263** | **Design of the incision** |

The patient should be placed in supine position, and the incision begin from the anterior and medial side of the ankle joint and continue along the tibialis anterior tendon to the navicular bone onto the cuneiform-metatarsal joint.

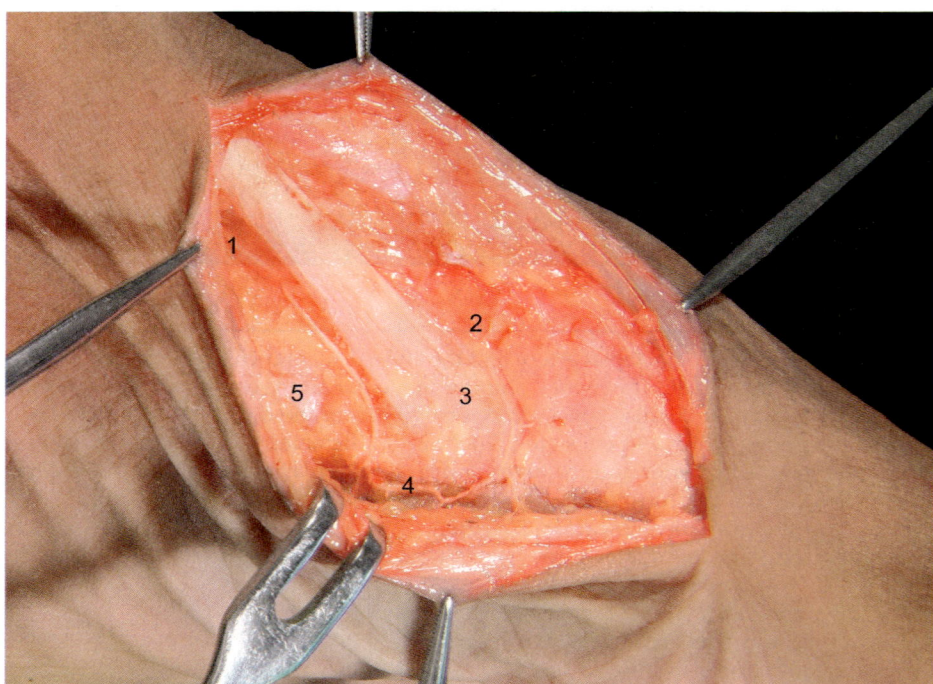

1. Medial anterior malleolar
   artery
2. Medial tarsal artery
3. Tibialis anterior tendon
4. Superficial branch of
   medial plantar artery
5. Tuberosity of navicular
   bone

| **Figure 3-264** | **Exposure of the vessels** |

The skin and the superficial fascia should be incised open and the tibialis anterior tendon pulled outwards to expose the trunk of the medial anterior malleolar artery, which is situated next to the medial tibialis anterior tendon on the connection plane between the ankles. The incision should then be traced to the dorsal navicular bone.

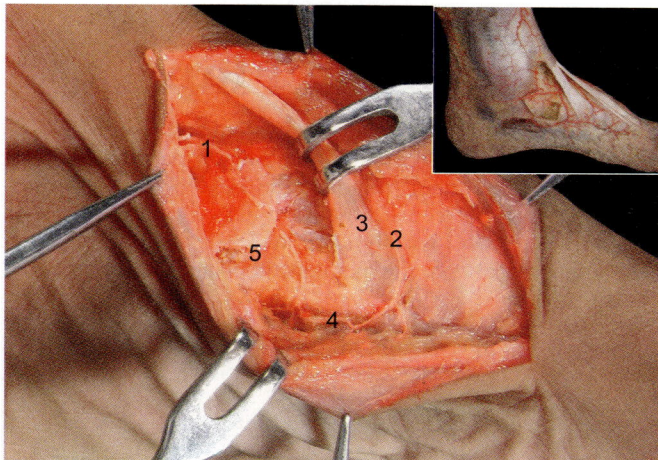

1. Medial anterior malleolar artery
2. Medial tarsal artery
3. Tibialis anterior tendon
4. Superficial branch of medial plantar artery
5. Donor site

Figure 3-265   **Harvest of the bone flap**

The border of the navicular bone should be identified before a periosteal flap is chiseled about 2×1.5 ×0.5cm in size.

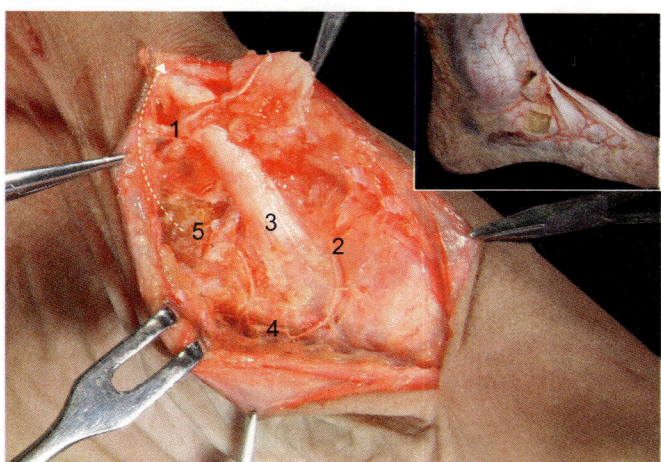

1. Medial anterior malleolar artery
2. Medial tarsal artery
3. Tibialis anterior tendon
4. Superficial branch of medial plantar artery
5. Donor site

Figure 3-266   **Transposition of the periosteal flap**

The fracture should be repositioned and internally fixed. A osseous slot should be chiseled on the medial neck and body of the talus before the periosteal flap is implanted into it.

Key points in applied anatomy

Firstly, there are three groups of vascular options in the donor site of the navicular periosteal flap, among which the anterior medial malleolus artery is the priority. It could be found along the medial tibialis anterior tendon. The medial tarsal artery might be taken into consideration if necessary and so might the superficial branch of the medial plantar artery. Secondly, the vascular pedicle should be found and the periosteal flap retrieved for further use. Then the talus articular capsule should be incised open and the fracture fixed internally. Thirdly, the medial tarsal artery, especially the one with the proper origin, might be chosen as a pedicle, and its origin should be identified. Fourthly, when the superficial branch of the medial plantar artery is chosen as a pedicle, the skin should be dissected to the navicular tuberosity to expose the superficial branch under the fascia and inside the musculus abductor hallucis. Then the muscles should be incised open and the incision traced to the arterial origin. Fifthly, it is preferable to retrieve periosteal flap at the anterior part of the dorsal superficial branch of the medial plantar artery and next to the navicular tuberosity. Sixthly, the residual cavity in the donor site should be properly managed.

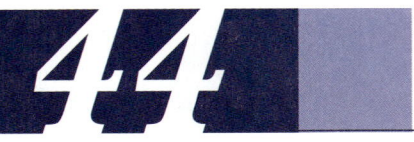

Metatarsal Periosteal Flap

The metatarsal periosteal flap with a vascular bundle has a complete blood supply system and many osteogenesis factors for the head necrosis of the metatarsal bone. The operation is easy to perform Treatment of the donor and the recipient sites with small subsequent trauma could be performed simultaneouly. There are two groups of vascular options that could be adopted as a pedicle clepending on the conditions. The operating procedures are considerably flexible. The metatarsal periosteal flap is suitable for the restoration of the ischemic necrosis of the metatarsal bone head.

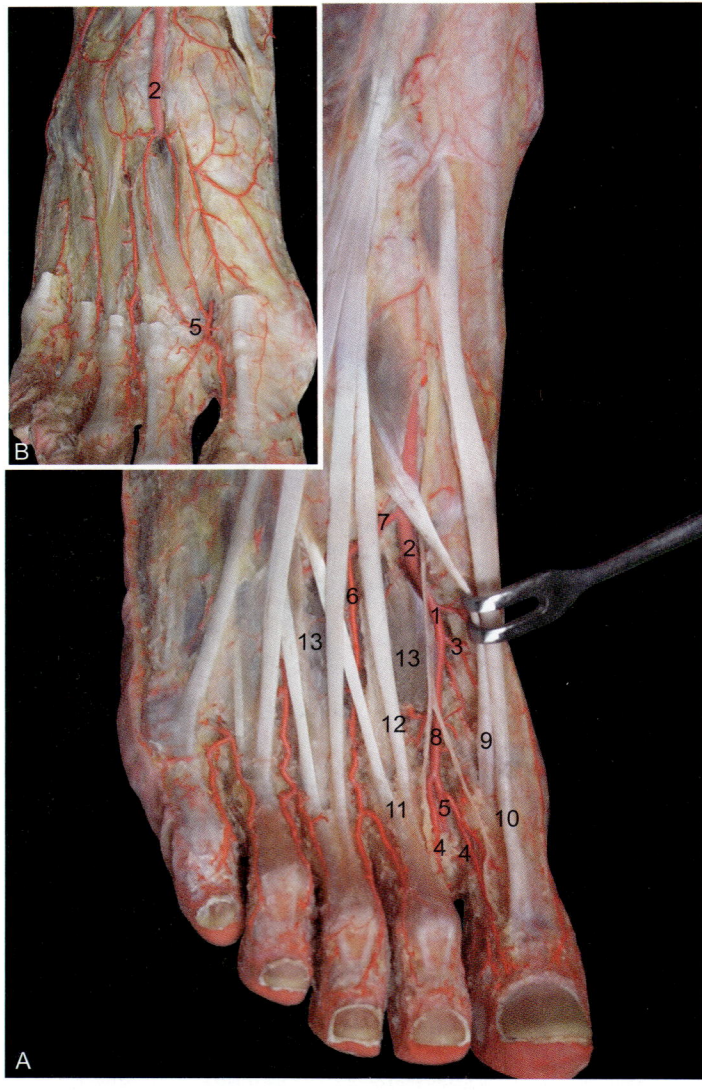

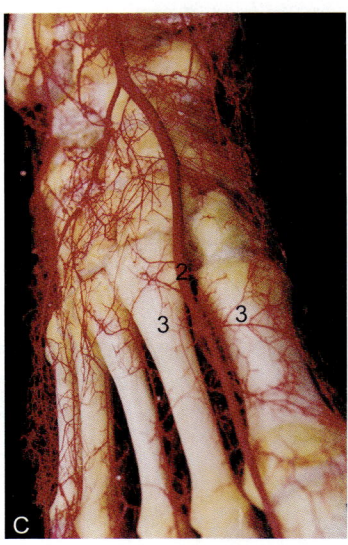

Figure 3-267   **Applied anatomy**

The metatarsal periosteal flap obtains its blood supply mainly from the dorsal metatarsal arteries. The 1st dorsal metatarsal artery is one of the terminal branches of the dorsal pedal artery. It runs through the interosseous space of the 1st metatarsal bone and gives periosteal branches bilaterally (Fig. C) to distribute on the lateral 1st metatarsal bone and the medial 2nd metatarsal bone. The 1st metatarsal artery extends for 1.6mm from the proximal 1st toe web and gives 2 dorsal digital arteries and perforating branches into the plantar thenar to anastomose with the 1st plantar metatarsal artery. This artery varies in depth while it runs through the intersection of the 1st metatarsal bone. There are three types of the artery: the superficial one (Fig. A), the deep one, and the slim and fragile one/the congenital absence (Fig. B). The 2nd metatarsal artery emerges from the dorsal pedal artery or the arcuate artery (Each accounts for 36.6%). In other cases (26.6%), it emerges from the thenar arterial arch. The artery extends forward in the space between the 2nd metatarsal bones and gives bilaterally 2-4 periosteal branches to distribute on the medial 2nd metatarsal bone and the lateral 3rd metatarsal bone. It continues to the 2nd toe web and gives 2 dorsal digital arteries and perforators.

1. 1st metatarsal artery
2. Dorsal pedal artery
3. Periosteal branch
4. Dorsal digital artery
5. Perforating branch
6. 2nd metatarsal artery
7. Arcuate artery
8. Deep peroneal nerve
9. Musculus extensor pollicis brevis tendon
10. Musculus extensor pollicis longus tendon
11. Extensor digitorum brevis tendon
12. Extensor digitorum longus tendon

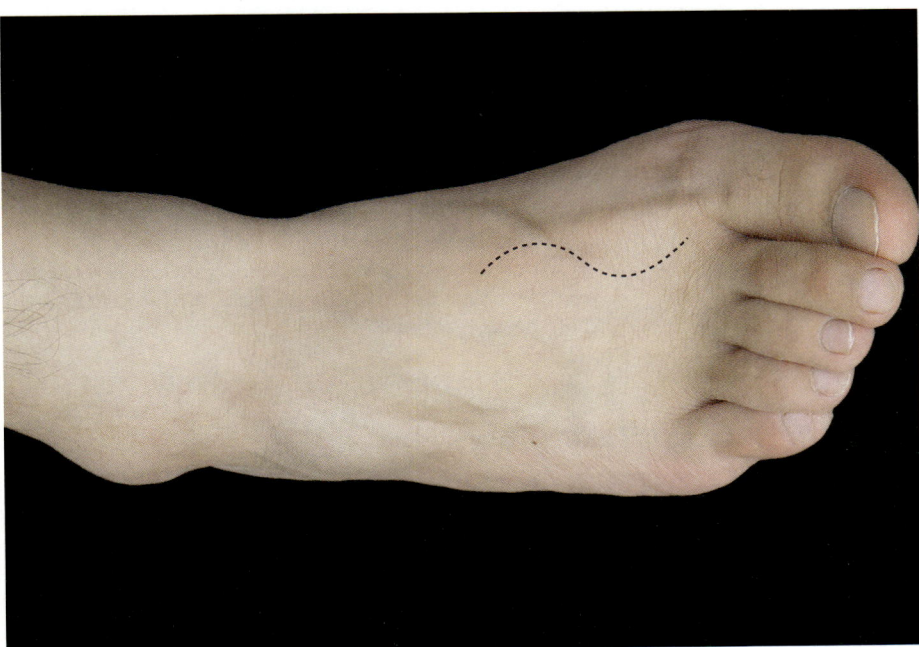

Figure 3-268   **Design of the incision**

The patient should be placed in supine position, and an S-shaped incision made with the 2nd metatarsal bone as its vertical axis. The proximal incision should begin with the 2nd plantar cuneiform-metatarsal joint and extend distally to the 2nd metatarsophalangeal joint to expose the interosseous space between the 1st and the 2nd metatarsal bones and the head of the 2nd metatarsal bone.

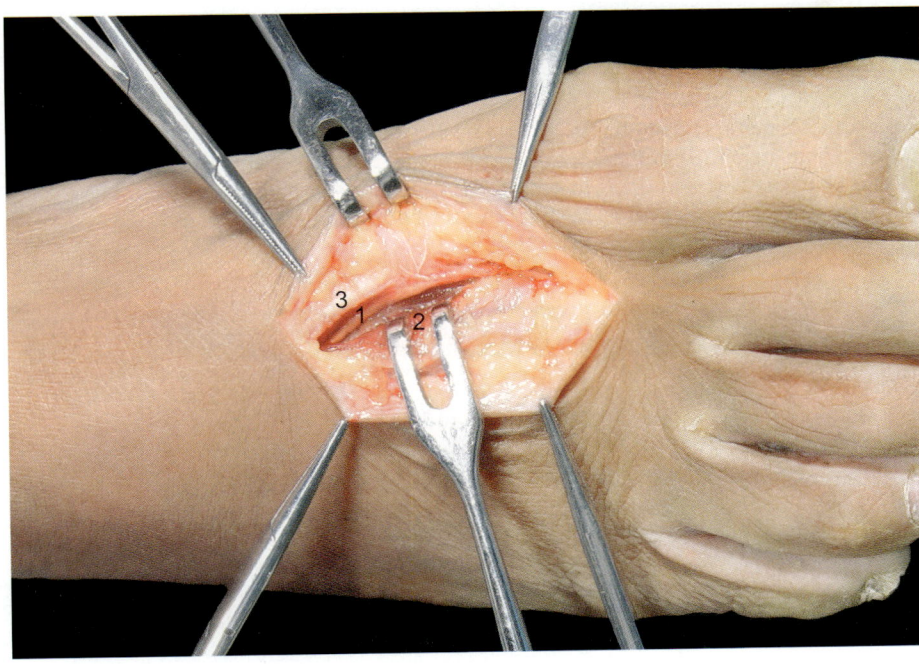

1. 1st dorsal metatarsal blood vessels
2. Dorsal interossei
3. Musculus extensor pollicis brevis tendon

Figure 3-269   **Exposure of the vessels**

The skin should be incised open to expose the 1st dorsal metatarsal artery on the surface of the interosseous muscle of the 1st metatarsal bone or in the superficial layer of the muscle. If the artery belongs to type Ⅰ, it might be chosen as a pedicle; if it belongs to type Ⅱ or type Ⅲ, the 2nd dorsal metatarsal artery should be adopted as an alternative.

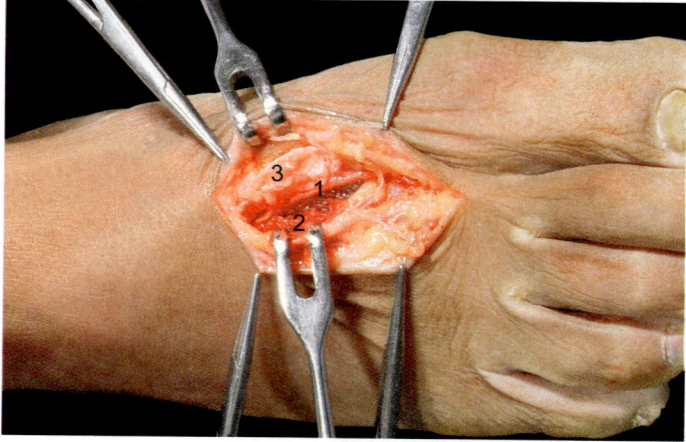

Figure 3-270   **Harvest of the bone flap**

The proximal dorsal lateral of the 1st metatarsal bone or the proximal dorsal medial of the 2nd metatarsal bone should be incised down to the periosteum before the periosteal flap is retrieved. The periosteum should be a bit larger than the periosteal flap.

1. 1st dorsal metatarsal blood vessels
2. Dorsal interossei
3. Periosteal flap

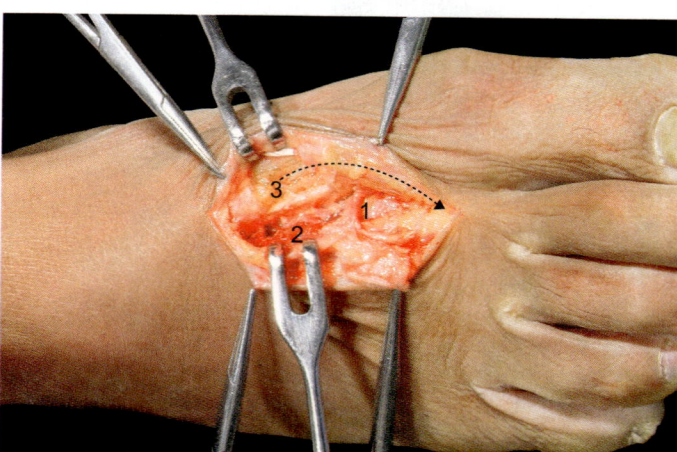

1. 1st dorsal metatarsal blood vessels
2. Dorsal interossei
3. Donor site

Figure 3-271   **Transposition of the periosteal flap**

The 2nd metatarsal bone should be exposed completely before an osseous slot is chiseled at the proximal dorsal greater tubercle of the 2nd metatarsal bone. The osseous slot should be extended inwards about 0.5mm. It should be 0.5cm in width and 1cm in length. The sequestrum and the granulation tissue in the head should be excavated and filled in with some cancellous bone chiseled from the metatarsal bone if necessary. And then the periosteal flap should be implanted into the osseous slot, and the periosteum sutured with the surrounding soft tissue.

Key points in applied anatomy

Firstly, a periosteal flap based on the proximal dorsal lateral segment of the 1st metatarsal bone or the proximal dorsal medial segment of the 2nd metatarsal bone should be retrieved with the 1st dorsal metatarsal blood vessels as its pedicle. It might be transferred retrogradely with its pivot point located at the point, where the dorsal perforating branch perforates through. It has its reverse blood supply. Secondly, a periosteal flap based on the proximal dorsal medial segment of the 2nd metatarsal bone should be retrieved with the 2nd dorsal metatarsal blood vessel as its pedicle. It might be transferred retrogradely with its pivot point located at the point, where the dorsal perforating branch perforates through. It has its reverse blood supply. Thirdly, the 2nd metatarsal bone should be taken as a vertical axis, and an S-shaped incision made to expose the interosseous space between the 1st and 2nd metatarsal bones and the 2nd head of metatarsal bone. Fourthly, the 1st dorsal metatarsal artery should be the priority as a pedicle, but if the artery belongs to the deep, the thin or congenital absence type (II or III), the 2nd dorsal metatarsal artery should be the alternative. Fifthly, the periosteal flap should be made about 1×0.5×0.5cm in size, and the bone osseous slot chiseled next to the dorsal greater tubercle of the 2nd head of metatarsal bone so that it could be large enough to accomodate the periosteal flap. Sixthly, the periosteum membrane flap should be a bit larger than the periosteum one so that it could be sutured and fixed with the nearby tissue.

Index

Saphenous nerve 87
Sartorius 149
Scapula 214, 217
Scapular flap 5
Scapular spinal 199
Spine of scapula 207, 211
Spine of scapula 203
Superficial circumflex iliac artery 60
Superficial epigastric artery 60
Superficial iliac circumflex artery 273
Superficial peroneal artery 99, 110
Superior ankle branch 318
Superior gluteal artery 145, 280
Superior ulnar 247
Superior ulnar collateral artery 18
Suprascapular artery 203, 211
suprascapular artery 207
Supraspinous branch 203
Sural flap 113
surgical neck of the humerus 221

T

Thoracoacromial artery 195, 199
thoracodorsal artery 217
Tibia 314, 318, 322, 326, 330, 335
transverse cervical artery 207
Trochiterian 283, 289, 293

U

Ulnar 259
Ulnar artery 142
ulnar artery 29
Ulnar forearm Flap 29

V

Vastus lateralis 154

W

Wrist fracture 255